# Surgical Treatment of Epilepsies

Josef Zentner

# Surgical Treatment of Epilepsies

## Diagnosis, Surgical Strategies, Results

Springer

Josef Zentner
Freiburg im Breisgau
Baden-Württemberg
Germany

ISBN 978-3-030-48747-8 ISBN 978-3-030-48748-5 (eBook)
https://doi.org/10.1007/978-3-030-48748-5



This Springer imprint is published by the registered company Springer Nature Switzerland AG
The registered company address is: Gewerbestrasse 11, 6330 Cham, Switzerland

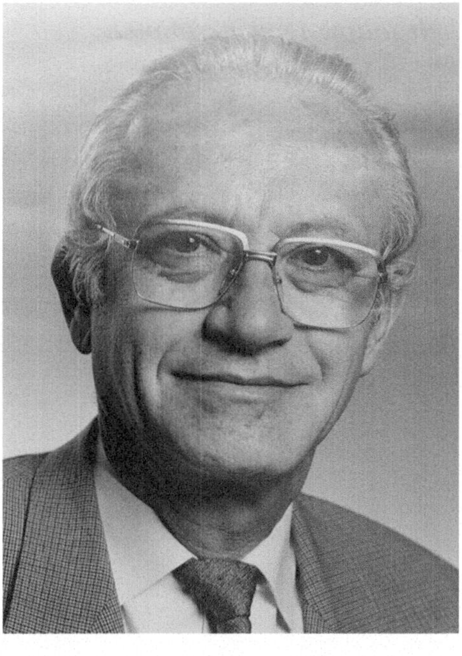

*This book is dedicated to my revered teacher of neurosurgery*
*Prof. Dr. med. Wolfgang Seeger*
*1929–2018*

*There is hardly anyone whose life was so identifiable with anatomy and microneurosurgery as Wolfgang Seeger. Pursuing his vision of anatomically guided surgery, he worked tirelessly to make functional anatomy and its evolutional basis understandable for neurosurgeons. His work supported by his enormous artistic abilities is reflected in 25 image atlases, the last of them he just finished the day before he passed away.*

*Wolfgang Seeger was one of the outstanding personalities pioneering the development of neurosurgery from a life-preserving to a function-preserving discipline.*

*In everyday clinical life, Wolfgang Seeger always convinced by his natural authority based on his tremendous work, his enormous knowledge and experience, his modest and friendly personality, and his open management style frankly addressing surgical errors, mistakes, and misadventures. In search for scientific truth, he never got tired of teaching his fellows to distinguish between assumptions and facts when discussing, always with compassion and deep respect for patients and for life. This philosophy will continue to live in his numerous neurosurgical scholars and their follow-up generation as well as in his textbooks.*

# Foreword

Living in a time in which the increase of medical scientific knowledge mutated to "exponential" and "medline" became the primary source for acquisition of medical information, a textbook written by one author seems to be out of time for many medical doctors and scientists. However, several thoughts should be considered. Firstly, epilepsy surgery is a field in which the so-called *evidence-based medicine* on a high level is based on a very small amount of data with very little information for the everyday life of doctors practically involved in this field. Power is a big issue due to the complexity of the patients and their variability concerning the basis used for scientific comparison. Secondly, the data given by numerous publications are difficult to value for those who are not so experienced because of a small number of treated patients. Finally, such a structured presentation of epilepsy surgery outside a multi-authored book is not available. This book here can be called exceptional concerning completeness, thoroughness, and readability.

Josef Zentner is a neurosurgeon with 30 years of experience in epilepsy surgery based on several thousand cases covering all types of surgical procedures. I had the fortune to have him as a surgical partner in Epilepsy for about one quarter of this time. All the intensive discussion we had showed that Josef has a deep understanding of the disease *epilepsy*, especially in its transformation into a sound epilepsy surgical concept with an ongoing evolution. Thus, who, but not him, is the candidate writing a monography on epilepsy surgery.

Whom would I recommend this book? First of all, neurosurgeons, neurologist, and neuropediatricians who want to enter this successful field of epilepsy treatment. They will find a systematic and complete information for their entry. Furthermore, experts, who look for a fast information, will never be disappointed. After all, the scientist will find a sound basis on which his work in epilepsy surgery will start easily. As a whole, I read it and will read it again.

Bonn, Germany Christian E. Elger

# Preface

Surgery is widely accepted as a valuable option for the treatment of patients with severe epilepsies. Milestones in this development were the Conference in Zurich in 1986 as well as the two Palm Desert Conferences in 1986 and 1992. With continuous refinement of presurgical work-up, sophisticated surgical strategies have been developed to remove the proper epileptogenic area avoiding additional neurological and neuropsychological deficits. However, successful operation of the epilepsy surgical program requires not only enormous investments for technical equipment, but also the availability of a highly specialized personnel. Epilepsy surgery constitutes a "window to the brain" for human neuroscience. It contributes to our understanding of the functional anatomy, electrophysiological relationships, and neuronal plasticity of the human brain. In addition, resective epilepsy surgery as most commonly practiced at present provides human material to basic science thus making important contributions to the solution of many outstanding problems of epileptogenesis and other neurological diseases. In all, there are good reasons to concentrate the epilepsy surgical program to a limited number of highly specialized centers.

During the last decades, a clear tendency towards epilepsy surgery in the pediatric age is witnessed. This trend reflects the insight that early intervention constitutes the only modifiable positive predictor for epileptological and developmental outcome. In addition, favorable long-term results after early surgical treatment are supported by the pronounced plasticity of young brains and their ability to compensate functional deficits. Therefore, it is necessary to convince general practitioners, neuropediatrists, and epileptologists to consider surgical options at an early stage of the disease and to refer affected children to epilepsy centers for further evaluation. In line with these insights, the 6$^{th}$ International Bethel-Cleveland Clinic Epilepsy Symposium 1995 has been specifically dedicated to epilepsy surgery in children. Moreover, the International League Against Epilepsy Subcommission and later Task Force for Epilepsy Surgery in Children have defined standards for referral and evaluation of children.

Actually, we face an increasing interest in minimally invasive strategies such as neurostimulation (vagal nerve stimulation, deep brain stimulation, responsive neurostimulation) pursuing palliative goals as well as thermoablation techniques (radiofrequency thermocoagulation, laser-induced thermotherapy) and stereotactic radiosurgery aiming at curative treatment of epilepsies. Although most of those techniques are not novel, they constitute promising tools that complement the surgical spectrum, particularly for patients with non-localizable seizure foci, failed resective surgery, and pathologies carrying high risks for resective approaches. Obviously, minimal invasiveness makes those strategies attractive both for patients and attending physicians, thus noticeably increasing the number of surgical candidates. In addition, development of efficient closed-loop intervention systems can be expected to change the appearance of epilepsy surgery during the next decades. In fact, the "window to the brain" offered by resective surgery seems to close more and more.

In contrast to the increasingly wider application and expansion of epilepsy surgery, respective training facilities for young neurosurgeons are limited. This reflects the facts that the epilepsy surgical program necessarily is restricted to highly specialized centers and that surgical techniques for epilepsies are not part of the neurosurgical training program. In consequence, neurosurgical monographs usually do not address those techniques. The literature on the surgical treatment of epilepsies refers more to the clinical results of surgery rather than to the proper surgical strategies. Moreover, surgical aspects presented in the literature usually reflect the individual institutional philosophy of the way to proceed. A monograph providing a comprehensive description of surgical techniques currently used including an overview on epileptological, neuroradiological, and pathological aspects, thus summarizing the epilepsy surgical program for the training of neurosurgeons is still lacking.

It is the aim of this book to fill the gap between the increasing demand for epilepsy surgical experience and limited training facilities on this area. Surgical strategies both for the adult and the pediatric age as currently available including resective and non-resective minimal invasive approaches independently of the practice at individual institutions are described. Essential aspects of various disciplines involved in the epilepsy surgical program are addressed for a better understanding of the complex matter of presurgical diagnostics and postoperative care. In addition, the author will provide his personal experience with epilepsy surgery acquired during a period of almost 30 years including tricks and pitfalls, thus preventing young neurosurgeons from learning by trial and error.

This book is primarily designed for neurosurgeons who want to get acquainted with the surgical treatment of epilepsies having completed their basic training program and passed the board examination. Therefore, it will be abstained from the presentation of basic surgical tools and techniques in favor of describing special aspects of epilepsy surgery. In particular, emphasis will be paid to techniques of functional localization, the definition of safe limits for resection, and the critical evaluation of results including complications. Epilepsy surgery is particularly rewarding for advanced neurosurgical training since it offers valuable lessons for functionally oriented and functionally guided approaches. In addition to the surgical training, this book may also provide useful information for neurologists, epileptologists, neuropediatrists, and members of other disciplines involved in the epilepsy surgical program for a better understanding of possibilities and limitations of surgical strategies.

I would like to express my thanks and acknowledgment to many colleagues who have contributed to this book. I am grateful to J. Schramm, the former head of the Department of Neurosurgery, Bonn, for facilitating my stay in the USA and Canada to get acquainted with epilepsy surgery, for confiding me the surgical part of the epilepsy surgical program in Bonn, and for his always valuable surgical advices. I would like to express my gratitude to C.E. Elger, the former head of the Department of Epileptology, Bonn, for the many years of trustful clinical and scientific collaboration, decisively contributing to my understanding of epileptological issues, and for supporting establishment of the epilepsy center in Freiburg. In addition, I highly appreciate his reviewing the manuscript of this book giving many valuable advices. Thanks are due to all colleagues of the epilepsy center Freiburg and cooperation partners in Kehl/Kork, Heidelberg, Mannheim, Kiel, and Stuttgart. In particular, I am grateful to A. Schulze-Bonhage, D. Altenmüller, M. Dümpelmann, K. Wagner, B. Metternich, M. Hirsch, and C. Gierschner, Epilepsy Center Freiburg, for their epileptological and neuropsychological comments. Special thanks I owe to H. Urbach, Department of Neuroradiology, for providing me comprehensive image material. I would like to thank S. Doostkam, Department of Neuropathology, who left me representative histopathological findings. Moreover, I am grateful to C. Haas, Experimental Epilepsy Research, J. Beck, M. Shah, O. Schnell, and B. Schmeiser, Department of Neurosurgery, V.A. Coenen and P. Reinacher, Department of Stereotactic and Functional Neurosurgery, S. Yang, Department of Neuroradiology, H.-J. Priebe, Department of Anesthesiology, P.T. Meyer, Department of Nuclear Medicine, A.L. Grosu, Department of Radiation Therapy, and G. Maio, Institute for Ethics and History in Medicine, for their suggestions and materials. I appreciate the contributions of G. Ramantani, Zürich, as well as comments and materials of P. Wolf, Copenhagen, H. Schneble, Kehl/Kork, J. Wellmer, Bochum, S. Fauser, Bethel-Bielefeld, and T. Gasser, Bonn. I am grateful to S. Freyberg, D. Devan, and A. Vishal from the Springer Publishing for accompanying the production process of this book. Finally, I would like to thank I. Vassilikos, M. Kniebühler, A. Wintermantel, and V. Leonhardt, Neurocenter Freiburg, for their help and technical assistance. I owe special thanks to all the patients I have treated for contributing to surgical skills and the understanding of functional localization. My major acknowledgment and gratitude is attributed to my wife Cilia who gave me the freedom during my entire professional life to dedicate care of patients entrusted to me.

Freiburg, Germany Josef Zentner

# Abbreviations

| | |
|---|---|
| AED | Antiepileptic drugs |
| AHE | Amygdalohippocampectomy |
| AHS | Ammon´s horn sclerosis |
| ANT | Anterior nucleus of thalamus |
| ASA | American Society of Anesthesiologists |
| ATL | Anterior temporal lobectomy |
| BBB | Blood brain barrier |
| CC | Corpus callosotomy |
| CEA | Cost-effectiveness analysis |
| CSF | Cerebrospinal fluid |
| CT | Computed tomography |
| DALY | Disability-adjusted life years |
| DNET | Dysembroplastic neuroepithelial tumor |
| DSA | Digital subtraction angiography |
| DTI | Diffusion tensor imaging |
| ECoG | Electrocorticogram |
| EEBB | European Epilepsy Brain Bank |
| EEG | Electroencephalogram |
| ELE | Extended lesionectomy |
| EPC | Epilepsia partialis continua |
| ESI | Electrical source imaging |
| ETE | Extratemporal epilepsy |
| FCD | Focal cortical dysplasia |
| FLE | Frontal lobe epilepsy |
| fMRI | Functional magnetic resonance imaging |
| FUS | Focused ultrasound |
| GABA | Gamma-aminobutyric acid |
| GG | Ganglioglioma |
| GK | Gamma Knife |
| HFO | High frequency oscillations |
| HH | Hypothalamic hamartoma |
| HRQOL | Health related quality of life |
| HS | Hippocampal sclerosis |
| IED | Interictal epileptic discharges |
| ILAE | International League Against Epilepsy |
| KH | Keyhole |
| LEAT | Long-term epilepsy-associated tumor |

| | |
|---|---|
| LINAC | Linear Accelerator |
| LITT | Laser induced thermal therapy |
| MCD | Malformation of cortical development |
| mMCD | mild Malformation of cortical development |
| MEG | Magnetic encephalography |
| MEP | Motor evoked potentials |
| MHT | Multiple hippocampal transections |
| MRI | Magnetic resonance imaging |
| MRS | Magnetic resonance spectroscopy |
| MSI | Magnetic source imaging |
| MST | Multiple subpial transections |
| MTLE | Mesial temporal lobe epilepsy |
| NPVH | Nodular periventricular heterotopia |
| OLE | Occipital lobe epilepsy |
| PCE | Posterior cortex epilepsy |
| PET | Positron emission tomography |
| PHFO | Pathological high frequency oscillations |
| PLE | Parietal lobe epilepsy |
| PGNT | Papillary glioneuronal tumor |
| PNES | Psychogenic non-epileptic seizures |
| PO | Parieto-occipital |
| PXA | Pleomorhic xanthoastrocytomy |
| QOL | Quality of life |
| QUALYs. | Quality-adjusted life years |
| RFTC | Radiofrequency thermocoagulation |
| RNS | Responsive neurostimulation |
| SEEG | Stereotactic electroencephalogram |
| SRS | Stereotactic radiosurgery |
| SAHE | Selective amygdalohippocampectomy |
| sSAHE | Subtemporal selective amygdalohippocampectomy |
| tSAHE | Transsylvian selective amygdalohippocampectomy |
| SEP | Somatosensory evoked potentials |
| SMA | Supplementary motor area |
| SPECT | Single-photon emission computed tomography |
| TLE | Temporal lobe epilepsy |
| TIVA | Total intravenous anesthesia |
| TO | Temporo-occipital |
| TPO | Temporo-parieto-occipital |
| TS | Tuberous sclerosis |
| VNS | Vagal nerve stimulation |
| WHO | World Health Organization |

# Contents

# History of Epilepsy Surgery

# 1

*History is who we are and why we are the way we are. History, despite its wrenching pain, cannot be unlived, but if faced with courage, need not be lived again. Those who cannot remember the past are condemned to repeat it.*

*David McCullough*

## Contents



History makes us better understand of what we do today. It makes us recognize that acting the way we do is based more on past developments than on our own merits, thus teaching us modesty and humility. Certainly, this is also true for the history of epilepsy surgery offering us the opportunity to understand our current approach and learn from past experience, both from successes and failures. Therefore, before reviewing strategies in epilepsy surgery, it seems appropriate to comprise their evolution in a brief overview.

## 1.1 Prehistoric Era

Trephinations are known since 10,000 years BC and have been performed in all Neolithic communities 4000 years ago [1]. In particular, numerous trephined skulls have been found in oriental and South American high cultures. In Europe, trephined skulls of the early bronze era found in hill graves are not known as well. It is thought that trephinations were based on the hypothesis of releasing evil spirits and demons as the cause of abnormal phenomena to which among others






J. Zentner, *Surgical Treatment of Epilepsies*, https://doi.org/10.1007/978-3-030-48748-5_1

epileptic symptoms may belong. A skull found in Hanstholm, a Danish harbor village at the North Sea, seems to be interesting. This skull which today may be seen in the archeological museum in Copenhagen shows a splinter impression fracture. The rectangular osteoclastic trephination defect is centered over the lesion. In contrast to the old fracture, no healing signs can be seen at the trephination rims. This case shows that in Europe experience with the elevation of impression fractures was already existing in the bronze era, and that the respective patient did not survive surgery for a long time. Splinting fractures, however, differ from usual laminary impression fractures by laceration of the dura leaving an atrophic brain-dura scar which is well known as a typical cause for focal epilepsies. Since the Hanstholm skull injury was localized over the left central area, it is not absurd to hypothesize that trephination in that case may have been done to ameliorate symptoms of epilepsy. It seems to be remarkable that none of the skulls found in the area of Hanstholm of patients who had survived trephination for a longer time as demonstrated by healing signs shows osteomyelitis as it is obvious in many trephined skulls found in Peru. Those Nordic ancestors used flintstone knifes milled in waveform for trephination, and it may be concluded that they had substantiated knowledge on hemostasis, since hematomas predispose to infection (W. Seeger, personal communication). From the Hanstholm case, the speculative conclusion may be drawn that prehistoric trephinations among other reasons may have been performed for the treatment of post-traumatic epilepsy.

## 1.2 Middle Ages

In the Middle Ages, epileptic phenomena have been interpreted as mysterious abnormalities or irreligious disorders. Accordingly, the treatment included magical or religious prayer, witchcraft, amulets labeled with holy incantations, and various types of fetishism. In addition, a variety of obscure diets, remedies, herbs, plants, and bloodletting were used [2]. The idea to create an outlet for pathogenic humors and vapors gave rise to surgical procedures such as scarification or arteriotomy [3] as it had been still advocated by Tissot in 1770 [4]. Relating epileptic phenomena to sexual activity, circumcision and castration have consequently been performed [3]. Moreover, removal of the irritative zone by cutting nerves, amputating fingers, or cauterization of the region involved has been suggested [4], approaches that were still advocated by Brown-Séquard in the middle of the nineteenth century [3]. Based on the theory, that closure of the larynx may play a major role in the development of a seizure, tracheotomy has been proposed [3]. Girvin [2] reviewed those surgical and non-surgical approaches for the treatment of epileptic disorders.

## 1.3 Nineteenth Century

In the nineteenth century, epilepsy, now called a falling sickness, began to be recognized as an organic disease [3]. Since the biological substrate of epilepsy was still unknown, different surgical procedures inside and outside the skull were proposed [5]. Alexander [6] supposed that ligature of the vertebral arteries might be a useful operation for the cure of epilepsy. Moreover, in 1898, Alexander introduced bilateral sympathectomy [7]. Trephination remained reserved to cases in which the disease followed an injury to the head. Dudley [8, 9] and Smith [10] reported early results of trephination for post-traumatic epilepsy.

On May 25, 1886, Victor Horsley removed a scar from the motor cortex in a patient presented by Hughlings Jackson [11, 12]. This 22-year-old male had focal motor seizures caused by a depressed fracture 15 years earlier, a case that reminds the abovementioned trephined skull found in Hanstholm. Postoperatively, the patient was seizure free. One month later, on June 22, 1886, Horsley operated another patient without traumatic injury. In this case, surgery was guided by seizure semiology pointing to the focus. This latter operation represents Horsley's first epilepsy surgical procedure in the proper sense

[13]. Unfortunately, the postoperative course of the patient remains unknown. Both operations demonstrate the principle of the surgical treatment of focal epilepsies on a strong neurophysiological basis. Horsley was influenced by the Jacksonian thinking, and Jackson himself had been influenced by the studies of the localization of function within the motor cortex by Hitzig [14]. Due to his neurophysiological approach, Horsley is acknowledged as the father of epilepsy surgery, and his operations are thought to indicate the beginning of modern epilepsy surgery. However, it should be mentioned that already in 1879, Macewen in Glasgow [15] had reported resection of an "invisible" lesion to treat epilepsy based on clinical seizure observations of Hughlings Jackson [16]. This report was followed by a series of cases published in 1881 [17]. Similar operations as performed by Horsley and Macewen which were named Horsley's operations were carried out at the same time by Keen [18], Nancrede [19], and Lloyd and Deaver [20]. O'Leary and Goldring [21] reviewed the early beginning of modern epilepsy surgery at the end of the nineteenth century.

## 1.4 Early Twentieth Century

In *Germany*, epilepsy surgery in the early twentieth century was pioneered by Fedor Krause in Berlin and Otfried Foerster in Breslau. Krause continued Jackson's view of focal epilepsy and extended the indication for the surgical treatment of Jacksonian epilepsy to different pathologies [22, 23]. In a first monograph he comprised 45 interventions for Jacksonian epilepsy [24] (Fig. 1.1). Based on the animal experiments of Schiff, Hitzig and Frisch, Sherrington and Grünaum, Horsley, and C. and O. Vogt, Krause localized the motor cortex by cortical stimulation and provided a detailed functional map. In 1932, Krause published a 900-page volume on epilepsy surgery together with his coworker Schum [26]. In this monograph, he summarized 400 cases operated for epilepsy during his career following the Jacksonian principle that only the excision of the "primary convulsing center" is a worthwhile

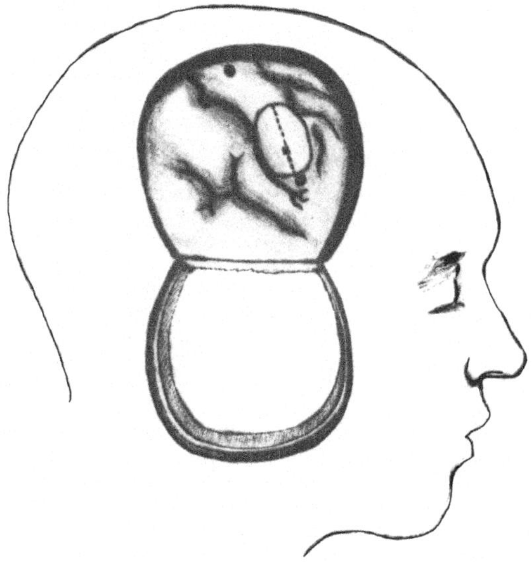

**Fig. 1.1** Drawing from F. Krause's [24] monograph demonstrating the situs of the patient who was operated on November 16, 1893, for epilepsy due to a postencephalitic subcortical cyst in the right precentral gyrus (from Wolf [25], with permission)

epilepsy surgical procedure. Krause and Schum also discussed interventions that have still been advocated at that time like lumbar puncture, pneumoencephalography, transcallosal puncture ("Balkenstich"), sympathectomy, carotidal ligature, adrenalectomy, transplantation of endocrine tissue, and peripheral operations for reflex epilepsy. However, apart from some exceptional situations they rejected all of them. In extension to Krause, Foerster focused on the semiology of seizures. He expanded localization of the epileptogenic focus to other areas outside the motor cortex and precisely described the cortical fields of seizure origin according to the semiology of seizures and results of cortical stimulation. While Krause advocated monopolar faradic stimulation, Foerster preferred galvanic stimulation [27–34]. Based on the cytoarchitectonic map of O. Vogt, Foerster and Penfield [35] developed a cortical map in which, however, the frontal and temporal lobes are spared to major parts (Fig. 1.2). Wolf [25] provided a detailed review on the history of the treatment of epilepsy in Europe. Lüders [36] appreciated the contributions of Fedor Krause and Otfried Foerster to epilepsy surgery.

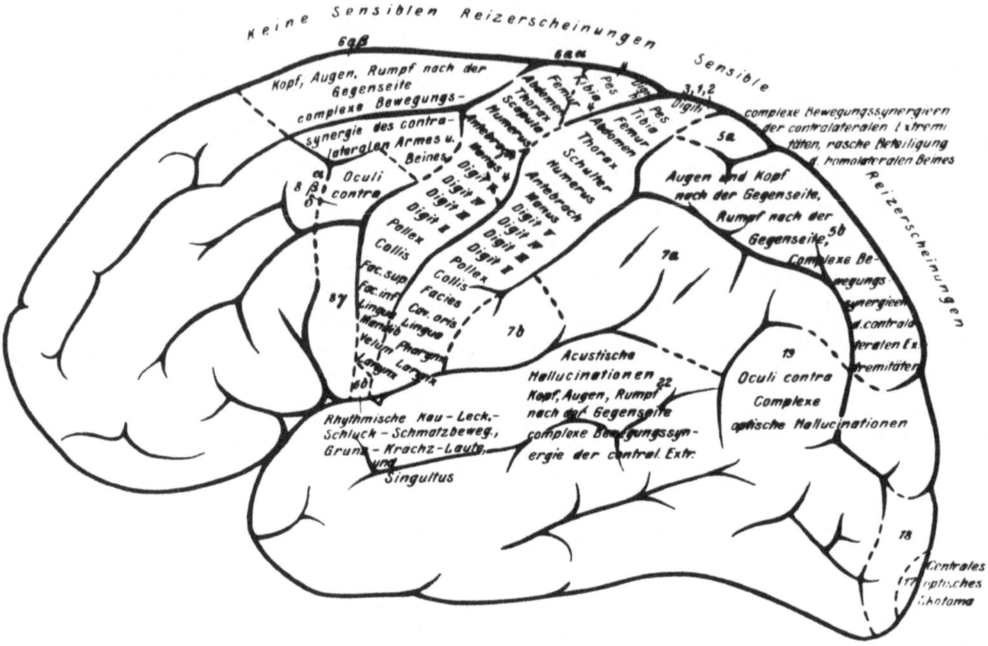


**Fig. 1.2** Cortical map of Foerster and Penfield [35], based on cytoarchitectonic studies of O. Vogt demonstrating results of electrical stimulation. The anterior frontal lobe and the anterior temporal lobe are still terrae incognitae (from Wolf [25], with permission)

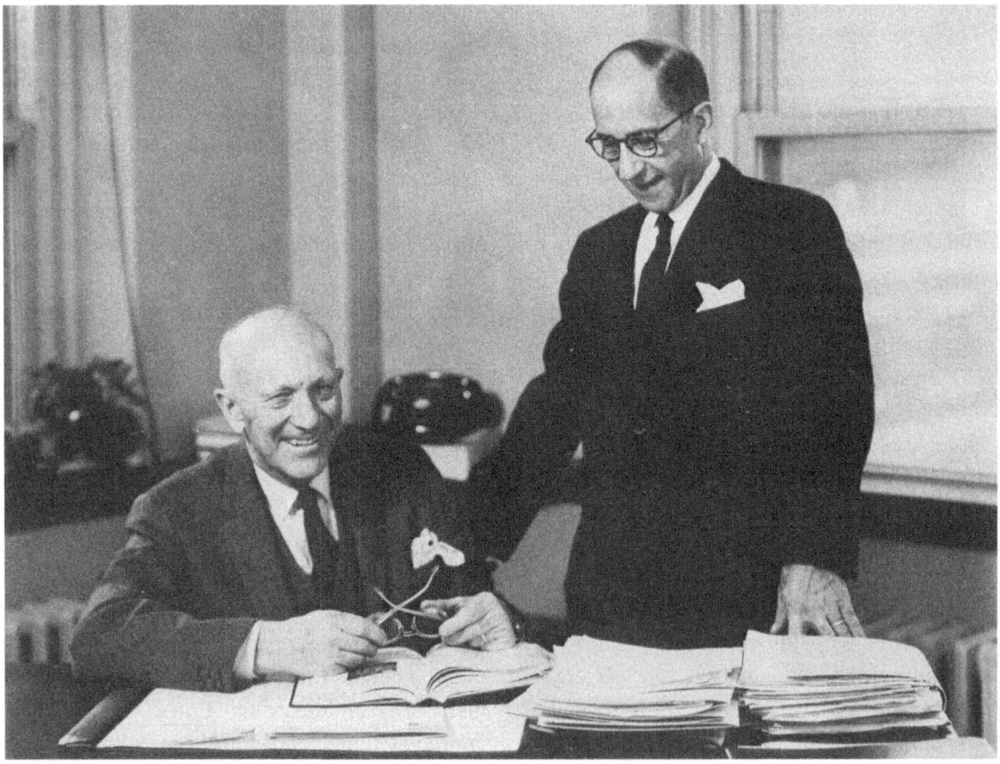

**Fig. 1.3** Wilder Penfield (neurosurgeon, left) and Herbert Jasper (neurophysiologist, right) at the Montreal Neurological Institute (MNI) (from Flanigin et al. [39], with permission)

In *North America*, epilepsy surgery was pioneered by the neurosurgeon Wilder Penfield and the neurophysiologist Herbert Jasper (Fig. 1.3). Wilder Penfield, after studying neurophysiology with Sherrington in Oxford and cerebral morphology with Hortega in Madrid, had trained with Foerster in Breslau. In 1928, he went back to *Montreal*, where he developed the Montreal School of Epilepsy Surgery. Continuing with cortical stimulation, Penfield described the cortical localization of the motor and sensory function in the pre- and postcentral gyri represented by the homunculus [37].

Based on the galvanometer of Einthoven, which allowed quantitative assessment of electrical phenomena in living structures, Berger in 1929 described for the first time recording of electrical activity from the human brain [38]. Recordings of epileptic activity from the scalp—electroencephalography (EEG)—and subsequently from the exposed cortex in the operating room—electrocorticography (ECoG)—constituted milestones in this era and provided the electrophysiological basis of epilepsy surgery (Figs. 1.4, 1.5, and 1.6). Impulses for refinement of EEG/ECoG shifted at that time from Europe to North America, especially to Montreal, where these techniques were of paramount importance for further development of epilepsy surgery.

Together with Jasper, Penfield performed extensive cortical recordings and detected temporal spike foci in a high number of epilepsy cases. A systematic description of electrocorticographical findings has been provided by Jasper [40, 41]. Thus, the focus of epilepsy surgery changed from the extratemporal to the temporal area, and temporal lobectomy has been inaugurated. In fact, these initial resections were corticectomies, and only approximately one-third of patients achieved seizure freedom [42].

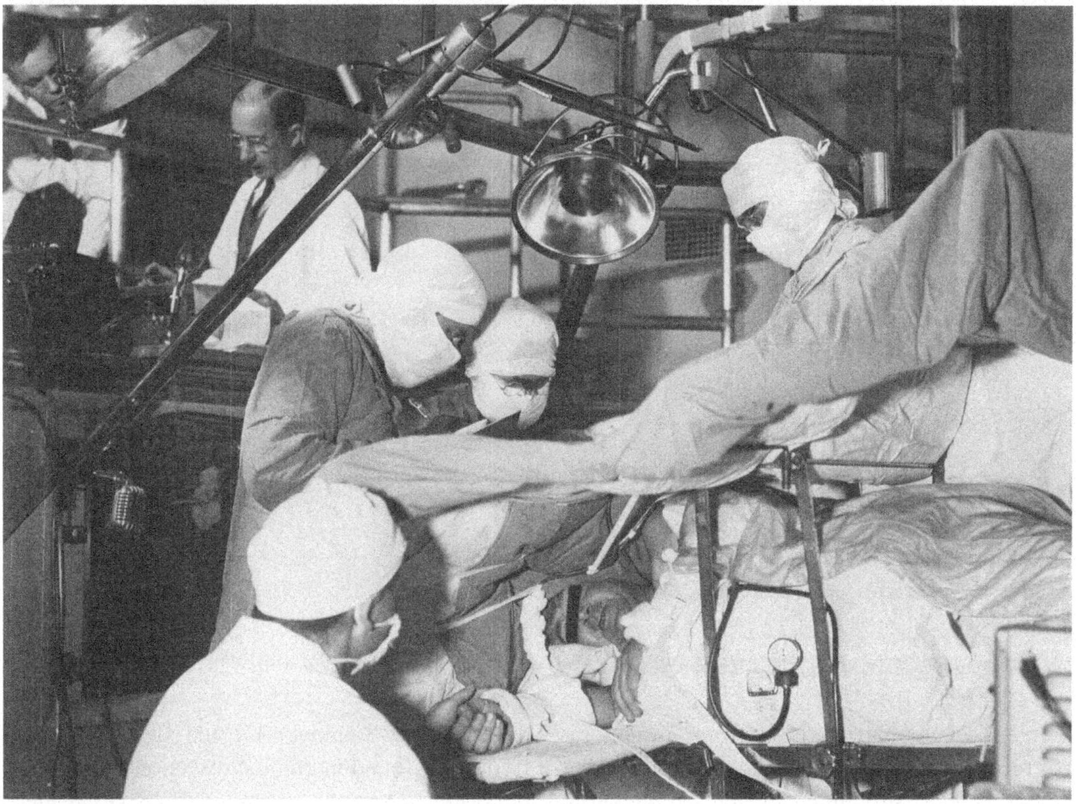

**Fig. 1.4** Operating theatre at the Montreal Neurological Institute (MNI). W. Penfield is operating, while H. Jasper is recording the EEG in the observation area (from Flanigin et al. [39], with permission)

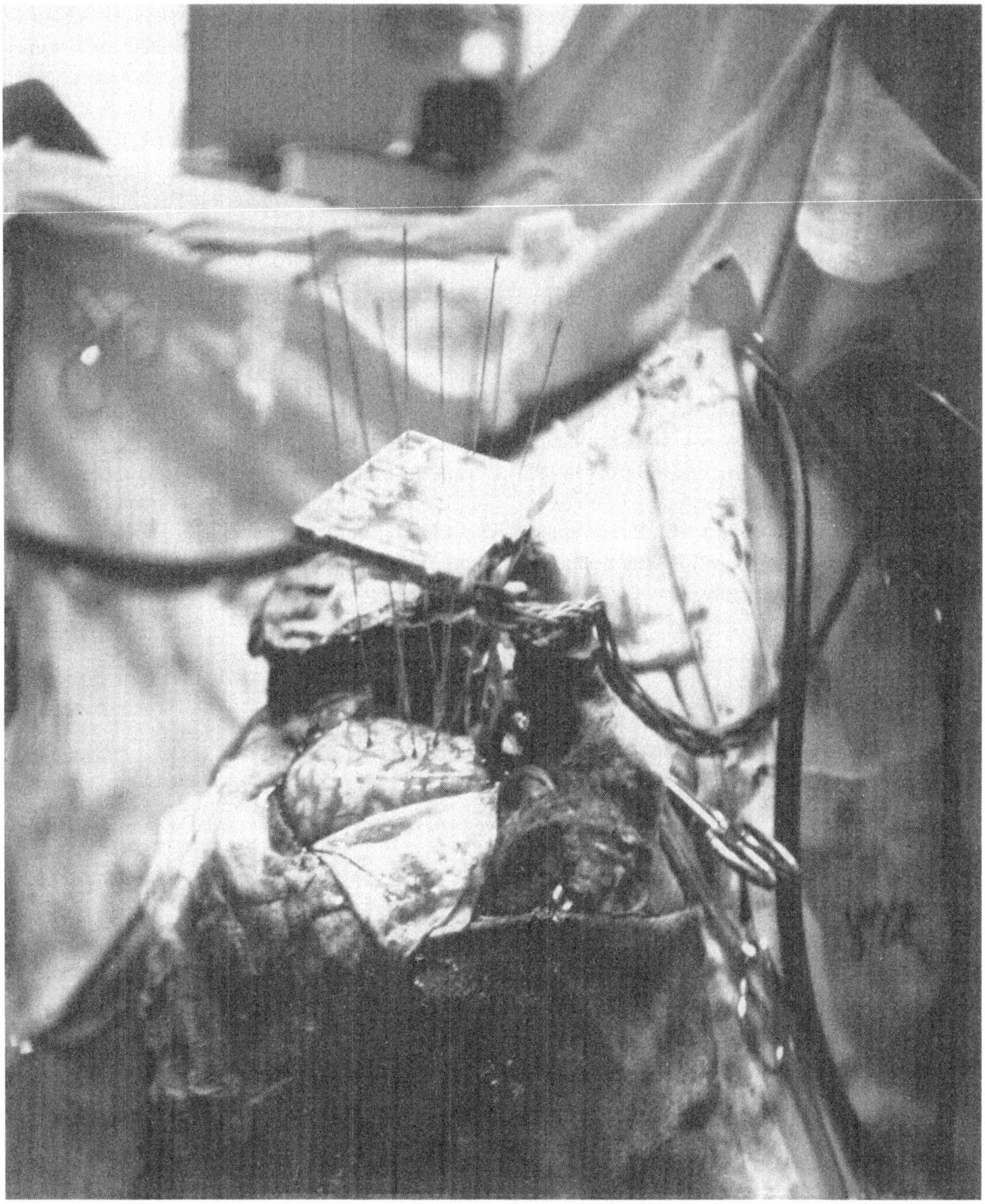

**Fig. 1.5** Intraoperative electrocorticography (ECoG) at the time of W. Penfield and H. Jasper at the Montreal Neurological Institute (MNI). The electrodes are placed on the exposed cortex (from Flanigin et al. [39], with permission)

It has been realized both from intraoperative recordings and from seizure semiology that temporomesial structures—uncus, amygdaloid body, and hippocampus—play an important role in epileptogenesis. Hippocampal sclerosis as first described by Sommer [43] and Bratz [44] was frequently found in en bloc resection of the temporal lobe. Over the course of the next decades, a number of other pathologies such as tumors, atrophic lesions, malformations of cortical

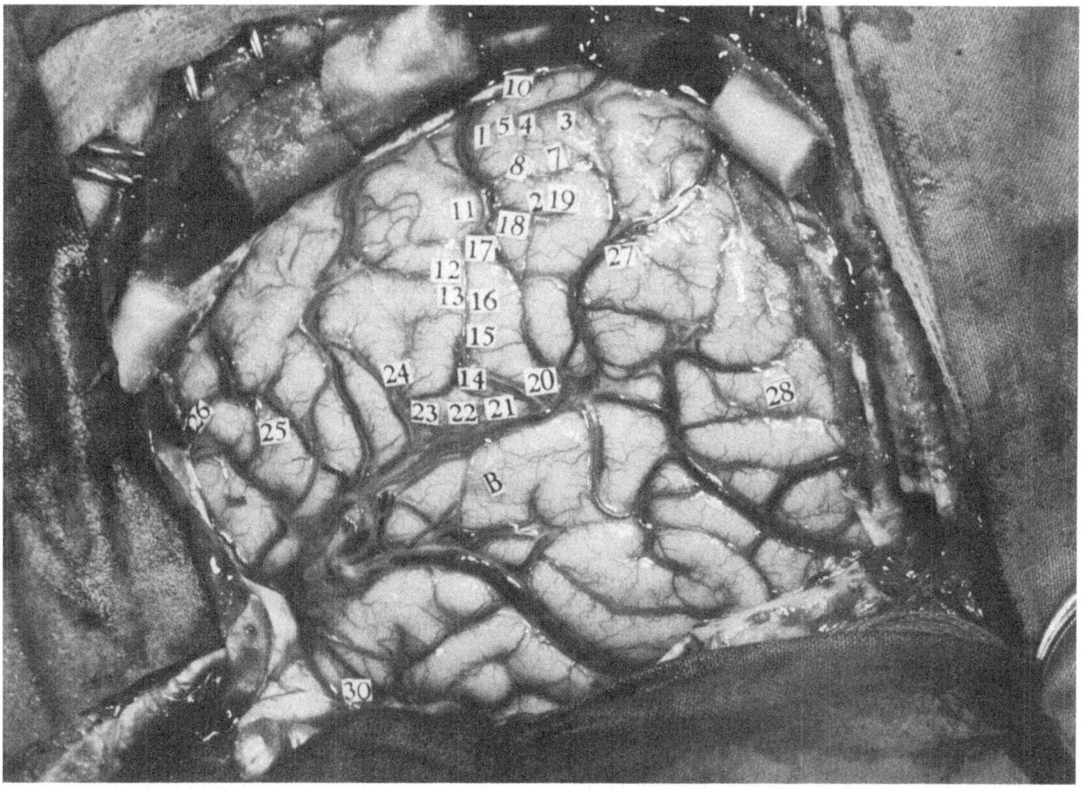

**Fig. 1.6** Identifying eloquent areas on the exposed cortex by stimulation at the time of W. Penfield and H. Jasper at the Montreal Neurological Institute (MNI) (from Flanigin et al. [39], with permission)

development, and Rasmussen's encephalitis have been described emphasizing the relevance of a localized pathology in epileptogenesis [45–48].

Parallel to Penfield in Montreal, Bailey and Gibbs [49, 50] and Sachs [51] initiated an epilepsy surgical program in *Chicago*. The Montreal [52] and Chicago [49, 50] schools dedicated to epilepsy surgery gained fundamental international importance in the middle of the last century. Over this era, trainees of those schools worldwide established epilepsy surgical centers, and a variety of publications outlined the contributions of surgery to the treatment of epilepsies. The influence of the Montreal school pioneered by Penfield, Jasper, and Rasmussen on the development of epilepsy surgery has been documented by O'Leary and Goldring [21], Feindel [53], Meador et al. [54], Feindel et al. [55], and Olivier [56]. A review on the significance of the Chicago school led by Baily and Gibbs for the increasing use of surgical options to treat epilepsies has been provided by Hermann and Stone [57].

The basic epilepsy surgical spectrum has been completed with the introduction of callosotomy in 1940 by Van Wagenen and Herren [58] and anatomical hemispherectomy by Krynauw in 1950 [59]. In the middle of the last century, epilepsy surgery has been promoted not only by advances in electrophysiological and surgical techniques, as well as by patho-anatomical studies, but also by new insights in the brain-behavior relationships. A striking experience was the case of H.M., who in 1954 underwent a bilateral temporal lobectomy for medically intractable seizures. This procedure was followed by a complete postoperative amnesia [60]. Certainly, H.M. was not the first case to undergo a bilateral temporal resection [61]. Milner and Penfield [62] described impaired memory function after unilateral resection of the hippocampal formation in the presence of bilateral temporomesial pathology, and Milner's systematic evaluations of surgical patients pointing to a critical role of the mesial temporal region for memory [63] have been widely recognized [42, 55]. Neuropsychological test patterns emerged providing significant information as to cognitive abilities, lateralization and localization of the epileptogenic focus, and prediction of the postoperative cognitive and psychosocial outcome [64]. In addition, the Wada test facilitated lateralization of speech and memory [65]. The history of epilepsy surgery in North America has been reviewed Flanigin et al. [39] and Girvin [2].

## 1.5 Late Twentieth Century

Prior to the early 1970s, only indirect methods such as ventriculography, pneumoencephalography, and angiography were available to demonstrate space-occupying lesions or abnormally vascularized areas, while benign morphological abnormalities without expansion or pathological vascularization were not detectable at all. The first technique facilitating direct imaging of the brain was computed tomography (CT) scanning [66]. Approximately 10 years later, the technique of magnetic resonance imaging (MRI) [67] emerged. The significance of MRI for further development of epilepsy surgery cannot be overemphasized, since this technique provided for the first time an effective tool to demonstrate the structural basis of epilepsies. By using blood oxygen level-dependent (BOLD) imaging, it was possible to show areas of high functionality such as the speech areas or the primary motor cortex, and to demonstrate the relationship between these areas and the structural lesion [68]. In addition, radionuclide imaging using positron-emission tomography (PET) detecting hypometabolic areas and ictal single-photon emission computed tomography (SPECT) demonstrating areas of increased perfusion during seizures has proven to be helpful for localizing the epileptogenic focus [69]. Thus, the three pillars of presurgical assessment of epilepsies, namely clinical and neuropsychological including neuropsychiatric evaluation, electrophysiological testing with both interictal and ictal recordings, as well as structural, functional, and radionuclide imaging, had been established. In 1978, H. Penin was appointed to the chair of epileptology in Bonn, which was the first such institution in Europe, succeeded by C.E. Elger in 1990. The epilepsy surgical program in Germany started around the same time in Bonn, Bethel, Berlin, and Erlangen.

In parallel, the second part of the twentieth century witnessed many advances in neurosurgery. An important milestone was the introduction of microsurgical operation techniques facilitating resection of seizure foci in or around areas of high functionality as well as gentle approaches to deep-seated lesions [70–74]. Development of refined electrophysiological techniques of intraoperative mapping and monitoring leading to improved neurological outcome refers to another milestone that may be called functionally guided surgery [75–77]. Multiple subpial transections (MST) have been proposed to treat seizure foci in eloquent areas without harm [78]. Neuronavigation enabled the surgeon to take advantage of anatomical and functional imaging data [79]. Functional hemispherectomy [80, 81] and its further modifications [82–85] facilitated hemispherical procedures with an acceptable morbidity. Isolated removal of the epileptogenic temporomesial area was rendered possible by the development of selective approaches using the transcortical [86], transsylvian [87, 88] and subtemporal [89] routes. In addition, histopathological and molecular classification of the pathological substrates of resective surgery [90] has been shown to provide useful information with respect to epileptogenesis and seizure outcome.

Besides resective and disconnective procedures, minimally invasive surgical strategies have gained increasing interest to treat seizure foci carrying high risks for resection or epilepsies without evidence of a distinct seizure-onset zone. These techniques have been stimulated by the introduction of stereotactic EEG (SEEG) by Talairach and Banceaud [91] and Crandall [92] from the 1950s onward. The pioneers of stereotaxy, Spiegel and Wycis [93], described the effects of coagulation of the dorsomesial nucleus of the thalamus. Umbach and Riechert [94] introduced fornicotomy including parts of the anterior commissure in temporal lobe epilepsy to prevent propagation of hippocampal discharges to the hypothalamus and to the contralateral hemisphere. This procedure as well as stereotactic amygdalotomy [95, 96] were motivated both for epileptological and for psychosurgical considerations [97].

Today, stereotactically guided lesioning including thermoablation (radiofrequency thermocoagulation and laser-induced thermotherapy) [98, 99] and stereotactic radiosurgery [100, 101] are increasingly used for the treatment of deep-seated lesions such as periventricular heterotopias, hypothalamic hamartomas, and temporomesial seizure foci. The most common form of neurostimulation in current use represents vagal nerve stimulation [102]. For deep-brain stimulation, a large number of targets have been proposed including the cerebellum [103], hippocampal structures [104], subthalamic nucleus [105], and centromedian thalamic nucleus [106]. The best investigated target is the anterior nucleus of the thalamus [107, 108]. Responsive stimulation techniques triggered by electrocorticographic patterns [109, 110] or tachycardia [111] indicative of impending seizures constitute first steps to the development of closed-loop intervention systems [112].

As noted by Wilson and Engel [42], the last decade of the twentieth century is marked by a conceptual change in the practice of epilepsy surgery. At the Conference on Presurgical Evaluation of Epileptics in Zurich in 1986 [113] and the first Palm Desert Conference on Surgical Treatment of the Epilepsies held in California in the same year [114], all of the epilepsy surgery programs around the world were presented and discussed to compare strategies and outcomes and to share experience. In consequence, most epilepsy surgery centers adopted approaches for different types of epilepsy not used so far. The follow-up Palm Desert conference in 1992 [115] confirmed that most centers were now applying similar strategies for presurgical evaluation and a large spectrum of surgical procedures [42]. Although conventional resective and disconnective procedures still dominate current epilepsy surgery, minimally invasive strategies are experiencing a huge upsurge. In fact, the future of epilepsy surgery may be expected in closed-loop systems acting in response to an arising seizure either by stimulation or by release of anticonvulsants.

## References


1. Fox WL. Chapter 1. Neurological surgery before Walter E Dandy: a brief introduction. In: Dandy of John Hopkins. Baltimore: Williams and Wilkins; 1984. p. 1–7.
2. Girvin JP. Operative techniques in epilepsy. Cham, Switzerland: Springer; 2015.
3. Temkin O. The falling sickness. 2nd ed. Baltimore: The John Hopkins Press; 1971.
4. Tissot SA. Traité de lépilepsie. Lausanne: Chapuis; 1770.
5. Billings JS. The surgical treatment of epilepsy. In: Williams D, editor. Modern trends in neurology, vol. 3. Washington: Butterworths; 1962. p. 125–37.
6. Alexander W. The treatment of epilepsy by ligature of the vertebral arteries. Brain. 1883;5:170–87.
7. Binswanger O. Die Epilepsie. Hölder: Wien; 1899.
8. Dudley BW. Observations on injuries of the head. Transylvania J Med. 1828;1:9–40.
9. Patchell RA, Young AB, Tibbs PA. Benjamin Winslow Dudley and the surgical treatment of epilepsy. Neurology. 1987;37:290–1.
10. Smith S. The surgical treatment of epilepsy, with statistical tables, comprising all recorded cases of ligature of the carotid artery; and also of trephining the cranium by American surgeons. NY J Med. 1852:220–42.
11. Horsley V. Brain-surgery. Br Med J. 1886;2:670–5.
12. Jackson H. Discussion of V. Horsleys paper. Br Med J. 1886;2:674–5.
13. Taylor DC. One hundred years of epilepsy surgery: Sir Victor Horsley's contribution. In: Engel J, editor. Surgical treatment of the epilepsies. New York: Raven Press; 1987. p. 7–11.
14. Hitzig E. Hughlings Jackson and the cortical motor centres in the light of physiological research. Brain. 1900;23:544–81.
15. Macewen W. Tumour of the dura mater removed during life in a person affected with epilepsy. Glasgow Med J. 1879;12:210.
16. Taylor J. Selected writings of John Hughlings Jackson, vol. 1. New York: Basic Books Inc.; 1958.
17. Macewen W. Intra-cranial lesions: illustrating some points in connexion with the localisation of cerebral affections and the advantages of aseptic trephining. Lancet. 1881;2:544–81.
18. Keen WW. The successful cases of cerebral surgery. Am J Med Sci. 1888;96:452–65.

19. Nancrede CB. Two successful cases of brain surgery. Med News. 1888;53:584–8.
20. Lloyd JH, Deaver JB. A case of focal epilepsy successfully treated by trephining and excision of the motor centres. Am J Med Sci. 1888;96:477–87.
21. O'Leary JL, Goldring S. Chapter 16. Role of neurological surgery in the treatment of epilepsy. In: Science and epilepsy: neuroscience gains in epilepsy research. New York: Raven; 1976. p. 227–50.
22. Krause F. Die operative Behandlung der Epilepsie. Med Klin Berlin. 1909;5:1418–22.
23. Krause F. Die Sehbahnen in chirurgischer Beziehung und die faradische Reizung des Sehzentrums. Klin Wschr. 1924;3:1260–5.
24. Krause F. Chirurgie des Gehirns und Rückenmarks nach eigenen Erfahrungen. Berlin, Wien: Urban, Schwarzenberg; 1911.
25. Wolf P. The history of surgical treatment of epilepsy in Europe. In: Lüders H, editor. Epilepsy Surgery. New York: Raven Press; 1992. p. 9–18.
26. Krause F, Schum H. Die spezielle Chirurgie der Gehirnkrankheiten, 2. Bd. Die epileptischen Erkrankungen. Stuttgart: Enke; 1932.
27. Foerster O. Zur Pathogenese und chirurgischen Behandlung der Epilepsie. Zentralbl Chir. 1925;52:531–49.
28. Foerster O. Zur Pathogenese und chirurgischen Behandlung der Epilepsie. Zentralbl Chir. 1929a;52:531–49.
29. Foerster O. Beiträge zur Pathophysiologie der Sehbahn und der Sehsphäre. J Psychol Neurol Lpz. 1929b;39:463–85.
30. Foerster O. Über die Bedeutung und Reichweite des Lokalisationsprinzips im Nervensystem. Verh Dtsch Ges Inn Med. 1934;46:117–211.
31. Foerster O, Altenburger H. Elektrobiologische Vorgänge an der menschlichen Hirnrinde. Dtsch Z Nervenheilkd. 1935;135:277–88.
32. Foerster O. Sensible Kortikale Felder. In: Bumke O, Foerster O, editors. Handbuch der neurologie, vol. 6. Berlin: Springer; 1936a. p. 1–448.
33. Foerster O. The motor cortex in man in the light of Hughlings Jackson's doctrines. Brain. 1936b;59:135–59.
34. Foerster O, Altenburger H. Elektrobiologische Vorgänge an der menschlichen Hirnrinde. Dtsch Arch Nervenheilk 1935;135:277–88
35. Foerster O, Penfield W. The structural basis of traumatic epilepsy and results of radical operation. Brain. 1930;53:99–120.
36. Lüders JC, Lüders HO. Contributions of Fedor Krause and Otfried Foerster to epilepsy surgery. In: Lüders HO, Comair YG, editors. Epilepsy surgery. Philadelphia: Lippincott William and Wilkins; 2001. p. 23–33.
37. Penfield W. Epilepsy and surgical therapy. Arch Neurol Psychiatry. 1936;36:449–84.
38. Berger H. Über das Elektrenkephalogramm des Menschen. Arch f Psychiatr 1929;87:527–70.
39. Flanigin HF, Hermann BP, King DW, et al. The history of surgical treatment of epilepsy in North America prior to 1975. In: Lüders H, editor. Epilepsy surgery. New York: Raven Press; 1992. p. 19–36.
40. Jasper HH. Electrical potentials from the intact human brain. Science. 1935;81:51–3.
41. Jasper HH. Electroencephalography. In: Penfield WE, editor. Epilepsy and cerebral localization. Springfield, IL: Charles C Thomas; 1941. p. 380–454.
42. Wilson SJ, Engel J. Diverse perspectives on developments in epilepsy surgery. Seizure. 2010;19:659–68.
43. Sommer W. Erkrankung des Ammonshorns als aetiologisches Moment der Epilepsie. Arch Psychiatr Nervenkr. 1880;10:631–75.
44. Bratz E. Ammonshornbefunde bei Epileptikern. Arch Psychiatr Nervenkr. 1889;32:820–35.
45. Penfield W, Jasper H. Epilepsy and the functional anatomy of the human brain. Boston: Little, Brown and Co; 1954. p. 896.
46. Polkey CE. The evolution of epilepsy surgery. Neurol India. 2017;65(Suppl 1):45–51.
47. Rasmussen T, Olszewski J, Lloyd-Smith D. Focal seizures due to chronic localized encephalitis. Neurology. 1958;8:435–45.
48. Taylor DC, Falconer MA, Bruton CJ, Corselius JAN. Focal dysplasia of the cerebral cortex in epilepsy. J Neurol Neurosurg Psychiatry. 1971;34:369–87.
49. Bailey P, Green JR, Amador L, Gibbs FA. Treatment of psychomotor states by anterior temporal lobectomy. A report of progress. Res Publ Ass Nerv Ment Dis. 1935;31:341–6.
50. Bailey P, Gibbs FA. The surgical treatment of psychomotor epilepsy. JAMA. 1951;145:365–70.
51. Sachs E. The subpial resection of the cortex in the treatment of Jacksonian Epilepsy (Horsley operation) with observations on areas 4 and 6. Brain. 1935;58:492–503.
52. Penfield W, Steelman H. The treatment of focal epilepsy by cortical excision. Ann Surg. 1947;126:740–62.
53. Feindel W. Electrical stimulation of the brain during surgery for epilepsy—historical highlights. Int Anesthesiol Clin. 1986;24:75–87.
54. Meador KJ, Loring DW, Flanigin HF. History of epilepsy surgery. J Epilepsy. 1989;2:21–5.
55. Feindel W, Leblanc R, Nogueira DE, Almeida A. Epilepsy surgery: historical highlights 1909–2009. Epilepsia. 2009;50:131–51.
56. Olivier A. Epilepsy surgery at the MNI: from Archibald to the creation of the Shirley and Mark Rayport fellowship in surgery of epilepsy. Epilepsia. 2010;51(Suppl. 1):97–100.
57. Hermann BP, Stone JL. A historical review of the epilepsy surgery program at the University of Illinois Medical Center: the contributions of Bailey, Gibbs, and collaborators to the refinement of anterior temporal lobectomy. J Epilepsy. 1989;2:155–63.
58. Van Wagenen WP, Herren RY. Surgical division of commissural pathways in the corpus callosum. AMA Arch Neurol Psychiat. 1940;44:740–59.
59. Krynauw RA. Infantile hemiplegia treated by removing one cerebral hemisphere. J Neurol Neurosurg Psychiatry. 1950;13:243–67.

60. Scoville WB, Milner B. Loss of recent memory after bilateral hippocampal lesions. J Neurol Neurosurg Psychiatry. 1957;20:11–21.
61. Baxendale S. Amnesia in temporal lobectomy patients: historical perspective and review. Seizure. 1998;7:15–24.
62. Milner B, Penfield W. The effect of hippocampal lesions on recent memory. Trans Am Neurol Assoc. 1955;80:42–8.
63. Milner B. Amnesia following operation on the temporal lobes. In: CMW W, Zangwill OL, editors. Amnesia. London: Butterworth; 1966. p. 109–33.
64. Rausch R. Psychological evaluation. In: Engel J, editor. Surgical treatment of the epilepsies. New York: Raven Press; 1987. p. 181–95.
65. Wada J, Rasmussen T. Intracarotid injection of sodium amytal for the lateralization of cerebral speech dominance: Experimental and clinical observations. J Neurosurg. 1960;17:266–82.
66. Ambrose J. Computerized X-ray scanning of the brain. J Neurosurg. 1974;40:679–95.
67. Holland GN, Moore WS, Hawkes RC. Nuclear magnetic resonance tomography of the brain. J Comput Assist Tomogr. 1980;4:1–3.
68. Belliveau JW, Kwong KK, Kennedy DN, Baker JR, Stern CE, Benson R, et al. Magnetic resonance imaging mapping of brain function. Human visual cortex. Investig Radiol. 1992;27(Suppl. 2):59–65.
69. Newton MR, Berkovic SF, Austin MC, Rowe CC, McKay WJ, Bladin PF. Postictal switch in blood flow distribution and temporal lobe seizures. J Neurol Neurosurg Psychiatry. 1992;55:891–4.
70. Kriss TC, Kriss VM. History of the operating microscope: from magnifying glass to microneurosurgery. Neurosurgery. 1998;42:899–908.
71. Seeger W. Atlas of topographical anatomy of the brain and surrounding structures. Wien: Springer; 1978.
72. Seeger W. Microsurgery of the brain. Anatomical and technical principles. Wien: Springer; 1984.
73. Yaşargil MG, Antic J, Laciga R, et al. Microsurgical pterional approach to aneurysms of the basilar bifurcation. Surg Neurol. 1976;6:83–91.
74. Yasargil MG. Microneurosurgery, vol. I. Stuttgart: Thieme; 1984.
75. Moller AR. Evoked potentials in intraoperative monitoring. Baltimore: Williams and Wilkins; 1988.
76. Schramm J, Moller AR, editors. Intraoperative neurophysiological monitoring in neurosurgery. Berlin, Heidelberg, New York: Springer; 1991.
77. Nuwer M. Intraoperative monitoring of neural function. Amsterdam: Elsevier; 2008.
78. Morrell F, Whisler WW, Bleck TP. Multiple subpial transection. A new approach to the surgical treatment of focal epilepsy. J Neurosurg. 1989;70:231–9.
79. Watanabe E, Watanabe T, Manaka S, et al. Three-dimensional digitizer (neuronavigator): new equipment for computerized tomography-guided stereotactic surgery. Surg Neurol. 1987;27:543–7.
80. Rasmussen T. Postoperative superficial cerebral hemosiderosis of the brain, its diagnosis, treatment and prevention. Am Neurol Assoc. 1973;98:133–7.
81. Rasmussen T, Andermann F. Hemispherectomy for seizures revisited. Can J Neurol Sci. 1983;10:71–8.
82. Adams CBT. Hemispherectomy—a modification. J Neurol Neurosurg Psychiatry. 1983;46:617–9.
83. Delalande O, Bulteau C, Dellatolas G, Fohlen M, Jalin C, Buret V, et al. Vertical parasagittal hemispherotomy: surgical procedures and clinical long-term outcomes in a population of 83 children. Neurosurgery. 2007;60(Suppl. 1):19–32.
84. Schramm J, Behrens E, Entzian W. Hemispherical deafferentiation: an alternative to functional hemispherectomy. Neurosurgery. 1995;36:509–15.
85. Villemure JG, Mascott CR. Peri-insular hemispherectomy: Surgical principles and anatomy. Neurosurgery. 1995;37:975–81.
86. Niemeyer P: The transventricular amygdala-hippocampectomy in temporal lobe epilepsy. In: Baldwin P (ed). Temporal Lobe Epilepsy. Charles C Thomas, Springfield, 1958;461–82.
87. Wieser HG, Yasargil MG. Selective amygdalohippocampectomy as a surgical treatment of mesiobasal limbic epilepsy. Surg Neurol. 1982;17(6):445–57.
88. Yasargil MG, Teddy PJ, Roth P. Selective amygdalo-hippocampectomy. Operative anatomy and surgical technique. In: Symon L, et al. editors. Advances and Technical Standards in Neurosurgery, vol. 12. Wien, New York: Springer; 1985. p. 93–123.
89. Hori T, Tabuchi S, Kurosaki M, Kondo S, Takenobu A, Watanabe T. Subtem- poral amygdalohippocampectomy for treating medically intractable temporal lobe epilepsy. Neurosurgery. 1993;33(1):50–6; discussion 56–7.
90. Vinters HV, Armstrong DL, Babb TL, et al. The neuropathology of human symptomatic epilepsy. In: Engel J, editor. Surgical treatment of the epilepsies. New York: Raven Press; 1993. p. 593–608.
91. Talairach J, Bancaud J, Szikla G, et al. Approche nouvelle de la neurochirurgie de l'épilepsie. Méthodologie stéréotaxique et résultants thérapeutiques. Neurochirurgie. 1974;20:92–8.
92. Crandall PH, Walter RD, Rand RW. Clinical applications of studies on stereotactically implanted electrodes in temporal lobe epilepsy. J Neurosurg. 1963;20:827–40.
93. Spiegel EA, Wycis HT, et al. Stereoencephalography. Proc Soc Exp Biol Med. 1948;69(1):175–7.
94. Umbach W, Riechert T. Elektrophysiologische und klinische Ergebnisse stereotaktischer Eingriffe im limbischen System bei temporaler Epilepsie. Nervenarzt. 1964;35:482–8.
95. Mundinger F, Becker P, Grolkner E. Late results of stereotactic surgery of epilepsy predominantly temporal lobe type. Acta Neurochir. 1976;23:177–82.
96. Schwab RS, Sweet WH, Mark VH, Kjellberg RN, Ervin FR. Treatment of intractable temporal lobe epilepsy by stereotactic amygdala lesions. Trans Am Neurol Assoc. 1965;90:12–9.

97. Bouchard G. Long term results of stereotactic fornicotomy and fornicoamygdalotomy in patients with temporal lobe epilepsy showing behavioral disturbances. In: Umbach W, editor. Special topics in stereotaxis. Stuttgart: Hippokrates; 1971. p. 53–63.
98. Parrent AG. Stereotactic radiofrequency ablation for the treatment of gelastic seizures associated with hypothalamic hamartoma. Case report. J Neurosurg. 1999;91:881–4.
99. Wilfong AA, Curry DJ. Hypothalamic hamartomas: optimal approach to clinical evaluation and diagnosis. Epilepsia. 2013;54(Suppl. 9):109–14.
100. Barcia-Solario JL, Barcia JA, Hernandez G, Lopez-Gomez L, Roldan P. Radiosurgery of epilepsy. Acta Neurochir Suppl. 1993;58:195–7.
101. Regis J, Peragui JC, Rey M, Samson Y, Levrier O, Porcheron D, et al. First selective amygdalohippocampal radiosurgery for mesial temporal lobe epilepsy. Stereotact Funct Neurosurg. 1995;64(Suppl 1):193–201.
102. Penry JK, Dean C. Prevention of intractable seizures by intermittent vagal stimulation in humans: preliminary results. Epilepsia. 1990;31(Suppl. 2):40–3.
103. Cooke PM, Snider RS. Some cerebellar influences on electrically induced cerebral seizures. Epilepsia. 1955;4:19–28.
104. Tyrand R, Seeck M, Pollo C, Boex C. Effects of amygdala-hippocampal stimulation on synchronization. Epilepsy Res. 2014;108:327–30. https://doi.org/10.1016/j.eplepsyres.2013.11.024.
105. Laxpati NG, Kasoff WS, Gross RE. Deep brain stimulation for the treatment of epilepsy: circuits, targets, and trials. Neurotherapeutics. 2014;11:508–26. https://doi.org/10.1007/s13311-014-0279-9.
106. Velasco AL, Velasco F, Jimenez F, Velasco M, Castro G, Carrillo-Ruiz JD, Fanghanel G, Boleaga B. Neuromodulation of the centromedian thalamic nuclei in the treatment of generalized seizures and the improvement of the quality of life in patients with Lennox-Gastaut syndrome. Epilepsia. 2006;47:1203–12. https://doi.org/10.1111/j.1528-1167.2006.00593.x.
107. Fisher R, Salanova V, Witt T, Worth R, Henry T, Gross R, et al. Electrical stimulation of the anterior nucleus of thalamus for treatment of refractory epilepsy. Epilepsia. 2010;51:899–908.
108. Salanova V, Witt T, Worth R, Henry T, Gross R, Nazzaro JM, et al. Long-term efficacy and safety of thalamic stimulation for drug-resistant partial epilepsy. Neurology. 2015;84:1017–25.
109. Morrell MJ. Group RNSSiES. Responsive cortical stimulation for the treatment of medically intractable partial epilepsy. Neurology. 2011;77:1295–304.
110. Morrell MJ. In response: the RNS System multicenter randomized double-blinded controlled trial of responsive cortical stimulation for adjunctive treatment of intractable partial epilepsy: knowledge and insights gained. Epilepsia. 2014;55:1470–1.
111. Boon P, Vonck K, van Rijckevorsel K, et al. A prospective, multicenter study of cardiac-based seizure detection to activate vagus nerve stimulation. Seizure. 2015;32:52–61.
112. Hartshorn A, Jobst B. Responsive brain stimulation in epilepsy. Ther Adv Chronic Dis. 2018;9(7):135–42.
113. Wieser HG, Elger CE. Presurgical evaluation of epileptics. Berlin, Heidelberg: Springer; 1987.
114. Engel J Jr. Surgical treatment of the epilepsies. New York: Raven Press; 1987. New York: Raven Press; 1975. p. 356
115. Engel J Jr. Surgical treatment of the epilepsies. 2nd ed. New York: Raven Press; 1993.

# 2 Epilepsy: Clinical, Epidemiological, and Therapeutical Aspects

*People think that epilepsy is divine simply because they don't have any idea what causes epilepsy. But I believe that someday we will understand what causes epilepsy, and at that moment, we will cease to believe that it's divine. And so it is with everything in the universe.*

*Hippocrates*

## Contents



Epilepsy is one of the most common neurological disorders affecting almost 1% of the population [1, 2]. According to the International League Against Epilepsy (ILAE), it is defined by any of the following conditions: (1) two unprovoked seizures occurring more than 24 h apart, (2) a single unprovoked seizure, if recurrence risk is high (at least 60% over the next 10 years), or (3) a diagnosis of an epilepsy syndrome [3]. Epilepsy has numerous neurobiological, cognitive, and psychosocial consequences [3]. In 1997, the WHO in conjunction with the ILAE and the International Bureau for Epilepsy launched the Global Campaign Against Epilepsy, which resulted in the 2015 World Health Assembly urging all states to address the specific needs of people with epilepsy [4, 5]. The classification and terminology of seizure types have been updated by the ILAE in 2017 [4, 6–8].

Epilepsy is characterized by a lasting predisposition to generate spontaneous epileptic seizures. The pathophysiological process of epileptogenesis is thought to result from an imbalance between excitatory and inhibitory activity within a neuronal network [4, 9]. In generalized epilepsies, epileptogenic networks are widely distributed, involving thalamocortical structures bilaterally [6, 7, 10], and most generalized epilepsies are thought to have a genetic basis [11]. For focal epilepsies, networks involve neuronal circuits in one hemisphere commonly including limbic or neocortical structures [6, 7]. Much of the understanding of focal epilepsies derives from animal models including epileptogenic brain


J. Zentner, *Surgical Treatment of Epilepsies*, https://doi.org/10.1007/978-3-030-48748-5_2

insult with proconvulsant agents, electrical stimulation, or traumatic brain injury [12, 13]. The best ascertained epileptogenic lesion is mesial temporal sclerosis [14–16] (see also Chap. 6).

## 2.1 Incidence and Prevalence

There is a bimodal distribution of epilepsy. The incidence presents a first peak in early life; it remains relatively high in childhood and adolescence, decreases between the third and sixth decades, and presents a second peak in older age [1, 17, 18] (Fig. 2.1). Risk factors vary between age groups. Malformations of cortical development are usually predominant in epilepsies developing during childhood. Trauma, infections, and tumors are mainly observed in epilepsies associated with the young adult age, while cerebrovascular disease is the most common risk factor in elderly people [19].

In high-income countries, incidence of epilepsy is consistent across different regions affecting around 50 people (range 40–70) per 100,000 of the population per year [1, 20–23]. The incidence of epilepsy is higher in low-income countries affecting 80–100 people per 100,000 of the population per year [4]. The prevalence of active epilepsy is usually between 4 and 12 people per 1000 of the population [1, 20–22]. Thus, epilepsy may affect over 70 million people worldwide [2, 4].

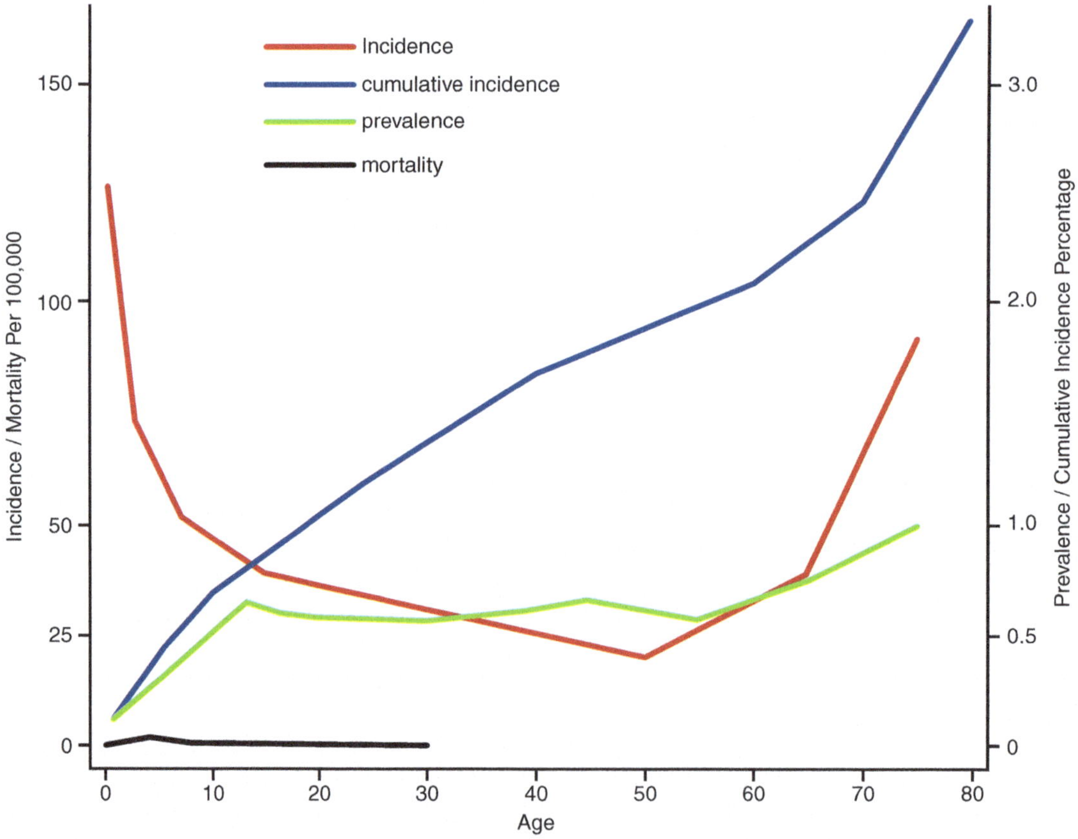


**Fig. 2.1** Incidence, cumulative incidence, prevalence, and mortality for epilepsy in Rochester, Minnesota, 1935–1974 (modified from Anderson et al. [17], with permission)

## 2.2 Psychosocial Consequences and Risk Factors

Patients with epilepsy suffer from restricted mobility, limited job options, and emotional stress arising from their disease and the associated stigmatization. More than 50% of people with epilepsy have one or several additional medical problems [24]. Psychiatric comorbidities (e.g., depression, anxiety, psychosis, autism) have been associated with epilepsy for a long time. More recently, somatic disorders (e.g., type I diabetes, arthritis, digestive tract ulcers, chronic obstructive pulmonary disease) have been linked to epilepsy as well [24].

Epilepsy patients are exposed to multiple risks: The annual incidence of status epilepticus is around 1% [25], and that of traumatic injury has been estimated as high as 27% [26]. Up to one-third of all premature deaths are either directly (e.g., status epilepticus, injuries, sudden unexpected death in epilepsy (SUDEP)) or indirectly (e.g., aspiration pneumonia, suicide, drowning) attributable to epilepsy [27]. Deaths due to external causes, e.g., accidents, seem to be more prevalent in low-income countries than in high-income countries [4, 27].

SUDEP is defined as a sudden and unexpected, nontraumatic and non-drowning death of epilepsy patients, without a toxicological or anatomical cause [28]. Ryvlin and Kahane [29] noted in a review a total of 154 SUDEP cases among 41,439 person years, resulting in a mean incidence of 3.7/1000/year. DeGiorgio et al. [30] amounted the incidence of SUDEP in adults to 1.2 per 1000 person years. Overall, SUDEP is thought to occur in about 1 of 1000 adults and 1 of 4500 children with epilepsy per year [31–33]. Proposed pathophysiological mechanisms include seizure-induced cardiac and respiratory arrests [34]. Uncontrolled generalized tonic-clonic seizures have been identified as the leading hazard factor predisposing to SUDEP [30]. These risks associated with epilepsy make it clear that therapeutic goals should aim at complete abolishment of seizures.

## 2.3 Pharmacotherapy and Pharmacoresistance

The primary treatment of epilepsy is the administration of an adequate medication. Even though pharmacotherapy has improved with the availability of new drugs, antiepileptic medication is frequently associated with side effects [35, 36]. Most frequent adverse effects refer to neuropsychiatric symptoms, e.g., fatigue, dizziness, unsteadiness, and irritability [37, 38]. Accepting those unintended side effects, antiepileptic medication suppresses seizures in up to two-thirds of all individuals. However, around one-third of all epilepsy patients (in Germany, more than 200,000 people) have persistent seizures despite optimal medical treatment [4]. If the patient's seizures fail to respond to the first two antiepileptic drugs that are tried, the probability of achieving a lasting seizure-free state with further changes in medication is only 5–10% [25, 39].

Drug-resistant epilepsy is assumed after the "failure of adequate trials of two tolerated, appropriately chosen and used antiseizure drug schedules (as monotherapies or in combination) to achieve sustained seizure freedom" [38]. It seems to be remarkable that despite the introduction of several new antiepileptic drugs (AEDs) over the past decades, the proportion of drug-resistant epilepsies remains constant at approximately 30–40% ([40, 41]). Drug-resistant epilepsy, however, leads to decreased life expectancy and impaired quality of life, and may imply devastating socioeconomic consequences [42, 43].

## 2.4 Surgical Options

In selected individuals with drug-resistant focal epilepsy, surgery has proven to be an effective option to achieve long-term seizure freedom. Patients might benefit from microsurgical removal or disconnection of a circumscribed brain region, or from minimally invasive stereotactic procedures. In addition to a large body of observational studies, two randomized controlled

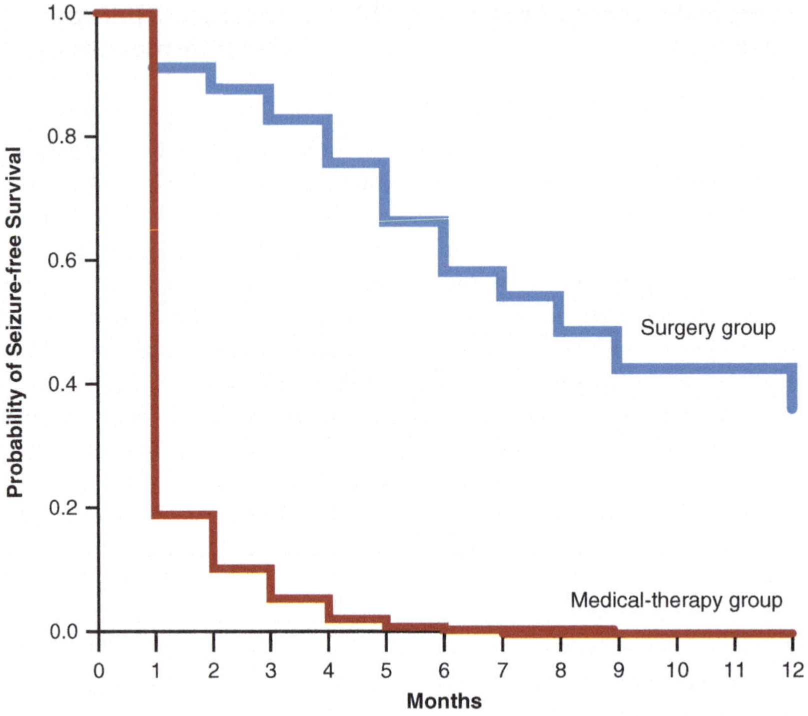


**Fig. 2.2** Single-center trial including 116 children and adolescents with drug-resistant epilepsy. Patients were randomly assigned to undergo surgery (surgical therapy group: 57 patients) or to a waiting list for surgery while receiving medical therapy alone (medical therapy group: 59 patients). At 12-month follow-up, seizure freedom occurred in 44 patients (77%) in the surgical therapy group, but only in 4 (7%) in the medical therapy group (p<0.001). In addition, children and adolescents who had undergone surgery had better scores with respect to behavior and quality of life than those who continued medical therapy alone (from Dwivedi et al. [45], with permission)

trials in adult patients with pharmacoresistant temporal lobe epilepsy provide grade I evidence for the superiority of epilepsy surgery to pharmacotherapy ([37, 44]; see also Chap. 6). Similarly, a randomized controlled study in children and adolescents with medically refractory temporal and extratemporal epilepsy demonstrated seizure freedom in 77% of the patients after surgery, but only in 7% with continuous medical therapy ([45]; see also Chap. 11) (Fig. 2.2). Thus, unlike with antiepileptic medication, epilepsy surgery offers the unique chance to cure epilepsy [46, 47]. Furthermore, it has been shown that surgery is associated with a reduction in mortality rate in drug-resistant epilepsy patients, when seizures are abolished or when at least a significant reduction of tonic-clonic seizure frequency is achieved [48].

Given that surgery has proven to be far superior to the best medical treatment in terms of seizure control and quality of life providing the unique chance to cure epilepsy, there is now an international consensus that patients in whom generation of epilepsy in a circumscribed, localizable area of the brain is suspected should be referred to an epilepsy center for presurgical evaluation, if their seizures have not responded to treatment with two drugs [38, 49].

## Concluding Remarks

- ***Incidence and pharmacoresistance of epilepsy.*** *The incidence of epilepsy presents a first peak in early life. It remains relatively high in childhood and adolescence, decreases between the third and sixth decades, and presents a second peak in older age. One-third of* *all epilepsy patients have persistent (drug resistant) seizures despite optimal medical treatment.*

- ***Psychosocial consequences and risks of epilepsy.*** *Patients with epilepsy suffer from restricted mobility, limited job options, and emotional stress. Comorbidities as observed in half of epilepsy patients include psychiatric and somatic disorders. Epilepsy patients are exposed to multiple risks including status epilepticus, traumatic injury, and sudden unexpected death in epilepsy (SUDEP).*
- ***Surgical options.*** *In selected individuals with drug-resistant focal epilepsy, surgery has proven to be an effective option providing the unique chance to cure epilepsy as demonstrated by three randomized controlled trials.*

## References


1. Fiest KM, Sauro KM, Wiebe S, et al. Prevalence and incidence of epilepsy: a systematic review and meta-analysis of international studies. Neurology. 2017;88:296–303.
2. Sander JW, Shorvon SD. Epidemiology of the epilepsies. J Neurol Neurosurg Psychiatry. 1996;61(5):433–43.
3. Fisher RS, Acevedo C, Arzimanoglou A, et al. ILAE official report: a practical clinical definition of epilepsy. Epilepsia. 2014;55:475–82.
4. Thijs RD, Surges R, O'Brien TJ, Sander LW. Epilepsy in adults. Lancet. 2019;393:689–701.
5. WHO. Global burden of epilepsy and the need for coordinated action at the country level to address its health, social and public knowledge implications. 2015: Resolution WHA68·20.
6. Fisher RS, Cross JH, French JA, et al. Operational classification of seizure types by the International League Against Epilepsy: position paper of the ILAE Commission for classification and terminology. Epilepsia. 2017;58:522–30.
7. Fisher RS, Cross JH, D'Souza C, et al. Instruction manual for the ILAE 2017 operational classification of seizure types. Epilepsia. 2017;58:531–42.
8. Scheffer IE, Berkovic S, Capovilla G, et al. ILAE classification of the epilepsies: Position paper of the ILAE Commission for Classification and Terminology. Epilepsia. 2017;58:512–21.
9. Fisher RS, van Emde BW, Blume W, et al. Epileptic seizures and epilepsy: definitions proposed by the International League Against Epilepsy (ILAE) and the International Bureau for Epilepsy (IBE). Epilepsia. 2005;46:470–2.
10. Crunelli V, Leresche N. Childhood absence epilepsy: genes, channels, neurons and networks. Nat Rev Neurosci. 2002;3:371–82.
11. Helbig I, Scheffer IE, Mulley JC, Berkovic SF. Navigating the channels and beyond: unravelling the genetics of the epilepsies. Lancet Neurol. 2008;7:231–45.
12. Fisher RS. Cellular mechanisms of the epilepsies. In: Hopkins A, Shorvon S, Cascino G, editors. Epilepsy. 2nd ed. London: Chapman & Hall; 1995. p. 35–58.
13. Sarkisian MR. Overview of the current animal models for human seizure and epileptic disorders. Epilepsy Behav. 2001;2:201–16.
14. Babb TL, Brown WJ, Pretorius J, Davenport C, Lieb JP, Crandall PH. Temporal lobe volumetric cell densities in temporal lobe epilepsy. Epilepsia. 1984;25:729–40.
15. Babb T, Brown W. Pathological findings in epilepsy. In: Engel J, editor. Surgical treatment of the epilepsies. New York: Raven Press; 1987.
16. Morimoto K, Fahnestock M, Racine RJ. Kindling and status epilepticus models of epilepsy: rewiring the brain. Prog Neurobiol. 2004;73:1–60.
17. Anderson VE, Hauser WA, Rich SS. Genetic heterogeneity in the epilepsies. In: Delgado-Escueta AV, Ward A, Woodbury DM, Porter RJ, editors. Advances in neurology, vol. 44. New York: Raven Press; 1986.
18. Hauser WA, Annegers JF, Kurland LT. Incidence of epilepsy and unprovoked seizures in Rochester, Minnesota: 1935-1984. Epilepsia. 1993;34(3):453–68.
19. Chen Z, Brodie MJ, Liew D, Kwan P. Treatment outcomes in patients with newly diagnosed epilepsy treated with established and new antiepileptic drugs: a 30-year longitudinal cohort study. JAMA Neurol. 2018;75:279–86.
20. Bell GS, Neligan A, Sander JW. An unknown quantity – the worldwide prevalence of epilepsy. Epilepsia. 2014;55:958–62.
21. Neligan A, Hauser WA, Sander JW. The epidemiology of the epilepsies. Handb Clin Neurol. 2012;107:113–33.
22. Ngugi AK, Kariuki SM, Bottomley C, Kleinschmidt I, Sander JW, Newton CR. Incidence of epilepsy: a systematic review and meta-analysis. Neurology. 2011;77:1005–12.
23. Zack MM, Kobau R. National and state estimates of the numbers of adults and children with active epilepsy—United States, 2015. MMWR Morb Mortal Wkly Rep. 2017;66:821–5.
24. Téllez-Zenteno JF, Matijevic S, Wiebe S. Somatic comorbidity of epilepsy in the general population in Canada. Epilepsia. 2005;46:1955–62.
25. Hauser WA. Status epilepticus: epidemiologic considerations. Neurology. 1990;40:9–13.
26. Beghi E, Cornaggia C. Morbidity and accidents in patients with epilepsy: results of a European cohort study. Epilepsia. 2002;43:1076–83.

27. Maguire MJ, Jackson CF, Marson AG, Nolan SJ. Treatments for the prevention of Sudden unexpected death in epilepsy (SUDEP). Cochrane Database Syst Rev. 2016;7:CD011792.
28. Terra VC, Cysneiros R, Cavalheiro EA, Scorza FA. Sudden unexpected death in epilepsy: from the lab to the clinic setting. Epilepsy Behav. 2013;26(3):415–20.
29. Ryvlin P, Kahane P. Does epilepsy surgery lower the mortality of drug-resistant epilepsy? Epilepsy Res. 2003;56:105–20.
30. DeGiorgio CM, Curtis A, Hertling D, et al. Sudden unexpected death in epilepsy: risk factors, biomarkers and prevention. Acta Neurol Scand. 2019;139(3):220–30.
31. Harden C, Tomson T, Gloss D, Buchhalter J, Cross JH, Donner E, French JA, Gil-Nagel A, Hesdorffer DC, Smithson WH, Spitz MC, Walczak TS, Sander JW, Ryvlin P. Practice guideline summary: Sudden unexpected death in epilepsy incidence rates and risk factors: Report of the Guideline Development, Dissemination, and Implementation Subcommittee of the American Academy of Neurology and the American Epilepsy Society. Neurology. 2017;88(17):1674–80.
32. Holst AG, Winkel BG, Risgaard B, et al. Epilepsy and risk of death and sudden unexpected death in the young: a nationwide study. Epilepsia. 2013;54:1613–20.
33. Schulze-Bonhage A. Der unerwartete Tod bei Epilepsiepatienten. Schweizerische Zeitschrift für Psychiatrie Neurologie. 2007;3:6–8.
34. Tolstykh GP, Cavazos JE. Potential mechanisms of sudden unexpected death in epilepsy. Epilepsy Behav. 2013;26(3):410–4.
35. Gaitatzis A, Sander JW. The long-term safety of antiepileptic drugs. CNS Drugs. 2013;27:435–55.
36. Perucca P, Gilliam FG. Adverse effects of antiepileptic drugs. Lancet Neurol. 2012;11:792–802.
37. Engel J Jr, McDermott MP, Wiebe S, the Early Randomized Surgical Epilepsy Trial (ERSET) Study Group, et al. Early surgical therapy for drug-resistant temporal lobe epilepsy: a randomized trial. JAMA. 2012;307:922–30.
38. Kwan P, Arzimanoglou A, Berg AT, et al. Definition of drug resistant epilepsy: consensus proposal by the ad hoc Task Force of the ILAE Commission on Therapeutic Strategies. Epilepsia. 2010;51:1069–77.
39. Kwan P, Brodie MJ. Early identification of refractory epilepsy. N Engl J Med. 2000;342:314–9.
40. Englot DJ. A modern epilepsy surgery treatment algorithm: Incorporating traditional and emerging technologies. Epilepsy Behav. 2018;80:68–74.
41. Engel J Jr. What can we do for people with drug-resistant epilepsy? The 2016 Wartenberg Lecture. Neurology. 2016;87:2483–9.
42. Baker GA, Jacoby A, Buck D, Stalgis C, Monnet D. Quality of life of people with epilepsy: a European study. Epilepsia. 1997;38(3):353–62.
43. Baker GA, Nashef L, van Hout BA. Current issues in the management of epilepsy: the impact of frequent seizures on cost of illness, quality of life, and mortality. Epilepsia. 1997;38(suppl 1):S1–8.
44. Wiebe S, Blume WT, Girvin JP, Eliasziw M, the Effectiveness and Efficiency of Surgery for Temporal Lobe Epilepsy Study Group. A randomized, controlled trial of surgery for temporal lobe epilepsy. N Engl J Med. 2001;345:311–8.
45. Dwivedi R, Ramanujam B, Chandra PS, et al. Surgery for drug resistant epilepsy in children. N Engl J Med. 2017;377:1639–47.
46. Schmidt D, Baumgartner C, Löscher W. The chance of cure following surgery for drug-resistant temporal lobe epilepsy. What do we know and do we need to revise our expectations? Epilepsy Res. 2004;60(2-3):187–201.
47. Schmidt D, Baumgartner C, Löscher W. Seizure recurrence after planned discontinuation of antiepileptic drugs in seizure-free patients after epilepsy surgery: a review of current clinical experience. Epilepsia. 2004;45(2):179–86.
48. Sperling MR, Barshow S, Nei M, Asadi-Pooya AA. A reappraisal of mortality after epilepsy surgery. Neurology. 2016;86:1938–44.
49. Kwan P, Schachter SC, Brodie MJ. Drug-resistant epilepsy. N Engl J Med. 2011;365:919–26.

# Presurgical Evaluation

# 3

*He who studies medicine without books sails an uncharted sea, but he who studies medicine without patients does not go to sea at all.*

*William Osler*

## Contents



The selection of appropriate candidates for surgical treatment requires comprehensive evaluation. It has to be confirmed that seizures fulfill the criteria of drug resistance, that the patient has been adequately treated, and that non-epileptic disorders are ruled out. The essential prerequisite for a resective surgical procedure is the evidence that seizures arise in a circumscribed area, known as the epileptogenic focus, and that this epileptogenic focus can be resected without harm. In addition, presurgical assessment has to evaluate the chances of controlling seizures and improve the patient's quality of life with surgery. Risks of surgery, especially regarding cognitive functions, have to be weighed up against the risks associated with continuous medical treatment [1–5].

The primary reason for patients to undergo epilepsy surgery, seizure freedom, includes several aspects. Concerns frequently voiced by patients refer to the acquisition of a driving license, independence, and employment, and getting rid of medication side effects and stigma. In all, patients anticipate psychosocial and psychological improvements and a better quality of life [6]. The prolonged nature of presurgical evaluation facilitates counselling of patients and



J. Zentner, *Surgical Treatment of Epilepsies*, https://doi.org/10.1007/978-3-030-48748-5_3

families at different points according to the actual data acquired. In particular, unrealistic expectations should be dampened, and the inevitable uncertainty of the individual outcome must be addressed. Epilepsy surgery provides the chance of seizure control with a certain statistical probability, but it cannot guarantee a better life, even when seizure freedom is achieved [6].

The main focus of presurgical evaluation is to accurately identify localization and extent of the epileptogenic zone which represents the area of the cortex that can generate epileptic seizures. By definition, total removal or disconnection of the epileptogenic zone is necessary to achieve seizure freedom. However, currently, no single method is available to accurately define this zone, which thus remains a hypothesis. Selection of surgical candidates constitutes a challenge to an interdisciplinary team. Evaluation of clinical history, seizure semiology, electroclinical features, and imaging data contribute to solve this problem and to formulate a hypothesis of the epileptogenic zone considering different cortical areas [4, 7] (Table 3.1).

This classical concept postulating that the epileptogenic zone categorically has to exceed limits of the structural abnormality may be questioned with respect to more recent reports on the efficacy of stereotactic lesioning techniques [8, 9] (see also Chap. 14). In fact, epilepsy primarily represents a clinico-electrophysiological phenomenon. For surgical treatment of focal epilepsy, however, the detection of its structural basis is of paramount importance, since the presence of a structural lesion will strictly guide the surgeon. Electrophysiological data serve to confirm the epileptogenicity of the structural abnormality and surrounding tissue, thus defining more clearly the total area to be resected. Overall, presurgical evaluation is based on three pillars: (1) *clinical, neuropsychological, and psychiatric assessment*; (2) *neuroimaging*; and (3) *electrophysiological diagnostics* [3, 4, 6, 10].

**Table 3.1** Classical concept of the epileptogenic zone which remains a hypothesis

| | |
|---|---|
| Irritative zone | Region of the cortex that generates interictal epileptiform discharges in EEG |
| Pacemaker (zone of seizure onset) | Region of the cortex from which the clinical seizures originate |
| Epileptogenic lesion | Structural lesion that is causally related to epilepsy |
| Ictal symptomatogenic zone | Region of the cortex that generates initial seizure symptomatology |
| Functional deficit zone | Region of the cortex that in the interictal period is functioning abnormally as assessed by neurological and/or neuropsychological examination |

This hypothesis can be formulated considering different cortical areas as shown (modified from Lüders and Awad [7], with permission)

## 3.1 Clinical, Neuropsychological, and Psychiatric Assessment

### 3.1.1 Clinical Assessment

Clinical data include patient's history, results of physical examination, social circumstances, and seizure manifestations (semiology). The semiology of the seizures can provide important information about the localization and lateralization of the ictal symptomatogenic zone. Unilateral ictal motor manifestations, e.g., version, clonic and tonic activity, unilateral epileptic spasms, dystonic posturing with preserved responsiveness, as well as ictal nystagmus, have been shown to have lateralizing value pointing to the contralateral hemisphere. Ictal speech usually indicates involvement of the nondominant hemisphere, while postictal sensoric aphasia is a common feature of seizures originating from the temporal lobe of the dominant hemisphere. Besides the lateralizing value, several localizing symptoms exist facilitating assignment to brain areas involved such as temporomesial structures with epigastric auras, temporo-occipital association areas with complex visual hallucinations, insular cortex with cardiac arrhythmias, and supplementary motor area with asymmetric posturing during the seizure (Table 3.2; Fig. 3.1). It is important to pay attention to seizure evolution rather than overemphasizing single seizure phenomena. Reviews of lateralizing and localizing signs have been provided by Loddenkemper and Kotagal [11], Stoyke et al. [12], Leutmezer and Baumgartner [13], and Rosenow and Lüders [4].

**Table 3.2** Lateralizing and localizing clinical signs of focal seizures

| Clinical sign | Seizure origin |
|---|---|
| Focal motor tonic or clonic with unclouded consciousness | Frontal area |
| Focal motor tonic or clonic with impaired consciousness | Temporal area |
| Focal motor with Jacksonian march | Precentral gyrus (with Todd's paralysis) |
| Focal sensory | Postcentral gyrus/insular |
| Tonic version | Frontodorsal including the premotor and supplementary motor cortex |
| Bilateral tonic posturing | Interhemispheric motor area |
| Asymmetric tonic limb posturing during bilateral tonic-clonic seizure ("figure-of-4 sign") | Contralateral hemisphere |
| Hypermotor seizures with crying | Anterior cingulate gyrus |
| Visual phenomena, elementary or complex | Temporomesial/basal or occipital |
| Vertiginous signs | Insular or parietal |
| Auditory symptoms | Heschl's gyrus/auditory belt |
| Epigastric sensations | Temporomesial |
| Olfactory auras | Amygdala/frontobasal |

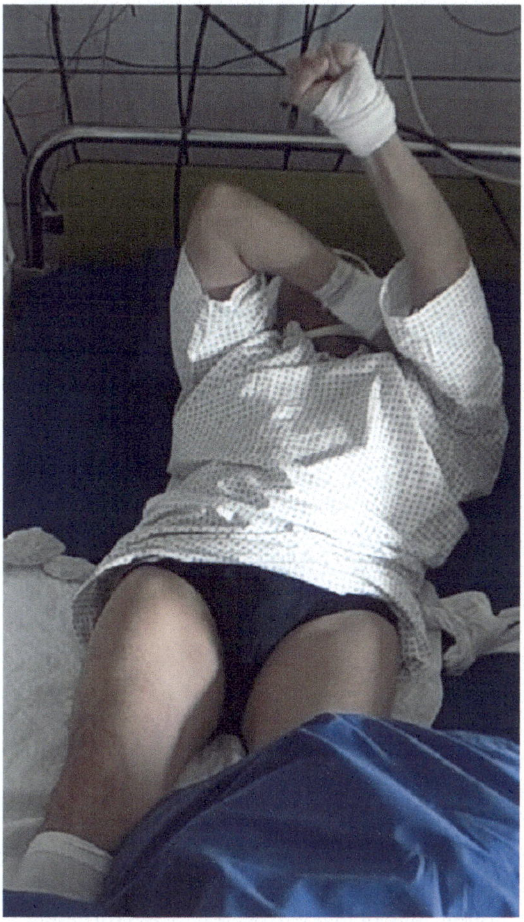

**Fig. 3.1** "Figure-of-4 sign" [14]: Asymmetric tonic limb posturing (extension of the arm contralateral to seizure onset and flexion of the opposite elbow) during the tonic phase of a bilateral tonic-clonic seizure (with courtesy of D.M. Altenmüller, Dpt. of Epileptology, Freiburg, and with permission of the patient)

### 3.1.2 Neuropsychological Assessment

Neuropsychological evaluation provides accessory information regarding the localization and lateralization of epilepsy-associated cognitive impairment. Preoperative neuropsychological profile is important when advising the patient about the cognitive risks of the proposed surgery. Evaluation of functional integrity of the structures to be resected and of the reserve capacities allows prediction of postoperative cognitive outcome [15–17]. Standardized neuropsychological test batteries are used to identify the site of dysfunction, estimate the functional risks of surgery, and assess hemispheric dominance. In addition, assessment of a patient's cognitive capabilities before and after epilepsy surgery is a useful tool for quality control which contributes to evaluation of effectiveness and safety of surgery. Neuropsychological evaluation of children poses special challenges due to limited cooperation capability and high prevalence of neuropsychological and behavioral disorders [18]. In 2012, the Neuropsychological Commission of the German Society for Epileptology (DGfE) has compiled a minimum standard for tests with regard to psychometric properties and evidence for seizure localization ([19]; Table 3.3).

#### 3.1.2.1 Temporal Lobe Epilepsy

In temporal lobe epilepsy, material-specific memory impairment can indicate lateralized temporal lobe dysfunction. Figural memory impairment can be seen in right temporal lobe

**Table 3.3** Tests recommended by the Neuropsychological Commission of the German Society for Epileptology (DGfE) (from Brückner [19], with permission)

| Function | Test procedure |
|---|---|
| Memory | Verbal learning and memory test (VLMT) |
| | Diagnosticum für Cerebralschädigung—Revised, DCS-R |
| | Verbal and visual memory spans |
| Language | Regensburger Wortflüssigkeitstest (RWT) |
| | Boston Naming Test (BNT) |
| Attention | Alertness, Go/Nogo (Testbatterie zur Aufmerksamkeitsprüfung) |
| | Divided attention |
| Spatial performance | Rey-Osterrieth Complex Figure Test (ROCFT) Copy |
| | Mosaic Test (WAIS-IV) |
| Executive functions | Flexibility (Testbatterie zur Aufmerksamkeitsprüfung) |
| | RWT (see above) |

epilepsy patients with hippocampal pathology [20]. In left temporal lobe epilepsy, qualitative and quantitative differentiation of mesial versus lateral temporal lobe functions may be possible based on the assessment of verbal learning and delayed free recall performances [16, 21]. Apart from memory impairment, naming difficulties are very common in left temporal lobe epilepsy [22, 23]. However, whereas there is a strong relation between the left temporal lobe and impairment of verbal memory [24], the relation between the right temporal lobe and figural visuospatial memory seems far less consistent [15, 16]. This can be explained partly by confounding factors like verbal memory strategies, atypical language dominance, or reorganization of memory functions [25, 26]. False lateralizing figural memory performance is more frequently seen in patients with left than with right temporal lobe epilepsy who show the expected figural visuospatial memory impairment [20]. Neuropsychological testing of the functional integrity of the hippocampus can be combined with imaging markers of its structural integrity [17]. fMRI for episodic memory is emerging as a predictor of verbal memory decline after temporal resection [27], and the risk of word finding difficulty after dominant temporal lobe resection can be estimated with fMRI [6, 28]. In addition, resting-state fMRI (rs-fMRI) seems to be a promising tool to investigate the functionality of memory networks [29].

#### 3.1.2.2 Extratemporal Epilepsies

Frontal deficits (attention, executive functions, working memory, and motor coordination) can be assessed using test batteries, while lateralization is challenging [16]. Dysfunction of frontal lobe capacities is often seen in temporal lobe epilepsy, and impaired memory is frequently observed in frontal lobe epilepsy. Thus, in clinical practice, the diagnosis of a frontotemporal dysfunction is common [15, 30]. Well-defined neuropsychological characteristics of parietal and occipital lobe epilepsies are not available. The classic parietal symptoms such as aphasia, alexia, agraphia, acalculia, agnosia, and neglect are very uncommon in chronic epilepsies. Impairments are diffuse and frequently mimic frontal or temporal lobe dysfunction [15].

### 3.1.3 Psychiatric Assessment

The prevalence of psychiatric disorders in patients with medically refractory epilepsy undergoing presurgical evaluation has been estimated to range between 40% and 80% [31]. Psychiatric comorbidities in epilepsy patients include interictal depression (5–50%), anxiety (0–48%), interictal psychosis (0–16%), and suicidality [32] with mood and anxiety (approximately 30%) being most common [33, 34] while psychotic disorders with a 7% prevalence in drug-resistant epilepsy cases are rather uncommon [35]. Structural brain damage, active epilepsy, and side effects of anti-seizure medication may contribute to these comorbidities [16]. In addition, psychiatric disturbances may be reactive to the epilepsy and associated psychosocial difficulties [6]. A history of psychiatric problems has been found to be associated with a lower chance of seizure freedom [36].

Pre- and postoperative psychiatric assessment is accomplished with the help of screening measures [6]. Preoperatively, it is important to identify risk factors for postoperative outcome [37]. Postoperative assessment is necessary in order to indicate adequate therapeutic options such as modification of antiepileptic medication, administration of antidepressants or neuroleptics, and psychotherapy [6, 38]. In addition, postoperative evaluation facilitates detection of de novo psychiatric symptoms and de novo psychogenic seizures [6].

## 3.2 Neuroimaging

About 60% of epilepsies are focal. The primary goal of *structural imaging* in epilepsy patients is to detect an epileptogenic lesion, defined as a radiological lesion that causes seizures [4]. When an epileptogenic lesion has been identified, *functional imaging* may be necessary in order to clarify spatial relationships of the lesion to eloquent cortex and white matter tracts. Advances in magnetic resonance imaging (MRI) as the gold standard of structural and functional imaging (functional MRI, fMRI) have improved the ability both to identify structural lesions causing focal epilepsy [39] and to define areas of high functionality [40]. If structural imaging studies have not revealed any potentially epileptic lesion, or if multiple lesions are present, *radionuclide imaging* has proven to be a useful tool to indicate the zone of seizure onset [41]. Figure 3.2 shows different imaging modalities frequently used.

### 3.2.1 Structural MR Imaging

Detection of an epileptogenic lesion is most important, since patients with an identified structural abnormality have 2.5 times higher odds of seizure freedom following surgery than those without [42]. However, structural imaging remains challenging, since even small lesions (down to a diameter of ≤5 mm) that often do not change during life can cause devastating epilepsy [43–47]. For detection of those subtle lesions which is particularly crucial, since most of the respective patients have excellent postsurgical outcome [48], special epilepsy-related MRI protocols and a high expertise of the neuroradiologist with epilepsy-associated lesions are necessary. Both for planning and evaluating of imaging, it is mandatory that the neuroradiologist is informed on the actual state of epileptological presurgical work-up including clinical data on the epilepsy syndrome and seizure semiology, as well as electrophysiological findings [49]. Von Oertzen et al. [50] found that with “nonexpert” reports of “standard” MRI scans, 61% of epileptogenic lesions remained undetected. Failure rate was reduced to 50% when expert neuroradiologists who were aware of the clinical focus hypothesis evaluated the “standard” MRI again. Contrarily, the application of an epilepsy-tailored MRI protocol plus reading by experienced neuroradiologists resulted in a failure rate of only 9% [50]. Similar observations have been reported by others [51]. Overviews on structural imaging have been given by Wellmer et al. [48] and Urbach et al. [40, 49, 52].

#### 3.2.1.1 MRI Techniques

High-field 3 T MR imaging has proven to be superior to 1.5 T MR imaging [39, 53] and is currently the state-of-the-art technique for the detection and characterization of epileptogenic lesions [40, 54]. In addition, new sequences and evaluation techniques have been implemented: three-dimensional fluid-attenuated inversion recovery (3D-FLAIR; [55]), susceptibility-weighted imaging (SWI; [56]), diffusion-weighted imaging (DWI; [57]), periodically rotated overlapping parallel lines with enhanced reconstruction (PROPELLER) sequences which reduce the extent of motion artifacts of moving patients [58], and MRI postprocessing [46, 47, 59]. Newer acquisitions include double-inversion recovery MRI and MP2RAGE, a variant of the well-known MPRAGE (magnetization-prepared rapid gradient echo) acquisition [60, 61]. Diffusional kurtosis imaging provides improved gray-white matter (GM-WM) contrast [62].

#### 3.2.1.2 The “Essential Six” Protocol

In a rank analysis of a large series comprising 2740 patients, Wellmer et al. [48] identified the spectrum of common epileptogenic lesions and determined

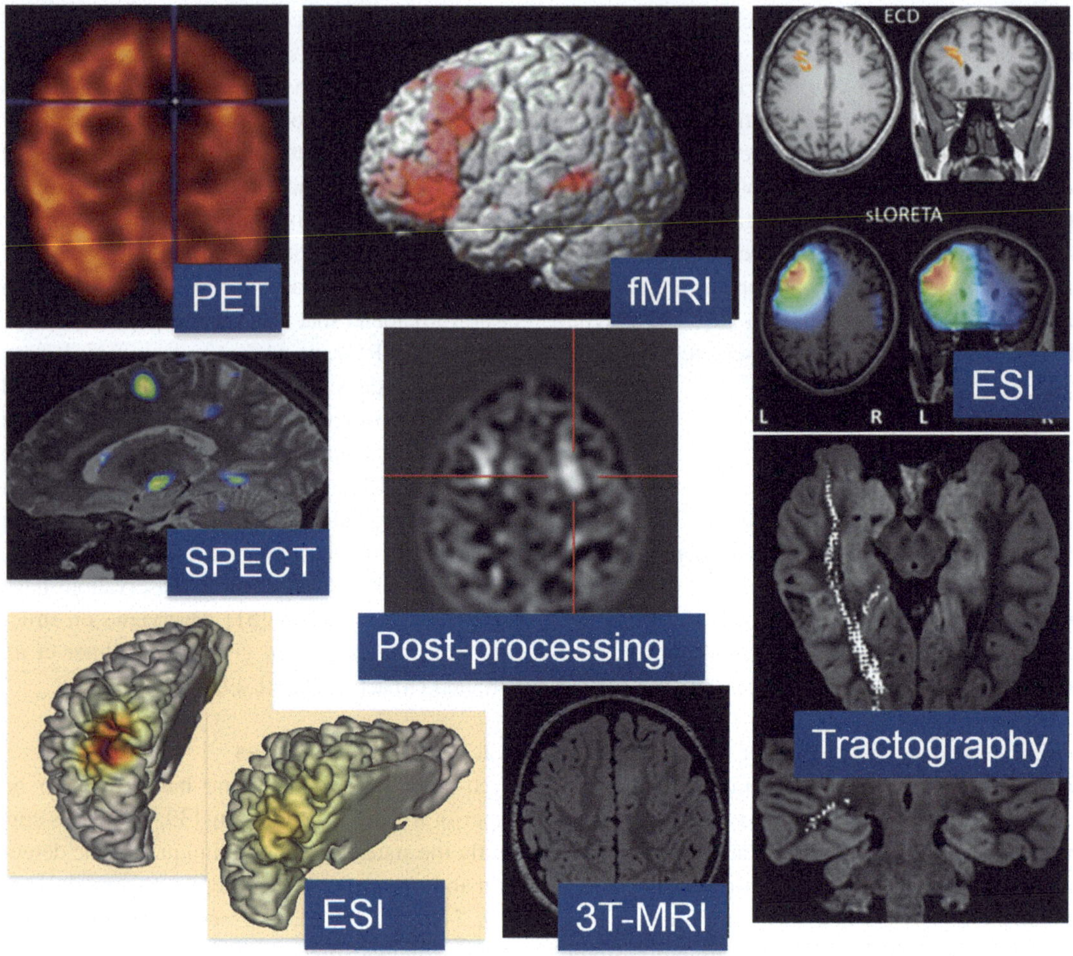


**Fig. 3.2** Overview on frequently used structural, functional, and radionuclide imaging modalities. *PET* positron-emission tomography; *SPECT* single-photon emission computed tomography; *ESI* electrical source imaging

the set of MRI sequences that are required for their reliable detection. Relying on a series of small, therapeutically relevant lesions they determined the required slice thickness, slice angulations, and orientations for an epilepsy-specific MRI protocol. The following parameters for an economic MRI protocol for the detection of epileptogenic lesions were identified: (1) 3D-T1-weighted images (1 mm isotropic; AC-PC angulation), (2) axial T2/STIR-weighted images (≤3 mm; HC angulation), (3) coronal T2/STIR-weighted images (≤3 mm; HC angulation), (4) axial inversion recovery (FLAIR) sequences (≤3 mm; HC angulation), (5) coronal FLAIR sequences (≤3 mm; HC angulation), and (6) axial hemo/calc sequences (≤3 mm; HC angulation). This protocol which was named "the essential six" allows the detection of almost all epileptogenic lesions [48] (Table 3.4). Cumulative percentages of lesion entities detected after the first to fifth sequence were 84.8% for FLAIR, 91.6% for coronal T2-weighted (w) fast spin-echo or STIR, 97.4% for T2*, 99.4% for T1-w or inversion recovery, and 100% for contrast-enhanced T1-w sequences. After FLAIR, T2/STIR, T2*, and T1-w sequences, 99.4% of all lesions and all lesion types were detected except for subtle pial angiomatosis [48].

The "essential six" protocol accords with most published recommendations for MRI protocols in demanding several sequences

**Table 3.4** The "essential six" MR imaging protocol for patients with focal epilepsies

| Sequence | | Orientation/slice thickness | Diagnostic yield |
|---|---|---|---|
| 3D T1-weighted (w) FFE or MPRAGE | | sag/1 × 1 × 1 mm$^3$ | Multiplanar reformation, voxel-based morphometry |
| 2D T2-w TSE | | ax/3–5 mm | Exact angulation |
| 3D FLAIR VISTA or SPACE | | sag/1 × 1 × 1 mm$^3$ | Focal cortical dysplasia, hippocampal sclerosis |
| Alternatively | 2D FLAIR-TSE | ax/2–3 mm | |
| | 2D FLAIR-TSE | cor/2–3 mm | |
| 2D T2-w TSE | | cor/2–3 mm | Hippocampal sclerosis |
| SWI or 2D-FFE | | ax/1.5–5 mm | Cavernoma, hemosiderin |
| 3D T1-w FFE or MPRAGE + Contrast | | sag/1 × 1 × 1 mm$^3$ | Long-term epilepsy-associated tumors |

*sag* sagittal; *ax* axial; *cor* coronal (modified from Urbach et al. [40], with permission)

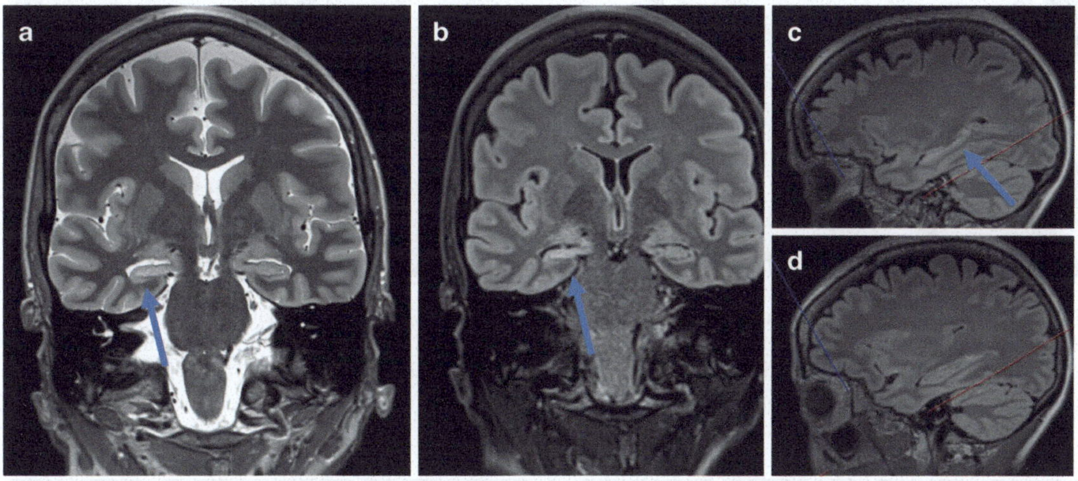


**Fig. 3.3** Right-sided hippocampal sclerosis. (**a**) Coronal T2-weighted fast spin-echo; (**b**) coronal FLAIR fast spin-echo; (**c**) sagittal 3D FLAIR SPACE images through the right; and (**d**) through the left hippocampus. Hippocampal sclerosis is characterized by atrophy and an increased T2 signal (with courtesy of H. Urbach, Dpt. of Neuroradiology, Freiburg)

and slice orientations, e.g., the 1997 protocol of the Commission on Neuroimaging of the International League Against Epilepsy (ILAE) [63, 64, 65]. The most obvious disadvantage of this protocol is that it requires more time than "standard brain" MRI. The pure scanning time for the "essential six" protocol is around 35–40 min in 1.5 T scanners [48]. Moreover, it should be noted that due to ongoing myelination, FLAIR sequences are of little value in the first 3 years of life. During this period, T1-w and T2-w sequences focusing on a high signal/noise ratio are preferred [40].

#### 3.2.1.3 Hippocampal Sclerosis

Hippocampal sclerosis (HS) as the most important pathology in adult temporal lobe epilepsy is characterized by atrophy and increased signal intensity on FLAIR and T2-weighted fast spin-echo images. This pattern is best visualized on thin (2–3 mm thick) coronal images (Fig. 3.3). Detection rate of HS depends on the exact angulation perpendicular to the hippocampal long axis, and the terms "epilepsy MRI" and "temporal angulation" are used synonymously. In contrast, in patients with extratemporal lobe epilepsies, perpendicular FLAIR slices through the anatomic region, from which the seizures are likely to originate according to clinical and EEG criteria, are preferred [49]. Nowadays, HS is detected with appropriate 3 T MRI protocols in almost all cases [40], and automated FLAIR analysis in patients undergoing selective amygdalohippocampectomy (SAHE) indicates that mild hippocampal sclerosis is either difficult to classify neuropathologically or does not exist [43, 45, 66, 67].

#### 3.2.1.4 Tumors, Non-tumorous Lesions

FLAIR sequences have proven to be sensitive for detection of focal cortical dysplasia (FCD) as the most important pathology in children, epilepsy-associated tumors, vascular malformations, inflammations, and scars (Figs. 3.4, 3.5, and 3.6; for tumors see also Chap. 9). In particular, very thin-sliced 3D-FLAIR images, e.g., with isotropic 1 mm voxel size, performed at 3 T devices, allow the detection of subtle cortical dysplasias [55, 56].

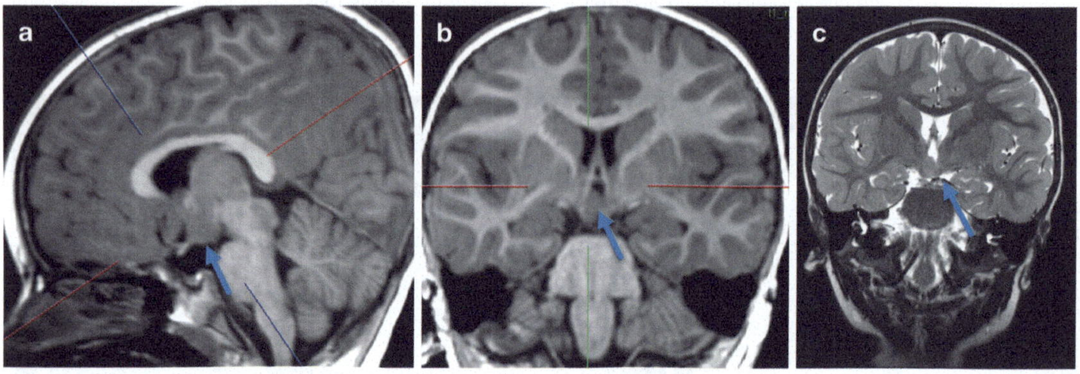


**Fig. 3.4** Hypothalamic hamartoma (Delalande type II). The hamartoma is located on the right side and closely connected to the right fornix and both mamillary bodies. (**a**) Sagittal T1-weighted gradient echo, (**b**) reformatted coronal T1-weighted gradient echo, (**c**) coronal T2-weighted fast spin-echo images (with courtesy of H. Urbach, Dep. Neuroradiology, Freiburg)

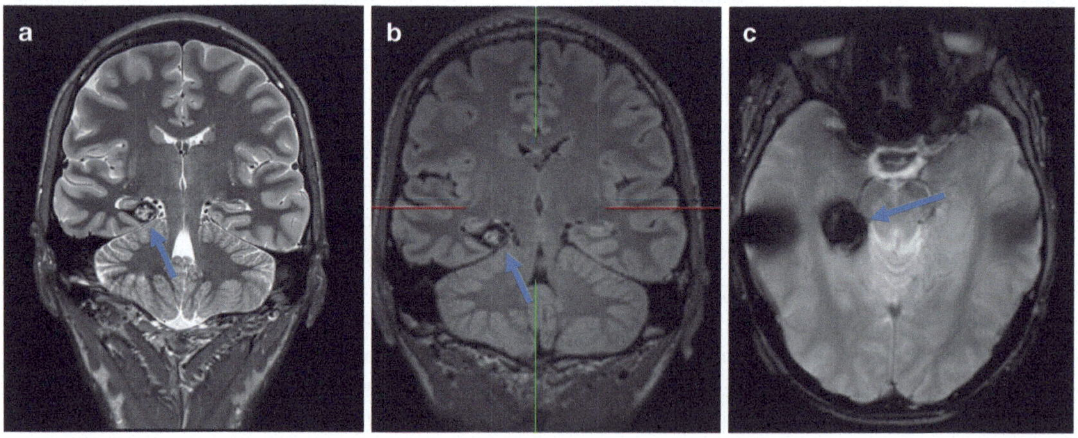


**Fig. 3.5** Cavernoma of the right parahippocampal gyrus. (**a**) Coronal T2-weighted fast spin-echo; (**b**) coronal FLAIR fast spin-echo; (**c**) axial T2* image. The cavernoma is depicted as a berrylike structure surrounded by a hemosiderin rim (**a**, **b**: arrow). The hemosiderin rim blooms up on T2-weighted gradient or SWI images (**c**: arrow) (with courtesy of H. Urbach, Dpt. of Neuroradiology, Freiburg)

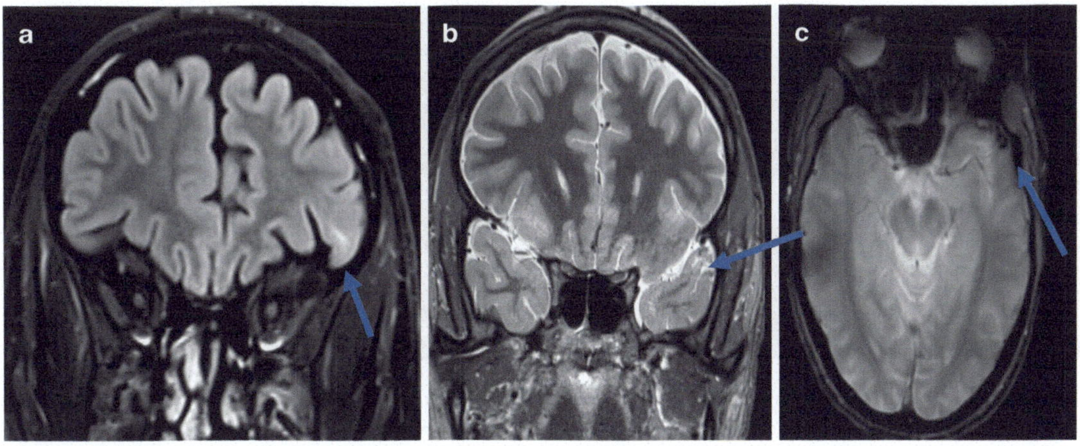


**Fig. 3.6** Post-traumatic changes (cortical contusions) of the left basal frontal lobe and the left anterior temporal lobe which represent predeliction sites for brain trauma (**a**, **b**: arrow). Note that due to susceptibility artifacts small lesions can be easily overlooked on T2-weighted gradient echo images (**c**: arrow) (with courtesy of H. Urbach, Dpt. of Neuroradiology, Freiburg)

This technique has noticeably increased the detection rate of FCD [1]. In addition, tensor-valued diffusion MRI has been found to improve delineation of malformations of cortical development (MCD) [68]. T2-weighted images are sensitive for the detection of cystic tissue components and the internal structure of the hippocampus. T1-weighted sequences display cortex-isointense structures, and a hemo/calc-sensitive sequence highlights lesions with calcification or hemosiderin deposits. The value of contrast-enhanced T1 sequences lies in tumor grading and differentiation from vascular lesions [40, 48, 52].

#### 3.2.1.5 Post-acquisition Processing Techniques

When an epileptogenic lesion has not been detected, but semiology of the seizures and EEG findings clearly point to a focal seizure onset, morphometric analysis of the 3D-T1-w (or 3D-T2-w) data sets may be helpful [40]. Computational post-processing techniques use statistical inference rather than visual inspection to identify abnormalities based on comparison with healthy controls. A variety of epilepsy-relevant features may be measured using a T1- or T2-weighted MRI scan: local gray matter volume, measured by voxel-based morphometry [69], cortical thickness [70], blurring of the boundary between gray and white matter in the cortex [71, 72], sulcal depth [73], or cortical gyrification [74] and texture [75, 76]. A combination of these features can be expected to be most sensitive for identifying relevant epilepsy-related areas [46, 47]. Moreover, post-processing methods can be applied to alternative imaging sequences, such as FLAIR imaging. In the study of [77], the application of voxel-based methods to FLAIR imaging identified structural changes in 11.4% of lesion-negative focal epilepsy cases. Post-processing techniques have also been applied to either confirmed cases of FCD or non-visible FCD. The latter seems to be important, as these techniques have been shown to identify 30% more patients who currently have no identifiable focal abnormality [72] (Figs. 3.7, 3.8, and 3.9). A review of Bernasconi et al. [78] discusses morphometric approaches for the detection of cryptogenic epileptic tissue in more detail.

#### 3.2.1.6 Diffusion Tensor Imaging (DTI)

DTI is an imaging technique that can provide insight into the structural integrity of the white matter through the measurement of water diffusion [79]. It allows generation of maps of quantitative diffusion measures [80]. DTI changes are particularly pronounced following seizures [81–84]. In addition, DTI studies have demonstrated bilateral white matter abnormalities in temporal lobe epilepsy that extend the temporal lobe, even in patients with unilateral hippocampal sclerosis

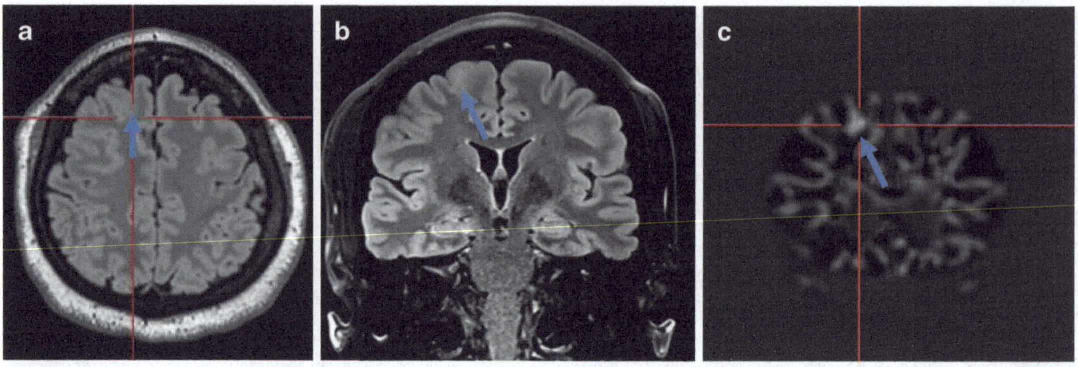


**Fig. 3.7** Focal cortical dysplasia (FCD) of the right superior frontal gyrus in a 35-year-old woman with a so far unclassified epilepsy. (**a**) Reformatted axial FLAIR; (**b**) reformatted coronal FLAIR; (**c**) post-processing with generation of a so-called junction image. The cortical thickening (**a**, **b**: arrows) was initially overlooked but well appreciated with the post-processing tool (with courtesy of H. Urbach, Dpt. of Neuroradiology, Freiburg)

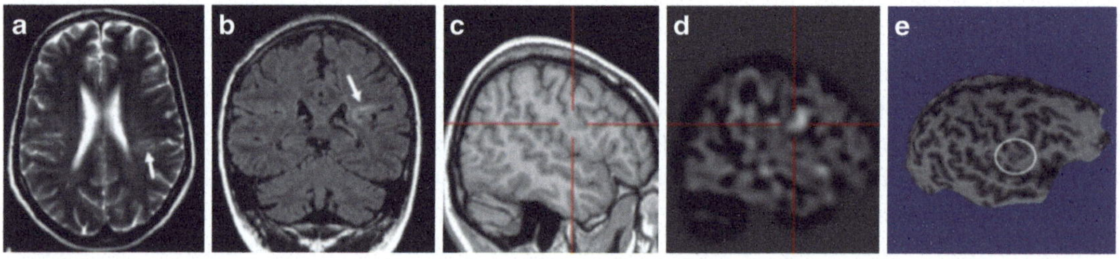


**Fig. 3.8** Axial T2-weighted TSE (**a**) and coronal FLAIR TSE (**b**) show a FCD with a transmantle sign extending from the bottom of the postcentral sulcus to the lateral ventricle. Sagittal MPRAGE (**c**), post-processed junction (**d**), and reformatted curvilinear images (**e**) reveal a circumscribed cortical thickening (with courtesy of H. Urbach, Dpt. of Neuroradiology, Freiburg)

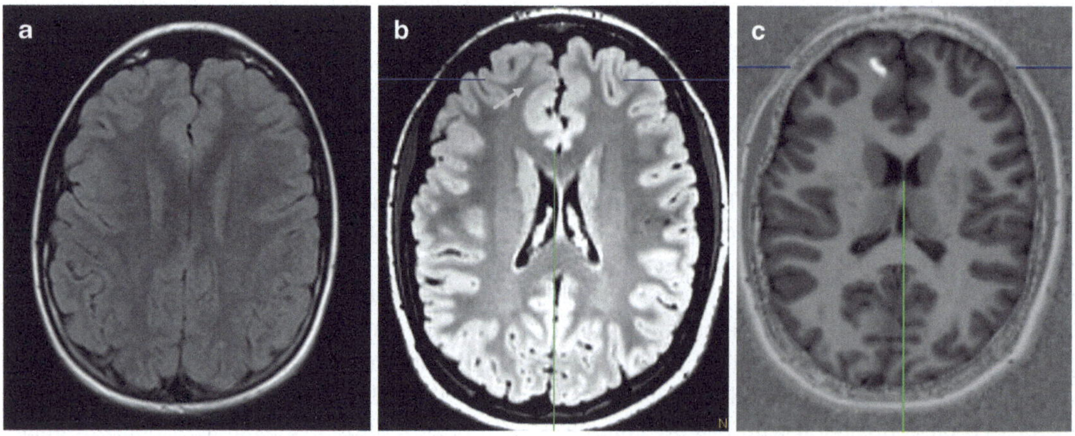


**Fig. 3.9** FCD of the right superior frontal gyrus. (**a**) Lesion not visible (3 mm thick 2D-FLAIR slice); (**b**) lesion poorly visible; the arrow points to a subtle transmantle sign (3D-FLAIR slice with 1 × 1 × 1 mm$^3$ voxel); (**c**) the lesion was identified via the morphometric analysis program and was co-registered to a MP2RAGE (with courtesy of H. Urbach, Dpt. of Neuroradiology, Freiburg)

indicating that abnormalities are not restricted to the ipsilateral hippocampus and temporal lobe white matter, but may involve an extensive bilateral network [79]. However, the role of the various involved structures in epileptogenesis and seizure propagation remains unclear [79]. Since water diffusion in white matter is reduced perpendicular to the white matter tracts, while parallel diffusion is relatively unimpeded [85], DTI can also provide 3D location of specific white matter tracts (DTI tractography) that are difficult to localize with other imaging techniques [79]. An approach called *apparent fiber density* allows diffusion differences to be detected in individual white fiber tracts within voxels that contain multiple fibers [86]. Such techniques may be useful to selectively cut fiber tracts, e.g., in callosotomy.

#### 3.2.1.7 Magnetic Resonance Spectroscopy (MRS)

MRS allows identification of areas of metabolic dysfunction in focal epilepsy similar to FDG-PET (see below). Proton spectroscopy ($^1$H-MRS) has proven to be sensitive to neuronal dysfunction or neuronal loss demonstrating reduced NAA (N-acetylaspartate) levels in focal epileptogenic areas irrespective of pathology. $^1$H-MRS abnormalities in epileptogenic temporal lobe regions with asymmetries in 70–80% of patients have been reported [87]. A study with 25 temporal lobe patients showed a mean reduction of 22% in the NAA signal ipsilateral to the seizure focus compared with control subjects [88]. On the basis of the NAA/creatine/choline ratio, correct localization of the seizure focus was achieved in 15 cases, with 3 incorrect [88]. Guye et al. [89] compared $^1$H-MRS imaging with electrophysiological abnormalities recorded by depth electrodes and with structural lesions in 25 temporal epilepsy patients. Results indicated that metabolic abnormalities were linked to ictal and interictal epileptiform activities rather than to structural alterations [89]. Thus, $^1$H-MRS may be useful in MRI-negative temporal lobe epilepsy. In addition, MRS studies have shown metabolic dysfunction of networks [90].

### 3.2.2 Functional MR Imaging

Functional MRI (fMRI) methods are based on the evaluation of temporal changes in oxygenated blood flow (blood-oxygenation-level-dependent [BOLD] imaging) and can be used to display important areas such as the language and motor cortex as well as the pyramidal and the optic tracts. An overview on functional imaging has been provided by Urbach et al. [40, 52].

#### 3.2.2.1 Language Area

For language MRI, a block-design experiment with at least two different tasks for language production and comprehension can be applied [40]. Handedness is usually assessed with the Edinburgh handedness score [91]. fMRI has been shown to demonstrate left lateralization of language in >90% of healthy volunteers, but only in approximately 78% of epilepsy patients. Bilateral (approximately 16%) or right (approximately 6%) representation of language is more common in epilepsy patients than in the general population, and these constellations are frequently associated with a lesion or brain injury at earlier age and a weaker right-hand dominance [92] (Fig. 3.10). Comparing fMRI with the Wada test as the gold standard for preoperative assessment of lateralization of language and memory function, a meta-analysis showed that fMRI and Wada test agreed in 94% of cases for typical language lateralization and in 51% for atypical language lateralization [93].

Thus, imaging is sufficient, if fMRI clearly shows left lateralization of language. It has to be kept in mind that lesions such as cavernomas, gliomas, and mass defects localized close to language areas may impair fMRI-based language lateralization [94]. If fMRI does not clearly show left-lateralized language or in other critical cases, it may be necessary to confirm localization of the language area with other techniques such as the Wada test or electrical stimulation mapping (see also Chap. 4) [40, 93]. Overall, the sensitivity and specificity of fMRI for language lateralization are between 80 and 90% and have replaced

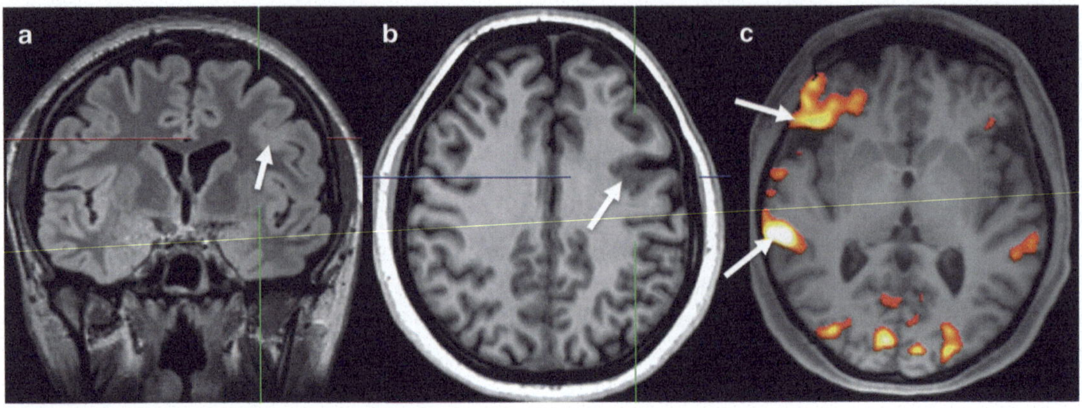


**Fig. 3.10** FCD of the left middle frontal gyrus (**a**, **b**: arrow). Language fMRI using a word generation paradigm shows strong activation of right-sided language areas (**c**: arrows) suggesting a right-hemispheric lateralization (with courtesy of H. Urbach, Dpt. of Neuroradiology, Freiburg)

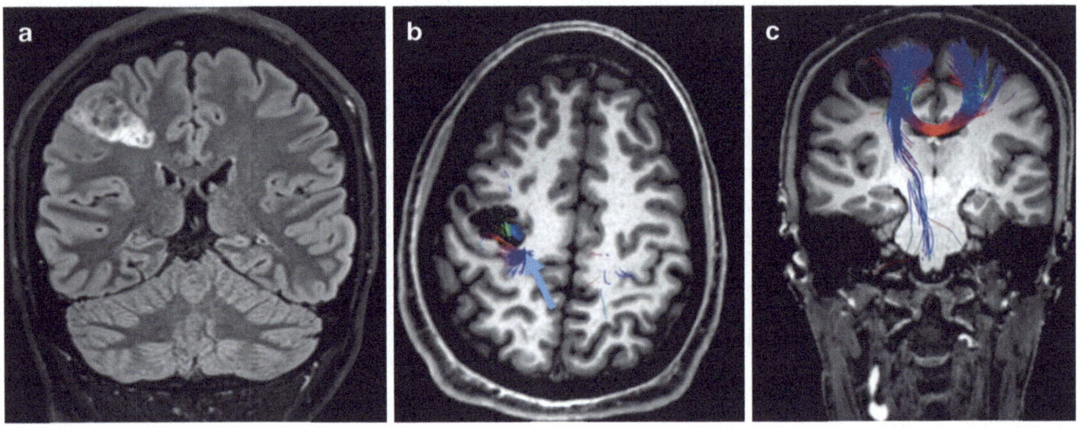


**Fig. 3.11** Dysembryoplastic neuroepithelial tumor (DNET) of the right anterior precentral gyrus. (**a**) Coronal FLAIR fast spin-echo, (**b**) reformatted axial, (**c**) reformatted coronal T1-weighted gradient echo images with co-registered right-sided corticospinal tract in blue. Note that tract is dorsal to the DNET (**b**: arrow) (with courtesy of H. Urbach, Dpt. of Neuroradiology, Freiburg)

the intracarotid sodium amobarbital procedure in most cases [93]. It should be kept in mind that fMRI indicates the cortical area actually used for language production that is rather more extensive compared to the proper language representation area (see also Chap. 4). In line, You et al. [95] suggested that the amount of the top 10% of language fMRI activation included in the resection area was the most significant predictor of postoperative change in naming ability.

### 3.2.2.2 Motor Cortex

The precentral gyrus can be identified via fMRI or automated parcellation with the FreeSurfer algorithm [96]. The pyramidal tract is calculated from a diffusion tensor imaging (DTI) sequence using two seed points in the precentral gyrus and ipsilateral crus cerebri [40]. DTI is increasingly used to detect white matter changes, and to identify important fiber tracts [97]. Ideally, activated voxel and calculated white matter tracts are co-registered to the 3D T1-w data set (Fig. 3.11) and stored into a neuronavigation system [40].

### 3.2.2.3 Optic Radiation

For identification of the optic radiation, two seed points in the pericalcarine cortex and lateral geniculate ganglion are selected (Fig. 3.12). The perical-

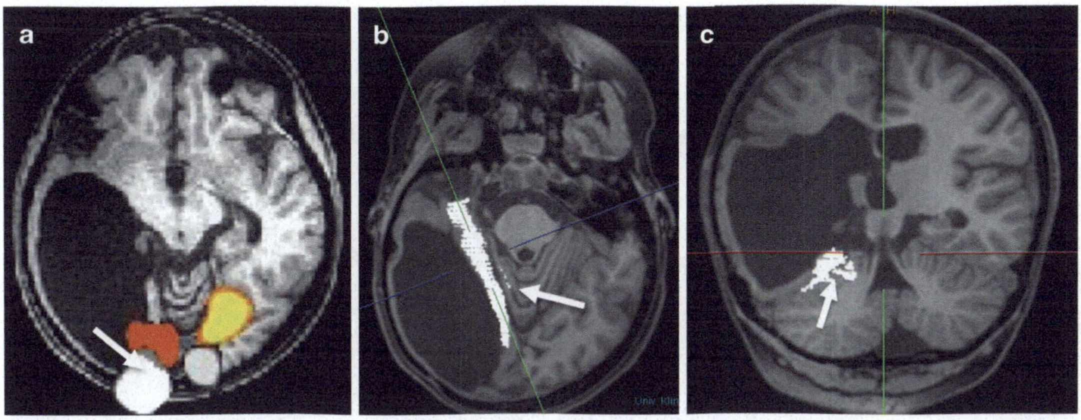


**Fig. 3.12** Porencephalic cyst in the right occipital lobe. (**a**) fMRI with chessboard stimulation was performed to display the visual cortex (**a**: arrow). The right visual cortex served as one seed point to calculate the optic radiation using the FACT algorithm. The optic radiation was co-registered to the MPRAGE data set and used for neuronavigation. Note that the optic radiation is displaced medially and caudally (**b**, **c**: arrow) (with courtesy of H. Urbach, Dpt. of Neuroradiology, Freiburg)

carine cortex is identified by a four-quadrant visual field stimulation paradigm. A probabilistic tracking algorithm is best suited to display the inferior or ventral bundle of the optic radiation [40]. This bundle known as Meyer's loop is located in the roof of the inferior horn and turns around the temporal horn of the lateral ventricle in a wide anterior and lateral loop [98]. In a series of ten patients, the mean distance between the temporal pole and the tip of the Meyer's loop was 34 mm with a range from 23.1 to 40.0 mm [40, 97] (see also Chap. 6).

### 3.2.3 Radionuclide Imaging

Two different techniques are commonly used: interictal positron-emission tomography (PET) of regional cerebral glucose metabolism and ictal single-photon emission computed tomography (SPECT) of regional cerebral blood flow (CBF), both of which reflect neuronal activity. The old term "metabolic imaging" seems to be insufficient, since only PET evaluates metabolic activity, while ictal SPECT reflects perfusion of the epileptogenic area. Thus, the term "radionuclide imaging" may be more appropriate for those modalities. PET and ictal SPECT have been primarily used in MRI-negative temporal lobe epilepsy, but they are now more frequently applied also in patients with MRI-negative extratemporal cases. In addition, ictal SPECT has proven to be helpful in patients with structural brain lesions that per se lead to reduced regional metabolism. In such cases, PET may not be able to differentiate between regional hypometabolism related to the lesion on the one hand and epileptogenic zone on the other hand, while ictal SPECT may accurately capture the seizure origin [99–101].

#### 3.2.3.1 PET

PET imaging is generally performed interictally. Hypometabolic areas as a marker of cortical dysfunction can be detected with FDG ([$^{18}$F] fluorodeoxyglucose)-PET (Fig. 3.13). FDG-PET has a sensitivity of up to 90% in temporal and 50% in extratemporal lobe epilepsy [102]. The region of hypometabolism detected by FDG-PET is generally larger than the epileptic zone and cannot be used to outline a surgical resection plan [6]. Anatomical information of FDG-PET can be improved by using statistical analysis methods, such as statistical parametric mapping (SPM), as well as by PET/MRI co-registration [103]. Overall, FDG-PET aids hemispheric lateralization and general lobar localization in cases with discordant scalp EEG and/or normal MRI [6]. The positive predictive value of a favorable seizure outcome evaluating FDG-PET in temporal lobe epilepsy was 77.5% when MRI, EEG, or both were non-concordant [6, 104].

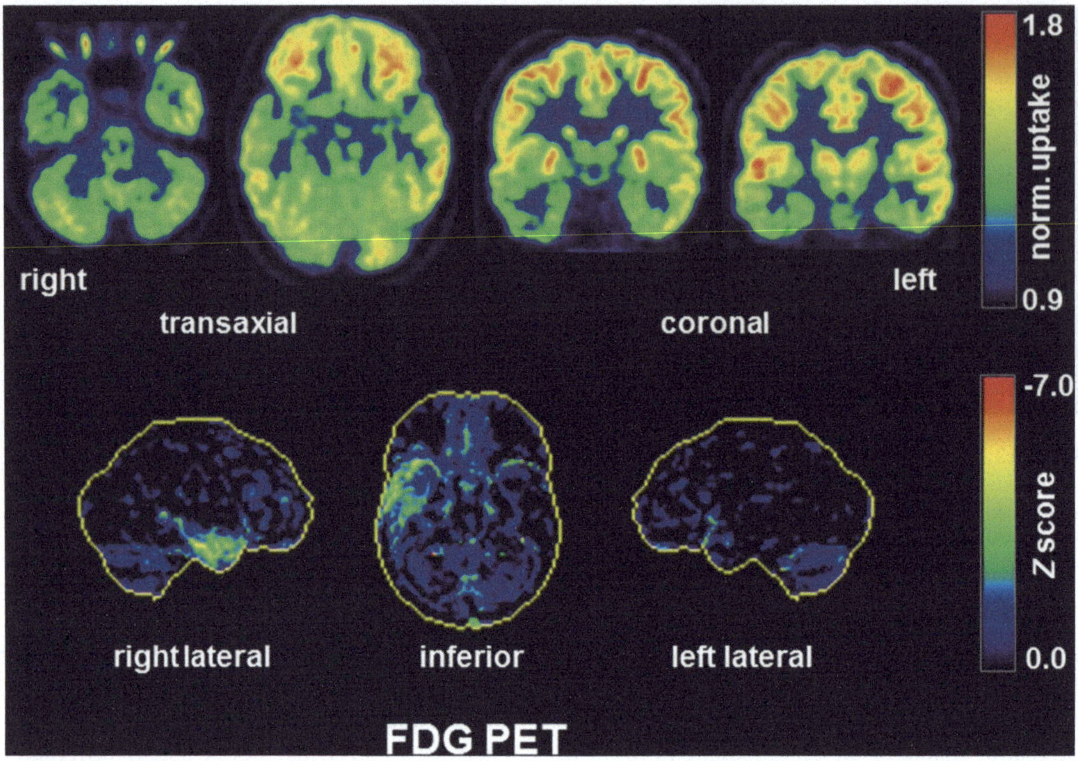


**Fig. 3.13** [[18F]]FDG PET in a patient with a right-sided temporal lobe epilepsy. The upper row shows images in axial and coronal views. The lower row demonstrates results of voxel-based statistical evaluation with Neurostat/3D-SSP depicting voxels with reduced metabolism on a 3D surface projection of the brain (color coded as negative *Z*-score compared to an age-matched normal collective). Note the hypometabolic area in the right temporal lobe (with courtesy of P.T. Meyer and J. Thurow, Dpt. of Nuclear Medicine, Freiburg)

It has been shown that PET imaging using GABA-A/benzodiazepine receptor radiotracers, such as $^{11}$C- or $^{18}$F-radiolabeled flumazenil can identify more restricted regions of abnormality in the epileptogenic zone and has a higher sensitivity in extratemporal location as compared to FDG-PET. Similarly, other PET receptor tracers have been tested, such as serotonin markers (5-$HT_{1A}$, [$^{18}$F]MPPF (4-(2′-methoxyphenyl)-1-[2′-[N-(2″-pyridinyl)-p-fluorobenzamido] ethyl]-piperazine), dopamine D2 receptors ([$^{18}$F]fallypride), glutamate/NMDA receptors ([$^{11}$C]-S-ketamine, [$^{11}$C]CNS 5161), and opioid receptors ([$^{11}$C]carfentanil) [41, 105]. However, these specific PET ligands for GABA-A, NMDA, opioid, and serotonin receptors have research applications and are not in widespread clinical use [104].

#### 3.2.3.2 SPECT

Ictal SPECT uses tracers like [$^{99m}$Tc]ECD or [$^{99m}$Tc]HMPAO (in its stabilized form) to demonstrate areas of increased cerebral blood flow (CBF) during seizures [106]. The tracer is injected within seconds after seizure onset under video-EEG monitoring (Fig. 3.14). Tracer administration as early into the seizure onset as possible is crucial to identify hyperperfusion associated with the seizure onset zone, since delayed administration visualizes areas that show hyperperfusion due to seizure propagation [6]. Ictal SPECT has been shown to have a 70% sensitivity compared to 78% with interictal FDG-PET [107]. When ictal and interictal SPECT are normalized and subtracted, the sensitivity of SPECT reached 87% [106]. In addition, the superposition of functional ("activation") data with three-dimensional MRI

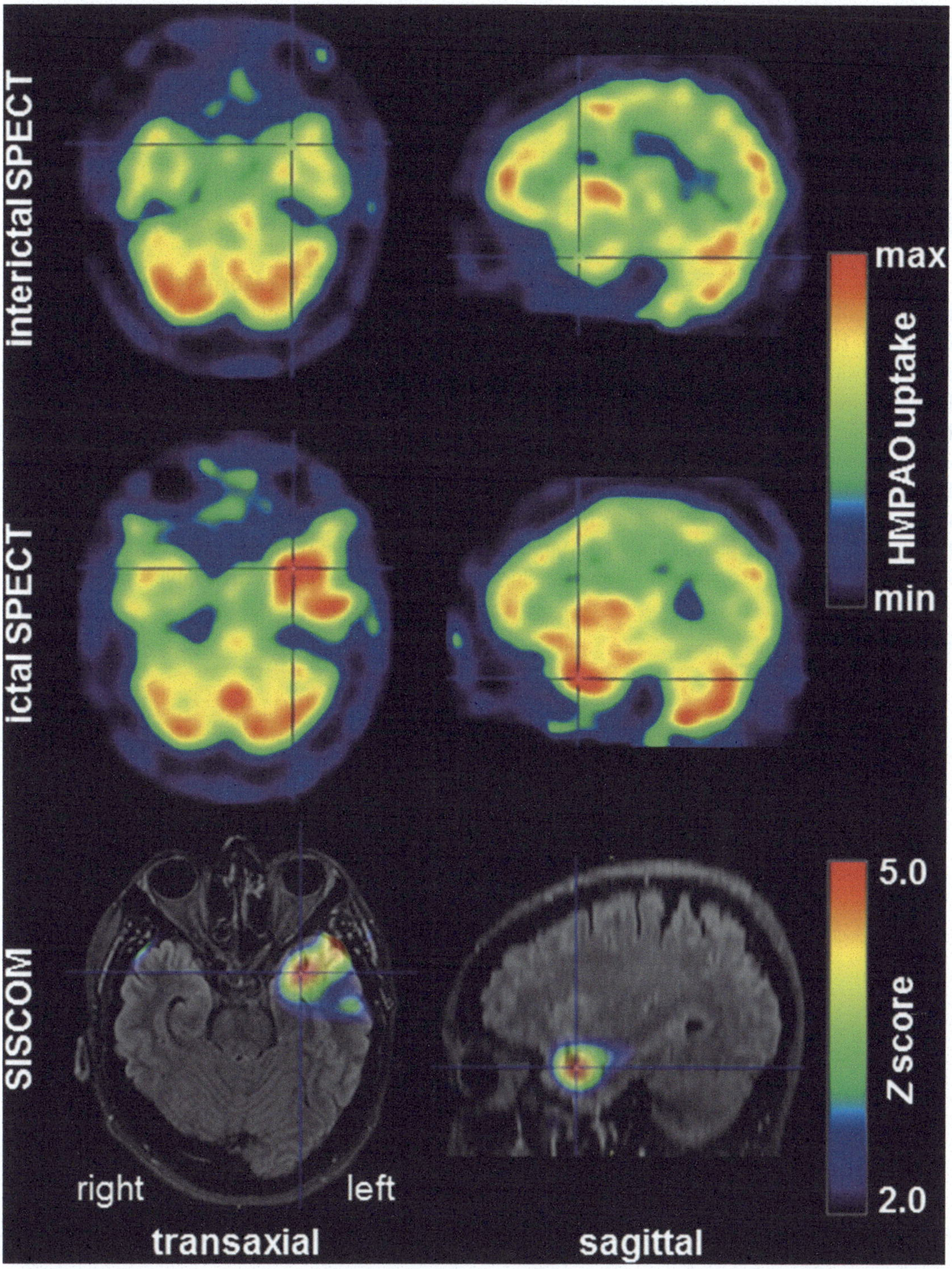


**Fig. 3.14** Patient with left-sided temporal lobe epilepsy. [$^{99m}$Tc]HMPAO SPECT shows a significant increase in perfusion in the left temporal lobe from the interictal (upper line) to the ictal (middle line) status (left, axial; right, sagittal). In the SISCOM analysis (lower line), voxels with a significant increase of cerebral blood flow (CBF) are color coded (Z score from interictal to ictal) and superimposed on MRI (FLAIR) of the patient (with courtesy of P.T. Meyer and J. Thurow, Dpt. of Nuclear Medicine, Freiburg)

data sets like SISCOM (subtraction ictal SPECT co-registered to MRI) has further increased the sensitivity and specificity of functional imaging for seizure focus localization [106], especially in comparison to ictal studies alone [101].

## 3.3 Electrophysiological Diagnostics

EEG recordings from electrodes placed according to the 10–20 system constitute the basis of electrophysiological diagnostics (Fig. 3.15). Evidence of focal seizure onset can be derived from regional EEG slowing or spikes. To record epileptic activity sensitively and completely, long-term EEG recordings are performed during periods of sleep and wakefulness. In general, the doses of antiepileptic drugs that suppress interictal spikes and seizures are lowered during recording. Long-term recording enables the analysis of interictal spikes and sharp waves, and high-density EEG recordings facilitate the localization of generators in relation to the patient's individual brain morphology [108].

### 3.3.1 Noninvasive Strategies

#### 3.3.1.1 Video-EEG Monitoring

The key point of electrophysiological assessment for epilepsy surgery is the recording of the patient's typical seizures with long-term video-EEG monitoring. Simultaneous video monitoring of the patient and recording of interictal and ictal EEG activity facilitate electroclinical correlation and allow a more precise classification of seizures (Fig. 3.16). Detailed analysis of seizure semiology in relation to electroencephalographic seizure patterns enables the individual

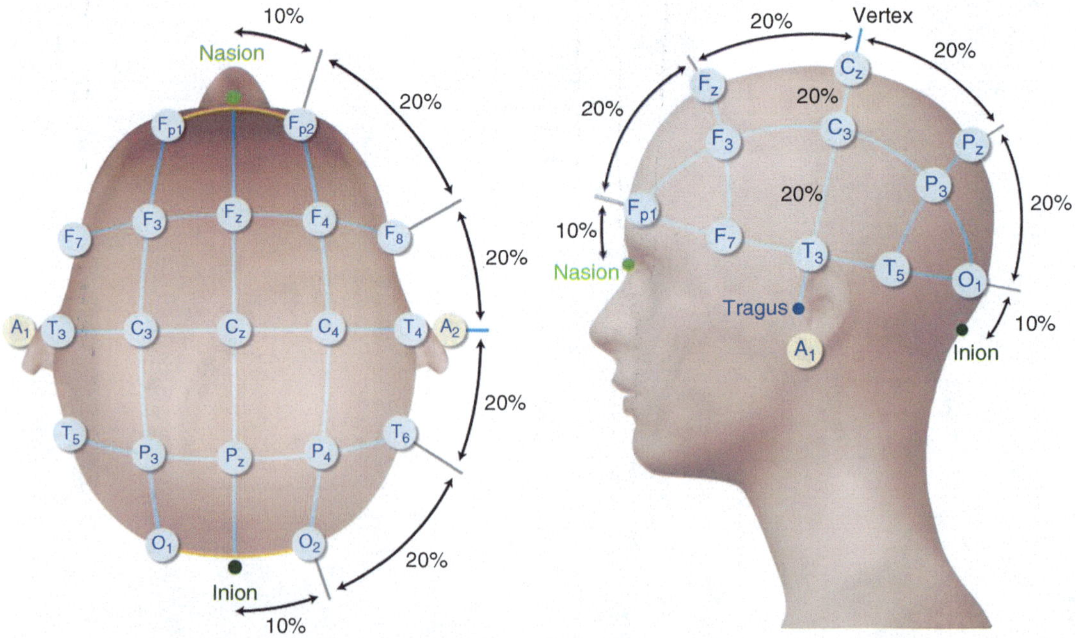


**Fig. 3.15** Schematic presentation of the 10–20 EEG system in axial (left) and sagittal (right) views. The length of the skull from the nasion to the inion and the distance between the two preauricular points A1 and A2 correspond to 100% and are divided into 10% and 20% sections. The electrodes are attached to the scalp according to these coordinates. Fp1/Fp2: gyrus frontalis superior (Brodmann area 10); F3/F4 = gyrus frontalis medius (Brodmann area 46); F7/F8: gyrus frontalis inferior (Brodmann area 45); C3/C4: gyrus praecentralis (Brodmann area 4); P3/P4: lobulus parietalis superior (Brodmann area 7), T3/T4: sulcus temporalis superior (Brodmann area 21/22); T5/T6: gyrus temporalis medius (Brodmann area 37); O1/O2: area lateral and above the occipital pole (Brodmann area 17) (with courtesy of R. Ott, Arcana Forum, Emmendingen)

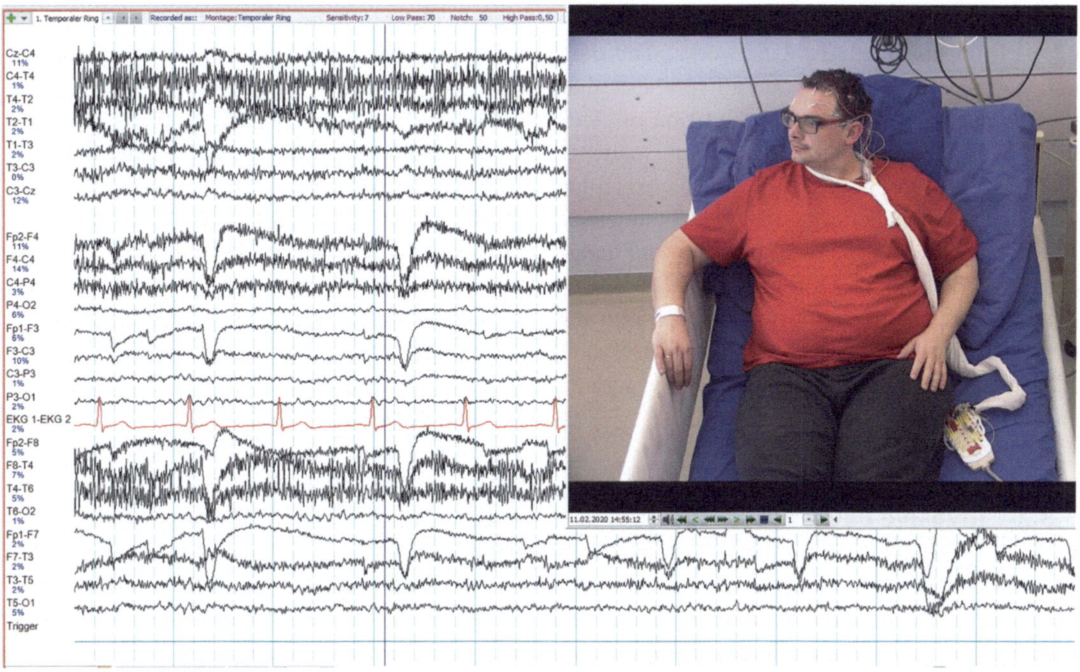


**Fig. 3.16** Video-EEG monitoring. Patient's seizure semiology and EEG are simultaneously recorded facilitating electroclinical correlation (with courtesy of D.M. Altenmüller, Dpt. of Epileptology, Freiburg, and with permission of the patient)

clinical features of a seizure to be ascribed to specific areas of the brain, e.g., complex visual hallucinations can be traced to temporo-occipital association areas, ictal changes of heart rate to the insular cortex, and asymmetrical posturing during the seizure to the supplementary motor cortex. In addition, video-EEG monitoring can be used to establish that the patient's seizures are indeed epileptic [108–110].

#### 3.3.1.2 EEG-fMRI

EEG-fMRI means that the EEG is recorded during fMRI acquisition. This technique can show hemodynamic changes associated with interictal epileptic discharges with a 30–40% sensitivity [111]. EEG-fMRI has been found to facilitate identification of epileptogenic zones in 55% of non-lesional epilepsy cases [112]. Kowalczyk et al. [113] noted that 50% of 118 EEG-fMRI studies were successful, and that 17% of the successful studies had a critical impact on the surgical decision.

#### 3.3.1.3 MEG

Magnetoencephalography (MEG) means the noninvasive measurement of magnetic fields produced by electrical currents in the brain that generate EEG signals. The spatial and temporal resolution of MEG is superior to scalp EEG, but is limited to dipoles on the cortical surface and less sensitive to deeper sources [6]. Thus, the role of MEG to define the epileptogenic zone is limited [6]. Diagnostic accuracy of MEG is significantly higher in extratemporal as compared to temporal epilepsies [114]. In patients in whom MEG signals were concordant with the resection area, long-term seizure-free outcome was 85%, compared to 37% when MEG signals were not concordant [115].

#### 3.3.1.4 ESI/MSI

*Electrical source imaging (ESI)* maps interictal epileptic discharges. MEG results can be co-registered to the patient's MRI which has been called *magnetic source imaging (MSI)* [116]. The current clinical place of these functional methods is to evaluate interictal networks. The data obtained may help to generate a hypothesis that may be useful for guiding implantation of electrodes for invasive recordings. Thus, patients requiring intracranial EEG to define the epileptogenic zone may benefit from these techniques [6, 114, 117–119]. In a systematic review and meta-analysis of 11 studies, Mouthaan et al. [120] suggested a summary sensitivity and specificity for overall source imaging modalities of 82% and 53%, respectively, with no statistically significant differences between ESI and MSI.

## 3.3.2 Invasive EEG Recordings

If noninvasive EEG studies remain inconclusive, additional invasive (intracranial) EEG recordings may be necessary, in particular under the following circumstances: (1) high-resolution imaging fails to detect a lesion, (2) noninvasive studies reveal discrepant findings due to the spread of epileptic activity, (3) there are multiple lesions or epileptic foci, and (4) a tailored resection is indicated in order to spare neighboring eloquent brain areas [6, 108]. Invasive recordings are necessary to localize the epileptogenic zone in around 30–40% of surgical candidates [121]. Chronic extraoperative recording is accomplished using subdural and/or intraparenchymal depth electrodes. In cases in whom the epileptogenic zone has been roughly defined by noninvasive strategies, intraoperative electrocorticography (ECoG) during the resective procedure using strip electrodes may be sufficient.

### 3.3.2.1 Subdural Electrodes

Subdural electrodes (stainless steel or MR-compatible platinum), embedded in strips or sheets (grids) of polyurethane or other synthetic material, are implanted over the suspected epileptogenic regions. Dependent on the individual needs, various electrode shapes are used (Figs. 3.17 and 3.18) [122].

- Strip electrodes are implanted as follows: An extended burr hole is created. The dura is coagulated and crosswide opened, and the electrode is gently inserted to the subdural space. The dura is roughly closed by single sutures, and

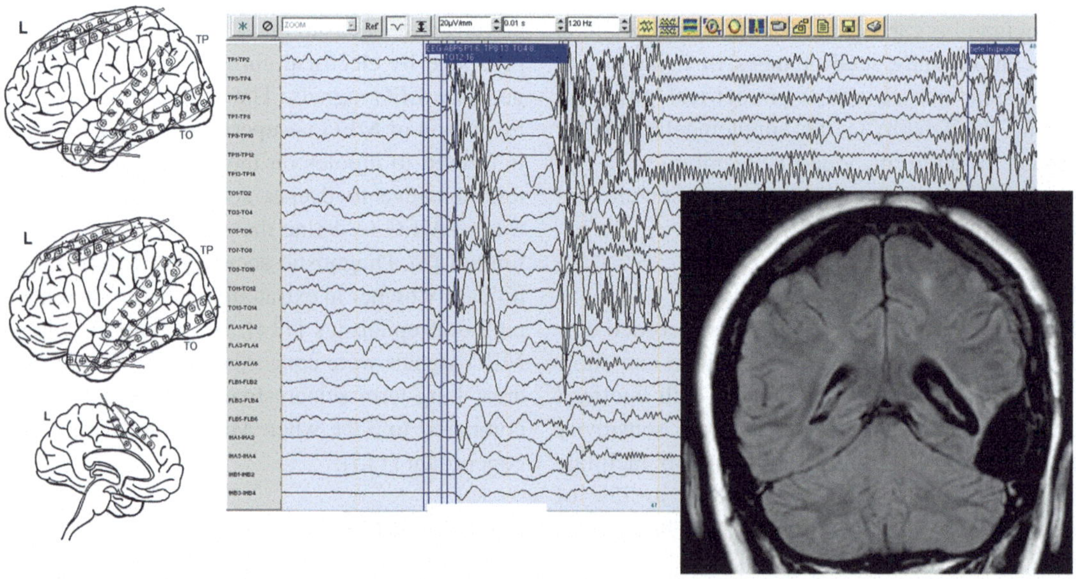


**Fig. 3.17** Patient with tuberous sclerosis and pharmacoresistant epilepsy. Due to multiple tubers and discordant noninvasive findings, multiple subdural electrodes were implanted (schematic illustration, left). Invasive EEG recordings (middle) pointed to the left temporodorsal tuber, removal of which (postoperative MRI, right) lead to seizure freedom (with courtesy of C.E. Elger, Dpt. of Epileptology, Bonn)

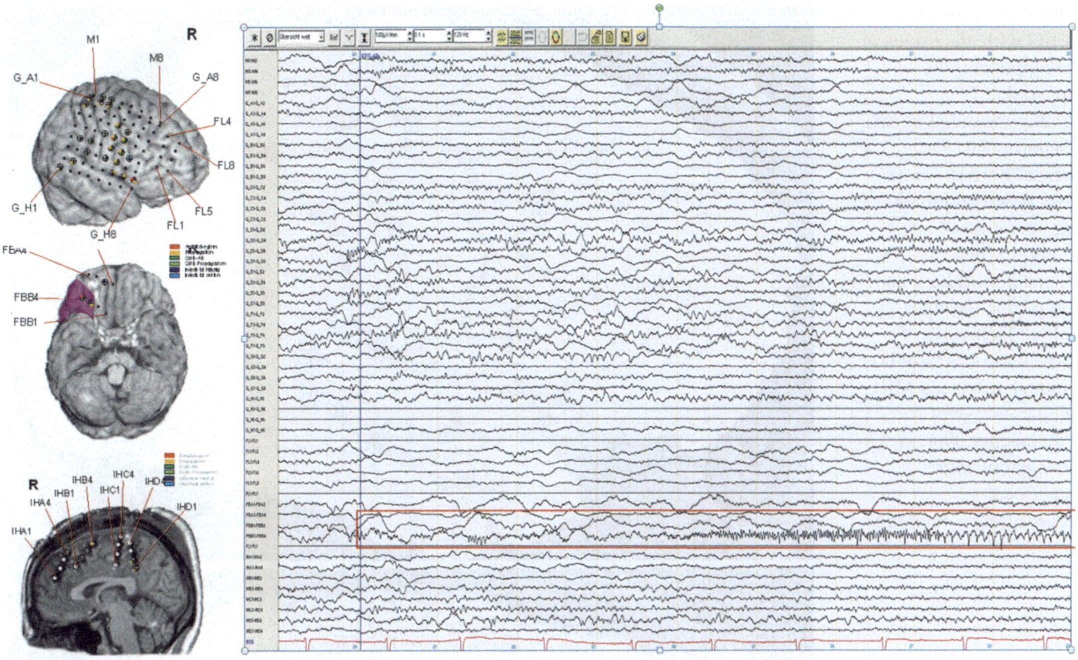


**Fig. 3.18** MRI-negative right frontal lobe epilepsy. Subdural recordings after implantation of grid and strip electrodes (left) demonstrate a circumscribed frontobasal seizure origin (right) (with courtesy of A. Schulze-Bonhage, Dpt. of Epileptology, Freiburg)

the burr hole is filled with spongy material such as Surgicel (Johnson and Johnson, Brussels, Belgium). The electrode lead is tunneled and fixed with a suture to the scalp.

- Implantation of grids requires an appropriate craniotomy. Care has to be taken in the parasagittal area with respect to bridging veins which may partially run in a dura duplication. In this location, craniotomy should expose the complete area to be covered by the grid. Folding of the grid predisposing to hemorrhage should be avoided. Tight closure of the dura is necessary to minimize CSF loss. After reimplantation of the bone flap, the leads are tunneled and fixed with sutures to the scalp.

The advantage of subdural electrodes is that they can cover large areas of the surface of the brain. Moreover, subdural electrodes are also highly suitable for functional mapping in order to define eloquent brain areas. This is accomplished by extraoperative electrical stimulation and/or recording of somatosensory evoked potentials (see also Chap. 4) [123–125]. Major disadvantage of subdural electrodes is that they fail to record epileptic activity from the depth.

#### 3.3.2.2 Depth Electrodes

Depth electrodes can be used for the detection of seizure generators in sulci or deeper structures such as the insula, the amygdala, or the hippocampus (stereotactic EEG, SEEG) (Fig. 3.19). Electrodes are available in various lengths and number of contacts depending on the specific brain area to be explored. For planning of electrode placement, computer-assisted algorithms have proven to be helpful [6, 126]. Implantation is mainly accomplished frame based [127], but may also be done robotic assisted [128] or navigation based [129]. Although subdural and depth electrodes have been used in parallel, both approaches can be combined, and electrodes may be placed frame based simultaneously [130].

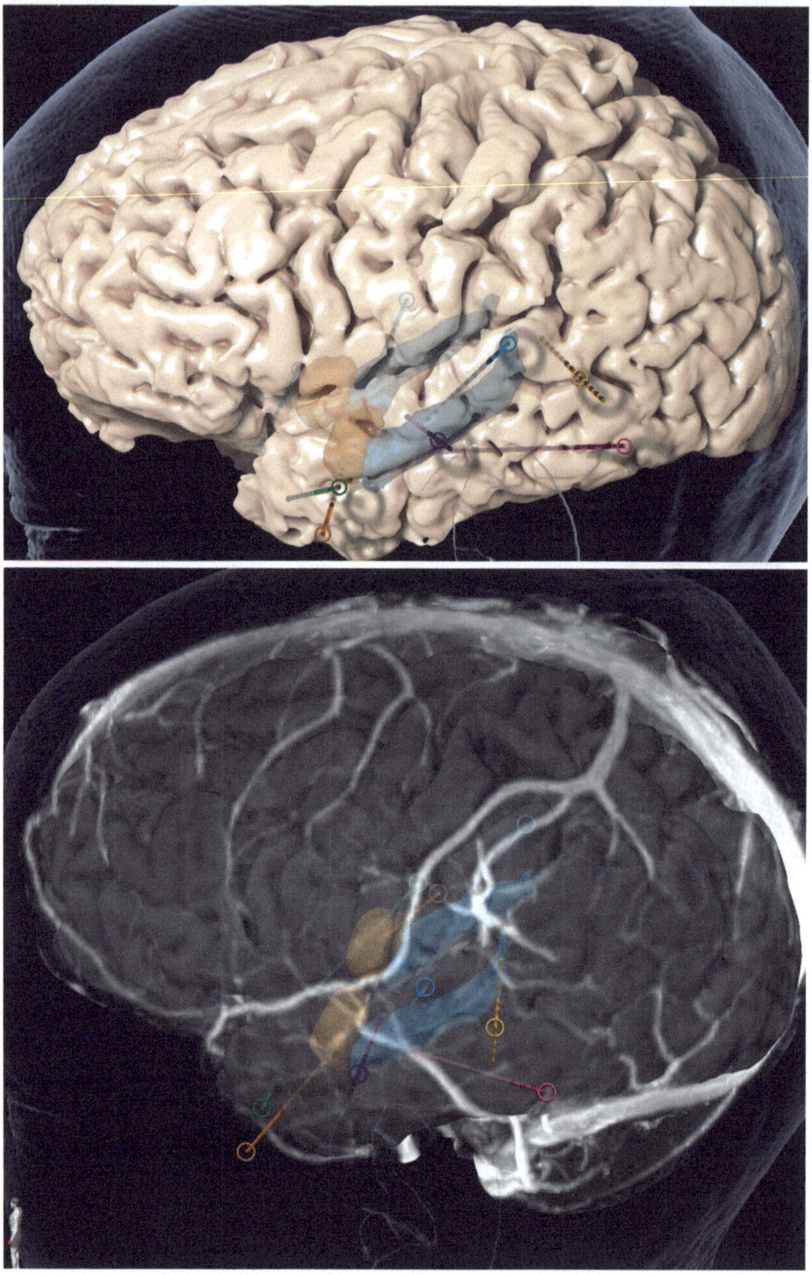

**Fig. 3.19** Typical SEEG with electrodes in the hippocampus, amygdala, parahippocampal gyrus, temporopolar, and parietal border. Above: MRI-based automatic segmentation of cerebrum (beige), hippocampi (blue), and amygdalae (orange). Below: Depiction of cortical vessels based on contrast-enhanced MRI (with courtesy of P. Reinacher, Dpt. of Stereotactic and Functional Neurosurgery, Freiburg)

- Frame-based electrode implantation is as follows: After computerized planning including imaging, the head is fixed. A spiral drill hole is created. The dura is coagulated and opened using a monopolar probe. A bolt is stereotactically guided screwed into the skull. After tunneling with a probe, the electrode is inserted through the bolt as planned and fixed to the bolt.

For extratemporal recordings, depth electrodes are implanted in orthogonal or oblique orientation [6, 122]. For recordings from the temporal lobe, electrodes can be inserted orthogonally through the middle temporal gyrus [131–133], or with a parieto-occipital entry point along the long axis of the hippocampus [134, 135]. Cardinale et al. [127] suggested a 3 mm safety margin from cerebral vessels. This may be facilitated by MR angiography or CT angiography, while others prefer digital subtraction catheter angiography (DSA).

Cardinale et al. [136] compared accuracy of robotic-assisted with Talairach frame-based implantation of depth electrodes in a meta-analysis. Robotic guidance achieved a median 0.78 mm entry point and 1.77 mm target point error, compared to a median 1.43 mm entry point and 2.69 mm target point error with manual Talairach frame placement. No significant differences in terms of accuracy and safety between the robotic-assisted and navigation-based implantation technique were observed [128]. Woolfe et al. [137] suggested a computer-assisted tool for the automated grading of the seizure activity recorded from depth electrodes. Processing seizures to extract biomarkers and evaluating their concentration have been shown to be a promising tool to identify the epileptogenic zone [137].

#### 3.3.2.3 Duration of Implantation

The duration of invasive monitoring depends on the seizure frequency, success of any planned stimulation, and patient compliance. It may take days to a few weeks. However, subdural grid recordings seldom extend beyond 10–14 days, as risks of infection and bleeding complications significantly increase with longer implantation duration.

#### 3.3.2.4 Strategies to Lower Risks

Increasing evidence suggests that SEEG procedures are safer than subdural recordings [127, 138]. In particular, a high complication rate has been noted with the use of grid electrodes [139] (see also Chap. 15). The number of electrode contacts as well as the number of burr holes or trephinations should be limited to what is necessary [125]. Moreover, it has been suggested that the duration of recording should be <2 weeks, and the electrodes should be tunneled far away from the point of dural entrance to prevent CSF leakage and to reduce the infection rate [134, 140–142]. In addition, patients should be adequately surveilled after implantation, since some reported major complications and even fatalities may be related to the lack of 24-h surveillance [143].

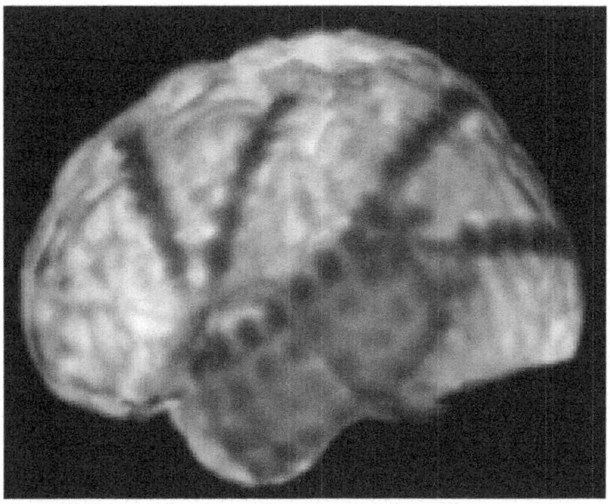

**Fig. 3.20** Visualization of subdural electrodes on postimplantation skull-stripped MRI as described by Kovalev et al. [144]. Female, 26 years; subdural grid covering the left temporal lobe and subdural strips covering frontal, parietal, and occipital regions of the left hemisphere are shown (with courtesy of D.-M. Altenmüller, Dpt. of Epileptology, Freiburg)

#### 3.3.2.5 Postoperative Visualization

Postoperative visualization of electrodes with respect to cortical and subcortical structures can be accomplished using a fully automated technique based on co-registration, normalization, optional cerebellum masking, and volume rendering of 3D MRI data (1.5 T MRI; T1-MPRAGE without contrast medium) taken before and after implantation. The skull-stripped preimplantation images are used as a mask to remove the skull on the postimplantation images. The extracted brain is depicted in 3D with the electrodes directly visible by their susceptibility artifacts [144] (Figs. 3.20 and 3.21). Others fuse postimplantation CT scans with preimplantation MRI data using special algorithms to depict subdural [145] and depth [146] electrodes.

#### 3.3.2.6 Efficiency of Subdural/Depth EEG

There are three reports analyzing the relative efficacy of SEEG and subdural EEG recordings with respect to seizure outcome. Tandon et al. [147] found favorable outcome (Engel I–II) in 57 of 75 (76.0%) SEEG cases and in 59 of 108 (54.6%) patients with subdurals. Considering

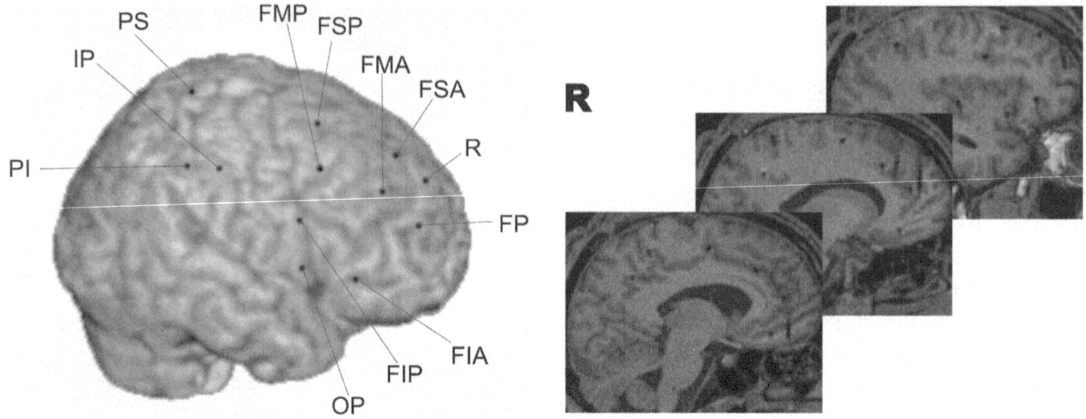


**Fig. 3.21** Visualization of the entry points (*left*, postimplantation skull-stripped MRI) and of selected intracerebral targets (*right*, sagittal postimplantation MRI slices) of 12 depth electrodes for extratemporal SEEG registration in the right hemisphere. Male, 29 years (with courtesy of D.-M. Altenmüller, Dpt. of Epileptology, Freiburg)

only non-lesional cases, favorable outcome was achieved in 27 of 39 SEEG (69.2%) versus 9 of 26 (34.6%) subdural cases. However, more patients underwent surgery after subdural recordings (91%) compared to SEEG (74%) [147]. In a systematic review and meta-analysis evaluating 16 articles including 974 procedures for SEEG and 19 articles including 1025 interventions for subdurals, Toth et al. [148] noted a seizure-free outcome (Engel I) rate of 64.7% after SEEG as compared to 55.9% after subdural recordings. Again, the proportion of patients selected for resective surgery was significantly higher following subdural compared to depth EEG monitoring (88.8% versus 79%). Yan et al. [149] analyzed 48 studies including 1973 SEEG and 2036 subdural EEG patients. Seizure-free outcome (Engel I) was found in 61.0% of patients undergoing SEEG versus 56.4% of cases after subdural EEG. Surgical resection rate was 81.6% with subdurals and 76.9% with SEEG.

In sum, all reports consistently found that SEEG was associated with a better seizure-free outcome yet with fewer resections, while subdural EEG facilitated more patients to undergo surgery yet with a lower seizure-free outcome rate. Major limitations of those studies relate to differences in cohorts assigned for SEEG and subdural recordings, respectively. In addition, differences may result from advances in MRI, since more SEEG than subdural EEG series have been published in the last years. Thus, overall efficiency of both invasive diagnostic modalities may be similar [147, 148]. Today, we face a clear trend towards SEEG in Europe, and there also seems to be a transition from subdural recordings towards SEEG in North America [147].

#### 3.3.2.7 Further Options

Invasive EEG recordings can be refined using *high-resolution (i.e., narrowly spaced) electrode grids* [108]. *Electrical source imaging (ESI)* based on spikes from invasive recordings may contribute to the demarcation of the spike origin [150, 151] (Fig. 3.22). Favorable seizure outcome was predicted by removal of highly epileptogenic areas derived from *mathematical models of interictal EEG functional connectivity* [6, 152]. A strong association between *pathological high-frequency oscillations (pHFOs)*, a biomarker for epileptogenicity recorded by noninvasive or invasive EEG or MEG [153] and epileptogenic tissue, has been demonstrated [153–156]. Dirodi et al. [157] showed that high-resolution surface EEG and MEG can localize cortical generators of high-frequency oscillations (HFOs) with high precision to the electrocorticography gold standard (92% for high-resolution EEG and 96% for MEG) in children suggesting that the need for invasive EEG recordings prior to surgery may be limited. The current place of HFOs has been reviewed by Thomschewski et al. [158].

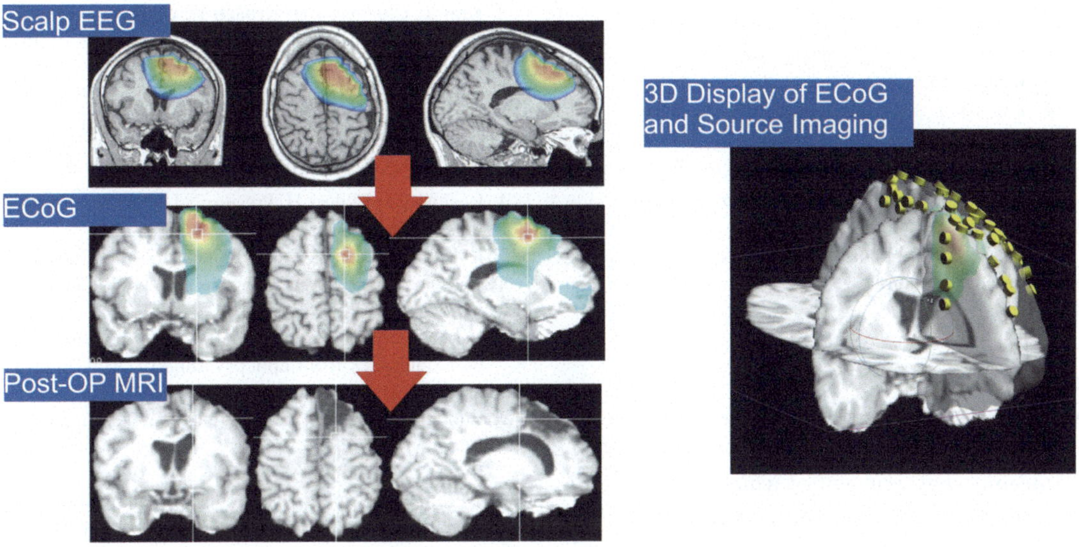


**Fig. 3.22** Contribution of electrical source imaging (ESI) to the delineation of the epileptogenic zone. Left side (from top to bottom): Source imaging based on spikes in noninvasive scalp EEG; subsequent source imaging based on spikes in ECoG allows a refined demarcation of the spike origin; postoperative MRI: crosshair indicates the position of the ECoG-based maximum source imaging. Right side: 3D display of MRI, ECoG electrodes on cortical surface, and results of source imaging. ECoG: Electrocorticogram (with courtesy of M. Dümpelmann and A. Schulze-Bonhage, Dpt. of Epileptology, Freiburg)

### 3.3.3 Seizure Outcome Scales

Classification systems are necessary in order to compare seizure outcomes between different studies. Most frequently, the Engel and the International League Against Epilepsy (ILAE) outcome scales are used. The Engel outcome scale arose out of the 1992 Palm Desert Conference on Epilepsy Surgery [159] and divides postoperative seizure outcomes into free of disabling seizures (class I), rare disabling seizures (class II), worthwhile improvement (class III), and no change (class IV) including subgroups for each class (Table 3.5). The ILAE scale is based on a proposal of Wieser [160, 161]. It classifies outcomes into six classes by percentage of seizure reduction (Table 3.6). The ILAE classification has been introduced to address some aspects missed in Engel's scale, e.g., to facilitate comparison of resective procedures with palliative ones and AED drug trials, which commonly use ≥50% seizure reduction as an end point, as well as to provide a simple system to better compare the data between different centers.

**Table 3.5** Engel's outcome scale

| |
|---|
| Class I: Free of disabling seizures |
| • IA: Completely seizure free since surgery |
| • IB: Non-disabling simple partial seizures only since surgery |
| • IC: Some disabling seizures after surgery, but free of disabling seizures for at least 2 years |
| • ID: Generalized convulsions with antiepileptic drug withdrawal only |
| Class II: Rare disabling seizures ("almost seizure free") |
| • IIA: Initially free of disabling seizures but rare seizures now |
| • IIB: Rare disabling seizures since surgery |
| • IIC: More than rare disabling seizures after surgery, but rare seizures for at least 2 years |
| • IID: Nocturnal seizures only |
| Class III: Worthwhile improvement |
| • IIIA: Worthwhile seizure reduction |
| • IIIB: Prolonged seizure-free intervals amounting to greater than half the follow-up period, but not less than 2 years |
| Class IV: No worthwhile improvement |
| • IVA: Significant seizure reduction |
| • IVB: No appreciable change |
| • IVC: Seizures worse |

**Table 3.6** ILAE outcome scale

| |
|---|
| • Class 1: Completely seizure free; no auras |
| • Class 2: Only auras; no other seizures |
| • Class 3: 1–3 seizure days per year; ± auras |
| • Class 4: 4 seizure days per year to 50% reduction of baseline seizure days; ± auras |
| • Class 5: Less than 50% reduction of baseline seizure days; ± auras |
| • Class 6: More than 100% increase of baseline seizure days; ± auras |

**Concluding Remarks**

- ***Tools for presurgical evaluation***. *Presurgical evaluation aims at the definition of the epileptogenic area, removal of which per definition leads to seizure freedom. It is based on clinical, neuropsychological and psychiatric assessment, neuroimaging, and electrophysiological diagnostics. MRI providing evidence of the structural basis of focal epilepsy has proven to be the key diagnostic tool guiding the surgeon, and removal of the structural abnormality has been shown to be the most important prognostic factor for postoperative seizure freedom.*
- ***Interdisciplinary epilepsy conference***. *Progress of diagnostic work-up is discussed in regular intervals in the interdisciplinary epilepsy conference consisting of a core team of epileptologists, neuropsychologists, neuropsychiatrists, neuroradiologists, EEG technicians, and neurosurgeons. Having reached consensus, the team formulates a detailed plan to proceed.*
- ***Proceeding with surgery***. *When all presurgical information points to a unifying location, i.e., when data from clinical, neuropsychological, and electrophysiological studies as well as from imaging modalities are congruent, the patient can proceed to surgical treatment.*

## References


1. Bien CG, Raabe AL, Schramm J, Becker A, Urbach H, Elger CE. Trends in presurgical evaluation and surgical treatment of epilepsy at one centre from 1988–2009. J Neurol Neurosurg Psychiatry. 2013;84:54–61.
2. Kral T, Clusmann H, Urbach H, et al. Preoperative evaluation for epilepsy surgery (Bonn algorithm). Zentralbl Neurochir. 2002;63:106–10.
3. Kwon C-S, Neal J, Tellez-Zenteno J, et al. Resective focal epilepsy surgery—Has selection of candidates changed? A systematic review. Epilepsy Res. 2016;122:37–43.
4. Rosenow F, Lüders H. Presurgical evaluation of epilepsy. Brain. 2001;124:1683–700.
5. Ryvlin P, Rheims S. Epilepsy surgery: eligibility criteria and presurgical evaluation. Dialogues Clin Neurosci. 2008;10(1):91–103.
6. Vakharia VN, Duncan JS, Witt J-A, et al. Getting the best outcomes from epilepsy surgery. Ann Neurol. 2018;83(4):676–90.
7. Lüders H, Awad I. Conceptual considerations. In: Lüders H, editor. Epilepsy surgery. New York: Raven Press; 1992. p. 51–62.
8. Wellmer J. Lesion focused radiofrequency thermocoagulation of bottom-of-sulcus focal cortical dysplasia type IIb: conceptional considerations with regard to the epileptogenic zone. Epilepsy Research 2018; https://doi.org/10.1016/j.eplepsyres.2018.02.009.
9. Grinenko O, Li J, Mosher JC, Wang IZ, Bulacio JC, Gonzalez-Martinez J, Nair D, Najm I, Leahy RM, Chauvel P. A fingerprint of the epileptogenic zone in human epilepsies. Brain. 2018;141(1):117–31.
10. Labiner DM, Bagic AI, Herman ST, Fountain NB, Walczak TS, Gumnit RJ, the National Association of Epilepsy Centers. Essential services, personnel, and facilities in specialized epilepsy centers–revised 2010 guidelines. Epilepsia. 2010;51:2322–33.
11. Loddenkemper T, Kotagal P. Lateralizing signs during seizures in focal epilepsy. Epilepsy Behav. 2005;7:1–17.
12. Stoyke C, Bilgin Ö, Noachtar S. Video atlas of lateralising and localizing seizure phenomena. Epileptic Disord. 2011;13:113–24.
13. Leutmezer F, Baumgartner C. Postictal signs of lateralizing and localizing significance. Epileptic Disord. 2002;4:43–8.
14. Kotagal P, Bleasel A, Geller E, Kankirawatana P, Moorjani BI, Rybicki L. Lateralizing value of asymmetric tonic limb posturing observed in secondarily generalized tonic–clonic seizures. Epilepsia. 2000;41:457–62.
15. Helmstaedter C. Neuropsychological aspects of epilepsy surgery. Epilepsy Behav. 2004;5:45–55.
16. Helmstaedter C, Witt J-A. Clinical neuropsychology in epilepsy: theoretical and practical issues. Handb Clin Neurol. 2012;107:437–59.
17. Witt J-A, Coras R, Schramm J, et al. Relevance of hippocampal integrity for memory outcome after surgical treatment of mesial temporal lobe epilepsy. J Neurol. 2015;262(10):2214–24.
18. Guerrini R, Scerrati M, Rubboli G, et al. Overview of presurgical assessment and surgical treatment of epilepsy from the Italian League Against Epilepsy. Epilepsia. 2013;54(Suppl. 7):35–48.

19. Brückner K. Standard der neuropsychologischen Testung in der prächirurgischen Epilepsiediagnostik. Z Epileptol. 2012;25:59–63.
20. Gleissner U, Helmstaedter C, Elger CE. Right hippocampal contribution to visual memory: a presurgical and postsurgical study in patients with temporal lobe epilepsy. J Neurol Neurosurg Psychiatry. 1998;65:665–9.
21. Helmstaedter C, Grunwald T, Lehnertz K, et al. Differential involvement of left temporolateral and temporomesial structures in verbal declarative learning and memory: evidence from temporal lobe epilepsy. Brain Cogn. 1997;35:110–31.
22. Hermann BP, Perrine K, Chelune GJ, Barr W, Loring DW, Strauss E, Trenerry MR, Westerveld M. Visual confrontation naming following left anterior temporal lobectomy: a comparison of surgical approaches. Neuropsychology. 1999;13(1):3–9.
23. Ives-Deliperi VL, Butler JT. Naming outcomes of anterior temporal lobectomy in epilepsy patients: a systematic review of the literature. Epilepsy Behav. 2012;24(2):194–8.
24. Frisk V, Milner B. The role of the left hippocampal region in the acquisition and retention of story content. Neuropsychologia. 1990;28(4):349–59.
25. Helmstaedter C, Kurthen M, Linke DB, Elger CE. Right hemisphere restitution of language and memory functions in right hemisphere language-dominant patients with left temporal lobe epilepsy. Brain. 1994;117(4):729–37.
26. Helmstaedter C, Pohl C, Elger CE. Relations between verbal and nonverbal memory performance: Evidence of confounding effects particularly in patients with right temporal lobe epilepsy. Cortex. 1995;31(2):345–55.
27. Sidhu MK, Stretton J, Winston GP, et al. Memory fMRI predicts verbal memory decline after anterior temporal lobe resection. Neurology. 2015;84(15):1512–9.
28. Bonelli SB, Thompson PJ, Yogarajah M, et al. Imaging language networks before and after anterior temporal lobe resection: results of a longitudinal fMRI study. Epilepsia. 2012;53(4):639–50.
29. Massot-Tarrús A, White K, Mirsattari SM. Comparing the Wada test and functional MRI for the presurgical evaluation of memory in temporal lobe epilepsy. Curr Neurol Neurosci Rep. 2019;19:31.
30. Shulman MB. The frontal lobes, epilepsy, and behavior. Epilepsy Behav. 2000;1:384–95.
31. Koch-Stoecker S. Personality disorders as predictors of severe postsurgical psychiatric complications in epilepsy patients undergoing temporal lobe resections. Epilepsy Behav. 2002;3:526–31.
32. Cleary RA, Baxendale SA, Thompson PJ, Foong J. Predicting and preventing psychopathology following temporal lobe epilepsy surgery. Epilepsy Behav. 2013;26(3):322–34.
33. Devinsky O, Barr WB, Vickrey BG, Berg AT, Bazil CW, Pacia SV, Langfitt JT, Walczak TS, Sperling MR, Shinnar S, Spencer SS. Changes in depression and anxiety after resective surgery for epilepsy. Neurology. 2005;65:1744–49.
34. Wrench JM, Wilson SJ, O'Shea MF, Reutens DC. Characterizing de novo depression after epilepsy surgery. Epilepsy Res. 2009;83:81–8.
35. Adams SJ, O'Brien TJ, Lloyd J, Kilpatrick CJ, Salzberg MR, Velakoulis D. Neuropsychiatric morbidity in focal epilepsy. Br J Psychiatry. 2008; 192:464–9.
36. Koch-Stoecker SC, Bien CG, Schulz R, May TW. Psychiatric lifetime diagnoses are associated with a reduced chance of seizure freedom after temporal lobe surgery. Epilepsia. 2017;58(6):983–93.
37. Gill SJ, Lukmanji S, Fiest KM, et al. Depression screening tools in persons with epilepsy: a systematic review of validated tools. Epilepsia. 2017;58(5):695–705.
38. Perucca P, Mula M. Antiepileptic drug effects on mood and behavior: molecular targets. Epilepsy Behav. 2013;26(3):440–9.
39. Knake S, Triantafyllou C, Wald LL, et al. 3T phased array MRI improves the presurgical evaluation in focal epilepsies: a prospective study. Neurology. 2005;65:1026–31.
40. Urbach H, Mast H, Egger K, Mader I. Presurgical MR imaging in epilepsy. Clin Neuroradiol. 2015;25(2):151–5.
41. Martinez A, Finegersh A, Cannon DM, Dustin I, Nugent A, Herscovitch P, Theodore WH. The 5-HT1A receptor and 5-HT transporter in temporal lobe epilepsy. Neurology. 2013;80:1465–71.
42. Téllez-Zenteno JF, Ronquillo LH, Moien-Afshari F, Wiebe S. Surgical outcomes in lesional and non-lesional epilepsy: a systematic review and meta-analysis. Epilepsy Res. 2010;89(2–3):310–8.
43. Bien CG, Szinai M, Wagner J, et al. Characteristics and surgical outcome of patients with refractory MRI-negative epilepsies. Arch Neurol. 2009a;66(12):1491–9.
44. Bien CG, Raabe AL, Schramm J, et al. Long-term developments in presurgical evaluation and surgical treatment of epilepsy at one tertiary center. Part II: Surgical outcome. Epilepsia. 2010;51(Suppl. 4):6.
45. Bien CG, Szinai M, Wagner J, Clusmann H, Becker AJ, Urbach H. Characteristics and surgical outcome of patients with refractory MRI-negative epilepsies. Arch Neurol. 2009b;66:1491–9.
46. Wagner J, Weber B, Urbach H, Elger CE, Huppertz HJ. Morphometric MRI analysis improves detection of focal cortical dysplasia type II. Brain. 2011a;134:2844–54.
47. Wagner J, Wellmer J, Urbach H, et al. Focal cortical dysplasia type IIb: completeness of cortical, not subcortical resection is necessary for seizure freedom. Epilepsia. 2011b;52(8):1418–24.
48. Wellmer J, Quesada CM, Rothe L, Elger CE, Bien CG, Urbach H. Proposal for a magnetic resonance imaging protocol for the detection of epilepto-

genic lesions at early outpatient stages. Epilepsia. 2013;44:1977–87.
49. Urbach H. Imaging of the epilepsies. Eur Radiol. 2005;15:494–500.
50. von Oertzen J, Urbach H, Jungbluth S, Kurthen M, Reuber M, Fernandez G, Elger CE. Standard magnetic resonance imaging is inadequate for patients with refractory focal epilepsy. J Neurol Neurosurg Psychiatry. 2002;73:643–7.
51. McBride MC, Bronstein KS, Bennett B, Erba G, Pilcher W, Berg MJ. Failure of standard magnetic resonance imaging in patients with refractory temporal lobe epilepsy. Arch Neurol. 1998;55:346–8.
52. Urbach H, editor. MRI in epilepsy. Berlin, Heidelberg: Springer; 2013.
53. Phal PM, Usmanov A, Nesbit GM, et al. Qualitative comparison of 3-T and 1.5-T MRI in the evaluation of epilepsy. AJR Am J Roentgenol. 2008;191(3):890–5.
54. Urbach H. High-filed magnetic resonance imaging for epilepsy. In: Willinek WA, editor. Applications of high-field MR imaging. Neuroimaging clinics of North America, vol. 22; 2012. p. 173–89.
55. Lummel N, Schoepf V, Burke M, Brueckmann H, Linn J. 3D fluid-attenuated inversion recovery imaging: reduced CSF artifacts and enhanced sensitivity and specificity for subarachnoid hemorrhage. AJNR Am J Neuroradiol. 2011;32:2054–60.
56. Saini J, Kesavadas C, Thomas B, Kapilamoorthy TR, Gupta AK, Radhakrishnan A, Radhakrishnan K. Susceptibility weighted imaging in the diagnostic evaluation of patients with intractable epilepsy. Epilepsia. 2009;50:1462–73.
57. Chatzikonstantinou A, Gass A, F€orster A, Hennerici MG, Szabo K. Features of acute DWI abnormalities related to status epilepticus. Epilepsy Res 2011; 97: 45–51.
58. Nyberg E, Sandhu GS, Jesberger J, Blackham KA, Hsu DP, Griswold MA, Sunshine JL. Comparison of brain MR images at 1.5T using BLADE and rectilinear techniques for patients who move during data acquisition. AJNR. 2012;33:77–82.
59. Huppertz HJ, Wellmer J, Staack AM, Altenmüller DM, Urbach H, KrÖll J. Voxel-based 3D MRI analysis helps to detect subtle forms of subcortical band heterotopia. Epilepsia. 2008;49(5):772–85.
60. Marques JP, Kober T, Krueger G, van der Zwaag W, Van de Moortele PF, Gruetter R. MP2RAGE, a self bias-field corrected sequence for improved segmentation and T1-mapping at high field. NeuroImage. 2010;49:1271–81.
61. Rugg-Gunn FJ, Boulby PA, Symms MR, Barker GJ, Duncan JS. Imaging the neocortex in epilepsy with double inversion recovery imaging. NeuroImage. 2006;31:39–50.
62. Bonhila L, Lee CY, Jensen JH, et al. Altered microstructure in temporal lobe epilepsy: A diffusional kurtosis imaging study. Am J Neuroradiol. 2015;36(4):719–24.
63. Serles W, Baumgartner C, Feichtinger M, Felber S, Feucht M, Podreka I, Prayer D, Trinka E. Richtlinien f€ur ein standardisiertes MRT- Protokoll für Patienten mit epileptischen Anfällen in Österreich. Mitteilungen der Österreichischen Sektion der Internationalen Liga Gegen Epilepsie. 2003;3:2–13.
64. Deblaere K, Achten E. Structural magnetic resonance imaging in epilepsy. Eur Radiol. 2008;18:119–29.
65. Jackson GD, Badawy RA. Selecting patients for epilepsy surgery: identifying a structural lesion. Epilepsy Behav. 2011;20:182–9.
66. Blümcke I, Thom M, Aronica E, Armstrong DD, Bartolomei F, Bernasconi A, Bernasconi N, Bien CG, Cendes F, Coras R, Cross JH, Jacques TS, Kahane P, Mathern GW, Miyata H, Moshé SL, Oz B, Özkara Ç, Perucca E, Sisodiya S, Wiebe S, Spreafico R. International consensus classification of hippocampal sclerosis in temporal lobe epilepsy: a task force report from the ILAE commission on diagnostic methods. Epilepsia. 2013;54:1315–29.
67. Urbach H, Huppertz HJ, Schwarzwald R, Becker AJ, Wagner J, Delsous Bahri M, Tschampa HJ. Is the type and extent of hippocampal sclerosis measurable on high-resolution MRI? Neuroradiology. 2014;56:731–5.
68. Lampinen B, Zampeli A, Björkman-Burtscher IM, et al. Tensor-valued diffusion MRI differentiates cortex and white matter in malformations of cortical development associated with epilepsy. Epilepsia 2020. https://doi.org/10.1111/epi.16605.
69. Colliot O, Bernasconi N, Khalili N, Antel SB, Naessens V, Bernasconi A. Individual voxel-based analysis of gray matter in focal cortical dysplasia. NeuroImage. 2006;29:162–71.
70. Bernhardt BC, Bernasconi N, Concha L, Bernasconi A. Cortical thickness analysis in temporal lobe epilepsy: reproducibility and relation to outcome. Neurology. 2010;74:1776–84.
71. Huppertz HJ, Grimm C, Fauser S, Kassubek J, Mader I, Hochmuth A, Spreer J, Schulze-Bonhage A. Enhanced visualization of blurred gray-white matter junctions in focal cortical dysplasia by voxel-based 3D MRI analysis. Epilepsy Res. 2005;67:35–50.
72. Thesen T, Quinn BT, Carlson C, Devinsky O, DuBois J, McDonald CR, French J, Leventer R, Felsovalyi O, Wang X, Halgren E, Kuzniecky R. Detection of epileptogenic cortical malformations with surface-based MRI morphometry. PLoS One. 2011;6:e16430.
73. Besson P, Andermann F, Dubeau F, Bernasconi A. Small focal cortical dysplasia lesions are located at the bottom of a deep sulcus. Brain. 2008;131:3246–55.
74. Ronan L, Murphy K, Delanty N, Doherty C, Maguire S, Scanlon C, Fitzsimons M. Cerebral cortical gyrification: a preliminary investigation in temporal lobe epilepsy. Epilepsia. 2007;48:211–9.
75. Bernasconi A, Antel SB, Collins DL, Bernasconi N, Olivier A, Dubeau F, Pike GB, Andermann F, Arnold DL. Texture analysis and morphological processing of magnetic resonance imaging assist detection

of focal cortical dysplasia in extra-temporal partial epilepsy. Ann Neurol. 2001;49:770–5.
76. De Oliveira MS, Betting LE, Mory SB, Cendes F, Castellano G. Texture analysis of magnetic resonance images of patients with juvenile myoclonic epilepsy. Epilepsy Behav. 2013;27:22–8.
77. Focke NK, Bonelli SB, Yogarajah M, et al. Automated normalized FLAIR imaging in MRI-negative patients with refractory focal epilepsy. Epilepsia. 2009;50(6):1484–90.
78. Bernasconi A, Bernasconi N, Bernhardt BC, Schrader D. Advances in MRI for 'cryptogenic' epilepsies. Nat Rev Neurol. 2011;7:99–108.
79. Gross DW. Diffusion tensor imaging in temporal lobe epilepsy. Epilepsia. 2011;52:32–4.
80. Widjaja E, Zarei Mahmoodabadi S, Otsubo H, Snead OC, Holowka S, Bells S, Raybaud C. Subcortical alterations in tissue microstructure adjacent to focal cortical dysplasia: detection at diffusion-tensor MR imaging by using magnetoencephalographic dipole cluster localization. Radiology. 2009;251:206–15.
81. Concha L, Kim H, Bernasconi A, Bernhardt BC, Bernasconi N. Spatial patterns of water diffusion along white matter tracts in temporal lobe epilepsy. Neurology. 2012;79:455–62.
82. Guye M, Ranjeva JP, Bartolomei F, Confort-Gouny S, McGonigal A, Régis J, Chauvel P, Cozzone PJ. What is the significance of interictal water diffusion changes in frontal lobe epilepsies? NeuroImage. 2007;35:28–37.
83. Hutchinson E, Pulsipher D, Dabbs K, Myers y Gutierrez A, Sheth R, Jones J, Seidenberg M, Meyerand E, Hermann B. Children with new-onset epilepsy exhibit diffusion abnormalities in cerebral white matter in the absence of volumetric differences. Epilepsy Res. 2010;88:208–14.
84. Oh JB, Lee SK, Kim KK, Song IC, Chang KH. Role of immediate postictal diffusion-weighted MRI in localizing epileptogenic foci of mesial temporal lobe epilepsy and non-lesional neocortical epilepsy. Seizure. 2004;13:509–16.
85. Beaulieu C. The basis of anisotropic water diffusion in the nervous system—a technical review. NMR Biomed. 2002;15:435–55.
86. Raffelt D, Tournier J-D, Rose S, Ridgway GR, Henderson R, Crozier S, Salvado O, Connelly A. Apparent Fibre Density: a novel measure for the analysis of diffusion-weighted magnetic resonance images. Neuroimage. 2012;59(4):3976–94.
87. Levin BE, Katzen HL, Maudsley A, Post J, Myerson C, Govind V, Nahab F, Scanlon B, Mittel A. Whole-brain proton MR spectroscopic imaging in Parkinson's disease. J Neuroimaging. 2014;24:39–44.
88. Connelly A, Jackson GD, Duncan JS. Magnetic resonance spectroscopy in temporal lobe epilepsy. Neurology. 1994;44(8):1411. https://doi.org/10.1212/WNL.44.8.1411.
89. Guye M, Fur YL, Confort-Gouny S, Ranjeva J-P. Metabolic and electrophysiological alterations in subtypes of temporal lobe epilepsy: a combined proton magnetic resonance spectroscopic imaging and depth electrodes study. Epilepsia. 2002;43(10):1197–209.
90. Pan JW, Spencer DD, Kuzniecky R, Duckrow RB, Hetherington H, Spencer SS. Metabolic networks in epilepsy by MR spectroscopic imaging. Acta Neurol Scand. 2012;126:411–20.
91. Oldfield RC. The assessment and analysis of handedness. Neuropsychologia. 1971;9:97–113.
92. Springer JA, Binder JR, Hammeke TA, Swanson SJ, Frost JA, Bellgowan PS, Brewer CC, Perry HM, Morris GL, Mueller WM. Language dominance in neurologically normal and epilepsy subjects. Brain. 1999;122:2033–45.
93. Bauer P, Reitsma JB, Houweling BM, Ferrier CH, Ramsey NF. Can fMRI safely replace the Wada test for preoperative assessment of language lateralisation? A meta-analysis and systematic review. J Neurol Neurosurg Psychiatry. 2014;85(5):581–8.
94. Wellmer J, Weber B, Urbach H, et al. Cerebral lesions can impair fMRI-based language lateralization. Epilepsia. 2009;50(10):2213–24.
95. You X, Zachery AN, Fanto EJ, et al. fMRI prediction of naming change after adult temporal lobe epilepsy surgery: activation matters. Epilepsia. 2019; https://doi.org/10.1111/epi.14656.
96. Destrieux C, Fischl B, Dale A, Halgren E. Automatic parcellation of human cortical gyri and sulci using standard anatomical nomenclature. NeuroImage. 2010;53:1–15. IEEE 2019
97. Anastasopoulos C, Reisert M, Kiselev VG, Nguyen-Thanh T, Schulze-Bonhaage A, Zentner J, Mader I. Local and global fiber tractography in patients with epilepsy. AJNR Am J Neuroradiol. 2014;35:291–6.
98. Winston GP, Daga P, Stretton J, Modat M, Symms MR, McEvoy AW, Ourselin S, Duncan JS. Optic radiation tractography and vision in anterior temporal lobe resection. Ann Neurol. 2012;71:334.
99. Kumar A, Chugani HT. The role of radionuclide imaging in epilepsy, Part 1: Sporadic temporal and extratemporal lobe epilepsy. JNMT. 2017a;45:114–21.
100. Kumar A, Chugani HT. The role of radionuclide imaging in epilepsy. Part 2: Epilepsy syndromes. JNMT. 2017b;45:122–9.
101. Kuzniecky RI, Knowlton RC. Neuroimaging of epilepsy. Semin Neurol. 2002;22:279–88.
102. Willmann O, Wennberg R, May T, et al. The contribution of 18F-FDG PET in preoperative epilepsy surgery evaluation for patients with temporal lobe epilepsy. A meta-analysis. Seizure. 2007;16(6):509–20.
103. Rubi S, Setoain X, Donaire A, Bargalló N, Sanmartí F, Carreño M, Rumià J, Calvo A, Aparicio J, Campistol J, Pons F. Validation of FDG-PET/MRI coregistration in nonlesional refractory childhood epilepsy. Epilepsia. 2011;52:2216–124.

104. Duncan JS, Winston GP, Koepp MJ, Ourselin S. Brain imaging in the assessment for epilepsy surgery. Lancet Neurol. 2016;15(4):420–33.
105. Picard F. New PET tracer in epilepsy. Epileptologie. 2007;24:66–72.
106. Desai A, Bekelis K, Thadani VM, et al. Interictal PET and ictal subtraction SPECT: sensitivity in the detection of seizure foci in patients with medically intractable epilepsy. Epilepsia. 2013;54:341–50.
107. la Fougère C, Rominger A, Förster S, et al. PET and SPECT in epilepsy: a critical review. Epilepsy Behav. 2009;15(1):50–5.
108. Schulze-Bonhage A, Zentner J. The preoperative evaluation and surgical treatment of epilepsy. Dtsch Arztebl Int. 2014;111:313–9.
109. Cascino GD. Video-EEG monitoring in adults. Epilepsia. 2002;43(Suppl. 3):80–93.
110. Cross JH, Jayakar P, Nordli D, Delalande O, Duchowny M, Wieser HG, et al. Proposed criteria for referral and evaluation of children for epilepsy surgery: recommendations of the Subcommission for Pediatric Epilepsy Surgery. Epilepsia. 2006 Jun;47(6):952–9.
111. Grouiller F, Thornton RC, Groening K, et al. With or without spikes: localization of focal epileptic activity by simultaneous electroencephalography and functional magnetic resonance imaging. Brain. 2011;134(Pt 10):2867–86.
112. Pittau F, Dubeau F, Gotman J. Contribution of EEG/fMRI to the definition of the epileptic focus. Neurology. 2012;78:1479–87.
113. Kowalczyk MA, Omidvarnia A, Abbott DF, et al. Clinical benefit of presurgical EEG-fMRI in difficult-to-localize focal epilepsy: a single-institution retrospective review. Epilepsia. 2019;
114. Rampp S, Stefan H, Wu X, et al. Magnetoencephalography for epileptic focus localization in a series of 1000 cases. Brain. 2019;142(10):3059–71.
115. Englot DJ, Nagarajan SS, Imber BS, et al. Epileptogenic zone localization using magnetoencephalography predicts seizure freedom in epilepsy surgery. Epilepsia. 2015;56(6):949–58.
116. Burgess R. Magnetoencephalography for localizing and characterizing the epileptic focus. In: Levin KH, Chauvel P, editors. Handbook of clinical neurology, Clinical neurophysiology: basis and technical aspects, vol. 160 (3rd series): Elsevier; 2019. https://doi.org/10.1016/B978-0-444-64032-1.00013-8.
117. Chaudhary UJ, Carmichael DW, Rodionov R, et al. Mapping preictal and ictal haemodynamic networks using video-electroencephalography and functional imaging. Brain. 2012;135(Pt 12):3645–63.
118. Thornton R, Vulliemoz S, Rodionov R, et al. Epileptic networks in focal cortical dysplasia revealed using electroencephalography-functional magnetic resonance imaging. Ann Neurol. 2011;70(5):822–37.
119. Van Houdt PJ, de Munck JC, Leijten FSS, et al. EEG-fMRI correlation patterns in the presurgical evaluation of focal epilepsy: a comparison with electrocorticographic data and surgical outcome measures. NeuroImage. 2013;75:238–48.
120. Mouthaan BE, Rados M, Boon P, et al. Diagnostic accuracy of interictal source imaging in presurgical epilepsy evaluation: a systematic review from the E-PILEPSY consortium. Clin Neurophysiol. 2019;130(5):845–55.
121. Zumsteg D, Wieser HG. Presurgical evaluation: current role of invasive EEG. Epilepsia. 2000;41(Suppl. 3):S55–60.
122. Chauvel P, Gonzales-Martinez J, Bulacio J. Presurgical intracranial investigations in epilepsy surgery. In: Levin KH, Chauvel P, editors. Handbook of clinical neurology, Clinical neurophysiology: diseases and disorders, vol. 161 (3rd series): Elsevier B.V; 2019. https://doi.org/10.1016/B978-0-444-64142-7.00045-X.
123. Behrens E, Zentner J, van Roost D, et al. Subdural and depth electrodes in the presurgical evaluation of epilepsy. Acta Neurochir. 1994;128:84–7.
124. Rosenbaum TJ, Laxer KD. Subdural electrode recordings for seizure focus localization. J Epilepsy. 1989;2:129–35.
125. Wellmer J, von der Groeben F, Klarmann U, Weber C, Elger CE, Urbach H, Clusmann H, von Lehe M. Risks and benefits of invasive epilepsy surgery workup with implanted subdural and depth electrodes. Epilepsia. 2012;53(8):1322–32.
126. Sparks R, Zombori G, Rodionov R, et al. Automated multiple trajectory planning algorithm for the placement of stereo-electroencephalography (SEEG) electrodes in epilepsy treatment. Int J Comput Assist Radiol Surg. 2016:1–14.
127. Cardinale F, Casaceli G, Raneri F, Miller J, Lo RG. Implantation of stereoelectroencephalography electrodes: a systematic review. J Clin Neurophysiol. 2016;33(6):490–502.
128. Kim LH, Feng AY, Ho AL, et al. Robot-assisted versus manual navigated stereoelectroencephalography in adult medically-refractory epilepsy patients. Epilepsy Res. 2020; https://doi.org/10.1016/j.eplepsyres.2019.106253.
129. Whiting AC, Catapano JS, Zavala B, et al. Doing more with less: a minimally invasive, cost-conscious approach to stereoelectroencephalography. World Neurosurg. 2019; https://doi.org/10.1016/j.wneu.2019.09.055.
130. Reinacher PC, Altenmüller D-M, Krüger M, et al. Simultaneous frame-assisted stereotactic placement of subdural grid electrodes and intracerebral depth electrodes. J Neurol Surg A. 2019;80:353–8.
131. Olivier A, Gloor P, Quesney F, Andermann F. The indications for and the role of depth electrode recording in epilepsy. Appl Neurophysiol. 1983;46:33–6.

132. Olivier A, Marchand E, Peters TM. Depth electrodes implantation at the Montreal Neurological Institute and hospital. In: Engel J, editor. Surgical treatment of the epilepsies. New York, NY: Raven Press; 1987. p. 595–602.
133. Olivier A, Boling W. Stereotactic intracranial recording (stereoencephalography). In: Schmidek HH, Sweet WH, editors. Operative neurosurgical techniques: indications, methods, and results. Philadelphia, PA: WB Sounders; 2000. p. 1511–28.
134. Ross D, Brunberg J, Drury I, Henry T. Intracerebral depth electrode monitoring in partial epilepsy: the morbidity and efficacy of placement using magnetic resonance image-guided stereotactic surgery. Neurosurgery. 1996;39:327–34.
135. Van Roost D, Solymosi L, Schramm J, et al. Depth electrode implantation in the length axis of the hippocampus for the presurgical evaluation of medial temporal lobe epilepsy: a computed tomography-based stereotactic insertion technique and its accuracy. Neurosurgery. 1988;43:819–27.
136. Cardinale F, Cossu M, Castana L, et al. Stereoelectroencephalography: surgical methodology, safety, and stereotactic application accuracy in 500 procedures. Neurosurgery. 2013;72(3):353–66.
137. Woolfe M, Prime D, Gillinder L, et al. Automatic detection of the epileptogenic zone: An application of the fingerprint of epilepsy. J Neurosci Methods. 2019;325:108347. https://doi.org/10.1016/j.jneumeth.2019.108347.
138. Arya R, Mangano FT, Horn PS, Holland KD, Rose DF, Glauser TA. Adverse events related to extraoperative invasive EEG monitoring with subdural grid electrodes: a systematic review and meta-analysis. Epilepsia. 2013;54(5):828–39.
139. Taussig D, Montavont A, Isnard J. Invasive EEG explorations. Clinical Neurophysiology. 2015; https://doi.org/10.1016/j.neucli.2014.11.006.
140. Burneo JG, Steven DA, McLachlan RS, Parrent AG. Morbidity associated with the use of intracranial electrodes for epilepsy surgery. Can J Neurol Sci. 2006;33:223–7.
141. Pilcher WH, Rusyniak WG. Complications of epilepsy surgery. Neurosurg Clin North Am. 1993;4:311–25.
142. Van Buren JM. Complications of surgical procedures in the diagnosis and treatment of epilepsy. In: Engel Jr J, editor. Surgical treatment of the epilepsies. New York: Raven Press; 1987. p. 465–75.
143. Wong CH, Birkett J, Byth K, Dexter M, Somerville E, Gill D, Chaseling R, Fearnside M, Bleasel A: Risk factors for complications during intracranial electrode recording in presurgical evaluation of drug resistant partial epilepsy. Acta Neurochir (Wien). 2009;151:37–50.
144. Kovalev D, Spreer J, Honegger J, Zentner J, Schulze-Bonhage A, Huppertz HJ. Rapid and fully automated visualization of subdural electrodes in the presurgical evaluation of epilepsy patients. AJNR Am J Neuroradiol. 2005;26:1078–83.
145. Sebastiano F, Di Gennaro G, Esposito V, et al. A rapid and reliable procedure to localize subdural electrodes in presurgical evaluation of patients with drug-resistant focal epilepsy. Clin Neurophysiol. 2006;117(2):341–7.
146. Arnulfo G, Narizzano M, Cardinale F, et al. Automatic segmentation of deep intracerebral electrodes in computed tomography scans. BMC Bioinformatics. 2015; https://doi.org/10.1186/s12859-015-0511-6.
147. Tandon N, Tong BA, Friedman ER, et al. Analysis of morbidity and outcomes associated with use of subdural grids vs. stereoelectroencephalography in patients with intractable epilepsy. JAMA Neurol. 2019; https://doi.org/10.1001/jamaneurol.2019.0098.
148. Toth M, Papp KS, Gede N, et al. Surgical outcomes related to invasive EEG monitoring with subdural grids or depth electrodes in adults: a systematic review and meta-analysis. Eur J Epilepsy. 2019;70:12–9.
149. Yan H, Katz JS, Anderson M, et al. Method of invasive monitoring in epilepsy surgery and seizure freedom and morbidity: a systematic review. Epilepsia. 2019:1–13. https://doi.org/10.1111/epi.16315.
150. Dümpelmann M, Jacobs J, Kerber K, Schulze-Bonhage A. Automatic 80–250 Hz "ripple" high frequency oscillation detection in invasive subdural grid and strip recordings in epilepsy by a radial basis function neural network. Clin Neurophysiol. 2012;123:1721–31.
151. Ryvlin P, Cross H, Rheims S. Epilepsy surgery in children and adults. Lancet Neurol. 2014;13:114–26
152. Sinha N, Dauwels J, Kaiser M, et al. Predicting neurosurgical outcomes in focal epilepsy patients using computational modelling. Brain. 2017;140(Pt 2):319–32.
153. Migliorelli C, Alonso JF, Romero S, et al. Automated detection of epileptic ripples in MEG using beamformer-based virtual sensors. J Neural Eng. 2017;14(4):46013.
154. Geertsema EE, van't Klooster MA, van Klink NEC, et al. Non-harmonicity in high-frequency components of the intra-operative corticogram to delineate epileptogenic tissue during surgery. Clin. Neurophysiology 2017; 128 (1): 153–164.
155. Holler Y, Kutil R, Klaffenbock L, et al. High-frequency oscillations in epilepsy and surgical outcome. A meta-analysis. Front Hum Neurosci. 2015;9:574.
156. Kerber K, Levan P, Dumpelmann M, et al. High frequency oscillations mirror disease activity in patients with focal cortical dysplasia. Epilepsia. 2013;54:1428–36.
157. Dirodi M, Tamilia E, Grant PE, et al. Noninvasive localization of high-frequency oscillations in children

with epilepsy: Validation against intracranial gold-standard. 978–1–5386-1311-5/19/$31.00; 2019.
158. Thomschewski A, Hincapié A-S, Frauscher B. Localization of the epileptogenic zone using high frequency oscillations. Front Neurol. 2019; https://doi.org/10.3389/fneur.2019.00094.
159. Engel J, van Ness PC, Rasmussen TB, Ojemann LM. Outcome with respect to epileptic seizures. In: Engel J, editor. Surgical treatment of the epilepsies. 2nd ed. New York: Raven Press; 1993. p. 615.
160. Wieser HG, Blume WT, Fish D, et al. ILAE Commission Report. Proposal for a new classification of outcome with respect to epileptic seizures following epilepsy surgery. Epilepsia. 2001;42(2):282–6.
161. Wieser HG. Proposal for a new classification of outcome with respect to epileptic seizures following epilepsy. Epilepsia. 2008;42:282–6. https://doi.org/10.1046/j.1528-1157.2001.35100.x.

# Surgical Tools and Techniques

# 4

*The brain is the organ of destiny. It holds within its humming mechanism secrets that will determine the future of the human race.*

*Wilder Penfield*

## Contents



Current neurosurgery is best characterized by the terms functionally oriented and functionally guided surgery. Microsurgical techniques, intraoperative electrophysiological monitoring, and neuronavigation, all introduced in the second half of the twentieth century and continuously refined up to now, facilitate neurosurgical interventions in most brain regions with calculable risks. The technique of subpial gyral emptying which is well known for many decades has proven to be particularly important for epilepsy surgical procedures in or around eloquent and highly vascularized areas. With all these tools available, it should be emphasized that functional anatomy remains the essential basis for all neurosurgical interventions.



J. Zentner, *Surgical Treatment of Epilepsies*, https://doi.org/10.1007/978-3-030-48748-5_4

## 4.1 Functional Anatomy

Traditional anatomical training of neurosurgeons is based on macroscopic dissections. Microsurgical operation techniques along with modern imaging have changed the surgeon's view facilitating spatial presentation of anatomical details. Therefore, conventional neuroanatomical depictions had to be renewed for the microneurosurgeon providing those topographical relationships that are faced under the operation microscope. It is the great merit of W. Seeger and others [1–3] to take up this challenge. Between 1978 [4] and 2018 [5], Seeger provided a comprehensive renewed depiction of neuroanatomy in 25 pictorial atlases. This tremendous work provides a detailed description of various regions and their corresponding vasculature with a particular focus on surgical approaches.

Thorough knowledge of neuroanatomy and of functional localization is even more critical in epilepsy surgery than in other fields of neurosurgery, since from the surgeon's view the epileptogenic zone to be removed frequently is not clearly distinguishable from normal and eloquent surrounding areas that have to be spared [6]. Technologies including neuronavigation cannot be a substitute for anatomical knowledge and surgical experience. On the other hand, epilepsy surgery provides a unique chance for the neurosurgeon to become acquainted with the intrinsic functional topographic anatomy of the brain and to learn to proceed with resection to acceptable limits in order to completely remove the area intended while avoiding neurological deficits.

Specific topographical relationships of different brain areas as described by W. Seeger and others that are important with respect to surgical approaches will be discussed in the respective chapters. Based on the extensive work of M.G. Yasargil, the following is limited to some general anatomical and functional aspects necessary for an understanding of seizure propagation and respective surgical intervention. Along with other neuroanatomical, neuroradiological, neurophysiological, and neuropathological studies [5, 7–13], Yasargil's anatomical depictions [2, 3] clearly demonstrate that the brain constitutes a unique functional unit consisting of an integrated, dynamic network of several subsystems.

### 4.1.1 Anatomy of Gyri

The large increase of cortical surface due to evolutional development without adequate increase in cranial volume was rendered possible by the invagination of over two-thirds of the cerebral surface into the depths resulting in the characteristic convolute shape of the gyral architecture. Although each hemisphere contains almost constantly three horizontal frontal and temporal gyri, respectively, two perpendicularly oriented central gyri (precentral and postcentral gyrus), four to five diagonal insular gyri, and two to three semicircular parieto-occipital lobules, there is a considerable variation in gyral-sulcal patterns both interindividually and between the hemispheres in the same subject. Therefore, attempts to identify structures at the surface by landmarks are limited [3, 14, 15].

In addition, delineation of individual gyri is only feasible at the surface. Already at a depth of a few millimeters, multiple connections between different gyri can be observed. This typical architecture has been named the *gyral continuum* [3, 14, 15]. The principle of gyral continuum has already been recognized by Broca who used the term "*plis de passage*" [16]. It means that gyri and sulci are joined each other by bridges, thus forming a continuum. During the last decades, gyral and sulcal continuum has been confirmed by MRI 3D reconstruction [14, 15].

On the lateral surface of the hemisphere, the frontal transverse gyri (F1, F2, and F3) are continuous with the precentral gyrus through three bridges, and the first temporal gyrus (T1) continues into the posterior limb of the supramarginal gyrus. The supramarginal gyrus caps the posterior ascending limb of the Sylvian fissure. Similar bridges exist at all lobes and aspects of both hemispheres [3, 14, 15] (Fig. 4.1). This fundamental anatomical principle is of great importance for the understanding of the dynamic process involved in the spread of cortical epileptic discharges as well as for the surgical technique of gyral emptying (see below). An overview on the concept of the gyral and sulcal continuum has been provided by Yasargil [3] and Olivier et al. [14, 15].

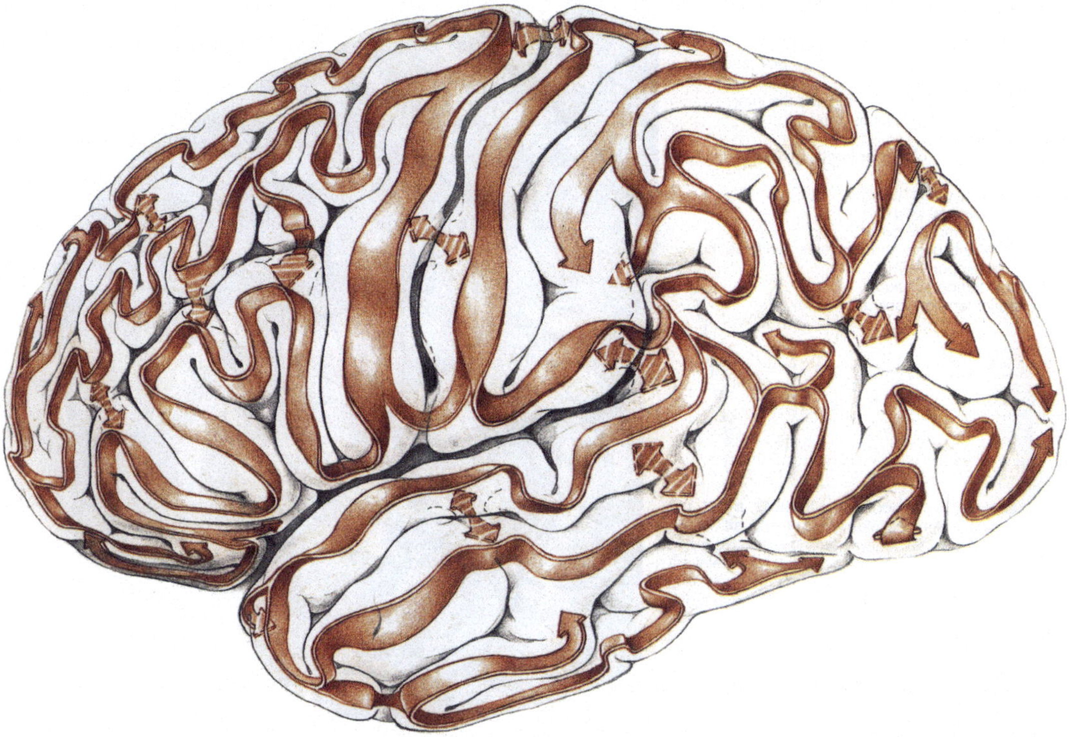

**Fig. 4.1** Schematic illustration of the gyral continuum of the left hemisphere. There is an uninterrupted connection between gyri within the hemisphere (from Yasargil [3], with permission)

### 4.1.2 Anatomy of White Matter

The white matter consists of myelinated commissural, association, and projection fibers, as well as of pathways for migration of neuroglia, vascularization, and cerebrospinal fluid. Commissural fibers (corpus callosum, anterior and posterior commissure, fornix, habenular commissure) connect corresponding regions of the left and right brain hemispheres. Association fibers include short fibers linking parts of a single gyral segment, and long fibers (cingulum, dorsal, medial, superior, and inferior longitudinal fasciculus, occipito-frontal and uncinate fasciculus) connecting cortical regions within the same hemisphere. Projection fibers connect the cortex with the basal ganglia, central nuclei, brainstem, and spinal cord [3] (Fig. 4.2). Knowledge of the white matter anatomy is useful for the understanding of seizure spread and its disruption, e.g., by multiple subpial transections (see also Chap. 14) and the semiology of seizures, as well as for safe resection of seizure foci in critical areas. Most of these fiber systems can be identified with MRI techniques (Fig. 4.3).

## 4.2 Neuronavigation

Image-guided surgery for the treatment of epilepsy started in the 1950s with the application of frames for the stereotactic placement of depth electrodes by Bancaud and Talairach [18, 19]. Favorable results led to more widespread use of frame-based stereotaxis for invasive EEG studies [20–22]. Stereotactic angiography has been used in some centers as an adjunct to avoid vascular injury during electrode placement [21]. The correlating of 3D defined image data sets with surgical stereotactic space as defined by a stereotactic frame has been pioneered by Kelly [23–25]. When data sets are acquired as a volume, paired common points in the image data set and

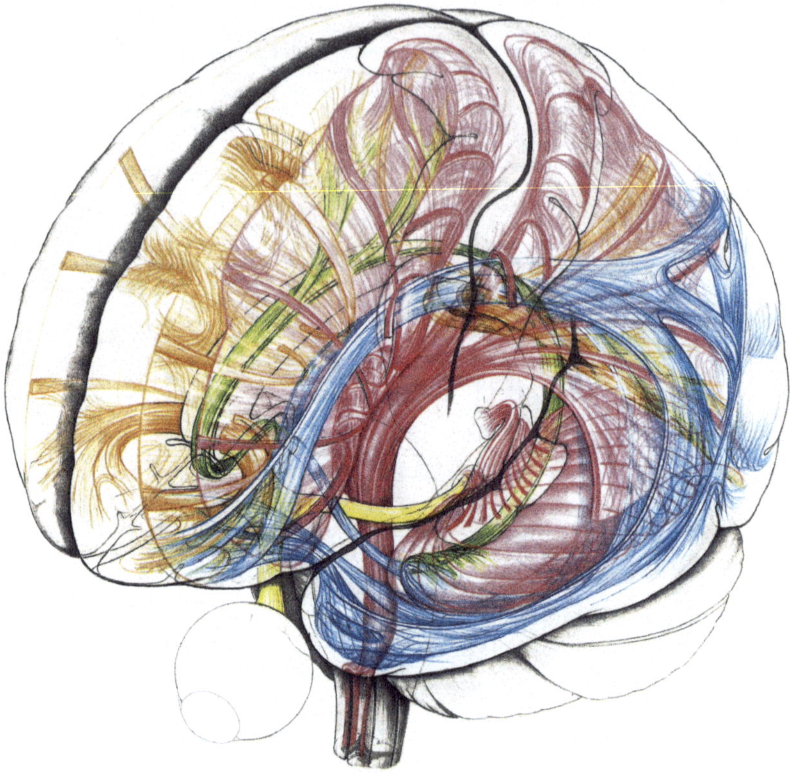

**Fig. 4.2** Artistic depiction of the organization of the white matter fibers. Red: projection fibers; blue: association fibers; yellow: commissural fibers; green: cingulate fibers (from Yasargil [3], with permission)

the real world can be used for registration. Thus, the *concept of frameless stereotaxis* was born [6, 26–28]. Since the development of this concept is closely related to epilepsy surgery, its realization for clinical practice as well as its actual application possibilities will be addressed in more detail following the overview given by Mascott [6].

### 4.2.1 Technical Principles

#### 4.2.1.1 Registration

Registration refers to the process correlating the anatomy on the images with the surgical anatomy of the patient. This is accomplished by matching defined points in image space with their counterparts in surgical space, the latter being defined within a frame of reference (e.g., by means of optical, magnetic, or mechanical triangulation) [29, 30]. The patient's head is immobilized, e.g., with a Mayfield clamp. A reference device, called tracking system, is used to determine the position of points in space with regard to a fixed reference [6]. Earlier forms of frameless registration used ultrasound or mechanical arms for tracking [31–33]. Most currently available image guidance systems use optical tracking with the patient reference device and instrument positions being defined within the reference of an optical camera system [29, 34–36]. After registration is completed, the patient reference device must not move in relation to the patient's head [6].

Connection of the patient with the computerized images can be achieved by co-registering a series of fiducial markers with homologous points on the patient's images. Nowadays, the patient's own anatomical landmarks (e.g., inner and outer canthi of both eyes, the glabella, and a point located above the tragus of both ears) are used instead of fiducial markers. In order to optimize accuracy, surface registration is accomplished matching a series of random points on the scalp and face with the surface-rendered MRI or CT. Alternatively, techniques

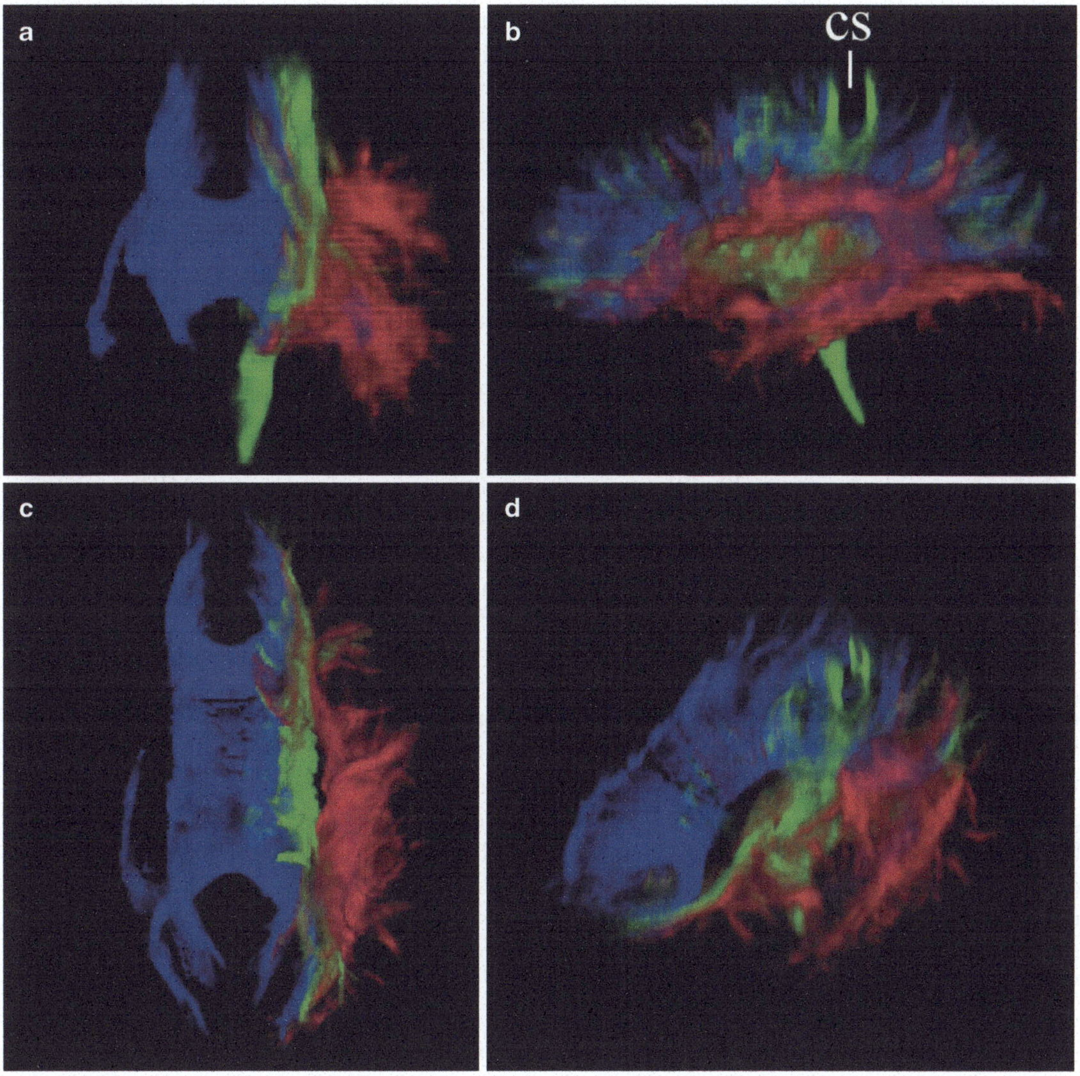


**Fig. 4.3** Three-dimensional presentation of projection (green), association (red), and callosal (blue) fibers. (**a**) coronal view; (**b**) left lateral view; (**c**) axial view; (**d**) oblique view. To demonstrate relative locations, different groups of fibers are depicted simultaneously. Note the dominant presence of projection fibers in cortical areas around the central sulcus (cs) (from Wakana et al., 2004, [17], with permission)

of laser scalp surface scanning and surface matching algorithms facilitate registration without the need for paired point registration [37]. Accuracy is confirmed by visual control using clearly definable anatomical landmarks such as the glabella, the outer ear canal, and the tip of the nose. The time required for intraoperative calibration of the system amounts to around 10 min [6, 26, 29, 30].

#### 4.2.1.2 Accuracy and Errors

The approach described above yields registration precision of 1–2 mm [38]. During surgery, accuracy of the system is repeatedly controlled using fixed structures such as landmarks at the surface, the skull base, or the midline. Knowledge of errors and limitations of the system is important. The most common cause of unexpected error is movement of the patient reference in relation to the head. In this case, correction can be tried by surface matching using free aspects of the skull or of the draped scalp. The other most important source of error refers to brain shift which constitutes the main limitation of computerized navigation, since the system is based on preoperative imaging data. Therefore, imprecision is unavoidable after release of CSF and during resection. In particular, after opening of the ventricular system or debulking of a space-occupying tumor, noticeable brain shift is inevitable. Due to brain shift, it is advisable to address any critical target early during surgery prior to shift effects [6]. Technologies available to compensate brain shift include ultrasound navigation [39, 40], or intraoperative MRI or CT [41, 42].

### 4.2.2 Applications in Epilepsy Surgery

#### 4.2.2.1 Application Fields

Neuronavigation in epilepsy surgery can be used for preoperative planning on a virtual basis. In addition, surgical approaches can be trained by young neurosurgeons [6, 14, 15]. Although depth electrodes are traditionally placed by means of stereotactic frames [21], some institutions use frameless neuronavigation [31, 43, 44]. Similarly, exact placement of subdural strip and grid electrodes may be facilitated by navigation [6]. During therapeutic procedures, navigation can be useful for exact skin incision and craniotomy. In temporal resections, particularly in selective amygdalohippocampectomy using the transsylvian, transcortical, transsulcal, or subtemporal route, it can be used to define the trajectory in order to identify the inferior horn [45]. Extratemporally, navigation may be useful to localize the central sulcus as well as the precentral and the postcentral gyrus. Moreover, epilepsy surgery frequently encounters small tumors not visible on the cortical surface and lesions such as cortical dysplasias that are not clearly identifiable. In these cases, navigation can facilitate planning of the trajectory to approach those lesions and to define resection borders [6, 14, 15, 31]. In addition, it can be helpful in disconnecting procedures such as corpus callosotomy to define the extent of section, and in hemispheric procedures (multilobectomy and hemispherectomy) to provide orientation. Finally, delineation of eloquent areas for multiple subpial transections (MST) may be supported by neuronavigation [6].

#### 4.2.2.2 Image Fusion

The correlation of different imaging sequences and modalities has proven to be useful. Most actual navigation systems have a software that performs image fusion between different data sets, e.g., based on mutual shared information algorithms including fMRI and tractography (Figs. 4.4 and 4.5). Moreover, co-registration of other non-MRI modalities can be facilitated by the workstation software. These include EEG source localization (electrical source imaging, ESI), magnetoencephalography (MEG), PET, and ictal SPECT. Thus, image fusion makes anatomical, functional, and radionuclide data available for the surgeon [35, 46–49]. Imaging protocols can be designed for both analysis and surgery, a cost-effective strategy to avoid repeat imaging [6]. Epilepsy surgery in the future may focus more on the disruption or disconnection of epileptogenic networks than on resective procedures. These networks can be expected to vary essentially between patients, and individualized surgical strategies may be required combining resective and disconnective approaches. Neuronavigation may be helpful to accurately access respective targets [6].

## 4.3 Intraoperative Imaging

Optimal preoperative imaging and complete resection of a structural abnormality have been demonstrated to be the most important predictors for seizure control in lesional epilepsies [50–53]. Accordingly, it has been shown that the main reason for failed surgery is too limited and incomplete resection of the epileptogenic lesion. On the other hand, the concept of minimalization of resection requires an individually tailored procedure. Although neuronavigation has proven to be a useful tool to define resection borders, it is based on preoperative imaging data, and brain

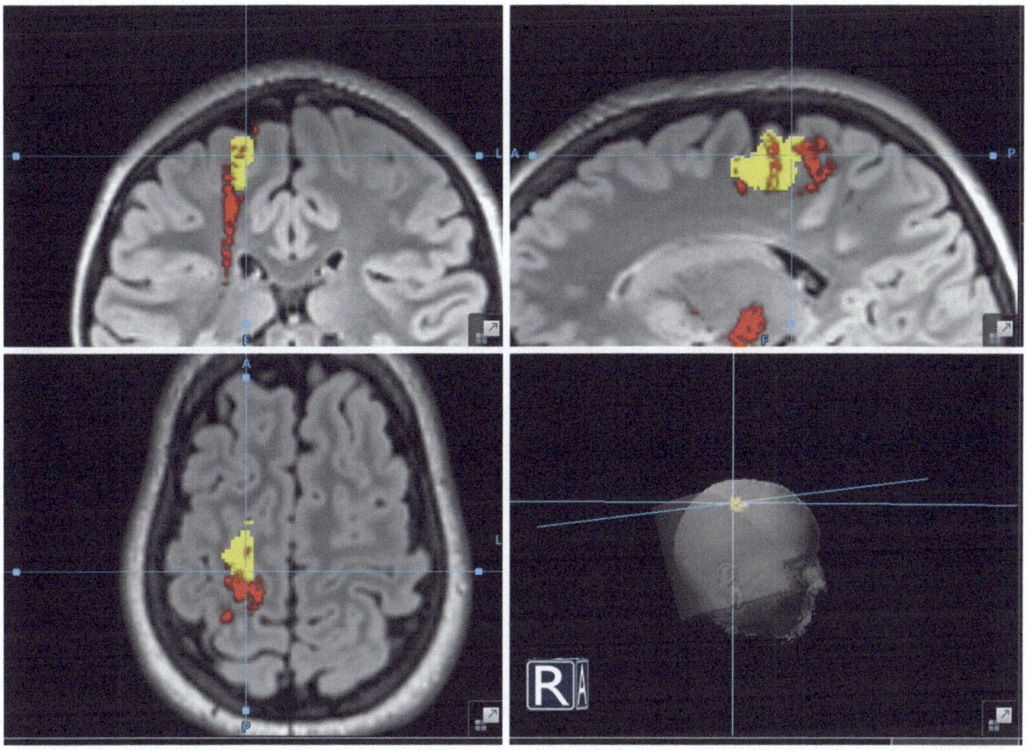


**Fig. 4.4** Fusion of anatomical and functional imaging data. MRI demonstrates a lesion of the central area with fiber tracking of the motor cortex and pyramidal tract. Yellow: lesion; red: motor cortex and pyramidal tract (with courtesy of M. Shah, Dpt. of Neurosurgery, Freiburg)

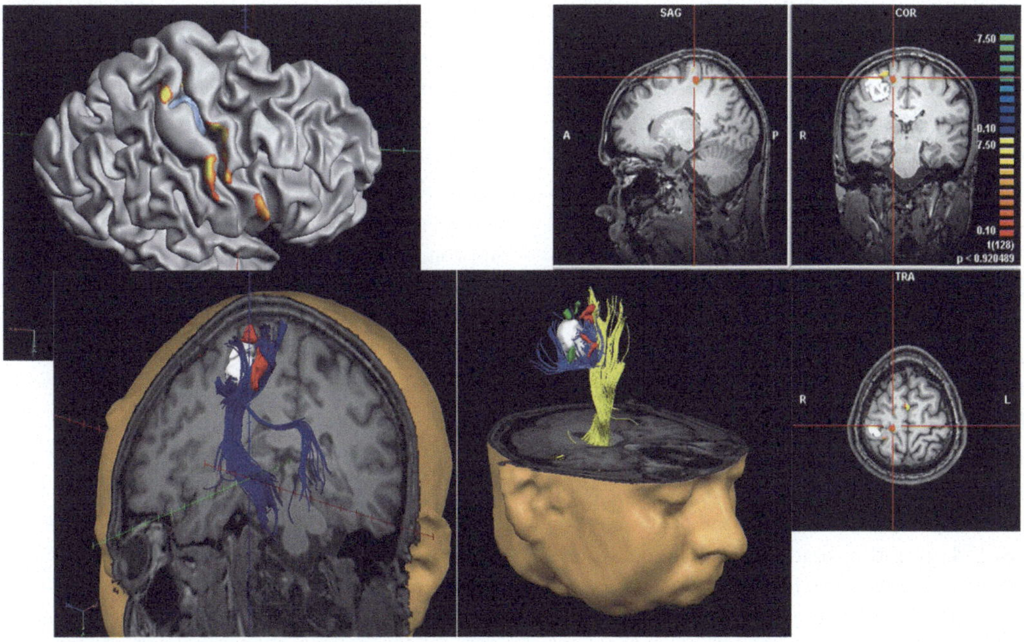


**Fig. 4.5** Tumor of the right central area. Image fusion and navigation make anatomical and functional data available for the surgeon

shift due to CSF release and decompression poses concerns towards its reliability during the ongoing procedure [54, 55]. Therefore, intraoperative imaging may be desirable for real-time guidance.

Different diagnostic imaging devices have been adopted to the operating room ranging from plain radiography to intraoperative computed tomography (iCT), intraoperative magnetic resonance imaging (iMRI), and intraoperative ultrasound (iUS). In addition, optical imaging (OI) may be used for visualization of blood flow or detection of tumor tissue [56]. The question arises whether and to what extent intraoperative imaging is necessary in epilepsy surgery. In temporal lobe epilepsies, resection boundaries are well defined by anatomic landmarks including mesial structures. Similarly, hemispheric procedures are standardized and guided by clearly visible landmarks. Extent of callosum sectioning can be best defined by neuronavigation. Thus, those procedures do not require intraoperative imaging. This holds also true for most extratemporal cortical resections, borders of which can accurately be defined by neuronavigation when applied just after dura opening before brain shift has occurred. However, there are poorly delimitable and subcortically extending lesions such as developmental malformations which are difficult to visualize and to delineate. Thus, intraoperative imaging may be desired for a subgroup of diffuse and subtle extratemporal pathologies. For these goals, iMRI (mainly 1.5 T) and iUS are available.

### 4.3.1 Intraoperative MRI (iMRI)

Kurwale et al. [57] evaluated 39 patients with extratemporal epilepsies. In the lesional group, iMRI modified operative strategy in 5 of 23 (21%) patients resulting in larger resections. Complete lesion resection was achieved in 87% of patients [57]. Analyzing 25 extratemporal cases, Sommer et al. [54] reported that 20% of patients underwent further resection based on iMRI findings. Sacino et al. [58] reviewing 12 pediatric cases with focal cortical dysplasia (FCD) noted that iMRI influenced intraoperative decision-making in 5 of 12 (42%) patients. Buchfelder et al. [59] found that iMRI caused a second look in 3 of 29 (10%) lesional cases increasing the rate of total lesion resection from 79% to 90%. In a large series of 88 patients, Roessler et al. [60] emphasized the beneficial effect of iMRI for resection of cortical malformations suggesting reduced morbidity and improved seizure control.

Overall, authors experienced with intraoperative MR imaging feel that this technique is a valuable adjunct in extratemporal lesional cases, particularly in malformations of cortical development, to achieve maximal and safe lesion resection [54, 57, 59–61]. However, some shortcomings of iMRI have been noted. It has been suggested that intraoperative MR data acquisition amounts to around 25% of the total anesthesia time, and that about the same time is required for preparing the operation room for the special needs of iMRI. Moreover, the iMRI head holder restricts positioning of patient's head, thus limiting optimal surgical access. The main limitation of iMRI, however, refers to the visualization of structural abnormalities: Visualization of subtle lesions such as focal cortical dysplasias (FCD), intraoperative assessment of which is most desired, is limited using 1.5 T MR scanners compared to preoperative optimized imaging based on 3 T scanners and epilepsy-specific protocols [57]. Considering advantages and disadvantages of iMRI, controlled prospective trials addressing iMR protocols, operation time, as well as impact of iMRI to modify surgical strategy and—most importantly—on the postsurgical outcome comparing different approaches (e.g., navigation-, iMRI-, and iUS-based resections) are required in order to define the value of iMRI in epilepsy surgery [57].

### 4.3.2 Intraoperative Ultrasound (iUS)

3D intraoperative ultrasound (iUS) is widely used for real-time monitoring in brain tumor surgery allowing the visualization of the tumor and neighbouring structures including vessels as well as to explore the postsurgical tumor cavity with respect to tumor remnants [62–64]

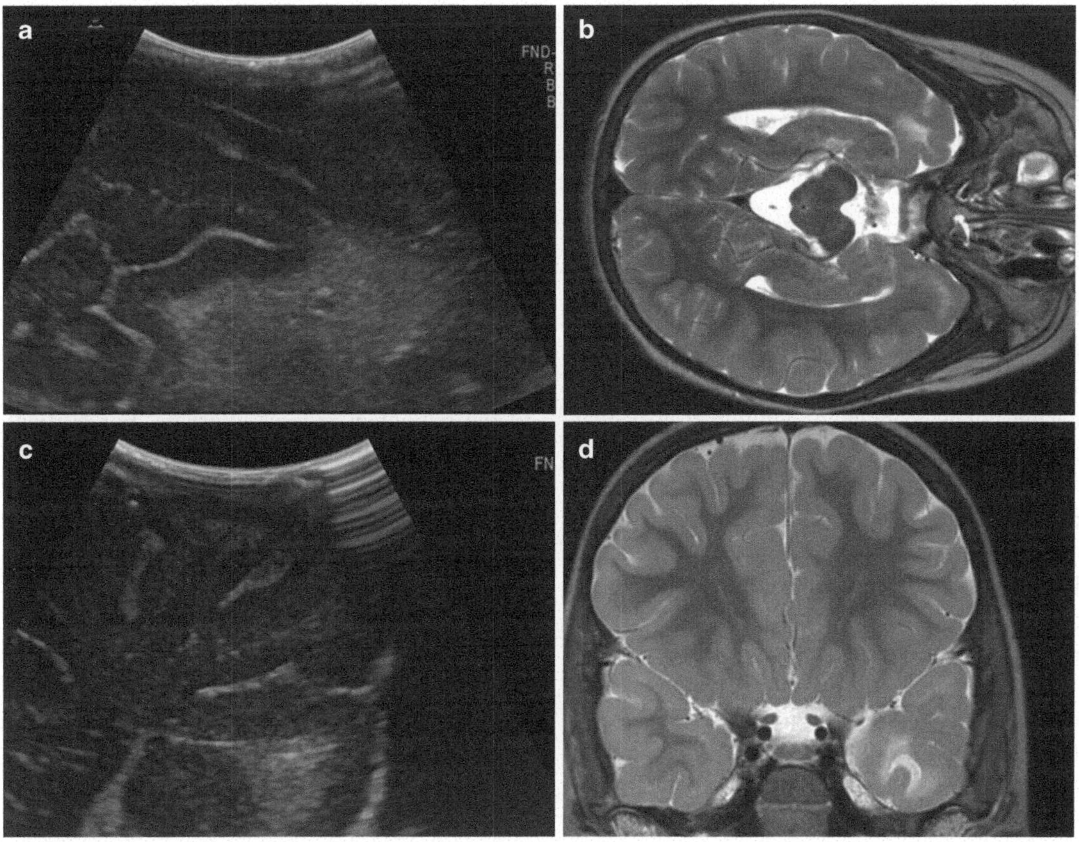


**Fig. 4.6** Left temporal ganglioglioma in a 3-year-old girl with pharmacorefractory epilepsy. iUS images (**a**, **c**) and preoperative T2-weighted MRI (**b**, **d**) are shown in corresponding section planes and orientation. iUS images clearly demonstrate a hyperechogenic lesion with a small cystic structure characteristic for a ganglioglioma corresponding to MR depiction of the lesion (with courtesy of M. Shah, Dpt. of Neurosurgery, Freiburg)

(Fig. 4.6). However, only a paucity of studies are available evaluating the sensitivity of iUS to detect subtle lesions such as FCD for which intraoperative imaging may be desired. In these studies, a high concordance of iUS with preoperative T2-weighted/FLAIR images has been demonstrated. In addition, it has been suggested that iUS may even allow a more clear demarcation of the gray-white matter junction as compared to preoperative MRI (and thus necessarily also to intraoperative MRI) [40, 65–68]. iUS facilitates spatial resolution of approximately 0.5 mm, and high temporal resolution leads to a reduction of partial volume effect [69]. Comparing iUS findings of five patients with type IIb FCD with preoperative MRI, Prada et al. [70] concluded that FCD was identified by iUS in all cases. In addition, borders of the lesion were more clearly demonstrated in iUS images than in MRI [70].

Overall, only preliminary results are available suggesting that iUS may constitute an efficient tool to guide surgical procedures for epilepsy when intraoperative imaging is desired, facilitating detection and delineation of subtle lesions such as FCD similar to preoperative MRI [70]. Contrast-enhanced iUS (CEUS) and elastosonography evaluation of lesions may provide even more detailed information [71]. In contrast to iMRI, iUS is widely available, relatively inexpensive, and less time consuming, and does not limit positioning of the patient's head. However, extensive experience is necessary to interpret findings and to be oriented towards the images acquired in oblique planes. Orientation may be facilitated combining iUS with MRI neuronavigation. In sum, iUS seems to be a promising tool, but its place for real-time guidance of epilepsy surgical procedures has still to be defined.

## 4.4 Mapping and Monitoring

**Mapping**. During resective procedures for epilepsy, eloquent cortical areas and respective pathways are frequently endangered. Mapping means the functional topographic definition of an eloquent area. This can be accomplished extraoperatively (in a separate procedure apart from the proper resection of the epileptogenic area), or intraoperatively (during the proper epilepsy surgical procedure). For mapping, electrical stimulation techniques still provide the standard that serve to validate more recent functional techniques [72–80].

**Monitoring**. Electrophysiological monitoring aims at the continuous intraoperative control of function using nerve or muscle action potentials or evoked potentials. Neurophysiological monitoring in epilepsy surgery is mainly limited to the recording of somatosensory and motor evoked potentials (SEP and MEP). However, intraoperatively, there is continuous crossover between mapping and monitoring.

### 4.4.1 Mapping

#### 4.4.1.1 Language Areas

**Intraoperative Stimulation Mapping**

Intraoperative mapping of language areas by electrical cortex stimulation requires awake craniotomy (see also Chap. 5). This procedure is known since the early beginning of epilepsy surgery about 100 years ago [81–83]. During the last decades, this technique has been reactivated [84–89]. Images of simple objects are shown to the patient in regular intervals. For cortical stimulation, a low-frequency paradigm consisting of short pulse trains with frequencies of 25–60 Hz is used. The most commonly applied frequencies are 50 Hz (Europe) and 60 Hz (North America). Cortical stimulation is applied prior to the presentation of each image and continued until there is a correct response or the next image is presented. Each preselected site is stimulated 3–4 times. Sites where stimulation produces consistent speech arrest or anomia are considered to be essential to language function [87, 88] (Fig. 4.7). An overview on language mapping in awake surgery has been provided by Szelényi et al. [90].

Ojemann and Dodrill [91] reported an 80% accuracy of intraoperative cortical stimulation

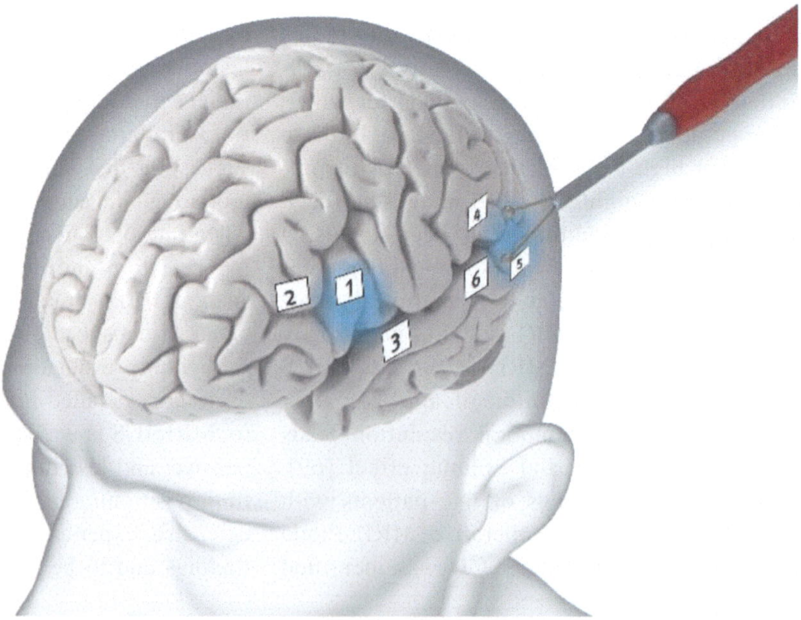


**Fig. 4.7** Schematic illustration of intraoperative stimulation mapping of language areas during awake surgery. Using a bipolar fork probe, the area in question is scanned. Stimulation of specific areas blocks language function. 1–3: Broca's area; 4–6: Wernicke's area (with courtesy of R. Ott, Arcana Forum, Emmendingen)

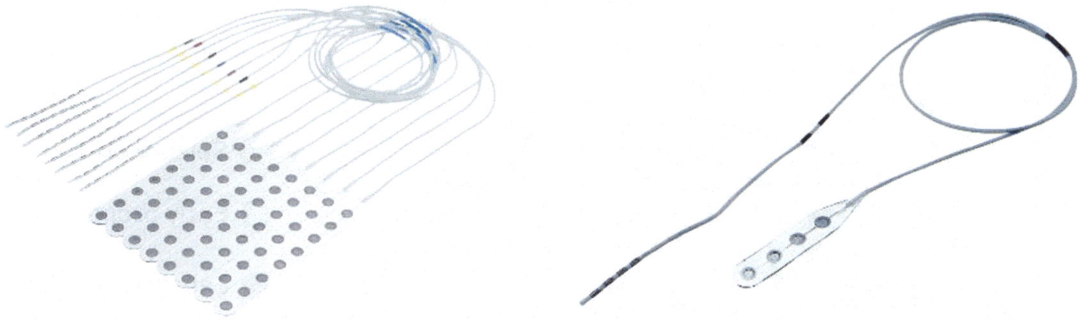

**Fig. 4.8** Subdural grid (left) and strip (right) electrode for extraoperative and intraoperative mapping and monitoring

mapping in predicting postoperative language performance. It has been demonstrated that resections within a 10 mm boundary zone of language cortex may lead to transient postoperative speech difficulties, while injury to essential language area can be expected to cause permanent deficits [87]. Intraoperative stimulation mapping revealed a highly variable topography of language areas from individuum to individuum [87]. Besides the typical Broca's and Wernicke's areas, three or more sites for language have been identified, including areas at the temporal base [87, 92, 93], particularly in the fusiform gyrus [94]. In an international survey, Hamberger et al. [95] noted that persistent postoperative language deficits were reported by 13% of centers after resecting basal temporal cortex defined as language areas. However, others did not find such additional language sites using similar stimulation protocols [96]. In patients familiar with more than one language, separate areas for each of their different languages have been described [88].

Effectivity of intraoperative stimulation mapping during awake surgery depends on a number of factors such as the anesthesia level, current leakage along the cortical surface depending on tissue hydration, and in particular the ability of the individual patient to cooperate under the tense conditions of the operating room. Certainly, intraoperative stimulation mapping in awake surgery cannot be used for patients sustaining attention deficits and hyperactivity problems, patients in a state of confusion, or very young patients (see also Chap. 5) [88]. Under these conditions, extraoperative stimulation mapping is preferred.

### Extraoperative Stimulation Mapping

Extraoperative mapping of the language areas can be accomplished using a grid electrode placed over the area in question (Fig. 4.8) [97–100]. The grid which can be combined with subdural electrodes is implanted in a first procedure. Usually, the electrodes serve initially for recording of epileptogenic activity, thus defining the epileptogenic area. Thereafter, they can be used for cortical stimulation to delineate language areas as well as the motor cortex, if required [97, 99–102] (Fig. 4.9). The proper resection of the epileptogenic zone is performed in a second operation. Thus, with extraoperative stimulation mapping, two surgical procedures are required.

The essential advantage of extraoperative mapping is that the procedure can be repeated on several days when the patient is at his/her best. This is particularly important for children. Thus, in principle, more reliable results can be expected as compared to the mapping procedure during awake surgery. However, Cervenka et al. [103, 104] noted that postoperative language performance was not clearly anticipated by extraoperative stimulation mapping in more than half of their cases. Duffeau [105] recommended extraoperative mapping in non-tumoral epilepsy surgery, while he found intraoperative mapping advantageous for surgical treatment of large gliomas facilitating identification of subcortical tracts.

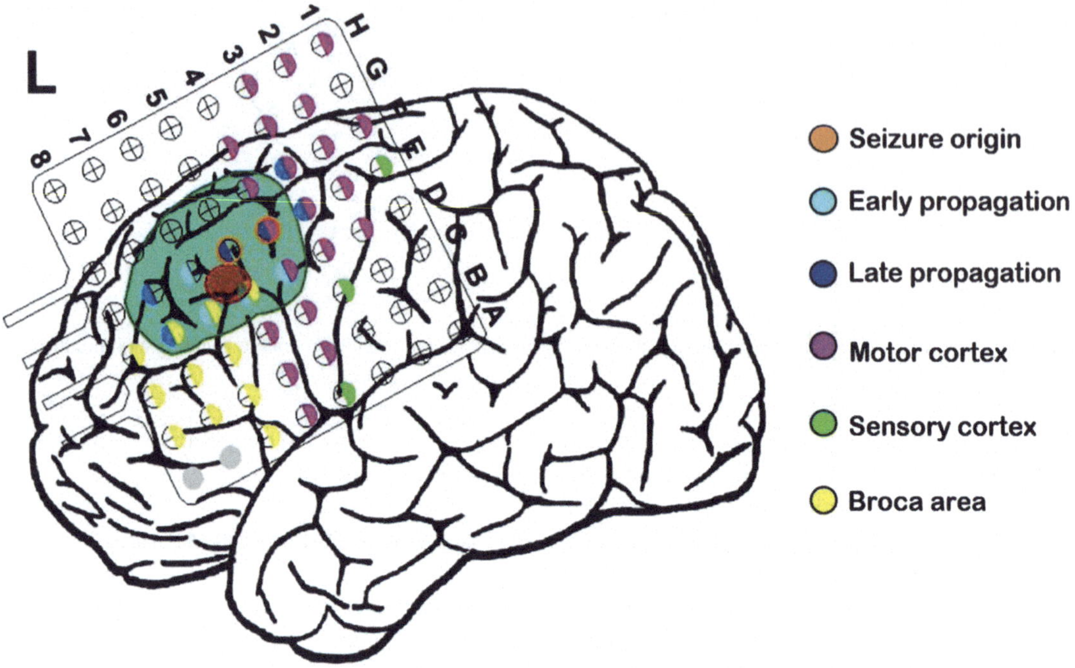


**Fig. 4.9** Patient with a left frontolateral lesion. Extraoperative recording of epileptogenic activity and mapping of language and motor areas are accomplished by placing a grid electrode over the area in question. Results of EEG recordings and mapping facilitate resection of the epileptogenic zone (green area) sparing areas of high functionality (with courtesy of C.E. Elger, Dpt. Epileptology, Bonn)

### Limitations of Intraoperative and Extraoperative Mapping

Evaluating results of intraoperative and extraoperative stimulation mapping, Hamberger et al. [106] concluded that sparing of visual naming sites as considered to be the gold standard for identifying essential language areas did not reliably prevent word-finding difficulties after temporal resections. Using auditory naming tasks, they observed a better correlation between removal of respective naming sites and postoperative naming decline. These results emphasize that the reliability of both extraoperative and intraoperative cortical stimulation for the prediction of postoperative language performance highly depends on the specific tasks used [106]. A survey of data from 56 epilepsy centers found marked variability in technical approaches, including stimulation parameters, language functions tested, definitions of errors, and size of resection margins, and most centers reported adverse language outcomes despite preserving all eloquent sites defined by the mapping procedure [95]. Reviewing 25 articles of intraoperative stimulation mapping, Rofes et al. [107] analyzed dissociations and associations between language functions to facilitate the understanding of which language functions are assessed with each task and how to best combine language tasks to tailor surgeries to individual needs.

It has to be kept in mind that blockade of language function primarily represents a stimulation phenomenon, and due to different spread of current depending on the individual tissue characteristics its correlation with the real topographical representation of language remains in question. Furthermore, a stimulation strength above the threshold value triggering afterdischarges may additionally activate more distant areas. Hermann et al. [108] concluded in their review of the results of eight centers involving more than 200 cases that neither intraoperative nor extraoperative cortical stimulation-guided surgeries are any more effective in reducing postoperative naming deficits than non-cortical stimulation-guided surgeries are. Despite these limitations, most authors are convinced of the benefits of intraoperative and extraoperative stimulation mapping [105, 109].

**Alternative Noninvasive Techniques**

During the last decade, functional magnetic resonance imaging (fMRI) as a noninvasive method has proven to be useful to delineate language areas [110–112]. Rolinski et al. [113] assessed the ability of fMRI to predict postoperative language decline (Broca's and Wernicke's area) compared to direct cortical stimulation using subdural electrodes. fMRI demonstrated 100% sensitivity and 46% specificity for outcome compared to 50% and 85%, respectively, for cortical stimulation. Thus, it has been suggested that fMRI identifying language areas via behavior-associated activation may be more sensitive but less specific than direct cortical stimulation acting by focal disruption [113]. Regions activated on fMRI were more extensive than those identified by cortical stimulation, which could lead to more conservative surgical decisions [113]. However, data available on the relative value of fMRI and cortical stimulation are limited, and differences between fMRI techniques and stimulation tasks and testing methods need to be considered when comparing results of both modalities [113]. The matter is all the more difficult because patients with epilepsy often demonstrate mixed or atypical patterns of language dominance [114].

In a study involving a small patient sample, Simos et al. [115] showed compatibility of cortical stimulation and magnetencephalography (MEG) for localizing receptive language-related cortical sites, as did Castillo et al. [116]. Similarly, a high degree of concordance between cortical stimulation and MEG localization of language-specific areas as well as between cortical stimulation, fMRI, and navigated transcranial motor stimulation (TMS) has been shown by Babajani-Feremi et al. [117]. Others demonstrated correlation of results of navigated TMS with those of cortical stimulation mapping [118, 119] as well as those of MEG [119]. Thus, a variety of noninvasive alternative techniques to intraoperative or extraoperative stimulation mapping for the definition of language areas are available [120]. Therefore, it has been suggested first to use noninvasive techniques for presurgical functional mapping of language areas, whenever they are available, and to consider invasive ones including awake surgery only if the combined results of noninvasive techniques remain ambiguous or unconvincing [120].

### 4.4.1.2 Motor and Sensory Cortex

**Intraoperative Stimulation Mapping**

Electrophysiological mapping of the motor and sensory cortex is of interest, since anatomical criteria even in combination with neuronavigation have been found to be insufficient to reliably localize these areas in every case. As with language, localization of the motor and sensory cortex by intraoperative stimulation mapping has been successfully practiced in awake surgery since more than a century [81–83, 121, 122]. Szélenyi et al. [123] provided an overview on current techniques used for intraoperative mapping of the motor cortex in awake surgery.

**Evoked Potentials**

Besides those techniques, evoked potentials are available which can be used both for extraoperative and for intraoperative localization of the central area under general anesthesia [88, 124–128]. The sensory cortex is defined by recording somatosensory evoked potentials (SEP) [88], while mapping of the motor cortex is accomplished by recording of motor evoked potentials (MEP), elicited by high-frequency (256–512 Hz) stimulation as proposed by Taniguchi et al. [129], a procedure, which has been named the train-of-five (TOF) technique.

**Phase Reversal of SEP**

In addition to the recording of SEP and MEP, phase reversal of SEP has proven to be an excellent electrophysiological tool to identify the central sulcus and thus the motor and sensory cortex during general anesthesia [130, 131] (Fig. 4.10). SEP phase reversal has been found to be successful in more than 90% of cases. However, the method may fail in patients with tumor etiol-

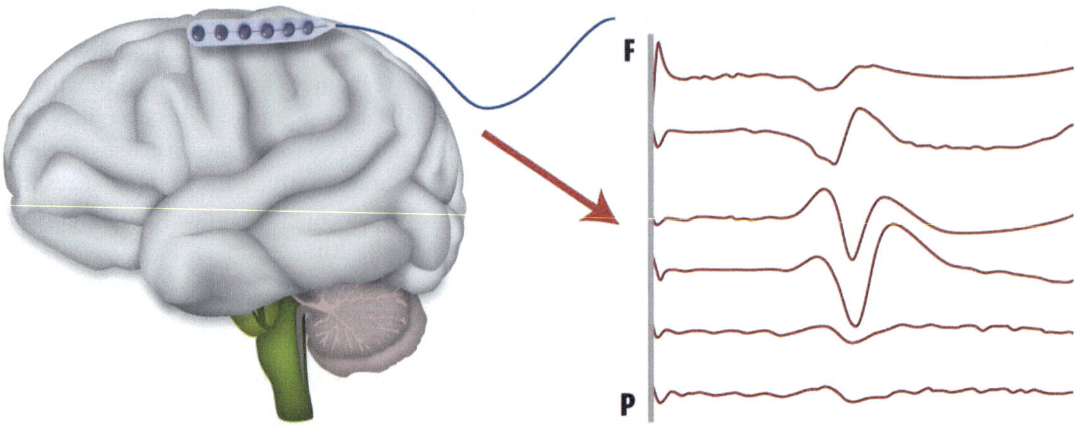


**Fig. 4.10** Phase reversal of SEP for localization of the central area. SEP are recorded using a strip electrode after contralateral median nerve stimulation at the wrist. Note phase reversal of SEP between the second and the third lines or electrode contacts corresponding to the location of the central sulcus. F: frontal; P: parietal (with courtesy of R. Ott, Arcana Forum, Emmendingen)

ogy in which the anatomical cortex structure is deranged [102, 130, 132].

Overall, electrophysiological techniques as available today allow reliable definition of the sensorimotor cortex during general anesthesia, and there is no need for awake craniotomy to define those areas. Using intraoperative or extraoperative electrical stimulation of the motor cortex, Branco et al. [133] found in a total of 43 maps from 36 patients variations in the organization of the primary motor cortex in 7 cases (19%) indicating that representation of motor areas in the homunculus may not be consistent in every case.

### Stimulation-Associated Seizures

Stimulation, particularly of the Rolandic area, may cause seizures, particularly in the presence of focal lesions [90]). Stimulation-associated seizures have been reported in 1.2% with the train-of-five (TOF) technique during general anesthesia [134]. However, no increased risk of seizures for patients with symptomatic epilepsy compared to those without has been found [134]. Goldstein et al. [135] evaluated the incidence of research stimulation-associated seizures in a large multi-institutional data set including 188 subjects across 10 institutions participating in 770 research stimulation sessions. The overall rate of stimulation-induced seizures in general anesthesia was estimated between 0.4% and 1.8% of sessions [135]. Jain et al. [136] compared intraoperative and extraoperative mapping of the motor cortex in pediatric patients. While extraoperative mapping could not be completed in 4 of 17 patients, intraoperative mapping during general anesthesia was successful in all 20 cases tested. In none of the individuals tested intraoperatively, seizures occurred, while extraoperative stimulation provoked seizures in 6 of 17 children [136]. Intraoperative seizures can easily be terminated by direct application of iced Ringer's solution onto the cortex [137].

### Alternative Noninvasive Techniques

fMRI has been shown to facilitate definition of the central area [12]. In addition, MEG responses evoked by electrical stimulation of the median nerve were found to be useful for localization of the central sulcus [138]. Säisänen et al. [139] recommended navigated TMS as a feasible tool for noninvasive preoperative localization of the motor cortex. Moreover, Tarapore et al. [119] demonstrated that the maps of the motor system generated with TMS correlate well with those generated by both MEG imaging and cortical stimulation mapping [120]. Thus, as with mapping of language areas, noninvasive alternative techniques are available to localize the central area.

#### 4.4.1.3 Pyramidal Tract

**Intermittent Mapping**

Subcortical stimulation may be necessary during resection of the epileptogenic area to localize the pyramidal tract. This can be accomplished intermittently with a hand probe [140, 141]. Using the monopolar train-of-five (TOF) technique, a motor threshold (MT)-to-distance relationship can be defined [142–146]. A meta-analysis based on 20 years of glioma surgery investigating more than 8000 cases demonstrated that the use of intraoperative mapping significantly decreased the rate of permanent neurologic deficits while increasing the extent of resection [109]. However, during tumor removal, the surgeon does not know exactly where and how critically the corticospinal tract is approached, unless the resection is stopped and the mapping probe is used to explore the resection cavity point by point.

**Continuous Dynamic Mapping**

Raabe et al. [147] provided a method allowing continuous dynamic mapping for localizing the exact site of the corticospinal tract using the mapping sucker (Fig. 4.11). By means of the monopolar train-of-five (TOF) technique, they found a safe corridor between 20 mA representing the highest stimulation intensity to start with and 5 mA at the lower range [148, 149]. The surgeon usually starts with a stimulation intensity of approximately 10–15 mA when neuronavigation indicates a distance of approximately 10–15 mm from the corticospinal tract. Approaching the corticospinal tract, MEP is triggered which can be coupled with an acoustic sound. At the MEP-positive site, the stimulus intensity is lowered in 2 mA steps and resection is continued [147]. The depth of tissue penetration is roughly proportional to the stimulation current (1 mA = 1 mm). The acoustic feedback and the ability to stimulate the tissue continuously and exactly at the site of tissue removal improve the accuracy of mapping, especially at low (<5 mA) stimulation intensities. Resection should latest be stopped, when a motor threshold of 1 mA is reached, that is, when at 1 mA MEP can be recorded [147–149]. This new technique increases the safety of surgery affecting descending motor pathways (Fig. 4.12).

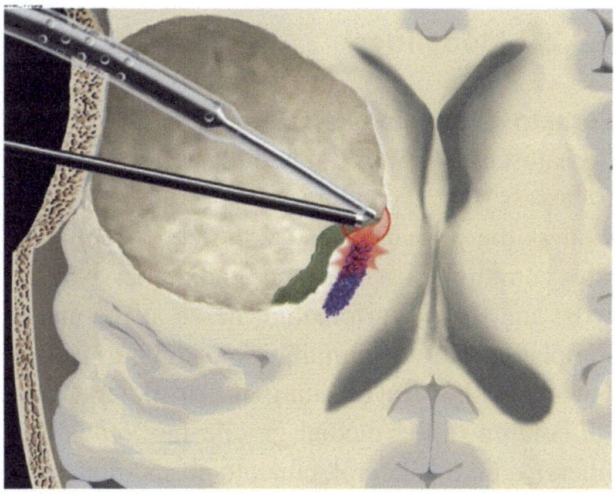

**Fig. 4.12** Schematic illustration of dynamic intraoperative mapping. After debulking of the most part of the tumor, further resection and ultrasonic aspiration of the tumor remnants (green) carry a high risk of damaging the corticospinal tract (CST = blue). The dynamic suction device is able to deliver the subcortical simulation paradigm (monopolar train-of-five pulses). The depth of tissue penetration of the stimulation current is proportional to the applied stimulation intensity (rough rule: 1 mA = 1 mm). Depending on the stimulation intensity (e.g., 8 mA), the CST is stimulated within a certain range (e.g., 8 mm as indicated by the red circle) and elicits a peripheral motor response (MEP). The motor response is indicated with a loud and clear BEEP sound serving as an alarm. The surgeon then reduces the stimulation threshold (e.g., to 5 and then 3 mA) or ceases resection. This dynamic intraoperative monitoring paradigm aims for maximum extent of resection and preservation of function (from Raabe et al. [147], with permission)

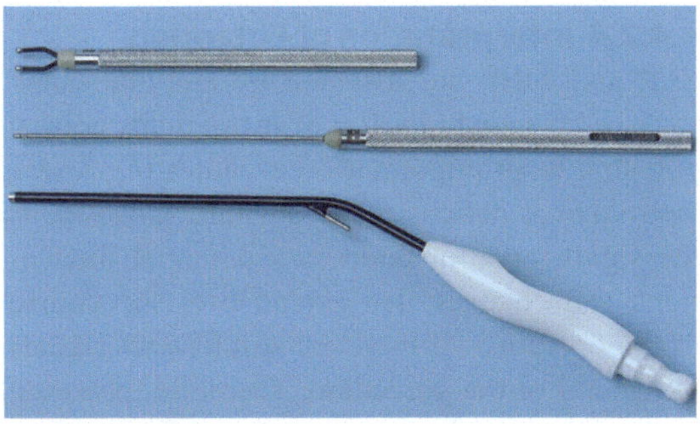

**Fig. 4.11** Devices for stimulation. Bipolar (top) and monopolar (middle) stimulation electrodes, as well as the monopolar dynamic suction device according to Raabe (below), are shown (modified from Raabe et al. [147], with permission)

### 4.4.2 Monitoring

#### 4.4.2.1 Monitoring Concept

In epilepsy surgery, intraoperative electrophysiological monitoring is accomplished by recording somatosensory and motor evoked potentials (SEP and MEP). Monitoring is based on the so-called monitoring concept [127, 128]. According to this concept, changed potentials should indicate impending neurological dysfunction, while unchanged potentials should reassure the surgeon regarding the harmlessness of the surgical steps undertaken so far. This means that monitoring can only be successful, if potential changes occur early at a reversible stage, i.e., a stage at which it is still possible to correct the surgical maneuvers in order to reverse both potential changes and associated impending functional impairment [127, 128, 150].

#### 4.4.2.2 Modalities

**Somatosensory Evoked Potentials (SEP)**

Somatosensory evoked potentials (SEP) are used to assess the ascending sensory pathways as well as the primary sensory cortex. Stimulation sites commonly used are the median nerve at the wrist and the posterior tibial nerve at the ankle. Peripheral nerve stimulation triggers action potentials that travel along the ipsilateral dorsal column to the medial gracile fasciculus (leg fibers) and the lateral cuneate fasciculus (arm fibers) and terminate in the gracile and cuneate nuclei of the medulla, respectively [151]. From there, second-order axons crossing the midline ascend the medial lemniscus to synapse in the ventral posterolateral thalamic nucleus [151]. Third-order axons ascend the posterior limb of the internal capsule and then fan out in the thalamocortical radiation to synapse in the primary sensory cortex, from where SEP are recorded by subdural strip or grid electrodes [151].

**Motor Evoked Potentials (MEP)**

Motor evoked potentials (MEP) are used to assess the primary motor cortex as well as the descending motor pathways. MEP are elicited by direct stimulation of the motor hand and/or leg area. Responses at the upper extremities are typically recorded from the pollicis brevis or the abductor digiti minimi muscles, and at the lower extremities from the anterior tibial, the gastrocnemius, or the abductor hallucis muscles. The signals travel from primary motor cortex in the corona radiata which converges at the internal capsule to a tightly bundled tract down the cerebral peduncle, pons, and medullar pyramid (hence the name "pyramidal tract") [152]. Crossing the midline at the pyramidal decussation (75–90% of fibers), corticospinal fibers descend mainly in the lateral corticospinal tract. In the anterior horn of the spinal cord, action potentials switch to second-order axons (alpha-motoneuron). From there, signals travel to the muscular end plate, excitation of which finally leads to contraction of the target muscle [152].

#### 4.4.2.3 Influence of Anesthesia

While recording of SEP is feasible with different anesthetic regimes [126, 151, 153], it has been found that single-pulse motor cortex stimulation usually does not provide sufficient muscle responses due to the depressant effects of general anesthesia on motoneuronal (alpha-motoneuron) transmission [154]. However, the train-of-five (TOF) technique allows reliable intraoperative recording of muscle responses during total intravenous anesthesia (TIVA) based on propofol and opioid infusion [129, 152, 155, 156]. Thus, TIVA is generally recommended when SEP and MEP recordings are required [151, 157].

#### 4.4.2.4 Interpretation of Potentials

SEP and MEP are assessed by amplitude and latency. Obviously, the loss of an originally normal potential is an important event indicating severe neurological deficits. Less obvious, however, is the significance of temporary potential fluctuations and changes that extend over the course of the operation, if there are still distinct signals at the end of the procedure. Therefore, potential findings have to be interpreted, and limit values must be defined which serve the surgeon as so-called warning or intervention criteria. However, although based on a lengthy experience, these criteria are arbitrarily defined. If the limits of accepted potential changes are set too narrowly, numerous false-positive results can be expected and the surgeon is unnecessarily warned. If, however, the limits are set too far, there is a danger of a false-negative correlation, which particularly is disastrous as the surgeon feels a supposed sense of safety. For clinical practice, the reduction of the amplitude by 50% and the increase of the latency by 10% of the baseline have proven to be reliable and useful criteria. With these limits, false-negative results are extremely rare, while false-positive correlations are more likely to be accepted [90, 150, 155, 158–164].

#### 4.4.2.5 Clinical Significance

##### Results

Both SEP and MEP fulfill the prerequisites of the monitoring concept. SEP monitoring has been successfully practiced for many decades [127, 128, 151, 153]. Meanwhile, also sufficient experience with supratentorial MEP monitoring exists clearly indicating the value of MEP to preserve motor function [126, 165, 166]. In a series of 182 patients, Neuloh et al. [150] found reliable MEP in 167 cases (91.8%). Significant MEP changes based on an acceptable reduction in the amplitude of maximal 50% occurred in 39% of patients, and 32% had new postoperative motor deficits. There was no false-negative correlation. Similar results have been observed by others [130, 167–169]. Weinzierl et al. [170] reported results of combined SEP and MEP monitoring. In 49 of 69 operations (71%), SEP and MEP were stable, and the patients remained neurologically intact. Critical MEP changes with stable SEP were noted in 18 cases, and in 12 of them MEP partially recovered after modification of the surgical strategy without significant clinical sequelae, while persistent potential changes beyond acceptable limits in the remaining 6 patients were followed by postoperative motor deficits in all of them [170].

Obviously, SEP cannot indicate impending motor deficits, if the sensory pathways are not involved and vice versa. Ascending sensory and descending motor pathways run in different tracts attributed to own vascular territories and thus may not be simultaneously affected by a given lesion. For monitoring of supratentorial subcortical structures, MEP have been shown to be superior to SEP reflecting functionality of the more critical motor pathways. However, both modalities provide complementary information and therefore are frequently used in combination [170]. Overall, SEP and MEP monitoring during supratentorial surgery may be helpful to maximize resection within the limits of preserved sensorimotor function. Failed monitoring is possible in very young patients due to insufficient myelinization of white matter tracts [166]. Typical monitoring cases are shown in Figs. 4.13 and 4.14.

##### Chances and Limits

SEP and MEP monitoring has proven to be a valuable tool providing the surgeon with feedback on the functional effects of surgical steps undertaken at a reversible stage, thus fulfilling requirements of the monitoring concept. In addition, monitoring has become an educational tool indicating which maneuvers may be dangerous and thus teaching to avoid them. Finally, if the surgeon is willing to include the information gained by monitoring in his/her surgical strategy, one can speak of a functionally guided surgery. However, there are also some limitations. Only circumscribed pathways can be monitored. Therefore, impending deficits can only be indicated if the respective pathways are involved in the operation field. In addition, the interpretation of the potential findings remains still unclear in certain cases. Overall, although not necessary in every patient, intraoperative electrophysiological monitoring has proven to be definitely valuable in selected patients [150].

## 4.5 Subpial Gyral Emptying

Traditionally, epileptogenic foci are treated by "en bloc" resection. During these procedures, blood vessels that traverse the resected area are coagulated and divided. Typical examples are

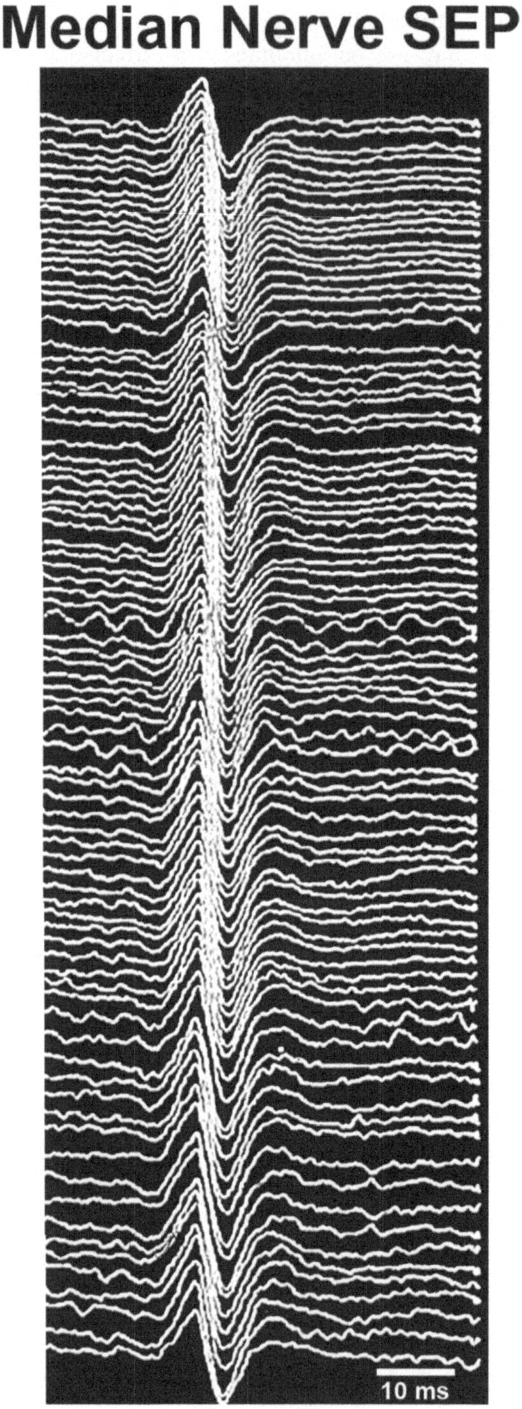


**Fig. 4.13** Intraoperative monitoring of the sensory cortex by somatosensory evoked potentials (SEP) elicited by median nerve stimulation. Stable potentials throughout the procedure indicate an uneventful postoperative sensory status

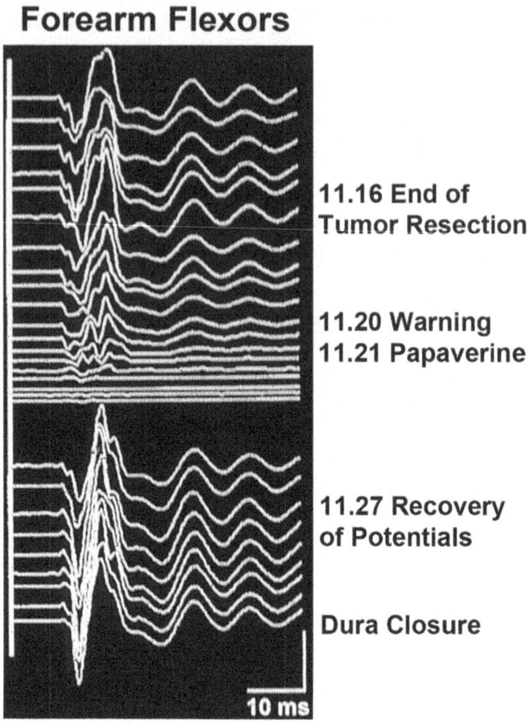


**Fig. 4.14** Intraoperative monitoring of motor pathways by motor evoked potentials (MEP) recorded from the forearm flexors during resection of an insular tumor. At the end of tumor resection, continuous reduction of the amplitudes up to loss of potentials was observed, and thus the surgeon was warned. Since no obvious cause for deterioration of potentials could be identified, the situs was irrigated with papaverine as a spasmolyitc under the hypothesis of vasospasms. In the further course, rapid recovery of potentials up to baseline values was observed. The postoperative neurological status was intact without additional deficits

frontal or temporal lobectomy. In these cases, some minor bypassing blood vessels can be divided without disadvantage, since resections roughly correspond to vascular territories without major vessels traversing the resection borders. However, with seizure foci in the fronto-parietal opercula, the central cortex, or the temporo-parieto-occipital transition area, en bloc resection may be critical causing infarctions in more distant territories. In these locations, resection strategies are required that focus on the removal of the epileptogenic tissue, leaving traversing vascular structures intact [14, 15].

### 4.5.1 Concept

Subpial gyral emptying is a fundamental technique for the resection of epileptic foci in highly vascularized areas, and a practical application of the anatomical principle of the gyral-sulcal continuum. This technique has already been applied by Horsley [171], and has later on been used for the treatment of Jacksonian epilepsies [172]. Subpial resection or subpial gyral emptying means selective removal of the epileptogenic tissue while leaving the pial and arachnoid banks between the gyri with their vascular elements that do not participate in the seizure process intact. The goal is to maintain vascular supply to areas that are not removed [14, 15]. Subpial gyral emptying can also be used in combination with en bloc resection.

### 4.5.2 Surgical Technique

The technique of subpial gyral emptying has been reviewed by Olivier et al. [14, 15]. Figure 4.15 demonstrates a typical case. The procedure includes the following steps:

- The zone of resection is identified and delineated with a thread.
- The intervascular areas at the midline of the gyri within the planned resection area are coagulated and opened with the tip of a sharp bipolar. Pial opening is enlarged with a microscissor.
- Emptying of the gyrus is best accomplished with the ultrasonic aspirator. The neighboring gyri which are connected by anatomical bridges are emptied in the same way.
- The cavities are joined together by dissecting in between, under, and around the pial and arachnoid boundaries. Thus, the bypassing blood vessels remain intact.

**Concluding Remarks**

- ***Anatomy***. *Knowledge of the anatomical concept of the gyral-sulcal continuum as well as of the architecture of white matter and the topographic anatomy of fiber tracts contributes to the understanding of seizure spread and semiology as well as to planning adequate resection strategies.*
- ***Neuronavigation***. *Fused structural and functional imaging data can be made available for the neurosurgeon by neuronavigation both for planning the approach and for setting boundaries of resection. It is advisable to address any critical target early during surgery prior to brain shift effects.*
- ***Intraoperative imaging***. *Real-time guidance of surgery by intraoperative imaging may be useful in selected cases, e.g., to delineate subtle lesions such as focal cortical dysplasias in extratemporal location. With respect to advantages and disadvantages of techniques available, ultrasound seems to be the most promising future tool. However, the place of real-time guidance of epilepsy surgical procedures has still to be defined.*
- ***Mapping***. *In principle, noninvasive techniques for presurgical mapping such as fMRI, MEG, and TMS, if available, should be applied before invasive ones are considered. Stimulation mapping to define language areas can be performed extraoperatively requiring a second procedure for resection, or intraoperatively during awake surgery. Additional language areas besides those of Broca and Wernicke, e.g., at the temporal base as observed with stimulation mapping, may represent stimulation artifacts rather than true functional zones and can be resected without disadvantage. Mapping of the central area as well as of the pyramidal tract is feasible in general anesthesia with electrophysiological techniques.*
- ***Monitoring***. *SEP and MEP have proven to be useful tools for intraoperative monitoring of the central area as well as ascending and descending pathways, and both modalities provide complementary information. Based on reduction of amplitudes of > 50% and increase in latencies of > 10% of baselines as warning or intervention criteria, SEP and MEP allow reliable prediction of the sensorimotor outcome in most cases. For supratentorial subcortical monitoring, MEP are*

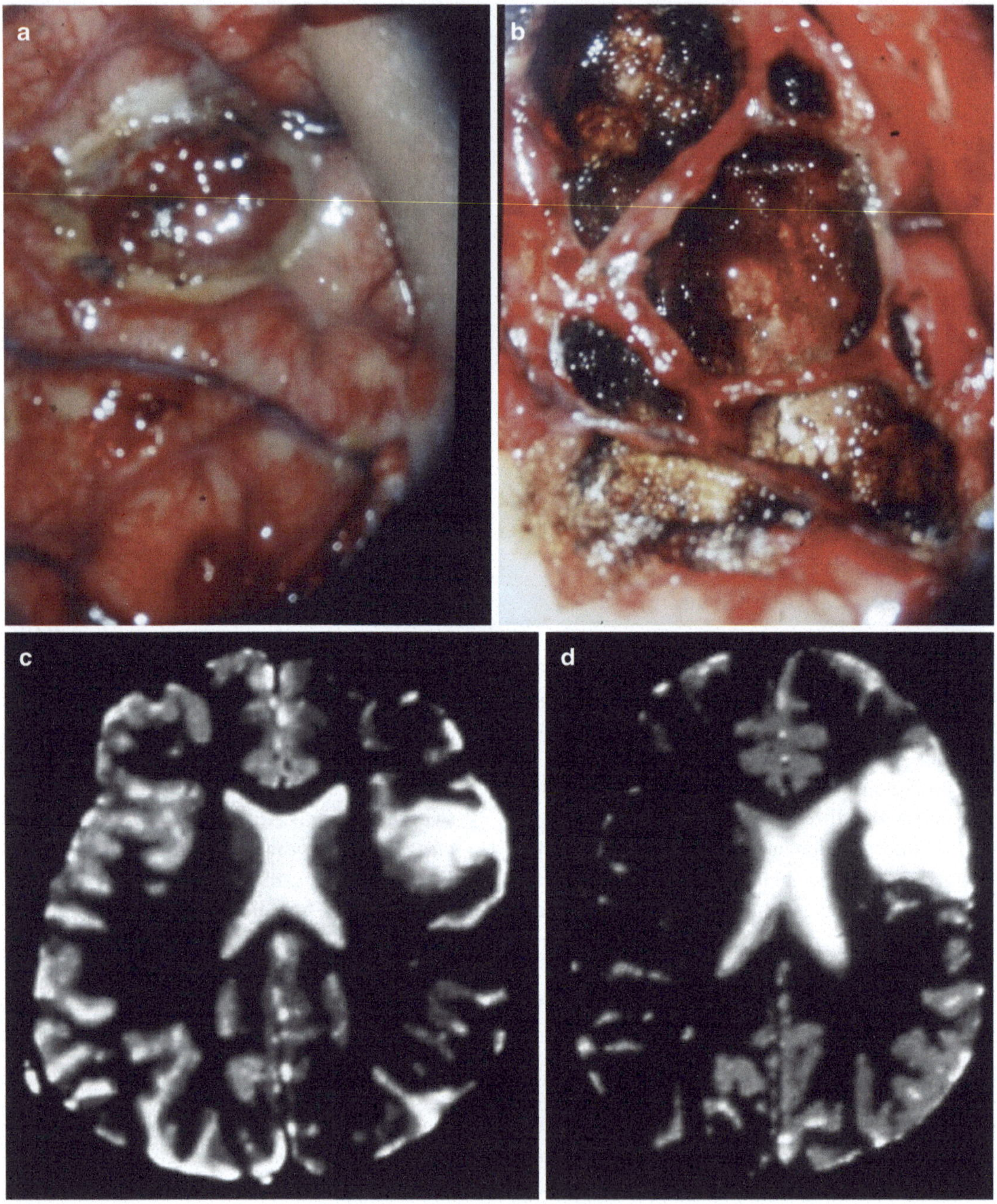


**Fig. 4.15** Technique of subpial gyral emptying (the same patient as shown in Fig. 4.9). Intraoperative view (**a**) and axial MRI (**c**) show the cystic defect and residual lesion in the left frontal operculum after the primary procedure several months ago. Reoperation with extended lesionectomy was indicated due to persistent seizures. Intraoperative view (**b**) and axial MRI (**d**) after reoperation demonstrate extended lesionectomy. Note that in (**b**) the resection cavities are joint together, while the pial and arachnoid boundaries of the gyri with their vascular structures are left intact. The postoperative course was uneventful without speech or motor deficits

*superior to SEP reflecting functionality of the more critical motor pathways.*

- ***Triggering a seizure***. *Cortical stimulation with high currents may elicit local or generalized seizure activity. Electrocorticography (ECoG) during stimulation mapping may be useful to define the afterdischarge threshold, thus keeping the current for stimulation below this level. If an epileptic seizure occurs triggered by direct cortical stimulation, it is recommended to immediately irrigate the brain with "ice water", e.g., 4 °C cold isotonic NaCl or Ringer's solution to interrupt seizure activity.*
- ***Gyral emptying***. *For gyral emptying, it is advisable to restrict the ultrasonic aspirator to half of its power and to limit the suction to a strength preserving the pial banks. Hemostasis is accomplished using hemostyptic agents such as Tabotamp (Johnson and Johnson Medical, 22,844 Norderstedt, Germany), or Surgicel (Johnson and Johnson, Brussels, Belgium), while coagulation should be avoided. Manipulation-induced vasospasms can be easily treated by application of spasmolytics such as papaverine during critical phases as well as at the end of the procedure.*

## References


1. Rhoton AL. The cerebrum. Neurosurgery. 2007;61(Suppl 1):37–119.
2. Yasargil MG. Microneurosurgery, Microsurgery anatomy of the basal cisterns and vessels of the brain, vol. I. Stuttgart, New York: Thieme; 1984.
3. Yasargil MG. Microneurosurgery. Stuttgart, New York: Thieme; 1994.
4. Seeger W. Atlas of topographical anatomy of the brain and surrounding structures. Wien: Springer; 1978.
5. Seeger W, Zentner J. Anatomical basis of cranial neurosurgery. Heidelberg: Springer; 2018.
6. Mascott RM. Image guidance and epilepsy surgery. In: Baltuch GH, Villemure J-G, editors. Operative techniques in epilepsy surgery. New York: Thieme; 2009. p. 3–19.
7. Cervos-Navarro J, Ferszt R. Klinische Neuropathologie. Stuttgart, New York: Thieme; 1989.
8. Kiernan JA. Anatomy of the temporal lobe. Epilepsy Res Treatment. 2012; https://doi.org/10.1155/2012/176157.
9. Seeger W. The microsurgical approaches to the target areas of the brain. Wien, New York: Springer; 1993.
10. Seeger W. Microanatomical aspects for neurosurgeons and neuroradiologists. Wine, New York: Springer; 2000.
11. Seeger W, Zentner J. Neuronavigation and neuroanatomy. Wien, New York: Springer; 2002.
12. Urbach H, editor. MRI in epilepsy. Berlin, Heidelberg: Springer; 2013.
13. Wen HT, Rhoton AL, et al. Microsurgical anatomy of the temporal lobe: Part 2—Sylvian fissure region and its clinical application. Neurosurgery. 2009;65(ONS Suppl. 1):ons1–ons36.
14. Olivier A, Boling WW, Tanriverdi T. Techniques in epilepsy surgery. Cambridge: University Press; 2012a. p. 41–53.
15. Olivier A, Boling WW, Tanriverdi T. Techniques in epilepsy surgery. The MNI approach. Cambridge, New York: Cambridge University Press; 2012b.
16. Broca P. Description élémentaire des circonvolutions cérébrales de l'homme. In: Reinwald C, editor. Mémoires sur le Cerveau de l'Homme et des Primates. Paris; 1888.
17. Wakana S, Jiang H, Nagae-Poetscher LM. Fiber tract-based atlas of human white matter anatomy. Radiology. 2004;230:77–87.
18. Bancaud J, Dell MB. Techniques and méthode de l'interfacing exploration fonctionnelle stéréotaxique des structures encephaliques chez l'homme (cortex, sous-cortex, noyaux gris centraux). Rev Neurol. 1959;101:213–27.
19. Talairach J, Bancaud J, Szikla G, et al. Approche nouvelle de la neurochirurgie de l'epilepsie: méthodologie stéréotaxique et résultats thérapeutiques. Neurochirurgie. 1974;20 Suppl:1–240.
20. Motti ED, Marossero F. Head-holder interfacing computed tomography with Talairach stereotactic frame. J Neurosurg Sci. 1983;27(3):219–23.
21. Olivier A, Bertrand G, Peters T. Stereotactic systems and procedures for depth electrode placement: technical aspects. Appl Neurophysiol. 1983;46(1–4):37–40.
22. Peters TM, Olivier A. C.T. aided stereotaxy for depth electrode implantation and biopsy. Can J Neurol Sci. 1983;10(3):166–9.
23. Kelly PJ, Sharbrough FW, Kall BA, et al. Magnetic resonance imaging-based computer-assisted stereotactic resection of the hippocampus and amygdala in patients with temporal lobe epilepsy. May Clin Proc. 1987;62(2):103–8.
24. Kelly PJ. State of the art and future directions of minimally invasive stereotactic neurosurgery. Cancer Control. 1995;2(4):287–92.

25. Kelly PJ. Computer-assisted stereotaxis: new approaches for the management of intracranial intra-axial tumors. Neurology. 1986;36(4):535–41.
26. Bucholz RD, McDurmont L. From discovery to design: image-guided surgery. Clin Neurosurg. 2003;50:13–25.
27. Roberts DW, Strohbehn JW, Hatch JF, et al. A frameless stereotaxic integration of computerized tomographic imaging and the operating microscope. J Neurosurg. 1986;65(4):545–9.
28. Watanabe E, Watanabe T, Manaka S, et al. Three-dimensional digitizer (neuronavigator): new equipment for computed tomography-guided stereotaxic surgery. Surg Neurol. 1987;27(6):543–7.
29. Mascott CR. Comparison of magnetic tracking and optical tracking by simultaneous use of two independent frameless stereotactic systems. Neurosurgery. 2005;57(4):295–301.
30. Mascott CR, Jean-Christophe S, Bousquet P, et al. Quantification of true in vivo (application) accuracy in cranial image-guided surgery: influence of mode of patient registration. Neurosurgery. 2006;59(1):146–56.
31. Olivier A, Alonso-Vanegas M, Comeau R, Peters TM. Image-guided surgery of epilepsy. Neurosurg Clin N Am. 1996;7:229–43.
32. Olivier A, Germano IM, Cukiert A, et al. Frameless stereotaxy for surgery of the epilepsies: perliminary experience. Technical note. J Neurosurg. 1994;81 (4):629–33.
33. Mascott CR, et al. Frameless stereotactic placement of depth electrodes for investigation of epilepsy. Meeting of the American Association of Neurological Surgeons, 1995.
34. Gumprecht HK, Widenka DC, Lumanta CB. BrainLab VectorVision neuronavigation system: technology and clinical experiences in 131 cases. Neurosurgery. 1999;44(1):97–104.
35. Hogan RE, Lowe VJ, Bucholz RD. Triple-technique (MR imaging, single-photon-emission CT, and CT) coregistration for image-guided surgical evaluation of patients with intractable epilepsy. AJNR Am J Neuroradiol. 1999;20(6):1054–8.
36. Mascott CR. In vivo accuracy of image guidance performed using optical tracking and optimized registration. J Neurosurg. 2006;105(4):561–7.
37. Raabe A, Krishnan R, Wolff R, et al. Laser surface scanning for patient registration in intracranial image-guided surgery. Neurosurgery. 2002;50:797–801.
38. Kato A, Yoshimine T, Hayakawa T, et al. A frameless, armless navigational system for computer-assisted neurosurgery. J Neurosurg. 1991;74:845–9.
39. Comeau RM, Sadikot AF, Fenster A, et al. Intraoperative ultrasound for guidance and tissue shift correction in image-guided neurosurgery. Med Phys. 2000;27:787–800.
40. Miller D, Knake S, Bauer S, Krakow K, Pagenstecher A, Sure U, et al. Intraoperative ultrasound to define focal cortical dysplasia in epilepsy surgery. Epilepsia. 2008;49:156–8.
41. Nimsky C, Ganslandt O, Fahlbusch R. 1.5 T: intraoperative imaging beyond standard anatomic imaging. Neurosurg Clin N Am. 2005;16(1):185–200.
42. Wirtz CR, Tronnier VM, Bonsanto MM, et al. Image-guided neurosurgery with intraoperative MRI: update of frameless stereotaxy and radicality control. Stereotact Funct Neurosurg. 1997;68:39–43.
43. Mehta AD, Labar D, Dean A, et al. Frameless stereotactic placement of depth electrodes in epilepsy surgery. J Neurosurg. 2005;192(6):1040–5.
44. Murphy MA, O'Brien TJ, Cook MJ. Insertion of depth electrodes with or without subdural grids using frameless stereotactic guidance systems—technique and outcome. Br J Neurosurg. 2002;16(2):119–25.
45. Oertel J, Gaab MR, Runge U, et al. Neuronavigation and complication rate in epilepsy surgery. Neurosurg Rev. 2004;27:214–7.
46. Duffner F, Freudenstein D, Schiffbauer H, et al. Combining MEG and MRI with neuronavigation for treatment of an epileptiform spike focus in the precentral region: a technical case report. Surg Neurol. 2003;59(1):40–6.
47. Gaillard WD, Bhatia S, Bookheimer SY, et al. FDG-PET and volumetric MRI in the evaluation of patients with partial epilepsy. Neurology. 1995;45(1):123–6.
48. Levesque MF, Zhang JX, Wilson CL, et al. Stereotactic investigation of limbic epilepsy using a multimodal image analysis system. Technical note. J Neurosurg. 1990;73(5):792–7.
49. Murphy MA, O'Brien TJ, Morris K, et al. Multimodality image-guided surgery for the treatment of medically refractory epilepsy. J Neurosurg. 2004;100(3):452–62.
50. Krsek P, Maton B, Jayakar P, et al. Incomplete resection of focal cortical dysplasia is the main predictor of poor postsurgical outcome. Neurology. 2009;72:217–23.
51. Rowland NC, Englot DJ, Cage TA, et al. A meta-analysis of predictors of seizure freedom in the surgical management of focal cortical dysplasia. J Neurosurg. 2012;116:1035–41.
52. Tripathi M, Singh MS, Padma MV, et al. Surgical outcome of cortical dysplasias presenting with chronic intractable epilepsy: a 10-year experience. Neurol India. 2008;56:138–43.
53. Wagner J, Urbach H, Niehusmann P, et al. Focal cortical dysplasia type IIb: completeness of cortical, not subcortical, resection is necessary for seizure freedom. Epilepsia. 2011;52:1418–24.
54. Sommer B, Grummich P, Coras R, et al. Integration of functional neuronavigation and intraoperative MRI in surgery for drug-resistant extratemporal epilepsy close to eloquent brain areas. Neurosurg Focus. 2013;34:E4.
55. Wurm G, Ringler H, Knogler F, Schnizer M. Evaluation of neuronavigation in lesional and non-lesional epilepsy surgery. Comput Aided Surg. 2003;8:204–14.
56. Fahlbusch R, Golby A, Prada F, et al. Introduction: utility of intraoperative imaging. J Neurosurg. 2016; https://doi.org/10.3171/2016.1.FOCUS1610.

57. Kurwale NS, Chandra SP, Chouksey P, et al. Impact of intraoperative MRI on outcomes in epilepsy surgery: preliminary experience of two years. Br J Neurosurg. 2015;29(3):380–5.
58. Sacino MF, Ho C-Y, Murnick J, et al. The role of intraoperative MRI in resective epilepsy surgery for peri-eloquent cortex cortical dysplasias and heterotopias in pediatric patients. Neurosurg Focus. 2016; 40(3):E16.
59. Buchfelder M, Ganslandt O, Fahlbusch R, Nimsky C. Intraoperative magnetic resonance imaging in epilepsy surgery. J Magn Reson Imaging. 2000;12(4):547–55.
60. Roessler K, Kasper BS, Heynold E, et al. Intraoperative MR imaging and neuronavigation during resection of FCD Type II in adult epilepsy surgery offers better seizure outcome. World Neurosurgery. 2017; https://doi.org/10.1016/j.wneu.2017.09.100.
61. Sacino MF, Ho C-Y, Murnick J, et al. Intraoperative MRI-guided resection of focal cortical dysplasia in pediatric patients: technique and outcomes. J Neurosurg Pediatr. 2016;17:672–8.
62. Mattei L, Prada F, Legnani FG, Perin A, Olivi A, DiMeco F, et al. Neurosurgical tools to extend tumor resection in hemispheric low-grade gliomas: conventional and contrast enhanced ultrasonography. Childs Nerv Syst. 2016;32(10):1907–14.
63. Prada F, Del Bene M, Casali C, Saladino A, Legnani FG, Perin A, et al. Intraoperative navigated angiosonography for skull base tumor surgery. World Neurosurg. 2015;84(6):1699–707.
64. Prada F, Vitale V, Del Bene M, Boffano C, Sconfienza LM, Pinzi V, Contrast-enhanced MR, et al. Imaging versus contrast-enhanced US: a comparison in glioblastoma surgery by using intraoperative fusion imaging. Radiology. 2017;285:242–9.
65. Chan HW, Pressler R, Uff C, Gunny R, St Piers K, Cross H, et al. A novel technique of detecting MRI-negative lesion in focal symptomatic epilepsy: intraoperative shear wave elastography. Epilepsia. 2014;55:30–3.
66. Lee C, Lin C, Yu H, Hung S, Shih Y, Hsu SPC. Applications of intraoperative ultrasound in epilepsy surgery for focal cortical dysplasia. J Med Ultrasound. 2014;22:43–6.
67. Miller D, Knake S, Menzler K, Krakow K, Rosenow F, Sure U. Intraoperative ultrasound in malformations of cortical development. Ultraschall Med. 2011;32(2):E69–74.
68. Tringali G, Bono B, Dones I, Cordella R, Didato G, Villani F, et al. Multimodal approach for radical excision of focal cortical dysplasia by combining advanced magnetic resonance imaging data to intraoperative ultrasound, electrocorticography, and cortical stimulation: a preliminary experience. World Neurosurg. 2018;113:e738–46.
69. Ng A, Swanevelder J. Resolution in ultrasound imaging. Contin Educ Anaesth Crit Care Pain. 2011;11:186–92.
70. Prada F, Gennari AG, Del Bene M, et al. Intraoperative ultrasonography (ioUS) characteristics of focal cortical dysplasia (FCD) type II b. Eur J Epilepsy. 2019;69:80–6.
71. Sidhu PS, Cantisani V, Dietrich CF, Gilja OH, Saftoiu A, Bartels E, et al. The EFSUMB guidelines and recommendations for the clinical practice of contrast-enhanced ultrasound (CEUS) in non-hepatic applications: update 2017 (short version). Ultraschall Med. 2018; https://doi.org/10.1055/s-0044-10125.
72. Braun V, Dempf S, Tomczak R, Wunderlich A, Weller R, Richter HP. Multimodal cranial neuronavigation: direct integration of functional magnetic resonance imaging and positron emission tomography data: technical note. Neurosurgery. 2001;48:1178–82.
73. Fandino J, Kollias SS, Wieser HG, Valavanis A, Yonekawa Y. Intraoperative validation of functional magnetic resonance imaging and cortical reorganization patterns in patients with brain tumors involving the primary motor cortex. J Neurosurg. 1999;91:238–50.
74. Krings T, Schreckenberger M, Rohde V, Foltys H, Spetzger U, Sabri O, Reinges MH, Kemeny S, Meyer PT, Moller-Hartmann W, Korinth M, Gilsbach JM, Buell U, Thron A. Metabolic and electrophysiological validation of functional MRI. J Neurol Neurosurg Psychiatry. 2001;71:762–71.
75. Lehericy S, Duffau H, Cornu P, Capelle L, Pidoux B, Carpentier A, Auliac S, Clemenceau S, Sichez JP, Bitar A, Valery CA, Van Effenterre R, Faillot T, Srour A, Fohanno D, Philippon J, Le Bihan D, Marsault C. Correspondence between functional magnetic resonance imaging somatotopy and individual brain anatomy of the central region: Comparison with intraoperative stimulation in patients with brain tumors. J Neurosurg. 2000;92:589–98.
76. Roberts TP, Ferrari P, Perry D, Rowley HA, Berger MS. Presurgical mapping with magnetic source imaging: comparisons with intraoperative findings. Brain Tumor Pathol. 2000;17:57–64.
77. Roux FE, Boulanouar K, Ibarrola D, Tremoulet M, Chollet F, Berry I. Functional MRI and intraoperative brain mapping to evaluate brain plasticity in patients with brain tumours and hemiparesis. J Neurol Neurosurg Psychiatry. 2000;69:453–63.
78. Roux FE, Boulanouar K, Ranjeva JP, Tremoulet M, Henry P, Manelfe C, Sabatier J, Berry I. Usefulness of motor functional MRI correlated to cortical mapping in Rolandic low-grade astrocytomas. Acta Neurochir. 1999;141:71–9.
79. Stapleton SR, Kiriakopoulos E, Mikulis D, Drake JM, Hoffman HJ, Humphreys R, Hwang P, Otsubo H, Holowka S, Logan W, Rutka JT. Combined utility of functional MRI, cortical mapping, and frameless stereotaxy in the resection of lesions in eloquent areas of brain in children. Pediatr Neurosurg. 1997;26:68–82.
80. Vinas FC, Zamorano L, Mueller RA, Jiang Z, Chugani H, Fuerst D, Muzik O, Mangner TJ. Diaz FG: [15O]-water PET and intraoperative brain map-

ping: a comparison in the localization of eloquent cortex. Neurol Res. 1997;19:601–8.
81. Foerster O. Zur Pathogenese und chirurgischen Behandlung der Epilepsie. Zentralbl Chir. 1925;52:531–49.
82. Penfield W, Boldrey E. Somatic motor and sensory representation in the cerebral cortex of man as studied by electric stimulation. Brain. 1937a;60:389–443.
83. Penfield W, Boldrey E. Somatic motor and sensory representation in the cerebral cortex of man as studied by electrical stimulation. Brain. 1937b;60:389–443.
84. Berger MS, Kincaid J, Ojemann GA, Lettich E. Brain mapping techniques to maximize resection, safety, and seizure control in children with brain tumors. Neurosurgery. 1989;25:786–92.
85. Berger MS. Minimalism through intraoperative functional mapping. Clin Neurosurg. 1996;43:324–37.
86. Ebeling U, Huber P. Localization of central lesions by correlation of CT findings and neurological deficits. Acta Neurochir. 1992;119:17–22. 14
87. Ojemann G, Ojemann J, Lettich E, Berger M. Cortical language localization in left, dominant hemisphere: an electrical stimulation mapping investigation in 117 patients. J Neurosurg. 1989;71:316–26.
88. Silbergeld DL. Cortical mapping. In: Lüders H, Comair YG, editors. Epilepsy surgery. Philadelphia: Lippincott William and Wilkins; 2001. p. 633–5.
89. Yingling CD, Ojemann S, Dodson B, Harrington MJ, Berger MS. Identification of motor pathways during tumor surgery facilitated by multichannel electromyographic recording. J Neurosurg. 1999;91:922–7.
90. Szelényi A, Hattingen E, Weidauer S, Seifert V, Ziemann U. Intraoperative motor evoked potential alteration in intracranial tumor surgery and its relation to signal alteration in postoperative magnetic resonance imaging. Neurosurgery. 2010;67:302–13.
91. Ojemann G, Dodrill CB. Verbal memory deficits after left temporal lobectomy for epilepsy. Mechanism and intraoperative prediction. J Neurosurg. 1985;62(1):101–7.
92. Lüders H, Lesser RP, Hahn J, et al. Basal temporal language area. Brain. 1991;114:743–54.
93. Ojemann GA. Cortical organization of language. J Neurosci. 1991;11(8):2281–7.
94. Schaffler L, Luders HO, Morris HH 3rd, et al. Anatomic distribution of cortical language sites in the basal temporal language area in patients with left temporal lobe epilepsy. Epilepsia. 1994;35:525–8.
95. Hamberger MJ, Williams AC, Schevon CA. Extraoperative neurostimulation mapping: results from an international survey of epilepsy surgery programs. Epilepsia. 2014;55:933–9.
96. Sanai N, Mirzadeh Z, Berger MS. Functional outcome after language mapping for glioma resection. N Engl J Med. 2008;358(1):18–27.
97. Behrens E, Zentner J, van Roost D, et al. Subdural and depth electrodes in the presurgical evaluation of epilepsy. Acta Neurochir. 1994;128:84–7.
98. Silbergeld DL. A new device for cortical stimulation mapping of surgically unexposed cortex: technical mote. J Neurosurg. 1993;79:612–4.
99. Wellmer J, von der Groeben F, Klarmann U, et al. Risks and benefits of invasive epilepsy surgery workup with implanted subdural and depth electrodes. Epilepsia. 2012;53:1322–32.
100. Wyler AR, Walker G, Somes G. The morbidity of long-term seizure monitoring using subdural strip electrodes. J Neurosurg. 1991;74:734–7.
101. Hedegard E, Bjellvi J, Edelvik A, et al. Complications to invasive epilepsy surgery workup with subdural and depth electrodes: a prospective population-based observational study. J Neurol Neurosurg Psychiatry. 2014;85:716–20.
102. Romstock J, Fahlbusch R, Ganslandt O, Nimsky C, Strauss C. Localisation of the sensorimotor cortex during surgery for brain tumours: feasibility and waveform patterns of somatosensory evoked potentials. J Neurol Neurosurg Psychiatry. 2002;72:221–9.
103. Cervenka MC, Boatman-Reich DF, Ward J, Franaszczuk PJ, Crone NE. Language mapping in multilingual patients: electrocorticography and cortical stimulation during naming. Front Hum Neurosci. 2011;5:13.
104. Cervenka MC, Corines J, Boatman-Reich DF, Eloyan A, Sheng X, Franaszczuk PJ, et al. Electrocorticographic functional mapping identifies human cortex critical for auditory and visual naming. NeuroImage. 2013;69:267–76.
105. Duffeau H. Brain mapping in tumors: intraoperative or extraoperative? Epilepsia. 2013;54(Suppl. 9):79–83.
106. Hamberger MJ, Seidel WT, McKhann GM 2nd, Perrine K, Goodman RR. Brain stimulation reveals critical auditory naming cortex. Brain. 2005;128(Pt 11):2742–9.
107. Rofes A, Mandonnet E, de Aguiar V, et al. Language processing from the perspective of electrical stimulation mapping. Cogn Neuropsychol. 2018; https://doi.org/10.1080/02643294.2018.1485636.
108. Hermann B, Davies K, Foley K, Bell B. Visual confrontation naming outcome after standard left anterior temporal lobectomy with sparing versus resection of the superior temporal gyrus: a randomized prospective clinical trial. Epilepsia. 1999;40(8):1070–6.
109. De Witt Hamer PC, Gil Robles S, Zwinderman A, Duffau H, Berger MS. Impact of intraoperative stimulation brain mapping on glioma surgery outcome: a meta-analysis. J Clin Oncol. 2012;30:2559–65.
110. Binder JR, Sabsevitz DS, Swanson SJ, Hammeke TA, Raghavan M, Mueller WM. Use of preoperative functional MRI to predict verbal memory decline after temporal lobe epilepsy surgery. Epilepsia. 2008;49(8):1377–94.
111. Bonelli SB, Powell RH, Yogarajah M, Samson RS, Symms MR, Thompson PJ, et al. Imaging memory in temporal lobe epilepsy: predicting the effects

of temporal lobe resection. Brain. 2010;133(Pt 4):1186–99.
112. Sabsevitz DS, Swanson SJ, Hammeke TA, Spanaki MV, Possing ET, Morris GL 3rd, et al. Use of preoperative functional neuroimaging to predict language deficits from epilepsy surgery. Neurology. 2003;60(11):1788–92.
113. Rolinski R, Austermuehle A, Wiggs E, et al. Functional MRI and direct cortical stimulation: Prediction of postoperative language decline. Epilepsia. 2019; https://doi.org/10.1111/epi.14666.
114. Berl MM, Zimmaro LA, Khan OI, et al. Characterization of atypical language activation patterns in focal epilepsy. Ann Neurol. 2014;75:33–42.
115. Simos PG, Breier JI, Maggio WW, Gormley WB, Zouridakis G, Willmore LJ, et al. Atypical temporal lobe language representation: MEG and intraoperative stimulation mapping correlation. Neuroreport. 1999;10(1):139–42.
116. Castillo EM, Breier JI, Wheless JW, Slater JD, Tandon N, Baumgartner JE, et al. Contributions of direct cortical stimulation and MEG recordings to identify "essential" language cortex. Epilepsia. 2005;46(S8):324. Abstract
117. Babajani-Feremi A, Narayana S, Rezaie R, Choudhri AF, Fulton SP, Boop FA, Wheless JW, Papanicolaou AC. Language mapping using high gamma electrocorticography, fMRI, and TMS versus electrocortical stimulation. Clin Neurophysiol. 2016;127(3):1822–36.
118. Picht T, Krieg SM, Sollmann N, Rosler J, Niraula B, Neuvonen T, et al. A comparison of language mapping by preoperative navigated transcranial magnetic stimulation and direct cortical stimulation during awake surgery. Neurosurgery. 2013;72(5):808–19.
119. Tarapore PE, Tate MC, Findlay AM, Honma SM, Mizuiri D, Berger MS, et al. Preoperative multimodal motor mapping: a comparison of magnetoencephalography imaging, navigated transcranial magnetic stimulation, and direct cortical stimulation. J Neurosurg. 2012;117(2):354–62.
120. Papanicolaou AC, Rezaie R, Narayana S, Choudhri AF, Babajani-Feremi A, Boop FA, Wehless JW. On the relative merits of invasive and non-invasive presurgical brain mapping: New tools in ablative epilepsy surgery. Epilepsy Res. 2018;142:153–5.
121. Cushing H. A note upon the faradic stimulation of the postcentral gyrus in conscious patients. Brain. 1909;32:44–53.
122. Penfield W, Jasper H. Epilepsy and the functional anatomy of the human brain. Boston: Little, Brown; 1954.
123. Szélenyi A, Bello L, Duffeau H, et al. Intraoperative electrical stimulation in awake craniotomy: methodological aspects of current practice. Neurosurg Focus. 2010;28(2):E7.
124. Deletis V, Shils J, editors. Neurophysiology in neurosurgery. A modern intraoperative approach. Amsterdam, London, New York: Academic Press, Elsevier; 2002.
125. MøllerAR. Intraoperative neurophysiological monitoring. New York, Heidelberg, London: Springer; 2011.
126. Nuwer M. Intraoperative monitoring of neuronal function. Amsterdam, Boston, Heidelberg, London, New York: Elsevier; 2008.
127. Schramm J, Moller AR. Intraoperative neurophysiological monitoring in neurosurgery. Berlin, Heidelberg, New York: Springer; 1991a.
128. Schramm J, Moller AR. Intraoperative neurophysiologic monitoring in neurosurgery. Berlin, New York: Srpinger; 1991b.
129. Taniguchi M, Cedzich C, Schramm J. Modification of cortical stimulation for motor evoked potentials under general anesthesia: technical description. Neurosurgery. 1993;32:219–26.
130. Cedzich C, Taniguchi M, Schafer S, Schramm J. Somatosensory evoked potential phase reversal and direct motor cortex stimulation during surgery in and around the central region. Neurosurgery. 1996;38:962–70.
131. Woolsey CN, Erickson TC, Gilson WE. Localization in somatic sensory and motor areas of human cerebral cortex as determined by direct recording of evoked potentials and electrical stimulation. J Neurosurg. 1979;51:476–506.
132. Salanova V, Morris HH 3rd., Van Ness PC, et al. Comparison of scalp electroencephalogram with subdural electrocorticogram recordings and functional mapping in frontal lobe epilepsy. Arch Neurol. 1993;50:294–9.
133. Branco DM, Coelho T, Branco BM, et al. Functional variability of the human cortical motor map: Electrical stimulation findings in perirolandic epilepsy surgery. J Clin Neurophysiol. 2003;20(1):17–25.
134. Szelényi A, Joksimovic B, Seifert V. Intraoperative risk of seizures associated with transient direct cortical stimulation in patients with symptomatic epilepsy. J Clin Neurophysiol. 2007;24(1):39–43.
135. Goldstein HE, Smith EH, Gross RE, et al. Risk of seizures induced by intracranial research stimulation: analysis of 770 stimulation sessions. J Neural Eng. 2019; https://doi.org/10.1088/1741-2552/ab4365.
136. Jain P, Whitney R, Strantzas S, et al. Intra-operative cortical motor mapping using subdural grid electrodes in children undergoing epilepsy surgery evaluation and comparison with the conventional extra-operative motor mapping. Clin Neurophysiol. 2018;129:2642–9.
137. Sartorius CJ, Berger MS. Rapid termination of intraoperative stimulation-evoked seizures with application of cold Ringer's lactate to the cortex. Technical note. J Neurosurg. 1998;88:349–51.
138. Ossenblok P, Leijten FS, de Munck JC, et al. Magnetic source imaging contributes to the presurgical identification of sensorimotor cortex in patients with frontal lobe epilepsy. Clin Neurophysiol. 2003;114:221–32.

139. Säisänen L, Könönen M, Julkunen P, et al. Noninvasive preoperative localization of primary motor cortex in epilepsy surgery by navigated transcranial magnetic stimulation. Epilepsy Res. 2010;92:134–43.
140. Berger MS, Hadjipanayis CG. Surgery of intrinsic cerebral tumors. Neurosurgery. 2007;61(Suppl 1):279–305.
141. Duffau H, Capelle L, Denvil D, Sichez N, Gatignol P, Tail-landier L, et al. Usefulness of intraoperative electrical subcortical mapping during surgery for low-grade gliomas located within eloquent brain regions: functional results in a consecutive series of 103 patients. J Neurosurg. 2003;98:764–78.
142. Kamada K, Todo T, Ota T, Ino K, Masutani Y, Aoki S, et al. The motor-evoked potential threshold evaluated by tractography and electrical stimulation. Clinical article. J Neurosurg. 2009;111:785–95.
143. Kombos T, Süss O, Vajkoczy P. Subcortical mapping and monitoring during insular tumor surgery. Neurosurg Focus. 2009;27(4):E5.
144. Nossek E, Korn A, Shahar T, Kanner AA, Yaffe H, Marcovici D, et al. Intraoperative mapping and monitoring of the corticospinal tracts with neurophysiological assessment and 3-dimensional ultrasonography-based navigation. Clinical article. J Neurosurg. 2011;114:738–46.
145. Ohue S, Kohno S, Inoue A, Yamashita D, Harada H, Kumon Y, et al. Accuracy of diffusion tensor magnetic resonance imaging-based tractography for surgery of gliomas near the pyramidal tract: a significant correlation between subcortical electrical stimulation and postoperative tractography. Neurosurgery. 2012;70:283–94.
146. Prabhu SS, Gasco J, Tummala S, Weinberg JS, Rao G. Intra-operative magnetic resonance imaging-guided tractography with integrated monopolar subcortical functional mapping for resection of brain tumors. Clinical article. J Neurosurg. 2011;114:719–26.
147. Raabe A, Beck J, Schucht P, Seidel K. Continuous dynamic mapping of the corticospinal tract during surgery of motor eloquent brain tumors: evaluation of a new method. J Neurosurg. 2014;120:1015–24.
148. Seidel K, Beck J, Stieglitz L, Schucht P, Raabe A. The warning-sign hierarchy between quantitative subcortical motor mapping and continuous motor evoked potential monitoring during resection of supratentorial brain tumors. Clinical article. J Neurosurg. 2013a;118:287–96.
149. Seidel K, Beck J, Stieglitz L, Schucht P, Raabe A. The warning-sign hierarchy between quantitative subcortical motor mapping and continuous motor evoked potential monitoring during resection of supratentorial brain tumors. J Neurosurg. 2013b;118:287–96.
150. Neuloh G, Schramm J. Intraoperative neurophysiological mapping and monitoring for supratentorial procedures. In: Deletis V, Shils JL, editors. Neurophysiology in neurosurgery. Amsterdam, Boston, London: Academic Press; 2002. p. 339–401.
151. MacDonald DB, Dong C, Qatrale R, et al. Recommendations of the International Society of Intraoperative Neurophysiology for intraoperative somatosensory evoked potentials. Clin Neurophysiol. 2019;130(1):161–79.
152. MacDonald DB, Skinner S, Shils J, et al. Intraoperative motor evoked potential monitoring—a position statement by the American Society of Neurophysiological Monitoring. Clin Neurophysiol. 2013;124(12):2291–316.
153. Nuwer M. Evoked potential monitoring in the operating Room. New York: Raven Press; 1986.
154. Zentner J, Kiss I, Ebner A. Influence of anesthetics—nitrous oxide in particular—on electromyographic response evoked by transcranial electrical stimulation of the cortex. Neurosurgery. 1989;24:253–6.
155. Pechstein U, Cedzich C, Nadstawek J, Schramm J. Transcranial high-frequency repetitive electrical stimulation for recording myogenic motor evoked potentials with the patient under general anesthesia. Neurosurgery. 1996;39:335–43. discussion 343–344
156. Taylor BA, Fennelly ME, Taylor A, Farrell J. Temporal summation: the key to motor evoked potential spinal cord monitoring in humans. J Neurol Neurosurg Psychiatry. 1993;56:104–6.
157. Scheufler KM, Zentner J. Total intravenous anesthesia for intraoperative monitoring of the motor pathways: an integral view combining clinical and experimental data. J Neurosurg. 2002;96:571–9.
158. Calancie B, Harris W, Brindle GF, Green BA, Landy HJ. Threshold-level repetitive transcranial electrical stimulation for intraoperative monitoring of central motor conduction. J Neurosurg. 2001;95:161–8.
159. de Haan P, Kalkman CJ. Spinal cord monitoring: somatosensory- and motor-evoked potentials. Anesthesiol Clin N Am. 2001;19:923–45.
160. Deletis V. Intraoperative monitoring of the functional integrity of the motor pathways. Adv Neurol. 1993;63:201–14.
161. Jacobs MJ, Meylaerts SA, de Haan P, de Mol BA, Kalkman CJ. Assessment of spinal cord ischemia by means of evoked potential monitoring during thoracoabdominal aortic surgery. Semin Vasc Surg. 2000;13:299–307.
162. Jones SJ, Harrison R, Koh KF, Mendoza N, Crockard HA. Motor evoked potential monitoring during spinal surgery: responses of distal limb muscles to transcranial cortical stimulation with pulse trains. Electroencephalogr Clin Neurophysiol. 1996;100:375–83.
163. Kothbauer K, Deletis V, Epstein FJ. Intraoperative spinal cord monitoring for intramedullary surgery: an essential adjunct. Pediatr Neurosurg. 1997;26:247–54.
164. Nuwer MR. Measuring outcomes for neurophysiological intraoperative monitoring. Clin Neurophysiol. 2015;127(1):3–4.

165. Mendiratta A, Emerson RG. Transcranial electrical MEP with muscle recording. In: Nuwer MR, editor. Intraoperative monitoring of neural function. Boston, Heidelberg, New York: Elsevier; 2008. p. 260–71.
166. Neuloh G, Pechstein U, Cedzich C, Schramm J. Motor evoked potential monitoring with supratentorial surgery. Neurosurgery. 2004;54:1061–72.
167. Kombos T, Suess O, Ciklatekerlio O, Brock M. Monitoring of intraoperative motor evoked potentials to increase the safety of surgery in and around the motor cortex. J Neurosurg. 2001;95:608–14.
168. Kothbauer KF, Deletis V, Epstein FJ. Intraoperative monitoring. Pediatr Neurosurg. 1998;29:54–5.
169. Zhou HH, Kelly PJ. Transcranial electrical motor evoked potential monitoring for brain tumor resection. Neurosurgery. 2001;48:1075–81.
170. Weinzierl MR, Reinacher P, Gilsbach M, et al. Combined motor and somatosensory evoked potentials for intraoperative monitoring: intra- and postoperative data in a series of 69 operations. Neurosurg Rev. 2007;30:109–16.
171. Horsley V. Brain-surgery. Br Med J. 1886;2:670–5.
172. Sachs E. The subpial resection of the cortex in the treatment of Jacksonian epilepsy (Horsley operation) with observations on areas 4 and 6. Brain. 1935;58:492–503.

# Anesthesia

# 5

*Life is pain and the enjoyment of love is an anesthetic*

*Cesare Pavese*

## Contents



Epilepsy surgery poses several considerable challenges to the anesthesiologist: (1) anticonvulsant therapy can adversely affect various organ systems, (2) effective intraoperative electrocorticography (ECoG) and electrophysiological mapping and monitoring require appropriate choice of anesthetics, and (3) extensive procedures like multilobectomy or hemispherectomy can be associated with homeostatic derangements, especially when performed during very early childhood. Anesthetic considerations in epilepsy surgery have been reviewed by Shetti et al. [1]. Koh et al. [2] addressed anesthesiological characteristics in the pediatric population. Overviews on surgery under local anesthesia have been given by Grivin [3] and Olivier [4].

**Anticonvulsants**. Anticonvulsant therapy may have relevant anesthetic implications [5]. Sodium valproate can cause dose-dependent thrombocytopenia and platelet dysfunction [6]. It should, therefore, be discontinued before intracranial surgery, and anticonvulsant medication be adjusted. As the hematologic effects of sodium valproate dissipate within 3–4 weeks, intracranial procedures can be scheduled about 4 weeks after its discontinuation. Carbamazepine can suppress the hematopoietic system and cause cardiac toxicity. Phenytoin may lead to gingival hyperplasia which can interfere with airway management [1]. In general, perioperative disruption of antiepileptic medication must be avoided. Patients should be advised to take their usual anticonvulsive medication on the morning of surgery. Regular



J. Zentner, *Surgical Treatment of Epilepsies*, https://doi.org/10.1007/978-3-030-48748-5_5

dosing should postoperatively be reinstituted as early as practicable.

**Electrophysiological Testing**. As the impact of anesthetics on excitatory and inhibitory neuronal activity is often dose dependent, reports on their proconvulsant and anticonvulsant effects vary. Thiopental and benzodiazepines are potent anticonvulsants suppressing EEG activity [7, 8]. While low-dose propofol activates the electrocorticogram, high doses can produce burst suppression [9]. Low-dose etomidate, methohexital, and ketamine increase EEG activity and can help localizing the zone of ictal origin [7].

Whereas a low-dose bolus or infusion of opioids has little clinically relevant effect on spike activity, high-dose bolus of synthetic opioids (i.e., fentanyl, sufentanil, alfentanil, and remifentanil) can provoke interictal spikes. An intravenous bolus of remifentanil has been found to induce spike activity in patients undergoing surgery for mesial temporal lobe epilepsy which may help to localize the epileptogenic zone [10]. The inhalational anesthetics isoflurane and desflurane have no proconvulsive properties [11]. As sevoflurane can elicit epileptogenic activity, especially at higher concentrations and in children, it is relatively contraindicated in epilepsy surgery [12]. Although nitrous oxide ($N_2O$) may itself not affect neuronal activity, in clinical practice, however, it is never administered alone. Overall evidence suggests that $N_2O$ may well suppress epileptiform activity when combined with baseline intravenous or inhalational anesthetics [13–15].

**Homeostasis**. There is a general trend towards surgical treatment of epilepsies during childhood, even as early as during the first months of life. However, young children frequently show large lesions which require extensive resections like multilobectomy or hemispherectomy. In other words, the younger the child, the larger the resection. The associated prolonged surgery time, elevated blood loss, and increased risk of hypovolemia, coagulopathy, and hypothermia pose considerable challenges to the anesthesiologist [15, 16]. Adequate intravenous access and blood products must be established and available at the time of skin incision. Frequent intraoperative monitoring of blood chemistry and coagulation variables is mandatory [2, 17].

## 5.1 History and Current Status

At the time of Victor Horsley and Fedor Krause at the transition from the nineteenth to the twentieth century, all procedures for epilepsy were performed under general anesthesia [18, 19]. Harvey Cushing was the first to report a series of patients operated on under local anesthesia [20]. Later on, Otfrid Foerster in Breslau performed his surgical procedures under local anesthesia with extensive cortical stimulation to map the sensorimotor cortex and to localize the seizure focus by provoking habitual seizure patterns. Penfield recognizing the potential of this approach took the technique of awake surgery to Montreal [21]. Facilitating stimulation mapping, awake craniotomy critically contributed to the understanding of the functional anatomy of the human neocortex. Besides mapping and monitoring, a major reason for awake surgery was undisturbed intraoperative electrocorticography (ECoG) for the localization of the epileptogenic focus [3, 4]. For this reason, epilepsy surgery under local anesthesia became standard practice at the Montreal Neurological Institute (MNI), and subsequently at many epilepsy surgical institutions at that time [3, 4, 22, 23].

Today, sophisticated electrophysiologic and anesthesiologic techniques enable reliable recording of epileptic activity as well as mapping and monitoring under general anesthesia. Total intravenous anesthesia (TIVA) with propofol in combination with opioids (mostly remifentanil) provides adequate conditions for reliable intraoperative ECoG as well as for functional mapping and monitoring by stimulation and recording somatosensory (SEP) and motor (MEP) evoked potentials and SEP phase reversal [24–28]. When detailed delineation of the speech areas is required, preoperative mapping by subdural grid electrodes is available which are implanted during a preceding procedure.

Proper resection of the epileptogenic area is completed in a second procedure. As effective methods are available to adequately manage epileptic lesions within or around areas of high functionality during general anesthesia, one could entirely forego surgeries under local anesthesia. Consequently, in most centers epilepsy surgery is performed under general anesthesia. Nevertheless, particularly for intraoperative language mapping, surgery under local anesthesia and sedation (referred to as "awake" craniotomy) has been reintroduced during the last decades, first for tumor surgery and subsequently also for epilepsy surgery [29].

## 5.2 Epilepsy Surgery Under General Anesthesia

Whereas awake craniotomy may be advantageous regarding functional testing of the language areas, general anesthesia offers the advantage of greater comfort, for both patient and surgeon [15, 30]. The overall anesthetic management for resection of epileptogenic foci and other epilepsy surgical procedures is similar to that for any craniotomy. Anesthesia is induced intravenously with a hypnotic (mostly propofol) and an opioid (e.g., remifentanil, sufentanil, or fentanyl). TIVA or inhalational anesthesia can safely be used for maintenance of anesthesia [1, 31, 32].

For cortical mapping and monitoring or ECoG-guided resection, TIVA with propofol is generally recommended [1]. Propofol is a hypnotic with a fast onset time and a short duration of action. In experienced hands, this enables good control of depth of anesthesia and reasonably fast recovery of consciousness upon its discontinuation. Because of its depressant effects on neural activity, propofol should be discontinued at least 15 min prior to ECoG, and anesthesia be maintained by a continuous infusion of opioids (preferably remifentanil because of its fast onset and offset times and its minimal effect on ECoG) or inhalational anesthetics. During ECoG, a bolus dose of methohexital can be administered to activate the epileptogenic zone, thereby guiding the extent of resection. Because of their potent anticonvulsant properties, premedication with benzodiazepines must be avoided when ECoG is planned [1, 2, 4].

## 5.3 Epilepsy Surgery in Awake Craniotomy

### 5.3.1 Anesthetic Management Principles

Irrespective of the specific management of awake craniotomy, some general principles always apply. Appropriate patient selection, comprehensive preoperative patient consultation and education, close communication between healthcare team and patient throughout the procedure, and an excellent anesthesiologist-patient rapport are crucial for achieving high-level patient satisfaction and procedural success [33].

#### 5.3.1.1 Patient Selection

Candidates for awake craniotomy are highly cooperative and motivated patients, while those with mental retardation, anxiety, claustrophobia, psychiatric disorders, and emotional instability are considered unsuitable [3]. Relative contraindications for awake craniotomy include patients with anticipated difficult airways, obesity, gastroesophageal reflux, and chronic cough. Moreover, obstructive sleep apnea may be considered a contraindication [29, 34]. However, patient refusal may be the only absolute contraindication to awake craniotomy.

#### 5.3.1.2 Pediatric Age

Different opinions exist towards awake craniotomy in the pediatric age regarding psychological fragility and vulnerability, cooperation, full understanding, and managing anxiety [35]. In particular, the cutoff limit for providing awake craniotomy to younger age groups remains unclear [36]. Klimek et al. [37] suggested in their case report of a 9-year-old boy that an awake craniotomy is feasible and can be performed safely even in very young patients refusing an age restriction. Others consider children below the age of 10 years as unsuitable for awake surgery

[3]. Lohkamp et al. [38] summarized the results of 18 studies including 50 pediatric cases. Median age was 15 years with the two youngest being 8 years old. Failure was noted in 4 cases: The awake phase had to be abandoned due to combative behavior in a 13-year-old patient, anxiety in an 8-year-old boy, intraoperative apnea in a 17-year-old female, and an anesthesiological complication in a 9-year-old child. A generalized seizure as observed in another child did not prevent the continuation of the awake episode. Postoperative neuropsychological assessment as available from 20 patients did not reveal signs of post-traumatic stress disorder in any case [38].

Overall, experience available suggests safety and feasibility of awake craniotomy in highly selected children and adolescents [38]. The psychological condition, temperament, and responsiveness of the individual patient may determine considering a child for awake surgery more than pure age [39, 40]. However, guidelines for standardized implementation of awake craniotomy in the pediatric age are pending and should include criteria of eligibility and psychological preparation [38].

#### 5.3.1.3 Preoperative Patient Preparation

Preoperative patient preparation includes detailed explanation of the various steps of the procedure and of the associated varying pain intensities at the different stages of the procedure. The patient must be informed that each intervention is communicated beforehand, and close communication between him/her and the surgeon as well as the anesthesiologist will be maintained throughout the procedure. Absence of this constant communication in a patient who is tense, waiting with fear for the next unannounced pain or crunching of bone, constitutes the main reason for failure of awake craniotomy [3]. The importance of a sensitive and experienced multidisciplinary operating room team (i.e., surgeons, anesthesiologists, nurses, and technicians) for a successful craniotomy under local anesthesia cannot be overemphasized. The operating room should be as quiet as possible [3].

#### 5.3.1.4 Anesthetic Techniques

A wide range of anesthetic management techniques for awake craniotomy exist. Most of them involve sedation or general anesthesia before and after intraoperative electrophysiologic mapping and surgical intervention. The capability of the anesthesiologist to reliably provide smooth and timely return of responsiveness upon discontinuation of the sedation or general anesthesia is crucial in allowing one or more intraoperative interventions to be performed in a responsive patient [41]. Thus, "craniotomy with intraoperative awakening" rather than "awake craniotomy" would probably be the more appropriate term [42].

### 5.3.2 Patient Positioning, Local Anesthesia, and Sedation

#### 5.3.2.1 Positioning of the Patient

As the patient may have to remain in the same position for a long period of time, establishing a comfortable and safe position is important. The supine, half-sitting, or lateral positions are most commonly used. To improve patient comfort and reduce the risk of nerve injury, soft pads need to be placed on the operating room table, and protective padding of hard surfaces or supports that may exert direct pressure to susceptible peripheral nerves be employed. Preferably, the head is fixed in a "sniffing" position because this reduces the risk of airway obstruction during sedation in the spontaneously breathing patient (particularly in the absence of a supraglottic airway device or an endotracheal tube), and it facilitates airway intervention if needed. Over-flexion or rotation of the head must be avoided because it promotes airway obstruction and hinders airway intervention. Free access to and view of the patient's face and extremities are important for safety reason, and for adequate sensory, motor, speech, and memory testing. Body temperature must continuously be monitored and protected by warmed blankets or, preferably, by a forced air warming blanket [34].

Spontaneous respiration is maintained throughout the procedure. Adequacy of spontaneous respiration must continuously be monitored by a nasal $CO_2$ sampling cannula. Supplemental oxygen is provided by face mask or nasal cannula. However, care must be taken to limit the local environmental oxygen concentration because the proximity of a high concentration of oxygen and electrocautery ("Bovie") increases the risk of fire and explosion [43]. The healthcare team must be prepared at all times to rapidly convert to general anesthesia if the situation demands.

#### 5.3.2.2 Local Anesthesia

Effective blockade of scalp sensation by local anesthetics is the cornerstone of any awake craniotomy technique. It importantly contributes to patient satisfaction. Local anesthesia is frequently performed under light sedation (mostly with propofol and/or remifentanil) [30, 44, 45]. It can be achieved by either direct blockade of each of the six nerves that innervate the scalp (i.e., auriculotemporal, zygomaticotemporal, supraorbital, supratrochlear, greater occipital, and lesser occipital nerves) (Fig. 5.1) or local anesthetic infiltration of the sites of surgical incision and Mayfield clamp pin. The direct nerve blocks are technically more demanding and possibly associated with more complications, but they require less amount of local anesthetic (approximately 40 ml of local anesthetic solution) and provide longer duration of analgesia [46]. Usually, a mixture of long-acting local anesthetics (0.25% bupivacaine, 0.2% ropivacaine, 0.25% levobupivacaine) is used. When the blocks are well performed, those long-acting local anesthetics can provide good and safe analgesia for up to 8 h. Nevertheless, additional intraoperative local infiltration of sensitive structures by the surgeon may at times be required. Epinephrine 1:200,000 is added to reduce systemic absorption and, thereby, the risk of systemic local anesthetic toxicity, to reduce bleeding during skin incision, and to prolong the duration of local anesthesia [47]. Despite routine use of scalp nerve blocks and potent opioids, pain remains a common complaint during awake craniotomy [3, 4, 48].

#### 5.3.2.3 Sedation

Providing the appropriate level of sedation during awake craniotomy requires considerable skill and experience. Oversedation may cause respira-

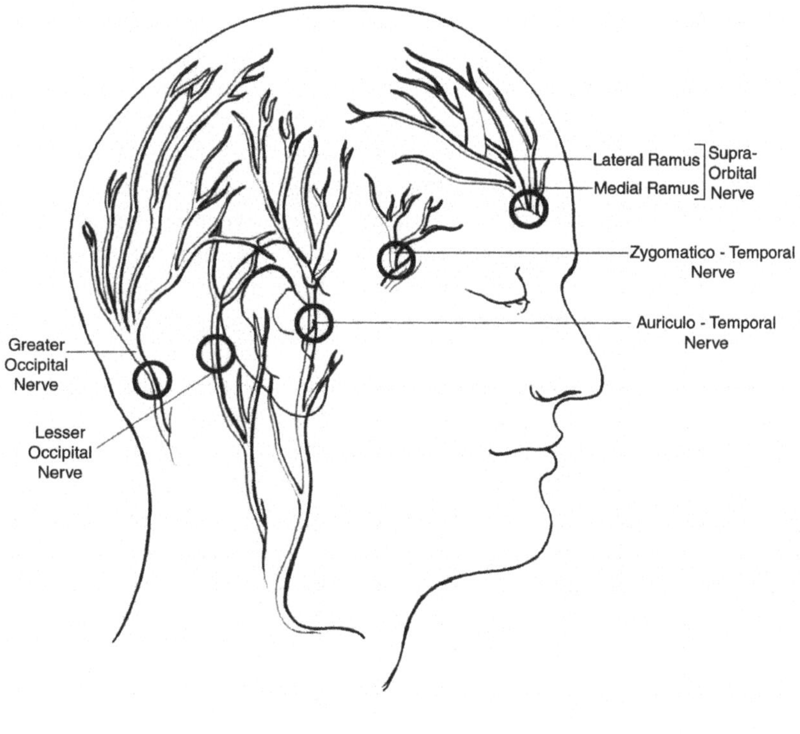


**Fig. 5.1** Illustration of the nerves innervating the scalp on the right side of the head. The sites of injection for blockade of scalp nerves with local anesthetics are marked with circles (from Girvin [3], with permission)

tory depression, airway obstruction, hypoxemia, and cardiovascular depression, and too little sedation may cause patient movement and anxiety. Sedation must not abolish the patient's ability to appropriately respond to verbal commands, either spontaneously or in response to light tactile stimulation. Sedation by a combination of propofol and remifentanil has become the standard technique. However, it is associated with an increased risk of respiratory depression [49]. Sedation by dexmedetomidine, a selective alpha-2-adrenoceptor agonist, demonstrated high efficacy and safety during awake craniotomy [48]. It provides anxiolysis, sedation, and analgesia, and has sympatholytic and opioid-sparing properties and very little effect on neuronal function. At low dose, the incidence of respiratory and circulatory depression is low. These characteristics make dexmedetomidine a rational alternative to propofol for sedation during awake craniotomy [50].

### 5.3.3 Combined General and Local Anesthesia

Awake craniotomy can be managed under local anesthesia combined with moderate sedation or by modifications combining general and local anesthesia. These combinations include the asleep-awake-asleep technique and the asleep-awake method [51–53]. The asleep-awake-asleep (AAA) technique consists of three phases, with periods of general anesthesia in the beginning and at the end, and a period of consciousness in between for mapping and monitoring. The latter requires effective local anesthesia, although less intense than that during "awake" craniotomy under sedation only.

Placement of an endotracheal tube for ventilation during the initial asleep phase was recommended in the early days of awake craniotomy. In today's practice, however, placement of a supraglottic airway device is the preferred technique by most anesthesiologists because of its ease of insertion, removal, and reinsertion without having to change the position of the patient and interrupt surgical activities, and because it requires a lesser depth of anesthesia which makes the wake-up more predictable and is associated with a lower risk of coughing and gagging on awakening [49, 54].

During the first phase of the asleep-awake-asleep technique, the patient is anesthetized. Shortly before phase 2, the depth of anesthesia is reduced to a degree of sedation which restores responsiveness to verbal command and spontaneous respiration. At this time, the supraglottic airway device (or more rarely in today's practice, the endotracheal tube) is removed and electrophysiologic mapping and monitoring are commenced. During phase 3, the patient is re-anesthetized, and the supraglottic airway device mask (or the endotracheal tube) reinserted [53].

### 5.3.4 Complications During Awake Craniotomy

Intraoperative complications during awake craniotomy may be related to anesthesia and surgical manipulation.

#### 5.3.4.1 Anesthesia-Related Complications

Anesthesia-related adverse events during awake craniotomy include respiratory and hemodynamic complications, desaturation and hypoxemia, nausea with or without vomiting, and pain [41]. Failure of awake craniotomy due to such events has been reported to occur in less than 2% of cases, irrespective of the anesthetic technique [55]. Comparing 332 propofol-based asleep-awake-asleep (AAA) craniotomies with unsecured airways and 129 craniotomies under general anesthesia with endotracheal intubation for epilepsy surgery, Skucas and Artru [56] found that the AAA technique was associated with a higher incidence of intraoperative respiratory and hemodynamic complications than the general anesthesia technique. However, as those adverse events were usually treated appropriately, in only one patient may the AAA technique have contributed to a poor clinical outcome because of intraoperative brain swelling and hemorrhage [56].

#### 5.3.4.2 Surgery-Related Complications

Among surgery-related complications, focal and generalized seizures during stimulation mapping in awake craniotomy are most feared, while other complications such as bleeding, brain swelling, or venous air embolism are rare [41]. As mentioned in the previous chapter, the incidence of stimulation-associated seizures during general anesthesia has been reported to range between 0.4% and 1.8% [57–59]. Contrarily, a higher incidence of intraoperative seizures between 0% and 32% has been observed during awake craniotomy for tumor surgery [41]. Analyzing 477 awake procedures, Nossek and Matot [60] noted that 60 patients (12.6%) experienced stimulation-induced seizures, and the procedure failed in 11 (2.3%) patients. A history of seizures, younger age, and frontal tumor location have been identified as risk factors [60]. Roca et al. [61] evaluated 39 publications (2000–2019) including one multicenter survey comprising 6085 patients and one meta-analysis including 2666 cases, all operated in awake craniotomy. The reported rates of stimulation-induced seizures ranged between 0% and 24% (mean: 7.7%). Frontal tumor location correlated with a higher risk, while no significant association was found between intraoperative seizure rate and preoperative seizure history as well as stimulation parameters used. Although intraoperative seizures might affect patients' postoperative status as well as the duration of hospital stay, they did not cause severe postoperative deficits [61]. Remifentanil seems to be associated with fewer seizures than other opioids [62]. Propofol has a protective effect against seizures but must be discontinued before cortical stimulation to not interfere with ECoG [41]. A higher incidence of seizures may be observed under neuroleptic analgesia [44]. As mentioned previously, irrigation of the cortex with iced NaCl or Ringer's solution will terminate an intraoperative seizure.

**Concluding Remarks**

- ***General anesthesia****. With availability of sophisticated tools for language mapping as well as for mapping and monitoring of sensorimotor functions, all surgical procedures for epilepsy can in principle be performed under general anesthesia. Overall, the anesthetic technique for epilepsy is similar to that for any craniotomy. However, cortical mapping, somatosensory and motor function monitoring, and ECoG-guided resections require modifications.*
- ***Awake craniotomy****. During the past decades, awake craniotomy has been reintroduced and has become an accepted technique for various neurosurgical interventions. Considerable progress in anesthetic techniques has facilitated this renaissance. The choice of a specific anesthetic regime for awake craniotomy still largely depends on the preference of the individual anesthesiologist. Special expertise is required to assure patient comfort and successful outcome. Provision of safe and effective local anesthesia and sedation, and of smooth and predictably rapid transition from unconsciousness to a cooperative state, remains a major anesthetic challenge. As the procedural demands are considerable, performance of awake craniotomy should be restricted to centers with sufficient experience.*

## References


1. Shetti A, Pardeshi S, Shah VM, Kulkarni A. Anesthesia considerations in epilepsy surgery. Int J Surg. 2015;36:454–9. https://doi.org/10.1016/j.ijsu.2015.07.006.
2. Koh JL, Egan B. Pediatric epilepsy surgery. Anaesthetic considerations. Anesthesiol Clin. 2012;30:191–206.
3. Girvin JP. Surgery under local anesthesia. In: Girvin JP, editor. Operative techniques in epilepsy. New York: Springer; 2015. p. 37–72.
4. Olivier A. Techniques in Epilepsy Surgery. The MNI Approach. Cambridge Medicine, 2012.

5. Manohar C, Avitsian R, Lozano S, et al. The effect of antiepileptic drugs on coagulation and bleeding in the perioperative period of epilepsy surgery: The Cleveland Clinic experience. J Clin Neurosci. 2011;18:1180–4.
6. Verrotti A, Greco R, Matera V, et al. Platelet count and function in children with epilepsy receiving valproic acid. Pediatr Neurol. 1999;21:611–4.
7. Modica PA, Tempelhoff R, White PF. Pro- and anticonvulsant effects of anesthetics (part II). Anesth Analg. 1990;70:433–44.
8. Schubert A, Lotto M. Awake craniotomy, epilepsy, minimally invasive and robotic surgery. In: Cottrell JE, Young WL, editors. Cottrell and young's neuroanesthesia. 5th ed. Mosby: Elsevier; 2010. p. 296–316.
9. Smith M, Smith SJ, Scott CA, Harkness WF. Activation of the electrocorticogram by propofol during surgery for epilepsy. Br J Anesthiol. 1992;76:652–4.
10. Grønlykke L, Knudsen ML, Høgenhaven H, Moltke FB, Madsen FF, Kjaer TW. Remifentanil-induced spike activity as a diagnostic tool in epilepsy surgery. Acta Neurol Scand. 2008;117:90–3.
11. Mirsattari M, Sharpe MD, Young GB. Treatment of refractory status epilepticus with inhalational anesthetic agents isoflurane and desflurane. Arch Neurol. 2004;61:1254–9.
12. Perks A, Cheema S, Mohanraj R. Anaesthesia and epilepsy. Br J Anaesth. 2012;108:562–71.
13. Artru AA, Lettich E, Colley PS, Ojemann GA. Nitrous oxide: suppression of focal epileptiform activity during inhalation, and spreading of seizure activity following withdrawal. J Neurosurg Anesthesiol. 1990;2:189–93.
14. Bindra A, Chouhan RS, Prabhakar H, Dash HH, Chandra PS, Tripathi M. Comparison of the effects of different anesthetic techniques on electrocorticography in patients undergoing epilepsy surgery—a bispectral index guided study. Seizure. 2012;21:501–7.
15. Bindra A, Chouhan RS, Prabhakar H, Chandra PS, Tripathi M. Perioperative anesthetic implications of epilepsy surgery: a retrospective analysis. J Anesth. 2015;29:229–34.
16. Basheer SN, Connolly MB, Lautzenhiser A, et al. Hemispheric surgery in children with refractory epilepsy: seizure outcome, complications, and adaptive function. Epilepsia. 2007;48:133–40.
17. Thudiuam MO, von Lehe M, Weeesling C, et al. Safety, feasibility and complications during resective pediatric epilepsy surgery: a retrospective analysis. BMC Anesthesiol. 2014;14:71–5.
18. Horsley V. Brain-surgery. Br Med J. 1886;2:670–5.
19. Krause F. Die operative Behandlung der Epilepsie. Med Klin Berlin. 1909;5:1418–22.
20. Cushing H. A note upon the faradic stimulation of the postcentral gyrus in conscious patients. Brain. 1909;32:44–53.
21. Foerster O, Penfield W. The structural basis of traumatic epilepsy and results of radical operation. Brain. 1930;53:99–120.
22. Penfield W, Steelman H. The treatment of focal epilepsy by cortical excision. Ann Surg. 1947;126:740–62.
23. Penfield W, Jasper H. Epilepsy and the functional anatomy of the human brain. Boston, MA: Little, Brown and Co.; 1954. p. 896.
24. Cedzich C, Taniguchi M, Schafer S, Schramm J. Somatosensory evoked potential phase reversal and direct motor cortex stimulation during surgery in and around the central region. Neurosurgery. 1996;38:962–70.
25. Neuloh G. Schramm J. Intraoperative neurophysiological mapping and monitoring for supratentorial procedures. In: Deletis V, JL S, editors. Neurophysiology in neurosurgery: a modern intraoperative approach. Amsterdam/Boston, MA: Academic Press; 2002. p. 339–401.
26. Pechstein U, Nadstawek J, Zentner J, Schramm J. Isoflurane plus nitrous oxide versus propofol for recording of myogenic motor evoked potentials after high frequency repetitive electric stimulation. EEG Clin Neurphysiol. 1998;108:175–81.
27. Scheufler KM, Zentner J. Total intravenous anesthesia for intraoperative monitoring of the motor pathways: an integral view combining clinical and experimental data. J Neurosurg. 2002;96:571–9.
28. Thees C, Scheufler KM, Nadstawek J, Pechstein U, Hanisch M, Juntke R, Zentner J, Hoeft A. Influence of fentanyl, alfentanil, and sufentanil on motor evoked potentials. J Neurosurg Anesthesiol. 1999;11:112–8.
29. Manninen PH, See JJ. Epilepsy, epilepsy surgery, awake craniotomy for tumor surgery, and intraoperative magnetic resonance imaging. In: Newfield P, Cottrell JE, editors. Handbook of neuroanesthesia. 4th ed. Philadelphia, PA: Lippincott William and Wilkins; 2007. p. 198–215.
30. Herrick IA, Gelb AW. Anesthesia for temporal lobe epilepsy. Can J Neurol Sci. 2000;27(Suppl 1):64–7.
31. Gignac E, Manninen P, Gelb AW. Comparison of fentanyl, sufentanil and alfentanil during awake craniotomy for epilepsy. Can J Anaesth. 1993;40:421–4.
32. Hans P, Bonhomme V, Born JD, Maertens de Noordhoudt A, Brichant JF, Dewandre PY. Target-controlled infusion of propofol and remifentanil combined with bispectral index monitoring for awake craniotomy. Anesthesia. 2000;55:255–9.
33. Potters JW, Klimek M. Awake craniotomy: improving the patient's experience. Curr Opin Anaesthesiol. 2015;28:511–6.
34. Erickson KM, Cole DJ. Anesthetic considerations for awake craniotomy for epilepsy and functional neurosurgery. Anesthesiol Clin. 2012;30:241–68.
35. Everett LL, van Rooyen IF, Warner MH, Shurtleff HA, Saneto RP, Ojemann JG. Use of dexmedetomidine in awake craniotomy in adolescents: report of two cases. Paediatr Anaesth. 2006;16:338–42.
36. Berger MS. The impact of technical adjuncts in the surgical management of cerebral hemispheric low-grade gliomas of childhood 1996. J Neurooncol. 1996;28:129–55.

37. Klimek M, Verbrugge SJ, Roubos S, van der Most E, Vincent AJ, Klein J. Awake craniotomy for glioblastoma in a 9-year-old child. Anaesthesia. 2004;59:607–9.
38. Lohkamp L-N, Mottolese C, Szathmari A, et al. Awake brain surgery in children—review of the literature and state-of-the-art. Childs Nerv Syst. 2019;35(11):2071–7. https://doi.org/10.1007/s00381-019-04279-w.
39. Beez T, Boge K, Wager M, Whittle I, Fontaine D, Spena G, Braun S, Szelenyi A, Bello L, Duffau H, Sabel M. Tolerance of awake surgery for glioma: a prospective European low grade glioma network multicenter study. Acta Neurochir. 2013;155:1301–8.
40. Milian M, Tatagiba M, Feigl GC. Patient response to awake craniotomy—a summary overview. Acta Neurochir. 2014;156:1063–70.
41. Piccioni F, Fanzio M. Management of anesthesia in awake craniotomy. Minerva Anesthesiol. 2008;74:393–408.
42. Lobo FA, Wagemakers M, Absalom AR. Anaesthesia for awake craniotomy. Br J Anaesthiol. 2016;116:740–4.
43. Jones TS, Black IH, Robinson TN, Jones EL. Operating room fires. Anesthesiology. 2019;130:492–501.
44. Herrick IA, Craen RA, Gelb AW, McLachlan RS, Girvin JP, Parrent AG, et al. Propofol sedation during awake craniotomy for seizures: electrocorticographic and epileptogenic effects. Anesth Analg. 1997a;84:1280–4.
45. Herrick IA, Craen RA, Gelb AW, Miller LA, Kubu CS, et al. Propofol sedation during awake craniotomy for seizures: Patient-controlled administration versus neurolept analgesia. Anesth Analg. 1997b;84:1285–91.
46. Potters JW, Klimek M. Local anesthetics for brain tumor resection: current perspectives. Local Reg Anesthiol. 2018;11:1–8.
47. Costello TG, Cormack JR. Anesthesia for awake craniotomy: A modern approach. J Clin Neurosci. 2004;11:16–9.
48. Kulikov A, Lubnin A. Anesthesia for awake craniotomy. Curr Opin Anaesthesiol. 2018;31:506–10.
49. Meng L, McDonagh DL, Berger MS, Gelb AW. Anesthesia for awake craniotomy: a how-to-guide for the occasional practitioner. Can J Anaesth. 2017;64:517–29.
50. Lin N, Vutskits L, Bebawy JF, Gelb AW. Perspectives on dexmedetomidine use for neurosurgical patients. J Neurosurg Anesthesiol. 2019;31(4):366–77. https://doi.org/10.1097/ANA.0000000000000554.
51. Huncke K, Van de Wiele B, Fried I, Rubinstein EH. The asleep-awake-asleep anesthetic technique for intraoperative language mapping. Neurosurgery. 1998;42:1312–6.
52. Olsen KS. The asleep-awake technique using propofol-remifentanil anesthesia for awake craniotomy for cerebral tumors. Eur J Anesthesiol. 2008;25:662–9.
53. Wang X, Wang T, et al. Asleep-awake-asleep regimen for epilepsy surgery: a prospective study of target-controlled infusion versus manually controlled infusion technique. J Clin Anesth. 2016;32:92–100.
54. Ghadhinglajkar S, Sreedhar R, Abraham M. Anesthesia management of awake craniotomy performed under asleep-awake-asleep technique using laryngeal mask airway: Report of two cases. Neurol India. 2008;56:65–7.
55. Sewell D, Smith M. Awake craniotomy. Anesthetic considerations based on outcome evidence. Curr Opin Anesthesiol. 2019;32:546–52.
56. Skucas AP, Artru AA. Anesthetic complications of awake craniotomies for epilepsy surgery. Anesth Analg. 2006;102:882–7.
57. Goldstein HE, Smith EH, Gross RE, et al. Risk of seizures induced by intracranial research stimulation: analysis of 770 stimulation sessions. J Neural Eng. 2019;16(6):066039. https://doi.org/10.1088/1741-2552/ab4365.
58. Szelényi A, Joksimoviã B, Seifert V. Intraoperative risk of seizures associated with transient direct cortical stimulation in patients with symptomatic epilepsy. J Clin Neurophysiol. 2007a;24:39–43.
59. Szelényi A, Joksimovic B, Seifert V. Intraoperative risk of seizures associated with transient direct cortical stimulation in patients with symptomatic epilepsy. J Clin Neurophysiol. 2007b;24(1):39–43.
60. Nossek E, Matot I. Intraoperative seizures during awake craniotomy: incidence and consequences—analysis of 477 patients. Neurosurgery. 2013;73(1):135–40. https://doi.org/10.1227/01.neu.0000429847.91707.97.
61. Roca E, Pallud J, Guerrini F, et al. Stimulation-related intraoperative seizures during awake surgery: a review of available evidences. Neurosurg Rev. 2020;43(1):87–93. https://doi.org/10.1007/s10143-019-01214-0.
62. Sarang A, Dinsmore J. Anaesthesia for awake craniotomy—evolution of a technique that facilitates awake neurological testing. Br J Anaesth. 2003;90:161–5.

# 6 Temporal Lobe Resections

*The best way to find yourself is to lose yourself in the service of others*

*Mahatma Gandhi*

## Contents



Based on clinical studies with cortical recordings by Penfield and Jasper at the Montreal Neurological Institute (MNI) [1–4] indicating temporal spike foci in a high number of epilepsy cases, temporal lobe resections for epilepsy have been started. In the first series of temporal lobectomies which were corticectomies, only approximately one-third of patients achieved seizure freedom. Further electrophysiological studies suggested that pure removal of the lateral temporal cortex was associated with unsatisfactory seizure outcome, and that removal of the limbic temporomesial structures as the proper epileptogenic substrates was required [1, 5–7]. Subsequently, temporal lobectomy including resection of amygdala and hippocampus, which



J. Zentner, *Surgical Treatment of Epilepsies*, https://doi.org/10.1007/978-3-030-48748-5_6

was found to be sclerotic in most cases, was promoted [6, 8–11]. Seizure freedom rates reported mainly ranged between 40% and 70% and marked reduction of seizure frequency between 60% and 90% [12–15]. Reviewing the MNI experience with temporal resections of 1102 patients by the end of 1978, Rasmussen [16] showed that at a mean follow-up of 11 years, 70% of patients experienced complete or nearly complete seizure freedom.

In 1954, William Scoville performed a bilateral mesial temporal lobe resection. Although the patient (H.M.) was seizure free after surgery, his memory was lost [17]. Stimulated by this report and other experiences demonstrating impairment of cognitive and verbal functions after resection of the dominant temporal lobe [18–21], neuropsychological testing has been attributed an important role in presurgical evaluation of patients with drug-resistant temporal lobe epilepsy (TLE). It has been shown that neuropsychological results are valuable both for lateralization of the seizure origin and for prediction of postoperative outcome [22–25]. In parallel, new technologies including video-EEG monitoring, MR imaging, as well as invasive EEG in the 1980s and 1990s improved understanding of epilepsy and contributed to selection of candidates; thus temporal resections could be offered to more complicated cases.

Nowadays, the syndrome of mesial temporal lobe epilepsy (MTLE) constitutes a well-known entity[26]. It accounts for 60–70% of focal epilepsies and for 90–95% of temporal lobe epilepsies [27, 28]. According to more actual surgical series, temporal resections are decreasing, but still amount to almost 60% epilepsy surgical procedures [29]. Various surgical techniques have been proposed all aiming at the complete removal of the epileptogenic zone without producing neurological or cognitive deficits. Anatomical standardized resections rely on the concept that TLE reflects a clinico-electrophysiological entity. In contrast, tailored resections emphasize individual pathophysiology [30]. Surgical approaches preferred in different centers reflect not only different pathology and pathophysiology, but also the history of epileptological and surgical concepts. Today, seizure control is achieved in 60–80% of patients after temporal resections [31–42] which is similar to the 1980 report of Rasmussen [16] demonstrating complete or nearly complete seizure freedom in 70% of patients.

## 6.1 Functional Anatomy

### 6.1.1 Surface

While sulci on the lateral surface of the temporal lobe delineating the superior, middle, and inferior temporal gyrus are largely constant, the sulci of the inferior surface are variable. Typically, the occipito-temporal sulcus separates the medial border of the inferior temporal gyrus from the lateral border of the fusiform or medial occipito-temporal gyrus. Medial to the fusiform gyrus is the collateral sulcus. The medial border of the inferior surface is formed by the parahippocampal gyrus.

The temporal lobe shows a smooth transition to the occipital and parietal lobes. The limits can be defined by arbitrary lines connecting anatomical landmarks. A line drawn from the parieto-occipital sulcus to the preoccipital notch which is an indentation in the inferior temporal gyrus, about 3 cm anterior to the occipital pole, defines the limit to the occipital lobe. From the midpoint of this line, a horizontal line passing forward to the lateral sulcus separates the temporal from the parietal lobe [43]. Figure 6.1 depicts essential anatomical aspects of the temporal lobe. Detailed reviews of the functional anatomy of the temporal lobe have been provided by Kiernan [43], Wen and Rhoton [44], Seeger 45–47], Yasargil [42, 48], Sindoue and Guenot [49], and Niewenhuys et al. [50].

### 6.1.2 Hippocampal Formation

#### 6.1.2.1 Components

The components of the hippocampal formation are the hippocampus which constitutes an enrolled gyrus adjacent to the parahippocampal gyrus, the dentate gyrus representing

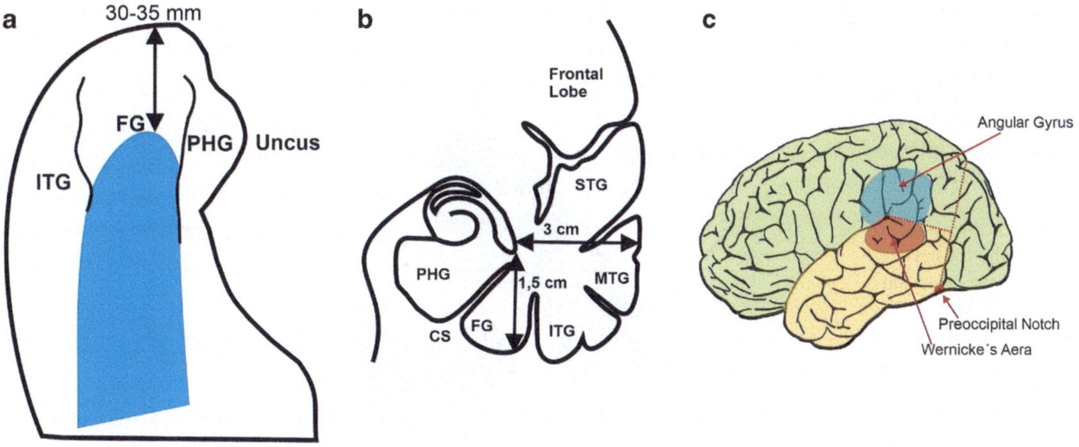


**Fig. 6.1** Schematic presentation of the left temporal lobe. (**a**) Axial view shows the distance from the temporal pole to the tip of the inferior horn (blue). (**b**) Coronal view demonstrates distances from the lateral and basal surface of the temporal lobe to the inferior horn. (**c**) Sagittal view illustrates limits of the temporal lobe to the parietal and occipital lobes. *STG* superior temporal gyrus, *MTG* middle temporal gyrus, *ITG* inferior temporal gyrus, *FG* fusiform gyrus, *PHG* parahippocampal gyrus, *CS* collateral sulcus

the free edge of the pallium, and the associated white matter, the alveus, fimbria, and fornix. The cortex adjacent to the hippocampus represents the entorhinal area which extends along the whole length of the parahippocampal gyrus [51]. The subiculum is a transitional zone between the entorhinal and hippocampal cortices. The most important function of the hippocampus is the consolidation of memory [43, 47].

#### 6.1.2.2 Development

The anatomy of the human hippocampal formation is best understood in the context of its development. The hippocampus and dentate gyrus become recognizable late in the embryonic stage in the edge of the pallium which results from a thin wall surrounding the ventricular system and later forms the cortex, white matter, and basal ganglia. Growth of the cortex and white matter pushes the hippocampal formation downward and forward to become the medial surface of the developing temporal lobe. The folding characterizing the hippocampal formation results from its bulging into the inferior horn of the lateral ventricle which is a characteristic feature of the human brain (Fig. 6.2).

#### 6.1.2.3 Anatomy

The hippocampus can be divided into the head (pes), the body, and the tail. It includes the Ammon's horn and the dentate gyrus which form two parallel interlocking cylinders. The Ammon's horn is covered by the alveus, a thin layer of white matter, which itself is covered by an ependymal membrane constituting the ventricular surface of the hippocampus [49]. The dentate gyrus shows a teeth-like surface as apparent on the surface of the hippocampus head. It continues posteriorly with the fasciolar gyrus and the indusium griseum which runs around the splenium of the corpus callosum [43, 47, 49, 52, 53]. The anatomy of the anterior hippocampal formation is illustrated in Fig. 6.3.

#### 6.1.2.4 Functional Aspects

The main pathways of the hippocampus are shown in Fig. 6.4. Projection fibers of the perforant pathway originating in the entorhinal cortex of the parahippocampal gyrus constitute the main cortical input to the hippocampus. In addition, signals from the contralateral hemisphere via commissural fibers merge to the dentate gyrus. Most of the glutamatergic ento-

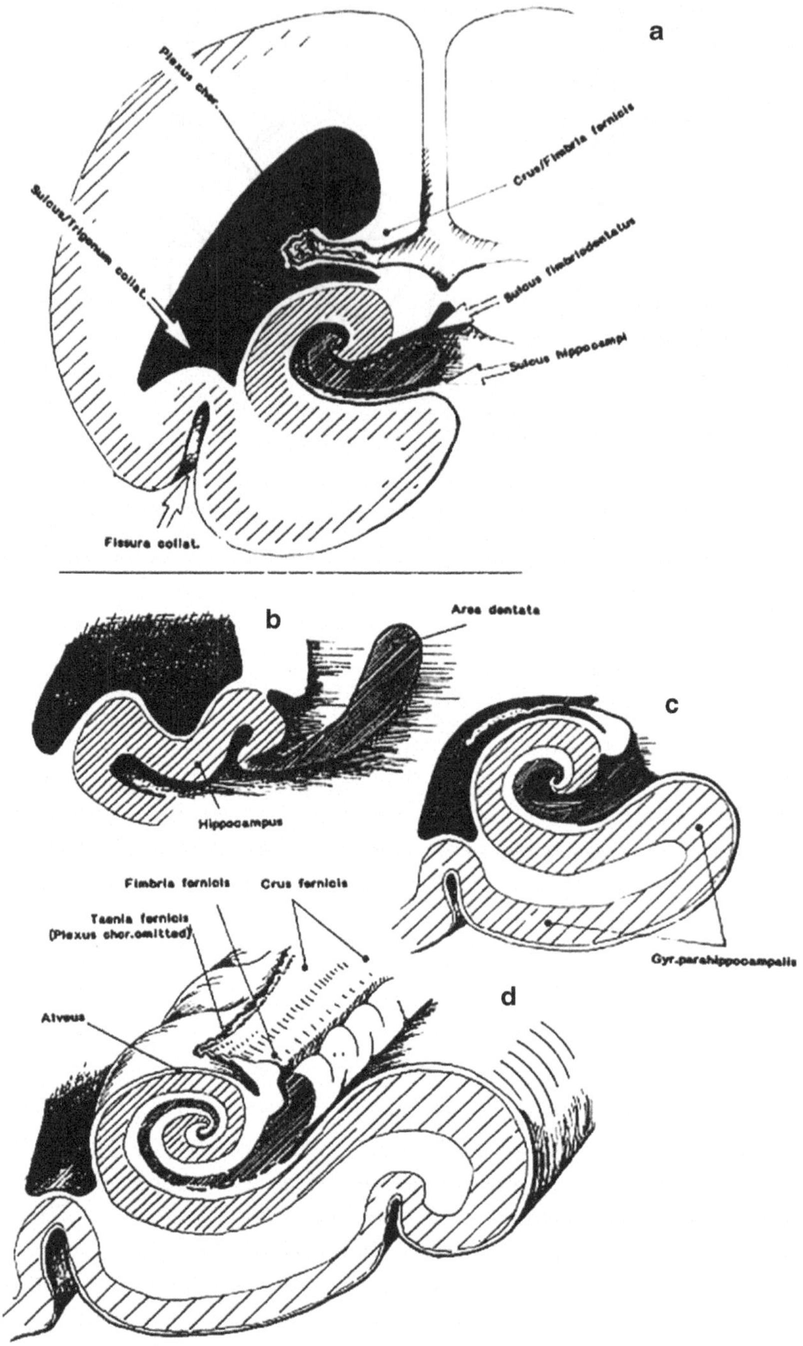


**Fig. 6.2** Development of area dentata, hippocampus, and parahippocampal gyrus (coronal view). (**a**) With growth of the cortex and white matter, the hippocampal formation is pushed downward to become the mesial aspect of the temporal lobe. (**b**–**d**) Further growth of the cortex and white matter results in the characteristic folding of the hippocampal formation and its bulging into the inferior horn (with courtesy of W. Seeger, Freiburg)

rhinal fibers synapse on granule cells of the dentate gyrus, while some terminate on dendrites of CA3 pyramidal cells. The axons of dentate granule cells, called mossy fibers, project to the pyramidal cells of the CA3 region, which in turn send their Schaffer collaterals to CA1 pyramidal cells. Excitation passes from the pyramidal cells of the CA1 subregion to the subiculum, the efferent fibers of which gather in the fimbria and fornix, respectively, constituting the main output of the hippocampal formation, and run back to the entorhinal cortex.

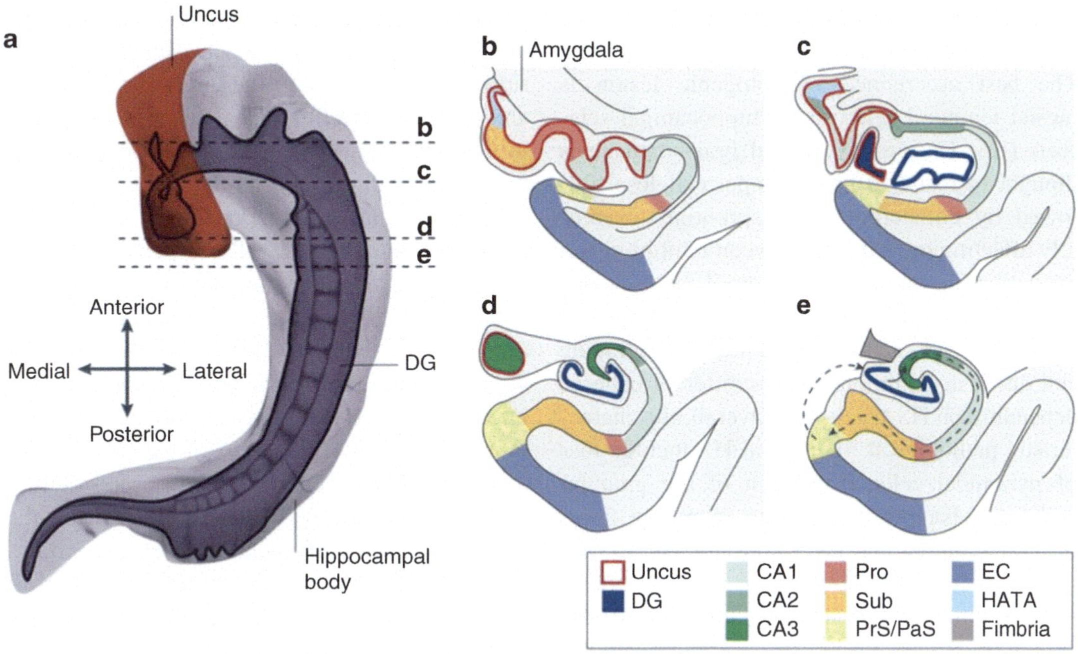


**Fig. 6.3** Schematic illustration of the anatomy of the anterior hippocampal formation. (**a**): Dorsal view of the uncus and hippocampus with the dentate gyrus (DG). (**b**–**e**): Coronal slices show the subfields in the anterior hippocampus with their typical cytoarchitecture. Arrows in **e** indicate the information flow in the hippocampal circuit. *EC* entorhinal cortex, *HATA* hippocampal–amygdaloid transition area, *Pro* prosubiculum, *PrS/PaS* presubiculum and parasubiculum (from Zeidman and Maguire [54], with permission)

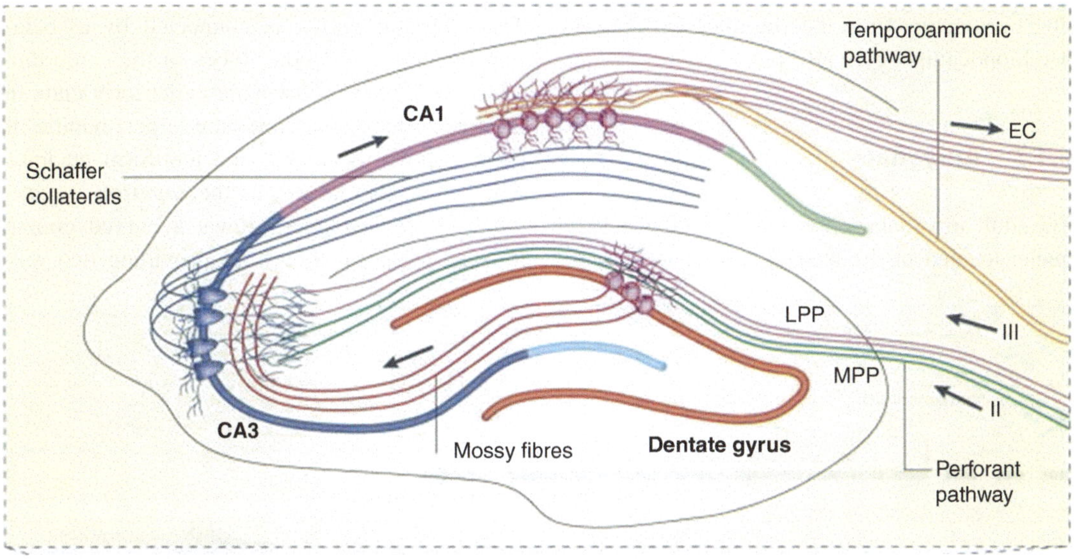


**Fig. 6.4** Schematic illustration of the hippocampal circuitry. The excitatory trisynaptic pathway (entorhinal cortex (EC)–dentate gyrus–CA3–CA1–EC) is depicted by black arrows. The axons of layer II neurons in the entorhinal cortex project to the granule cells of the dentate gyrus through the perforant pathway, including the lateral perforant pathway (LPP) and medial perforant pathway (MPP). The granule cells send their axons (mossy fibers) to the pyramidal cells in CA3, which relay the information to CA1 pyramidal neurons through Schaffer collaterals. CA1 pyramidal neurons send back projections into deep-layer neurons of the EC. CA3 also receives direct projections from EC layer II neurons through the PP. CA1 receives direct input from EC layer III neurons through the temporoammonic pathway (TA) (modified from Deng et al. [55], with permission)

#### 6.1.2.5 Hippocampal Sclerosis and Epilepsy

The best ascertained epileptogenic lesion is mesial temporal sclerosis or hippocampal sclerosis (HS) [56–58]. An initial brain damage is thought to result in hippocampal cell loss, followed by collateral axonal sprouting, eventually affecting the balance between inhibition and excitation in limbic circuits until spontaneous seizures ensue (Fig. 6.5). Mossy fiber sprouting correlates with neuronal cell loss and granule cell dispersion [59] and shows different patterns depending on HS types [60]. Overall, the characteristic pathological findings in HS include loss of pyramidal cells, dispersion of the granular cell layer, backward sprouting of mossy fibers into the granular cell layer and molecular layer, and synaptic reorganization, as well as alterations in glial function and structure [56, 61–64] (Fig. 6.6). Sclerosis and other common pathologies of the hippocampus on MRI are demonstrated in Fig. 6.7. Focusing on white matter tracts of the Papez circuit, it has been shown by diffusion tensor imaging (DTI) that in patients with intractable TLE unilateral HS is associated with a bilateral reduction of cingulum association fibers projecting from the cingulate gyrus to the parahippocampal gyrus [65].

### 6.1.3 Amygdala

The adult amygdala constitutes a group of several nuclei located in the medial part of the temporal pole, anterior to and partly overlapping the hippocampal head. It is attached medially, anteriorly, and inferiorly to the uncus. At its mesial and superior aspect there is no clear demarcation to the claustrum, the infralenticular region, and the globus pallidus. Posterolaterally, the amygdala bulges into the temporal horn of which it constitutes the anterior wall and parts of the roof [49]. The nuclei of the amygdala are organized in three groups (Fig. 6.8): corticomedial nuclei in the anterior part receive afferent fibers from the olfactory tract; basolateral nuclei comprising the inferolateral two-thirds of the amygdala receive input from association cortex of the visual, auditory, and somatosensory systems; and central nuclear group receives afferent fibers from the other two groups of nuclei. The extensive connections with sensory association cortex support the general role of the amygdala in mediating emotional responses to sensations [43].

### 6.1.4 White Matter

#### 6.1.4.1 Association and Projection Fibers

The temporal cortex is connected by association fibers with all other lobes of the cerebrum. The *arcuate fasciculus* which anteriorly ends in the frontal lobe constitutes the largest bundle. It passes above the insula and lentiform nucleus, where it is also known as the *superior longitudinal fasciculus*, and follows a curved course into the temporal lobe, thus providing two-way

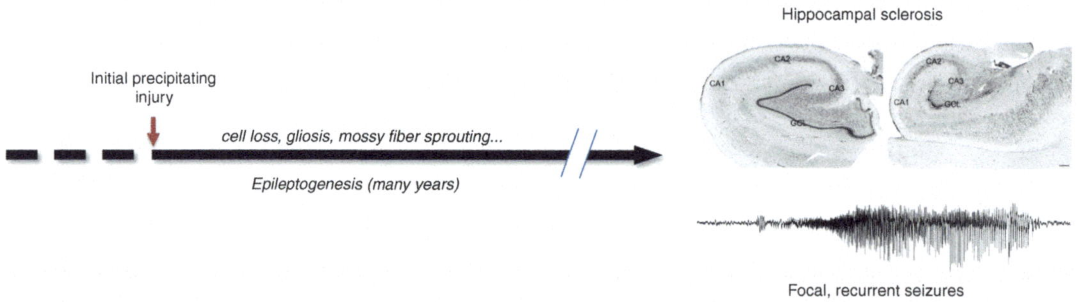


**Fig. 6.5** Simplified model of hippocampal sclerosis and epileptogenesis. An initial precipitating injury causes cell loss, gliosis, and mossy fiber sprouting in the hippocampus resulting in hippocampal sclerosis and epilepsy (with courtesy of C.A. Haas, Dep. of Neurosurgery, Freiburg)

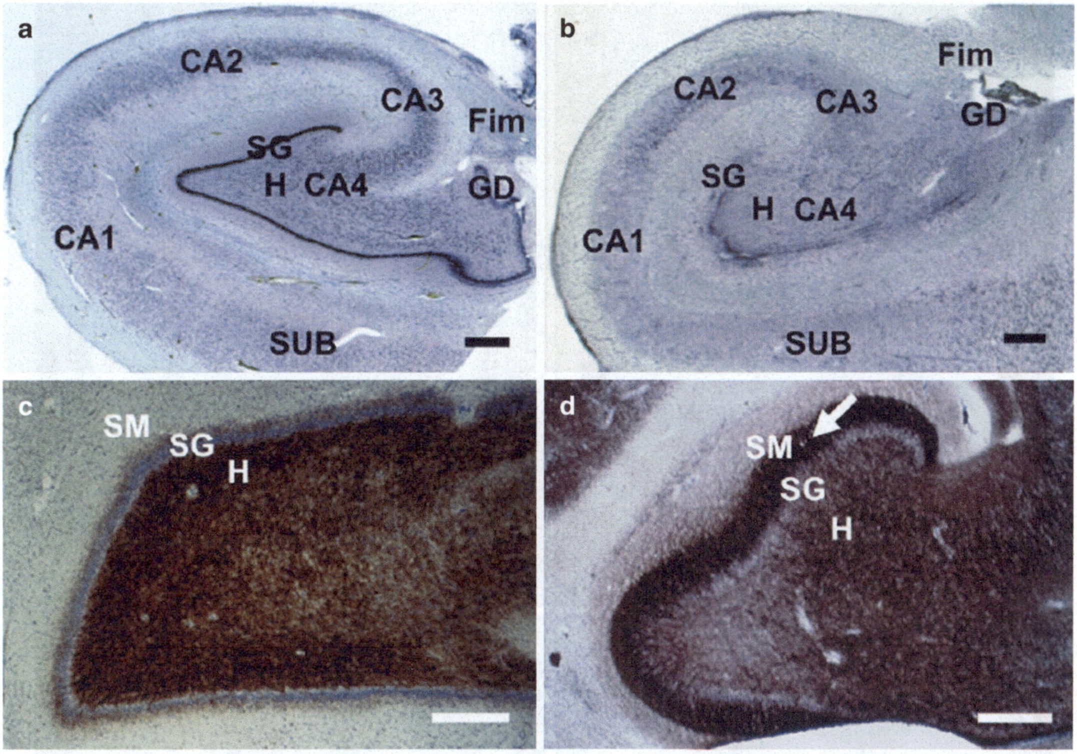


**Fig. 6.6** Sectional view of the human hippocampus with normal anatomy and hippocampal sclerosis. (**a**): Nissl staining shows normal anatomy of the hippocampus. The pyramidal cell layer is visible in the subiculum (Sub) and the subregions of the cornu ammonis (CA) from CA1 to CA4 (hilus, H). The granule cell layer (stratum granulare, SG) is dark due to high cell density. *Fim* fimbria, *GD* gyrus dentatus. (**b**) Typical hippocampal sclerosis with selective loss of pyramidal cells in CA1, CA3, and CA4, and dispersion of the granular cell layer. (**c**) Timm staining shows normal anatomy of the gyrus dentatus. Axons of the granule cells (mossy fibers; brown colored) are only found in the hilus. *SM* stratum moleculare. (**d**) Typical hippocampal sclerosis: backward sprouting of mossy fibers into the granular cell layer and molecular layer (stratum moleculare, SM) with broadened dark band above the granule cell layer (with courtesy of C. A. Haas and T.M. Freiman, Dep. of Neurosurgery, Freiburg)

communication between frontal cortex, including Broca's expressive speech area and Wernicke's receptive language area. Another frontotemporal association bundle is the hooklike *uncinate fasciculus*, which connects the prefrontal cortex to the temporal pole, the parahippocampal gyrus, and the anterior part of the insula through the limen insulae. Projection fibers afferent to the temporal cortex include those from the mesial geniculate body to the primary auditory area of the transverse temporal gyri [43].

#### 6.1.4.2 Meyer's Loop

An important pathway located in the roof of the inferior horn is *Meyer's loop* of the *geniculocalcarine tract*. This loop which noticeably differs between individuals with regard to its anterior and mesial extent carries signals arising from the upper quadrants of the contralateral visual fields to the corresponding primary visual cortex of the anterior half of the inferior bank of the calcarine sulcus. Contrarily, optic fibers representing the inferior visual field are located posteriorly of the lateral geniculate nucleus [43, 67]. Therefore, damage to Meyer's loop causes homonym superior quadrantanopia [43, 46]. Mean distance from the temporal pole to Meyer's loop measures 27±3.5 mm [68]. However, tractographic and dissection studies have shown considerable variability in the anterior extent of Meyer's loop, ranging from 20 to 50 mm from the temporal pole [69]. In addition,

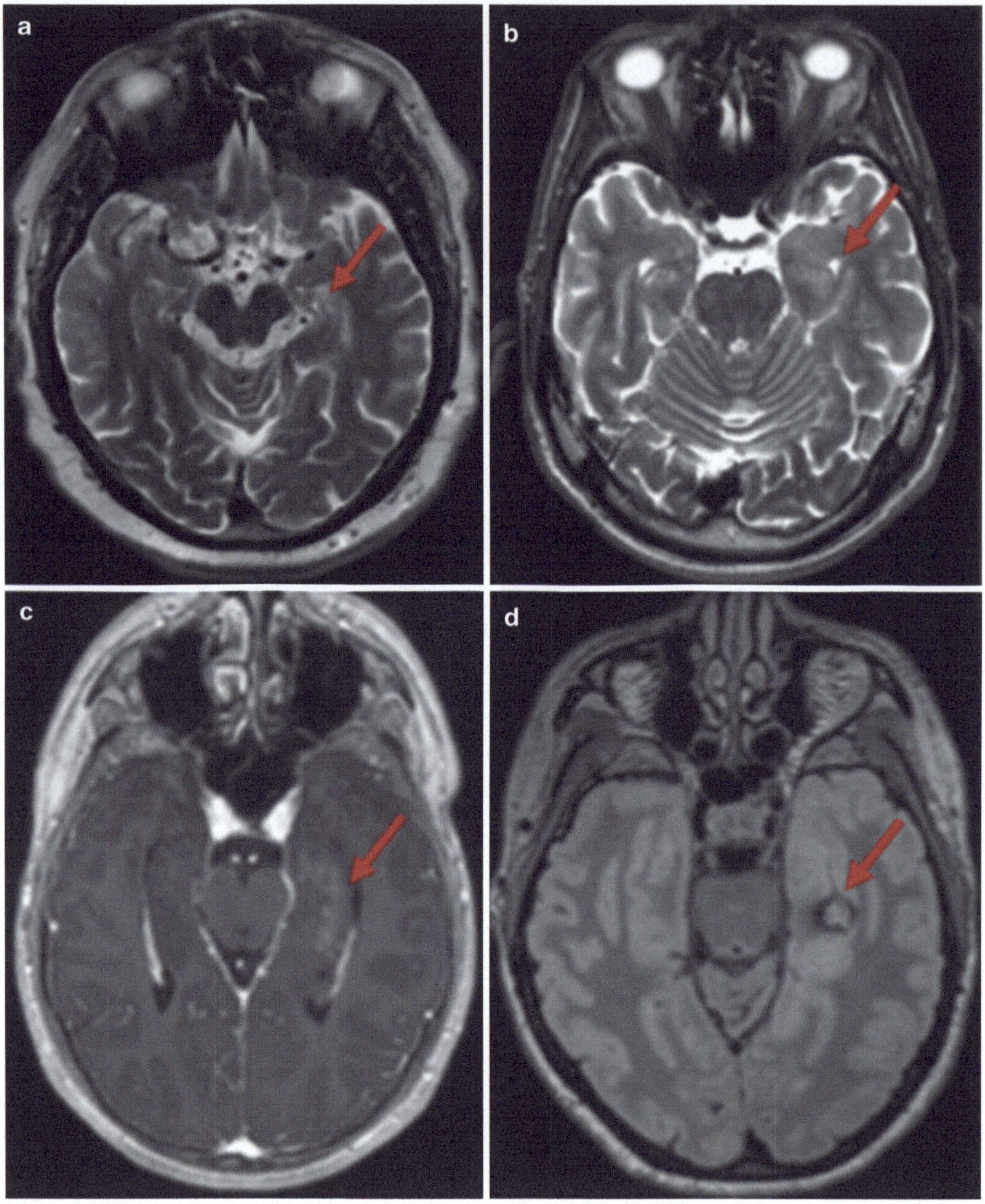


**Fig. 6.7** Common pathologies of the left hippocampal formation (red arrows). (**a**) Hippocampal sclerosis (T2w TSE); (**b**) FCD 1 (T2 TSE); (**c**) ganglioglioma (T1w MPRAGE); (**d**) cavernoma (T2w FLAIR) (with courtesy of H. Urbach, Dep. Neuroradiology, Freiburg)

it has been shown that the distance of Meyer's loop to the temporal pole is shorter in the left hemisphere as compared to the right side. Thus, Meyer's loop may particularly be endangered in left-sided temporal resections [70, 71].

Postoperative visual field deficits preclude up to 50% of patients from driving, even when seizure free [72]. As driving constitutes one of the key goals and motivations of patients to undergo surgery, preservation of visual fields is of para-

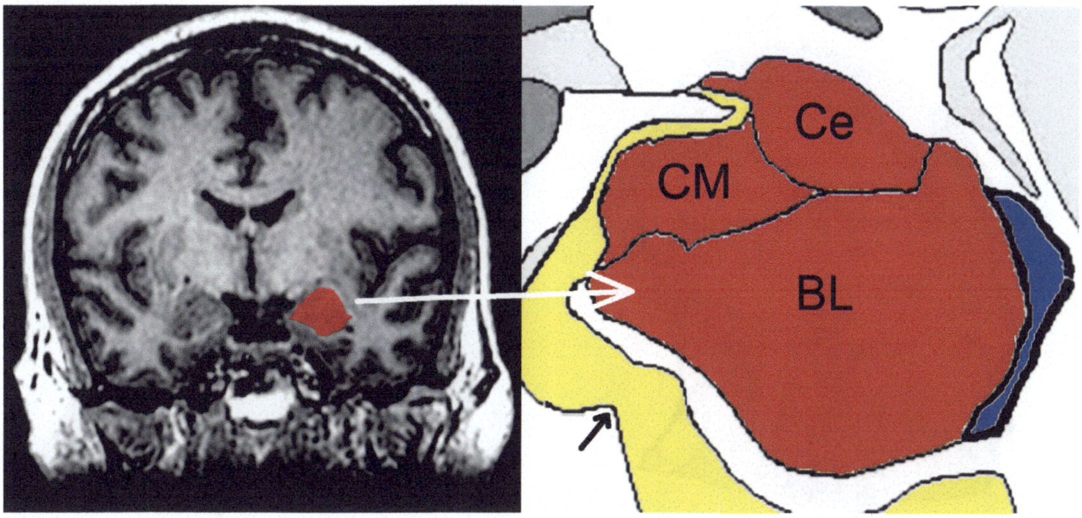


**Fig. 6.8** Left: MRI in coronal section at the level of the amygdala. Right: Illustration of the positions of the three nuclear groups of the amygdala: corticomedial (CM), basolateral (BL), and central (Ce). Red: amygdala; blue: inferior horn; yellow: uncus (mesial) and fusiform gyrus (basal); arrow: entorhinal sulcus (uncal notch) (modified from Inman et al. [66] (left) and Kiernan [43] (right), with permission)

mount importance. To get a diving license for passenger cars in Germany, a binocular vision field of 120° horizontal diameter and intact central 20° without homonymous absolute scotomata is necessary. Presenting the tractographic representation of the optic radiation into the surgical microscope has been found to reduce visual field deficits [73]. Figure 6.9 depicts the geniculocalcarine tract in a single patient. An illustration of variants of Meyer's loop is given in Fig. 6.10.

### 6.1.5 Vascular Structures

#### 6.1.5.1 Arterial Supply

The temporal lobe receives blood from both the carotid and the vertebrobasilar system. The supraclinoidal segment of the *internal carotid artery* is in close contact with the antero-mesial aspect of the uncus which is in part supplied by tiny uncal arteries. The middle cerebral artery (MCA) enters the Sylvian fissure at its basal aspect and divides after about 20 mm at the limen insulae into two (bifurcation), three (trifurcation), or even more terminal branches to supply the lateral temporal, frontal, and parietal cortex. Perforating arteries arise from the proximal trunk of the middle cerebral artery as well as from the carotid bifurcation and pass to the substantia perforata anterior to supply major parts of the striatum and the external as well as the internal capsule [43]. The anterior end of the parahippocampal gyrus, the uncus, the amygdala, and the choroid plexus in the temporal horn are supplied by the anterior choroid artery. Two to four temporal branches of the *posterior cerebral artery* supply the inferior surface of the temporal lobe. The anterior choroid artery and the p2 segment of the posterior cerebral artery are closely related to the mesial structures of the temporal lobe within the crural and the ambient cisterns, respectively. The border between these cisterns is marked by the point where the anterior choroid artery enters the temporal horn through the choroid point (see also below) [43, 46, 49]. Figure 6.11 demonstrates the arteries of the crural and ambient cisterns and their connections.

#### 6.1.5.2 Venous Drainage

The main venous drainage of the temporal lobe follows the superficial Sylvian veins and the inferior

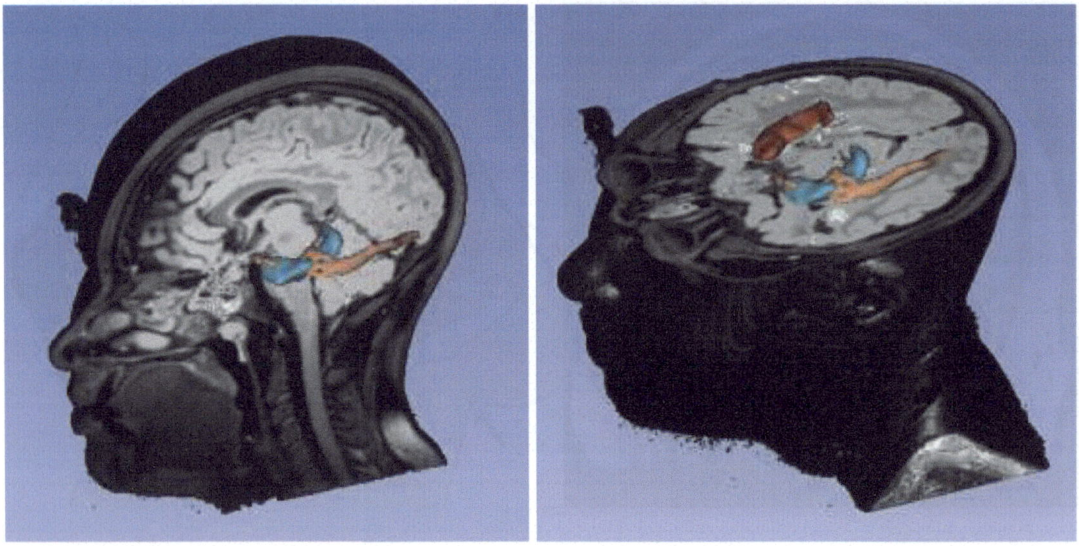

**Fig. 6.9** Depiction of the geniculocalcarine tract in a single case in sagittal (left) and axial (right) views. This subject was scanned using spin-echo for diffusion imaging and T1-MPRAGE for structure imaging. Diffusion-weighted images followed a global approach for tractography [74]. B0 image of diffusion-weighted images was co-registered to T1 image, and the corresponding Meyer's loop was transformed to T1 image space. The right and left hippocampus from LPBA-atlas [75] were inversely transformed to T1 image space which was subjected to SPM12 segmentation. Orange: Left geniculocalcarine tract and Meyer's loop; blue: left hippocampus; red: right hippocampus (with courtesy of S. Yang, Dpt. of Neuroradiology, Freiburg)

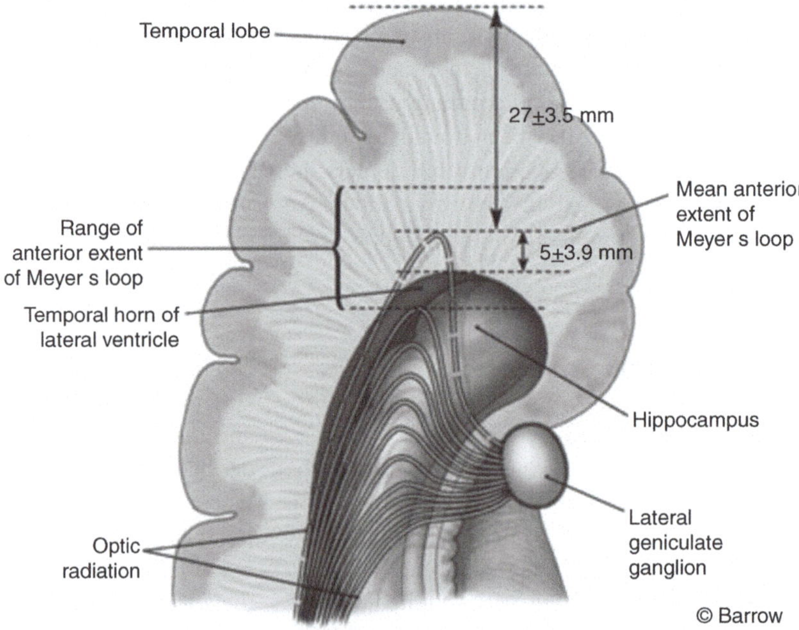


**Fig. 6.10** Axial illustration of the left anterior temporal lobe showing the variation in the course of Meyer's loop relative to the temporal horn and tip of the temporal lobe (from [68], with permission)

anastomotic vein (Labbé) connecting the superficial middle cerebral vein with the transverse sinus. *Sylvian veins* are covered by an adhesive arachnoid layer; thus they are hardly freed from the temporal lobe. Blood from interior temporal lobe, including the amygdala, hippocampus, and fornix, flows into the posterior choroid vein along the choroid plexus of the lateral ventricle joining

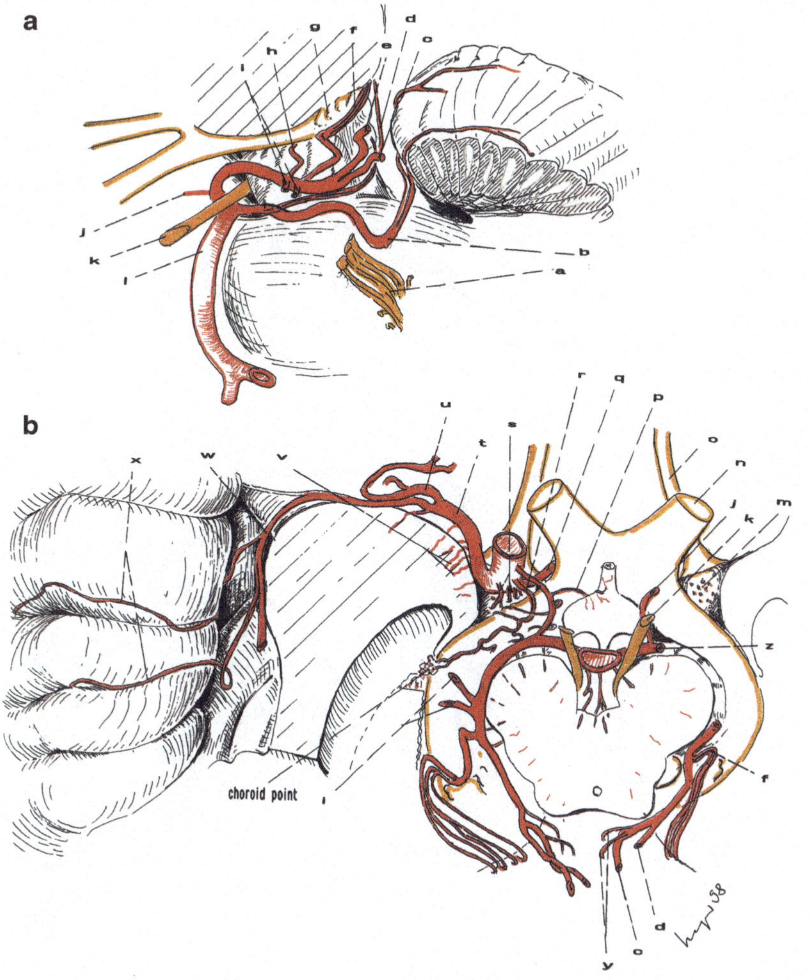


**Fig. 6.11** Arteries of the crural and ambient cisterns and their connections. (**A**) Lateral view; (**B**) axial view. N. V (a); A. cerebelli superior (b); A. calcarina (c); choroid branches (d); A. parieto-occipitalis (e); A. choroidea posterior (f); corpus geniculatum laterale (g); A. thalamogeniculata (h); Rr. temporales of A. cerebri posterior (i); A. communicans posterior (j); N. III (k); A. basilaris (l); substantia perforata anterior (m); N. II (n); N. I (o); hypothalamic branch of A. communicans posterior (p); A. cerebri anterior (q); A. choroidea anterior (r); perforating branches for substantia perforata anterior (s); A. cerebri media, main trunk (t); A. operculofrontalis ("candelabra"), main branch of A. cerebri media (u); Aa. lenticulostriate (v); A. cerebri media, distal trunk (w); parietal branches of A. cerebri media (x); Aa. splenii (y); A. cerebri posterior (z) (from Seeger [46], with permission)

the thalamostriate vein behind the interventricular foramen to form the internal cerebral vein. In the depth of the Sylvian fissure, a nearly constant small vein bridges the Sylvian fissure between the frontal lobe and the uncus connecting the inferior tip vein, the deep Sylvian veins, the veins in the roof of the inferior horn and of the choroid plexus, and the basal cisternal veins to a venous network that continues in a singular or network-formed *V. basalis (Rosenthal)* (Fig. 6.12). The choroid point is defined as the anterior end of choroid plexus of the inferior horn. This area represents the origin of V. basalis Rosenthal and the end of the anterior choroid artery with its plexus branches. Location of the choroid point in anterior-posterior direction is quite variable (Fig. 6.13) ([46, 47]; Kienan 2012).

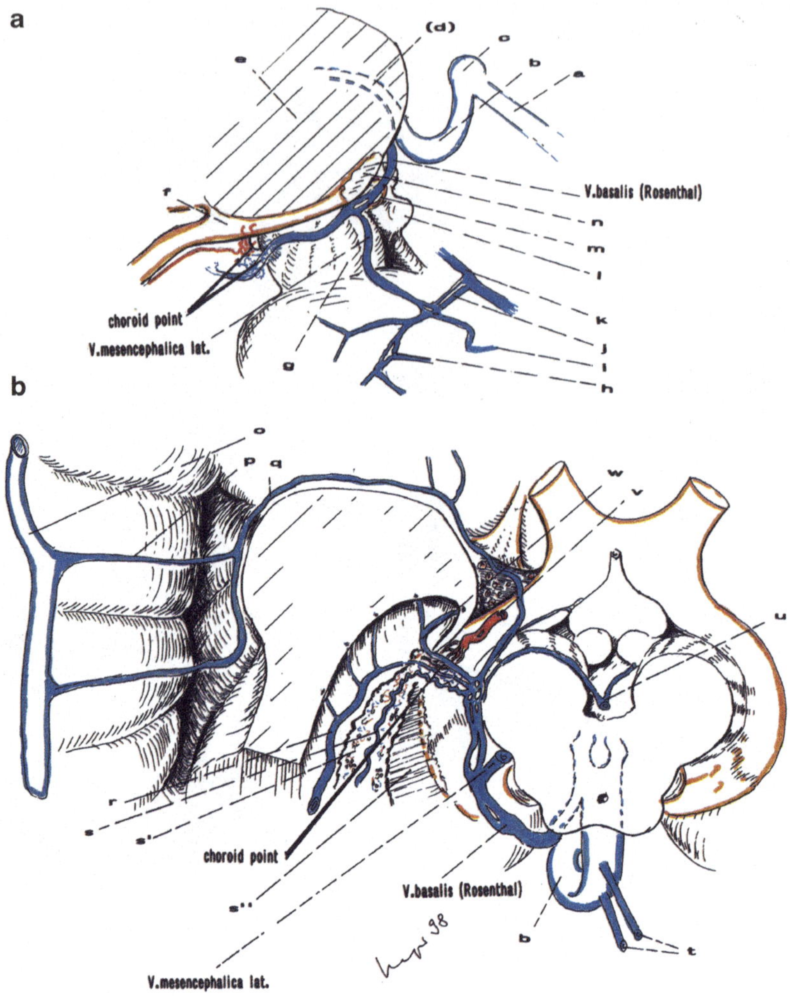


**Fig. 6.12** Veins of crural and ambient cisterns and their connections. (**A**) Lateral view; (**B**) axial view. Sinus rectus (a); V. magna Galeni (b); galenic point (c); V. cerebri interna, projection (d); thalamus (e); tractus opticus (f); crus cerebri (g); pontine vein (h); cerebellar vein (i); V. petrosa superior (k); colliculus inferior (l); corpus geniculatum mediale (m); corpus geniculatum laterale (n); superficial Sylvian vein (o); connecting vein (p); deep Sylvian vein (q); inferior ventricular vein (r); plexus vein (s); plexus choroideus (s´); taenia choroidea (s´´); cerebellar veins (t); V. interpeduncularis (u); A. choroidea anterior (v); inferior tip vein (w) (from Seeger [46], with permission)

## 6.2 Resection Strategies

The primary surgical goal is to completely resect the epileptogenic zone. Therefore, it is the major task of presurgical work-up to distinguish between a lateral cortical, a mesiotemporal, and a combined lateral and mesial epileptogenic zone, if necessary by means of long-term invasive recordings with subdural and/or depth electrodes, while the role of intraoperative electrocorticography (ECoG) is largely controversial [76, 77]. Incomplete resection of the epileptogenic zone strongly correlates with seizure recurrence in the long term [78–82]. On the other hand, extending the resection to intact medial temporal structures carries the risk of neuropsychological deterioration. It should be noted that dual pathology, that means the combination of hippocampal sclerosis (HS) with an extrahippocampal pathology, does not confer an inferior outcome compared to HS alone, provided that complete resection of the epileptogenic zone is achieved [41, 81].

Based on the results of presurgical evaluation, different options for surgical treatment of temporal lobe epilepsy (TLE) are available: (1) anterior temporal lobectomy (ATL), (2) keyhole (KH) approach to mesiotemporal structures, (3) extended lesionectomy (ELE), and (4) selective amygdalohippocampectomy (SAHE). For many decades, ATL combining extensive resection of the lateral cortex as well as of amygdala and hip-

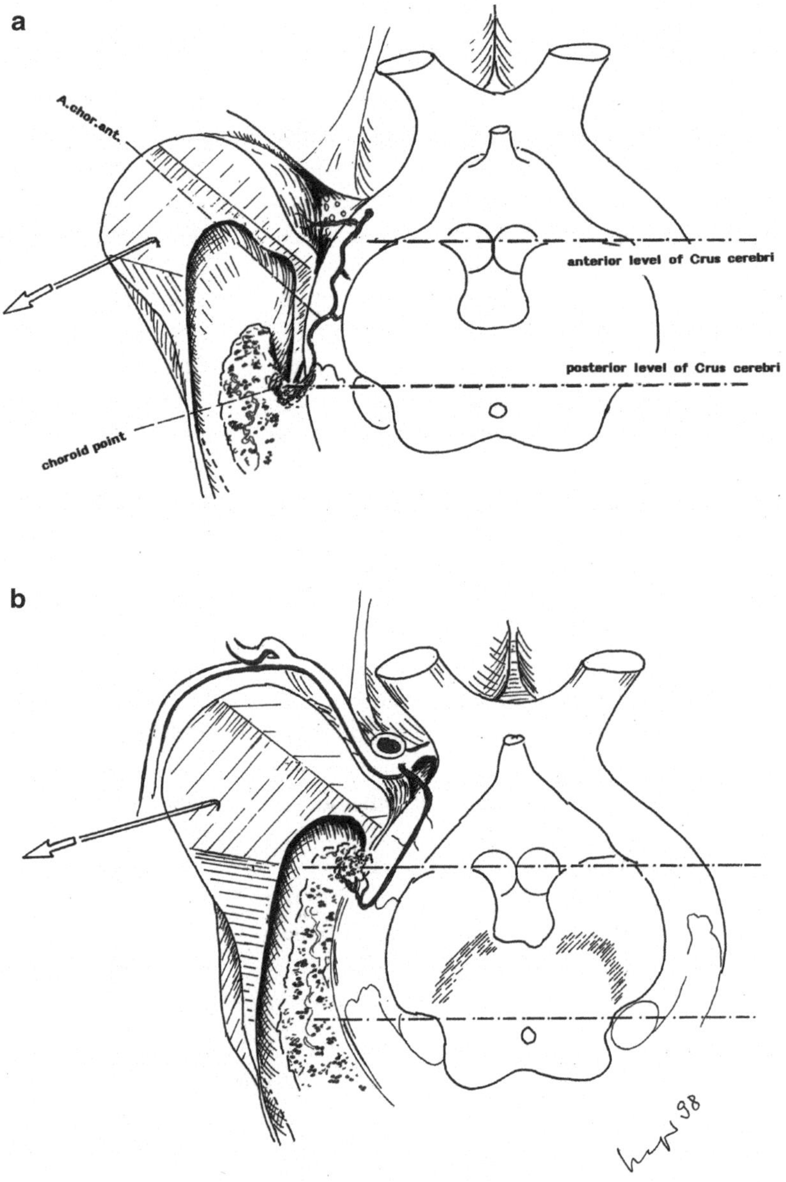


**Fig. 6.13** Variants of the choroid point defined as the anterior end of plexus choroideus of the inferior horn representing the origin of V. basalis Rosenthal and the end of A. choroidea anterior with its plexus branches. (**a**) Elongation of the inferior horn and posterior displacement of the choroid point. (**b**) Anterior location of the choroid point. Both variants (**a** and **b**) constitute common findings (from Seeger [46], with permission)

pocampal formation represented the gold standard for temporal procedures [1, 83, 84]. Advances in neuroimaging as well as in electrophysiological work-up allowed a more precise localization of the epileptogenic focus [15, 85–89]. This led to a better understanding of the pathophysiology of mesiotemporal lobe epilepsy (MTLE) as an own entity and a more precise selection of surgical candidates opening the option for more selective resections [26, 90–93]. Thus, ATL has been modified sparing parts of the neocortex [94], and eventually, SAHE has been introduced based on the hypothesis that cognitive functions may be better by preserving the temporal neocortex [95–99] while providing similar favorable epileptological results compared to ATL.

### 6.2.1 Anterior Temporal Lobectomy (ATL)

The classical procedure is standard anterior temporal lobectomy (ATL), frequently called anterior two-thirds lobectomy, which usually is combined with amygdalohippocampectomy (AHE). This procedure has been introduced in the early area of epilepsy surgery [1, 5, 9, 10], when tools for presurgical evaluation were limited. However also today, ATL with AHE represents the most frequently used procedure for TLE in many centers, since one can achieve good seizure results without the necessity to distinguish between purely mesial TLE, lateral neocortical TLE, and TLE affecting mesial and lateral structures. Moreover, this procedure provides an excellent overview on the temporal anatomy and can be recommended for any group starting with epilepsy surgery. Differences in ATL with AHE refer to the extent of lateral and mesial resection. Some surgeons leave main parts of the superior temporal gyrus intact so that cortical resection comprises only the middle and inferior temporal gyrus.

**Surgical Steps (Figs. 6.14 and 6.15)**

- The patient is positioned supine with the shoulder elevated. The head is turned (around 60°), and the vertex is lowered. Temporal craniotomy is performed exposing at least the Sylvian fissure and the superior and middle temporal gyri.
- After opening the dura, the distance from the temporal pool is measured along the first temporal gyrus which is incised at a length of 5.0 cm on the nondominant and 4.5 cm on the dominant hemisphere, respectively. At the posterior resection margin, incision curves inferiorly across the middle to the inferior temporal gyrus which is incised at a length of 5.5 cm (nondominant hemisphere) and 5 cm (dominant hemisphere).
- The superior temporal gyrus is dissected subpially along the Sylvian fissure with an ultrasound aspirator, and dissection is continued down to the floor of the middle fossa in a plane just lateral to the inferior horn. Thus, the major part of the lateral temporal lobe can be removed en bloc.
- Dissection plane is continuously shifted medially until the inferior horn is reached. The inferior horn is widely opened sparing its roof in order to avoid visual field deficits as far as possible. Now, the choroid plexus, the amygdala, and the hippocampal body are identified.
- The temporal pole is removed, and the uncus is emptied. Thus, the anterior circumference of the brainstem with the third nerve, the anterior communicating artery, the posterior cerebral artery, the anterior choroid artery, and the vein of Rosenthal covered by arachnoid are exposed.
- The bulging parts of the amygdala are removed. The hippocampal formation is disconnected laterally and mobilized medially to the vessels of the hippocampal sulcus. The disconnection of the hippocampus is continued at its mesial and anterior aspects. Posterior disconnection of the hippocampal formation is done at the length of 25–35 mm. Care is taken to transect the radial arteries of the hippocampal sulcus just at the hippocampal site and before the specimen is taken out en bloc.
- If requested, residual parts of the hippocampal formation can now be resected to the level of the colliculi, thus completely exposing the circumference of the brainstem. In addition, resection of the amygdala just mesially to the

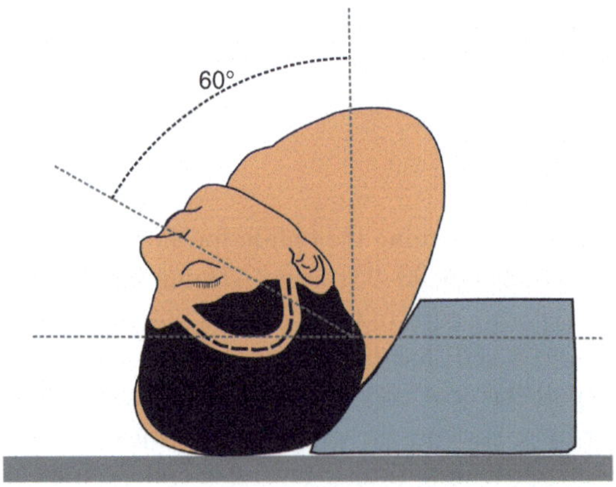


**Fig. 6.14** Position of the patient for ATL. The shoulder is elevated, and the head is turned (around 60°) with the vertex lowered

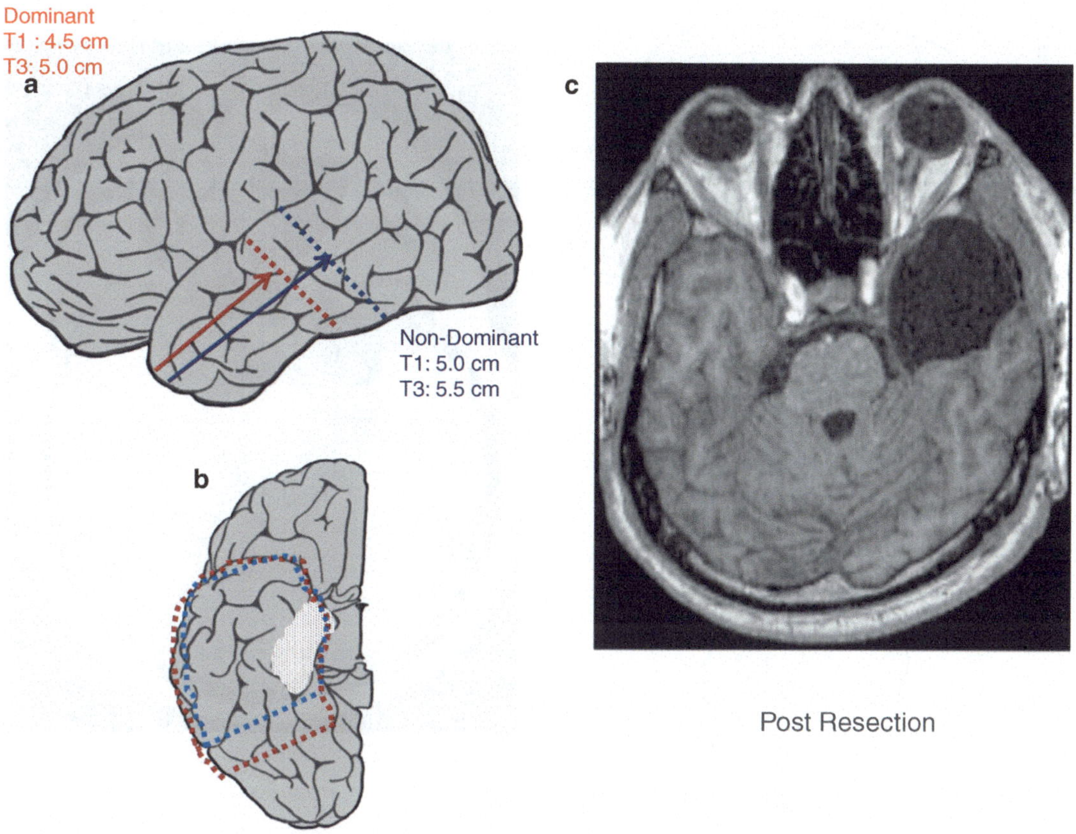


**Fig. 6.15** Anterior temporal lobectomy (ATL). Schematic representation of resection in sagittal (**a**) and axial (**b**) views including measures in the dominant and nondominant temporal lobe. (**c**) Result of resection on postoperative MRI in a single case (axial view)

tip of the plexus is completed. Hemostasis is accomplished by oxidized cellulose gauze and irrigation.

A special aspect of classical ATL refers to the handling of the vein of Labbé. Location of this vein is highly variable. In approximately 60% of cases, the vein is located in the middle temporal area, in 30% posterior, and in 10% more anterior [100]. In principle, it is advisable to preserve the vein of Labbé whenever possible to prevent edema or hemorrhagic infarction. However, with its anterior location, the resection area may extend dorsally to the vein. It has been shown that the vein of Labbé can be included in the resection in these cases without any harm [101].

### 6.2.2 Keyhole (KH) Approach

Based on the hypothesis that by minimizing the extent of lateral resection one could possibly reduce cognitive impairment, combined temporal pole and mesial resection has been introduced [94]. This procedure has been termed the keyhole (KH) approach to mesial structures, anterior one-third lobectomy combined with amygdalohippocampectomy, or anteromesial temporal lobectomy. The rationale of this procedure is to preserve major parts of the lateral temporal neocortex while providing sufficient access to mesiotemporal structures. It can also be used if a lesion in the pole area has to be removed along with mesial structures.

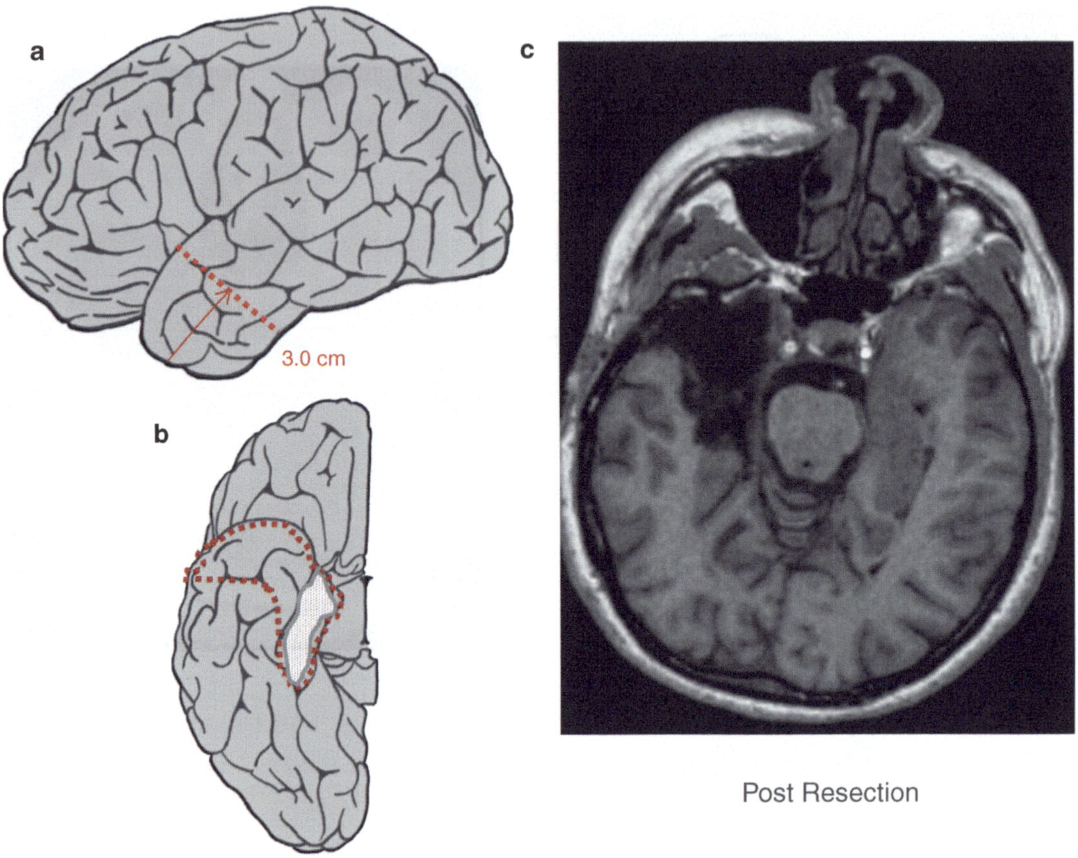


**Fig. 6.16** Keyhole (KH) approach to the mesiotemporal area. Schematic representation of resection in sagittal (**a**) and axial (**b**) views including measures. (**c**) Result of resection on postoperative MRI in a single case (axial view)

**Surgical Steps (Fig. 6.16)**

- The patient is positioned supine with elevated shoulder. It is important to turn the head only to 45° and to lower the vertex more as compared to ATL in order to get optimal access to temporomesial structures. Temporal craniotomy must almost reach the pole area.
- Cortical incision is made in the superior temporal gyrus 3–3.5 cm from the tip. At the posterior margin, incision curves inferiorly and slightly posteriorly across the middle to the inferior temporal gyrus.
- The anterior part of the superior temporal gyrus is dissected subpially with an ultrasound aspirator, and dissection is continued down to the floor of the middle fossa in a plane just lateral to the tip of the inferior horn. Thus, the anterior part of the lateral temporal lobe can be removed en bloc.
- Dissection plane is continuously shifted medially and posteriorly until the tip of the inferior horn is opened. Exposure of the inferior horn is only widened to its middle aspect. The choroid plexus, the amygdala, and the hippocampal body are identified.
- Removal of uncus and dissection of mesial structures is followed as described above.

Since major retraction of lateral temporal lobe has to be avoided, the access to the inferior horn of the lateral ventricle is limited. However, by positioning the head as described and gradually lowering the vertex during the procedure the more mesial and dorsal structures are dissected,

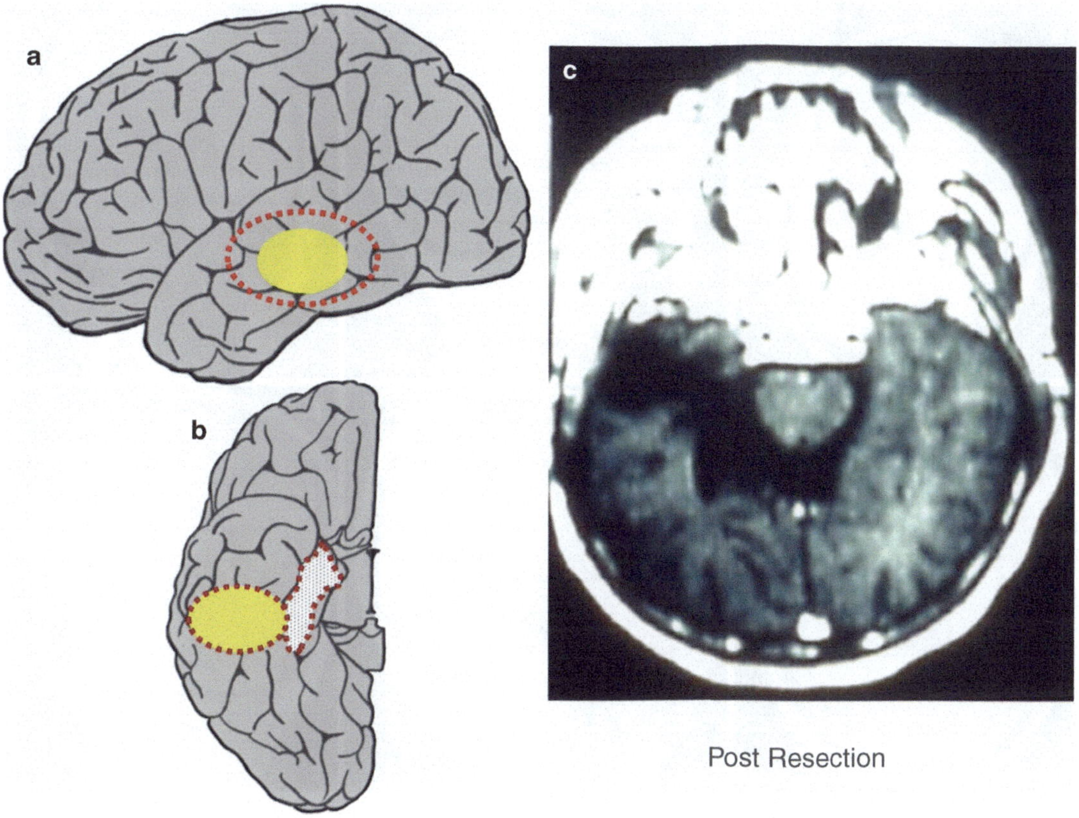


**Fig. 6.17** Extended lesionectomy (ELE) combined with amygdalohippocampectomy (AHE). Schematic representation of resection in lateral (**a**) and axial (**b**) views. (**c**) Result of resection on postoperative MRI in a single case (axial view)

the complete hippocampal formation can be visualized and resected as posteriorly as intended.

## 6.2.3 Extended Lesionectomy (ELE)

Extended lesionectomy (ELE) is applied for circumscribed neocortical lesions [102]. These lesions may include glial or glioneuronal tumors, cortical dysplasias, or vascular malformations. Experience has shown that lesionectomy alone may not be sufficient to achieve seizure control [103, 104]. Thus, a rim of 0.5–1.0 cm intact cortex around the lesion may additionally be removed (extended lesionectomy; see also Chap. 9). If the lesion attaches to amygdala or hippocampus, the bordering part of mesial structures may also be included in the resection. In other cases with lesions largely involving mesiotemporal area, extended lesionectomy can be combined with amygdalohippocampectomy.

**Surgical Steps (Figs. 6.17 and 6.18)**

- The patient is positioned, and craniotomy is performed according to the location of the lesion and the additional ictogenic areas to be resected.
- In a first step, the neocortical lesion is completely removed (lesionectomy). This is followed by resection of an intact margin of 0.5–1.0 cm around the borders of the lesion (extended lesionectomy). The white matter in the core of the temporal lobe can be left behind. Major arterial branches crossing the resection area are isolated and spared, similarly larger veins.
- If required, mesiotemporal structures can additionally be removed in part or completely as described above.

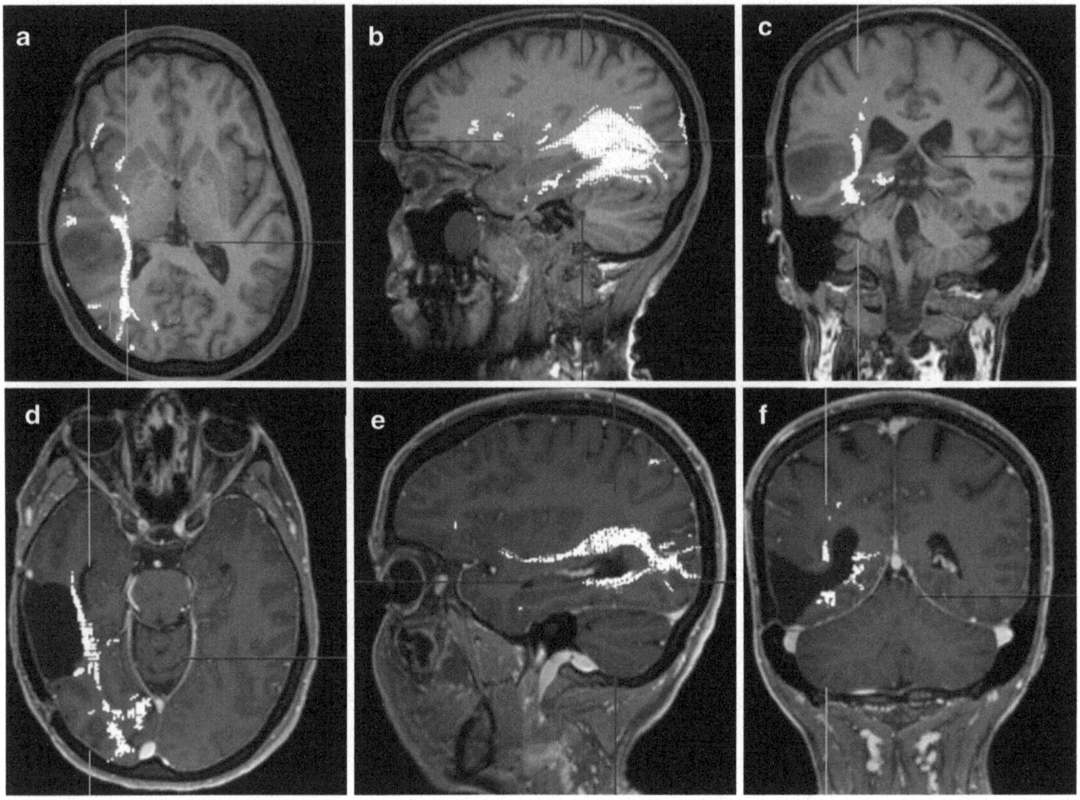


**Fig. 6.18** Extended lesionectomy (ELE) sparing temporomesial structures. 42-Year-old female patient with epilepsy and a slightly contrast-enhancing tumor right temporodorsal (astrocytoma WHO grade III). Upper sequence: Preoperative T1-weighted MRI with fiber tracking of optic pathways in axial (**a**), sagittal (**b**), and coronal (**c**) views. The tumor reaches optic pathways which are slightly bulged (**a** and **c**). Lower sequence: Postoperative MRI (**d–f**) demonstrates complete removal of the MR-visible tumor with intact optic pathways. Note that the bulge of optic pathways has disappeared (**d**). Postoperatively, visual fields remained completely intact

### 6.2.4 Selective Amygdalohippocampectomy (SAHE)

Selective amygdalohippocampectomy (SAHE) aims at the removal of mesial structures—amygdala, hippocampus, and parahippocampal gyrus—sparing the neocortex. Based on the principle that resection should be as radical as necessary, yet at the same time as selective as possible, indications for SAHE include patients with clear evidence of mesial temporal lobe seizure foci without involvement of lateral structures. Different approaches to selectively remove the epileptogenic mesiotemporal structures are available (Fig. 6.19).

#### 6.2.4.1 Transcortical/Transsulcal Approach

In 1958, Niemeyer [97] introduced the transcortical approach through an incision in the middle temporal gyrus (T2), providing access to the temporal horn. Rougier et al. [105] and Olivier et al. [106] reached the inferior horn by a transsulcal approach between the anterior parts of first and the second temporal gyri (T1/T2). Olivier [107] described a modification of Niemeyer's technique opening the temporal horn by passing through the anterior part of the superior temporal gyrus (T1). However, Olivier later reverted to the original Niemeyer approach. Sarmento et al. 108] proposed a minimally invasive approach via an

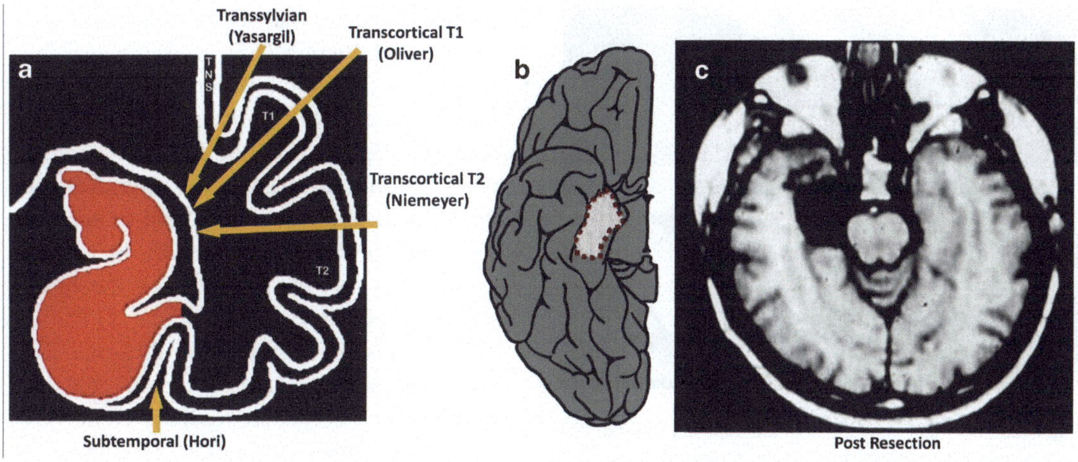


**Fig. 6.19** Selective amygdalohippocampectomy (SAHE). (**a**) Schematic illustration of different approaches for SAHE in coronal view. (**b**) Schematic illustration of amygdalohippocampectomy in axial view. (**c**) Result of resection using the transsylvian route on postoperative MRI in a single case (axial view)

enlarged burr hole through the middle temporal gyrus. Shimizu et al. [109] suggested an approach to the temporal horn through the inferior temporal gyrus (T3). A similar but minimalistic approach through the inferior temporal gyrus by a 2 × 3 cm trephine craniotomy above the zygoma has been described by Duckworth et al. [110]. It should be noted that the lateral transcortical/transsulcal approaches unavoidably produce injury to the temporal neocortex. Moreover, the disadvantage of the approaches through or between T1 and T2 is the necessity to dissect in close vicinity to optic radiation (Meyer's loop) which is located in the roof of the inferior horn.

#### 6.2.4.2 Transsylvian Approach

The transsylvian approach was pioneered by Wieser and Yasargil [99] and Yasargil et al. [111]. This approach took advantage of previous refinements in aneurysm surgery using the so-called pterional (i.e., frontotemporal) approach. Mayanagi [112] proposed the transsylvian "en bloc" resection which is very similar to Yasargil's technique, but adds resection of the uncus to amygdalohippocampectomy. With the transsylvian approach, the temporal neocortex is completely spared. However, the temporal stem and in particular the uncinate fascicle at the limen insulae have partly to be disconnected. The transsylvian approach provides an excellent overview on anteriorly located temporomesial structures and pathologies, while dissection of the posterior part of the hippocampal formation is more difficult. Moreover, the disadvantage of this approach is the necessity to dissect the Sylvian vessels with the risk of vascular infarcts [113]. It must be emphasized that the transsylvian approach is extremely confined and the space for dissection is limited. Considerable microsurgical experience and familiarity with the regional anatomy are required to safely perform this procedure, and only a few larger series on transsylvian SAHE are available [39, 99, 111, 114], while most studies present a limited number of cases [115–118].

#### 6.2.4.3 Subtemporal Approach

Hori et al. [95] described the subtemporal approach through the fusiform gyrus also named as T4. The primary rationale for this approach as also advocated by others [119] is to spare the lateral temporal neocortex (T1–T3), to avoid incision of the temporal stem, and to minimize visual field deficits. The presumed advantage of this basal approach for language function could not be supported [118]. The disadvantages of the subtemporal approach include retraction of the temporal lobe and danger for basal veins, especially the vein of

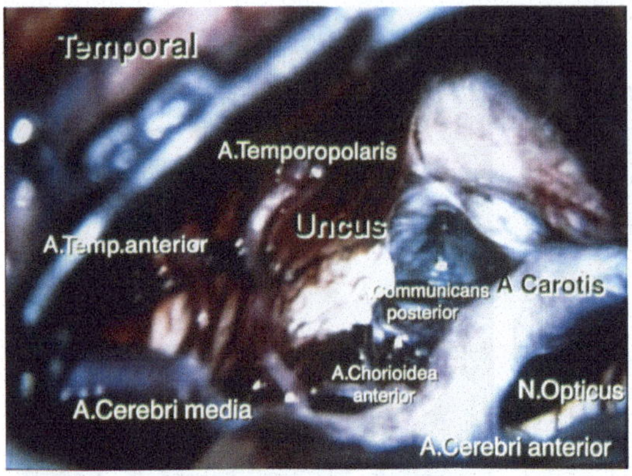


**Fig. 6.20** Surgical view through the exposed Sylvian fissure of the left temporal lobe to the temporal stem. The temporal stem (white) has been incised sparing major vessels. It is important to cut minor vessels of the temporal stem at its superior-lateral, i.e., temporal aspect, and to push them downward and mesially along with the arachnoid to expose the temporal stem

Labbé. Moreover, surgical orientation on where to enter the temporal lobe at its inferior surface is rather unclear and depends to a major part on the venous architecture [120]. While resection of the anterior aspects of temporomesial structures, e.g., uncus and amygdala, is somewhat difficult, the subtemporal approach provides an excellent overview on the posterior temporomesial area.

**Surgical Steps: Transsylvian SAHE (Figs. 6.20 and 6.21)**

- The patient is positioned supine with the shoulder elevated. The head is turned to 30–45°, and the vertex is lowered. A pterional (i.e., frontotemporal) craniotomy centered over the Sylvian fissure is performed.
- After opening of the dura, the Sylvian fissure is dissected. Splitting of the arachnoid starts at the frontal aspect of the superficial veins close to pars orbitalis of the inferior frontal gyrus. Dissection of the Sylvian fissure extends from the carotid bifurcation to about 2 cm distally to the bi- or trifurcation of the middle cerebral artery, thus exposing the limen insulae with the inferior circular sulcus and the anterior third of the insular cortex. Papaverine is applied to the Sylvian vessels to prevent vasospasm and ischemia.
- Incision of the temporal stem is made sparing major vessels. The inferior horn which is reached after 12–15 mm is widely opened, thus exposing the plexus, the amygdala, and the hippocampus. It is important to approach the ventricle more basolaterally in order to avoid to bypass the ventricle on the medial side entering the basal ganglia.
- The uncus is emptied with the ultrasonic aspirator. The bulging parts of the amygdala and the entorhinal cortex are resected. Removal of the hippocampal formation is similar as described above.

**Surgical Steps: Transcortical SAHE**

- The position of the head is similar to that used for anterior temporal lobectomy. Since a smaller craniotomy is needed, only a linear or slightly curved incision in front of the tragus may be performed. Neuronavigation is helpful to plan the craniotomy centered over the middle temporal gyrus as well as to plan the trajectory to the ventricle.
- The middle temporal gyrus is incised at a length of 2–3 cm. While dissecting in mesial direction, it is important to avoid damage to the roof of the ventricle endangering the optic radiation. In order to optimize overview, cortical incision may be extended anteriorly.
- Removal of uncus, amygdala, and hippocampal formation is similar as mentioned above, always leaving the mesial arachnoid intact.

**Surgical Steps: Subtemporal SAHE (Fig. 6.22)**

- The patient is placed in the lateral position. It is very important to significantly lower the vertex and to administer mannitol; thus the temporal lobe is relaxed and sinks back by gravity. Skin incision may be curvilinear temporal, linear or slightly curved in front of the tragus, or rectangular at the temporal base. A basal craniotomy over the inferior temporal gyrus (5 × 3 cm) is done. Opened mastoid cells are closed with wax.
- The temporal base is exposed and the venous anatomy is appreciated. It is important to plan

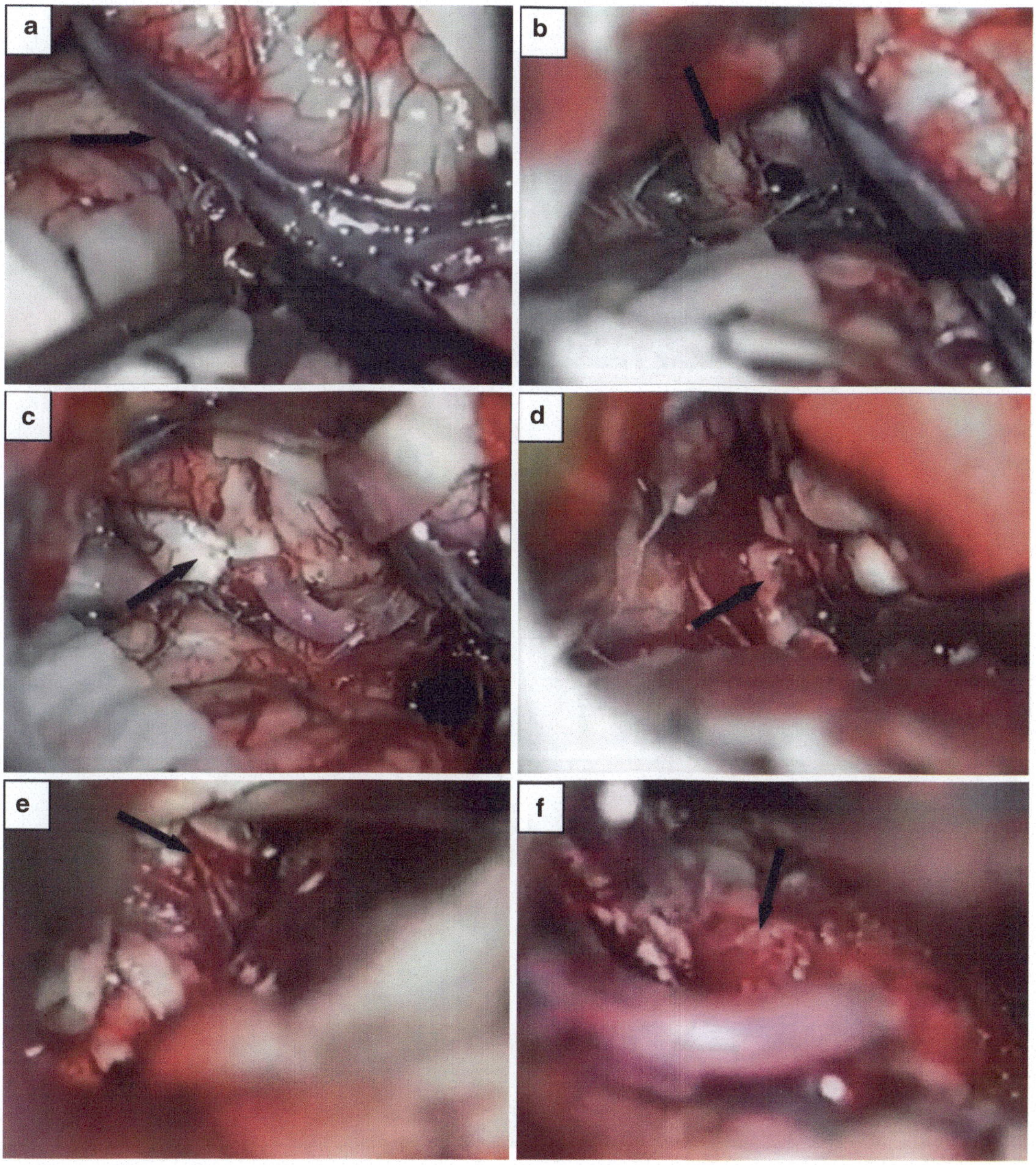

**Fig. 6.21** Surgical steps of transsylvian SAHE demonstrated from intraoperative view (right temporal lobe): (**a**) Starting dissection of the Sylvian fissure; (**b**) the right optic nerve is visible (arrow); (**c**) dissection of the Sylvian fissure is completed, and the temporal stem is visualized (arrow); (**d**) blunt dissection of the hippocampus (arrow); (**e**) vessels of the hippocampus (hippocampal sulcus) are coagulated and divided (arrow); (**f**) the hippocampus has been removed en bloc, thus exposing the circumference of the brainstem (arrow)

the entry into the ventricle depending on the individual venous architecture avoiding to cut major basal veins. Thus, a transcortical approach through the fusiform gyrus, a transsulcal approach through the collateral sulcus, or even a narrow transcortical tunnel through the inferior temporal gyrus may be used. All these approaches aim to enter the ventricle at its basolateral aspect. The challenge is to find the ventricle lumen preserving major veins and

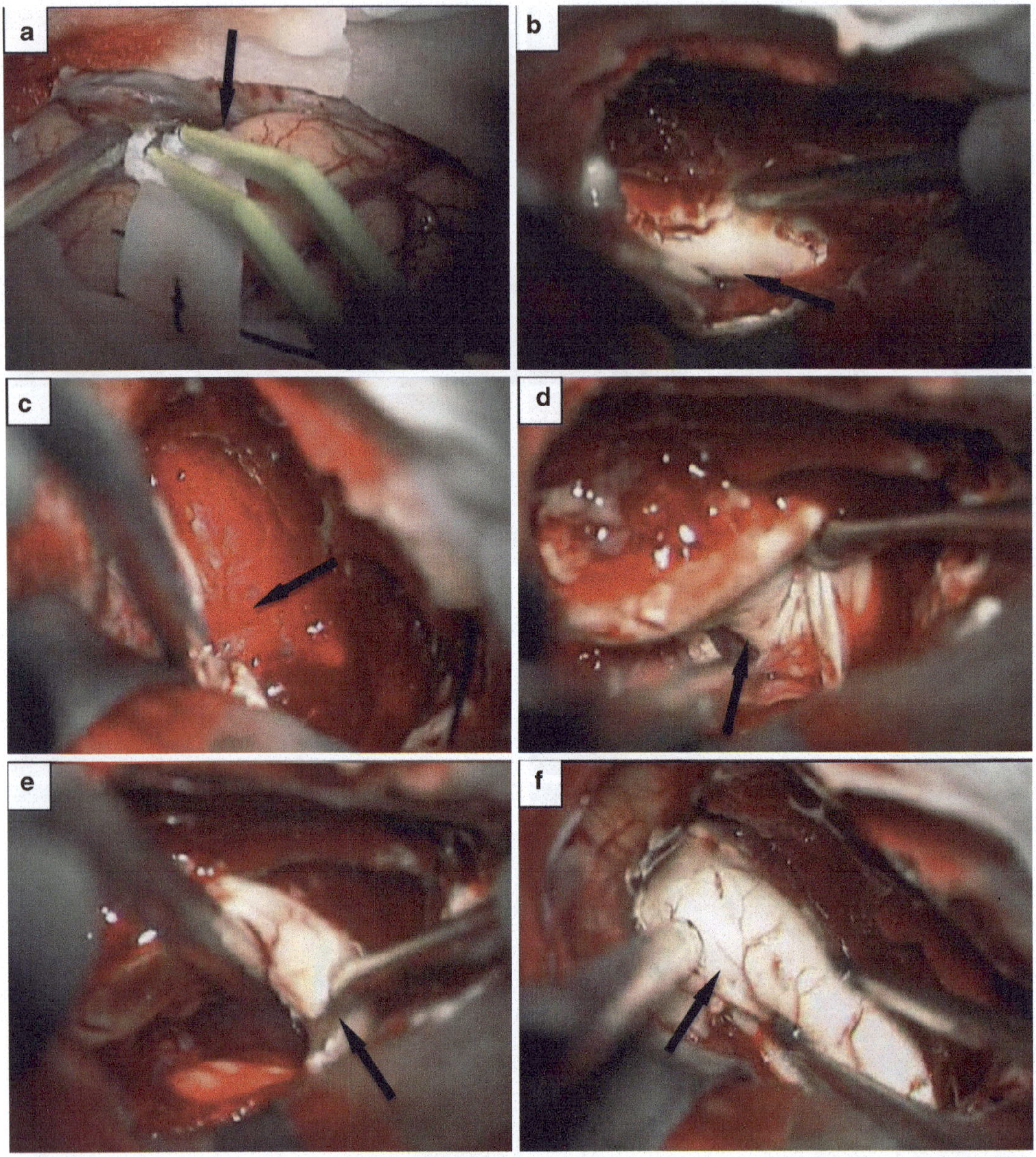


**Fig. 6.22** Surgical steps of subtemporal SAHE demonstrated from intraoperative view (right temporal lobe): (**a**) Dissection of the temporal base (arrow); (**b**) the inferior horn is opened, and the hippocampus is exposed (arrow); (**c**) lateral dissection of the hippocampus, the arachnoid of the ambient cistern is visualized (arrow); (**d**) mesial dissection of the hippocampus (arrow); (**e**) posterior disconnection of the hippocampus (arrow); (**f**) the hippocampus is being removed en bloc (arrow)

keeping temporal lobe retraction within limits. Neuronavigation may be useful for this step.

- Once the ventricle is entered, the cortical incision may be extended providing a good overview on mesial structures. Removal of uncus, amygdala, and hippocampal formation is performed similar to the description mentioned above.

Pitskhelauri et al. [121] suggested to perform subtemporal SAHE via a burr hole trephination.

The burr hole placed above the posterior part of the zygoma is cone shaped with a superficial diameter of 14 mm and an inner diameter of 18 mm [121].

## 6.3 Results

### 6.3.1 Seizure Outcome

#### 6.3.1.1 Randomized Controlled Trials (RCTs)

There are seven RCTs assessing seizure outcome after temporal resections [122–129]. In the trials of Wiebe et al. [128] and Engel et al. (2011), 80 and 38 patients, respectively, were randomized to either surgery or continued medical therapy. In a technical study, Wyler et al. [129] randomized 70 patients to partial hippocampectomy (to the level of the cerebral peduncle) or to total hippocampectomy (to the level of the superior colliculus). In another randomized study comprising 207 patients, Schramm et al. [125, 126] assigned 104 patients to a 2.5 cm and 103 patients to a 3.5 cm hippocampus and parahippocampus resection. A further technical study performed by Hermann et al. [123] randomized 30 patients with TLE to resection versus sparing of the first temporal gyrus. In the fourth technical study reported by Lutz et al. [124], 80 patients were randomized to receive SAHE by the transsylvian and the transcortical route, respectively. The fifth technical study provided by Vogt et al. [127] randomized 47 patients for subtemporal versus transsylvian SAHE (for results of RCTs, see below).

#### 6.3.1.2 ATL

Analyzing 80 patients, Wiebe et al. [128] noted in a RCT seizure freedom in 58% of patients with surgery and 8% with medical therapy at 1-year follow-up. The RCT of Engel et al. [122] showed seizure freedom in 73% (11 of 15 individuals) after surgery, but in none of 23 cases with medical therapy at 2-year follow-up. Both RCTs clearly demonstrate superiority of surgery compared to continued medical therapy in terms of seizure outcome. A RCT of 30 patients comparing resection versus sparing of the first temporal gyrus did not show any differences in seizure outcome between both groups [123].

In 1993, Engel collecting data on 3579 patients who underwent ATL reported seizure freedom in 68% of the cases, and 24% were improved [130]. A review of studies with 1–5-year follow-up demonstrated seizure freedom in 63.2% of cases [130]. Téllez-Zenteno et al. [131] found in a meta-analysis of 40 studies including 3895 patients seizure freedom in 66% of temporal resections. Evaluating systematic reviews and meta-analyses, multicenter studies, and large single-center studies, Jobst and Cascino [132] found seizure freedom rates between 34% and 76% after surgery. The median of seizure-free outcome across all studies was 62.5% [132].

Observational studies showed seizure freedom after ATL in 60–80%, in the mean around 70% of patients [32–37]. A two-thirds rate of seizure freedom following ATL has been reported by others [40, 133–139].

#### 6.3.1.3 Selective Resections

Following transsylvian SAHE, seizure freedom (Engel I) rates between 60% and 80% have been shown in observational studies [31, 38, 40–42]. In the Freiburg series comprising 162 consecutive transsylvian SAHE procedures, seizure freedom (Engel I) was achieved in 73.1% of patients at 1 year and in 68.0% at a mean observation time of 59 months [114].

Lutz et al. [124] compared in a RCT the transsylvian (41 patients) with the transcortical (39 patients) route. No differences were found at 1-year follow-up with 77% seizure-free patients using the transcortical and 73% seizure-free cases using the transsylvian route. Comparing subtemporal versus transsylvian SAHE, the RCT of Vogt et al. [127] showed no significant differences: 59% of individuals were seizure free after subtemporal and 64% after transsylvian SAHE. Similarly, no significant differences in seizure outcome were observed in observational studies comparing transsylvian with subtemporal SAHE [39] and the transsylvian with the transcortical [140] route.

#### 6.3.1.4 ATL/Selective Resections

Numerous studies addressing the question, whether neocortical resection is necessary to obtain satisfying seizure control, compare results of ATL with selective resections.

A meta-analysis including 1203 patients in 14 studies suggested improved seizure outcome with ATL over transcortical SAHE, with an 8% increased likelihood of seizure freedom [141]. Similar results have been found in another meta-analysis [142]. However, Kuang et al. [143] did not find in their meta-analysis statistically significant differences in seizure control rates at 1 year after surgery comparing SAHE with ATL. In line, the survey of the Second Palm Desert Survey in 1992 evaluating results of several centers showed a seizure-free rate of 68.8% for selective limbic resections and of 67.9% for ATL [130].

Some observational studies show a better seizure control after ATL with seizure freedom rates of 60–70% versus 40–60% following selective procedures [144–147]. Schmeiser et al. [39] analyzed seizure outcome with different surgical approaches in the Freiburg series of 458 patients. Overall, 72.9% of patients were seizure free at 1-year follow-up. In particular, seizure freedom rate was 72.8% after ATL, 76.9% after KH, 84.4% after ELE, 70.3% after transsylvian SAHE, and 59.1% after subtemporal SAHE. There were no statistically significant differences in seizure outcome, neither at short nor at long-term follow-up. The relatively low proportion of seizure-free patients after subtemporal SAHE is most probably related to the small number of patients within this group [39]. These results are in line with others who found no differences in seizure outcome comparing different resection strategies [38, 40, 85, 133, 138, 148–155].

In sum, SAHE seems to be as effective as more extensive resections. With all resection strategies, similar seizure-free outcomes between 60% and 80% can be achieved [31, 39–41, 59, 60, 85, 114, 133, 138, 149, 151, 156–158].

#### 6.3.1.5 Extent of Hippocampal Resection

The relationship between the extent of hippocampal resection and seizure outcome is controversially discussed in the literature.

Wyler et al. [129] assigned in a RCT 70 patients to partial or total hippocampectomy. They found a much better seizure outcome with extensive mesial resection: 38% of patients with partial but 69% with total hippocampectomy achieved seizure freedom. However, in this study the true extent of hippocampal resection was not controlled by postoperative MRI. A RCT published by Schramm et al. [125, 126] evaluating results of short (2.5 cm) versus long (3.5 cm) hippocampal and parahippocampal resections in a total of 207 patients revealed no statistically significant differences in seizure outcome: 74% of patients with short and 72.8% with long resections were seizure free at 1-year follow-up [126]. In contrast to the trial of Wyler et al. [129], the extent of mesial resection was controlled by postoperative MRI and volumetry in the study of Schramm et al. [126].

In an observational study, Nayel et al. [159] concluded that larger extent of mesial resection controlled by MRI was the most important positive prognostic factor for seizure control. Similarly, Siegel et al. [160] noted in their MRI-controlled study that a larger resection of the parahippocampal gyrus correlated with favorable seizure outcome. More favorable results with extended mesial resections have also been reported by others [161–163]. In a voxel-based MRI study, Bonilha et al. [164] emphasized removal of the entorhinal cortex and found that the extent of mesial resection showed a significant linear correlation with improved seizure outcome. Contrarily, Wolf et al. [165] found no statistically significant differences in seizure outcome for smaller (<2 cm) versus larger (>2 cm) mesial resections which is in line with the results reported by Son et al. [166]. Similarly, other studies did not find that extensive mesial resections are advantageous for seizure outcome [140, 165, 167–170].

Overall, there is no evidence that maximal mesial resection is necessary to achieve optimal seizure control [125, 126, 140, 167–170].

#### 6.3.1.6 Multiple Hippocampal Transections (MHT)

The technique of multiple subpial transections (MST) (see also Chap. 14) has been applied for the treatment of MTLE, a procedure that is called multiple hippocampal transections (MHT) [171]. The rationale of MHT is to avoid cognitive deficits. Warsi et al. [172] reported a total of 114 patients across five studies who underwent MHT. Engel class I seizure outcome across all studies ranged from 64.7% to 94.7%. On the average, seizure freedom (Engel I) was achieved in 84 of the 114 patients (74%). However, the durability of this effect over a long time period requires further studies [172].

#### 6.3.1.7 Prognostic Factors

The following positive predictors for seizure outcome after temporal resections have been identified in meta-analyses and observational studies: MRI-detectable lesion [162, 163, 173–179], complete resection of the lesion [162, 163, 173–178], well-localized EEG [131, 162, 163, 176], history of febrile seizures [163], absence of secondary generalized seizures [173, 174, 178, 180], absence of seizures within the first month after surgery [162, 178], and absence of epilepsy typical potentials at 3 months after surgery [178].

Lack of generalized seizures has also been identified as a positive predictor for seizure outcome in a meta-analysis of pediatric TLE series [174]. Conversely, the presence of generalized seizures may be appreciated as a measure of epilepsy chronification and has been linked to more significant mesial temporal atrophy [181] and postoperative seizure recurrence [78, 182, 183]. Similarly, preoperative bilateral ictal foci have been found to be a negative predictor for seizure outcome, while interictal epileptic discharges (IED) exceeding the affected temporal lobe in the ipsilateral hemisphere or even bilateral IED were compatible with a favorable seizure outcome, if seizure onset was strictly limited to the affected temporal lobe [157].

In a systematic review and meta-analysis, Bjellvi et al. [184] reported that patients with shorter epilepsy duration are more likely to be seizure free at follow-up. Similarly, younger age at surgery and shorter epilepsy duration were predictors for a favorable outcome in MTLE patients in the series of Schmeiser et al. [178]. However, the significance of these factors on seizure outcome has been questioned by others emphasizing excellent results in elderly patients [173, 185–187]. O'Dwyer et al. [188] concluded that age should not play a determining role in the decision-making process.

Barba et al. [180] distinguished between "pure" TLE and "temporal plus epilepsy" (in which primary temporal lobe epileptogenic zone is extended to neighboring regions, such as the insula, the suprasylvian operculum, the orbitofrontal cortex, and the temporo-parieto-occipital junction). They found the presence of a pure TLE to be the strongest positive predictor for seizure control [180].

In a long-term follow-up study of 325 temporal cases (mean follow-up: 9.6 years), McIntosh et al. [173] noted that patients with two seizure-free postoperative years had a 74% probability of seizure freedom by 10 postoperative years. Late seizure recurrence was not associated with any identified risk factors. Postoperative reduction in drug load has not been found to increase the risk for seizure relapse [173, 189], nor did increase in drug dosage led to improved seizure outcome in patients with persisting seizures [189].

#### 6.3.1.8 Children/Adults

In a study comparing children and adults with TLE matched for pathology, epilepsy onset, and side and type of surgery, children had a trend towards a better seizure outcome: 80% children, but only 63% adults were seizure free 1 year after surgery [190]. This is in line with the results of a meta-analysis reporting a trend to better seizure outcomes in children compared to adults following temporal resections [179].

Long-term follow-up has demonstrated relatively stable seizure outcome at 1–2 years after surgery in children [80]. In addition, similar postsurgical rates of seizure freedom have been found from early childhood through to adolescence [78, 80, 191–194].

#### 6.3.1.9 Pathology

In a review of the European Epilepsy Brain Bank (EEBB) comprising 9523 patients including 6847 temporal resections [195], at 1 year after surgery seizure freedom was achieved in 61.4% of the cases with hippocampal sclerosis, 68.4% with tumors (79.9% of children; 63.5% of adults), and 57.6% with malformations of cortical development (59.9% of children; 54.6% of adults). Moreover, seizure freedom was observed in 64.8% of patients with vascular malformations (73.0% of children; 63.4% of adults), and in 50.2% of patients without evidence of a structural lesion (55.2% of children; 48.7% of adults).

Similarly, others observed varying rates of seizure freedom ranging from 58% to 85% depending on the etiologic substrate in pediatric series [78, 80, 191–194]. Contrarily, Schmeiser et al. [39] did not find statistically significant differences in seizure outcome with respect to the histopathological diagnosis and the presence or absence of a dual pathology in an adult series.

#### 6.3.1.10 Gray/White Matter Abnormalities (GWMA)

GWMA are found in patients with HS with a frequency ranging from 32% to 75%, mainly around 50%, and have been associated with earlier epilepsy onset [196–200], while no differences between patients with and without GWMA were found in gender, presence or type of initial precipitating injury, history of secondary generalized seizures, seizure frequency before surgery, neuropsychological evaluation, and presence or lateralization of presurgical interictal epileptiform discharges [199]. It has been suggested that GWMA are caused by seizure-related insults during the critical period of cerebral myelination, and that GWMA may help lateralize the epileptogenic zone [199].

While Choi et al. [197] found a significant higher proportion of seizure-free patients in the group with GWMA, most studies failed to show significant differences in seizure outcome between patients with and without GWMA [196, 201–203]. Naves et al. [199] noted in a series of 122 consecutive HS cases postoperative seizure freedom in 73% of patients with GWMA and 69% without GWMA. As stated by Naves et al. [199], the major limitation of the studies that have investigated the impact of GWMA on postoperative outcome is that in most of them the temporal pole has been resected, whether GWMA is present or not. Schijns et al. [200] compared outcomes after ATL and transsylvian SAHE in 58 patients with HS and GWMA with 58 HS patients without GWMA. Seizure freedom (Engel I) was achieved in 76% of patients with GWMA and in 81% without. In particular, there were no significant differences in seizure outcome between patients with and without GWMA regarding the procedure (ATL versus transsylvian SAHE).

Overall, data available do not allow any conclusion as to the best suitable approach in the presence of GWMA [199, 200].

#### 6.3.1.11 Postoperative MRI Signal Alterations

Renowden et al. [140] reported on a 53% rate of postoperative signal alterations on MRI, particularly T2 hyperintensity, surrounding the resection cavity indicating gliosis in the residual temporal lobe. In line, postoperative gliosis was observed in 61.2% of patients by others [39]. Robinson et al. [204], however, noted signal alterations on MRI in only 30% of their patients after subtemporal SAHE. It has been speculated whether these abnormalities are caused by temporal lobe retraction, or whether they may be referred to Wallerian degeneration of the axons rather than to tissue damage [140, 204]. The influence of postoperative gliosis on the seizure outcome is still under discussion. Renowden et al. [140] and Robinson et al. [204] did not observe a relationship between seizure outcome and gliosis. The Freiburg data confirm these results [39].

#### 6.3.1.12 Selection Bias

It seems to be remarkable that in the randomized controlled trial of Wiebe et al. [128] seizure freedom was achieved in only 58% of patients, while other randomized trials noted seizure freedom rates of 69% [129], 73% [122], 74% [125, 126], and 75% [124]. Similarly, variable seizure-free outcome rates ranging from 34% to 85% have been found in observational studies [132, 200, 205].

As shown, the surgical strategy itself does not significantly influence seizure outcome [38–40, 85, 130, 133, 138, 148–155]. In fact, seizure outcome mainly reflects the selection of candidates. The stricter the selection of patients based on favorable prognostic criteria (e.g., MRI evidence of a distinct resectable unilateral structural abnormality), the better the seizure outcome and vice versa [162, 163, 174–179, 206, 207]. The influence of the selection bias on seizure outcome raises the question as to which patients are called appropriate surgical candidates, or—in other words—which patients with a limited prognosis should still be given the chance of at least a significant improvement of the seizure situation by surgery.

### 6.3.2 Cognitive Outcome

The temporal lobe plays a pivotal role in memory functions, and deterioration of memory performance may be a sequelae, particularly after resection of the dominant temporal lobe [40, 62, 136, 208–210]. Diagnostic tests can roughly predict memory outcomes from surgery. It has been shown that patients with a good preoperative performance are at the greatest risk for a postoperative deterioration [31, 38, 40, 98, 211]. However, reliable tools to accurately predict an individual's long-term potential for functional improvement or decline after resective surgery are still lacking [212]. Obviously, seizure control plays an important role in postoperative cognitive functions. However, the influence of individual factors such as age, seizure characteristics, functional status of the epileptogenic cortex, and surgical measures is not sufficiently understood [212]. As it has been shown, resection of the temporal neocortex as well as maximum resection of temporomesial structures are not necessary to achieve favorable seizure outcome. Conversely, the question arises whether the hypothesis to introduce selective approaches, namely that sparing of the neocortex, and limited temporomesial resection provide better neuropsychological results, holds true.

#### 6.3.2.1 Randomized Controlled Trials (RCTs)

There are four RCTs assessing neuropsychological outcome after temporal resections [123, 124, 127, 129]. Wyler et al. [129] randomized 70 patients to partial hippocampectomy (to the level of the cerebral peduncle) or to total hippocampectomy (to the level of the superior colliculus). The study performed by Hermann et al. [123] evaluating language by naming randomized 30 patients with TLE to resection versus sparing of the first temporal gyrus. Another study reported by Lutz et al. [124] evaluated neuropsychological functions in patients who were randomized to receive SAHE by the transsylvian and the transcortical route, respectively. The fourth study provided by Vogt et al. [127] analyzed neuropsychological outcome of patients randomized for subtemporal versus transsylvian SAHE (for results of RCTs, see below).

#### 6.3.2.2 ATL

A meta-analysis of 22 studies showed a decline in verbal memory in 44% of patients with left temporal resections and in 20% with right temporal resections [213]. Hermann et al. [123] evaluated in a RCT visual confrontation naming in 30 patients undergoing ATL randomized to resection versus sparing of the superior temporal gyrus. No differences in language function between the both procedures were found.

#### 6.3.2.3 Selective Resections

Deterioration of cognitive functions after selective resections has been shown in observational studies as well as in randomized controlled trials (RCTs).

Morino et al. [38] noted in a series of 32 patients verbal memory decline after left-sided transsylvian SAHE and improvement after right-sided operations which may in part be due to learning effects. The Freiburg series of 162 transsylvian SAHE cases [114] demonstrated decline of verbal memory (verbal learning and absolute delayed recall), especially after left-sided operations. Conversely, visual memory declined after right-sided SAHE in some cases 114] which is in line with other studies [214, 215]. Yet, there were no differences between left- or right-sided surgeries in verbal delayed memory loss (relative to learning success), visual learning and memory, or selective attention [114]. Considerable decline in verbal memory after left-sided SAHE has also been shown in previous reports [40, 214, 216–220]. Von Rhein et al. [118] found decline in verbal memory after subtemporal and transsylvian SAHE with verbal recognition memory being more affected by left transsylvian SAHE and nonverbal memory more by subtemporal SAHE irrespective of the side of surgery.

In the RCT of Vogt et al. [127], 47 patients were assigned to transsylvian (25 patients) or subtemporal (22 patients) SAHE. Verbal recognition memory declined irrespective of the approach. The subtemporal approach was associated with a worse outcome for verbal learning and delayed free recall as well as for semantic fluency. However, no approach was found to show significant superiority in cognitive outcome [127]. Lutz et al. [124] evaluated neuropsychological functions in a RCT including 80 patients who were assigned to receive SAHE by the transsylvian (41 patients) or the transcortical (39 patients) approach. Decline and partial improvement of neuropsychological functions were similar in both groups at 6-month and 1-year follow-up with the exception of better preserved phonemic fluency with the transcortical route.

#### 6.3.2.4 ATL/Selective Resections

Ambiguous results exist to the question whether and, if so, how far the extent of neocortical resection influences cognitive outcome.

Some studies observed better preservation of cognitive performance after tailored resections and SAHE as compared to ATL [31, 38, 40, 99, 145, 146, 150, 155, 209, 221, 222]. In line, Tanriverdi and Olivier [151] noted better recall after SAHE as compared to ATL. Similar results have been described by others [117, 148, 149, 223, 224]. Moreover, transsylvian SAHE has been shown to provide better results in terms of total IQ as well as verbal and performance IQ as compared to ATL [38, 117, 140]. The risk of severe global memory deficits has been found to be absent in SAHE [225], whereas this risk was reported as high as 1–5% in ATL cases [31]. Giovagnoli et al. [226] did not find any differences in verbal or visual memory after lesionectomy irrespective of the side of surgery as has also been noted by Beaton et al. [115] following transsylvian SAHE. Comparing three resection types (ATL, SAHE, and ELE), Helmstaedter et al. [224] found some advantage of SAHE over ATL and the best outcome for pure cortical ELE. These results seem to support the hypothesis that reduced cognitive outcome in ATL can be referred to more extensive resection of non-lesional functional tissue [227, 228].

Contrarily, other studies demonstrated similar neuropsychological deficits comparing SAHE and ATL [129, 138, 152, 153, 165, 229–232]. A meta-analysis did not find statistically significant differences in memory function after 1 year between ATL and SAHE [143]. In a prospective study comparing SAHE with anterior one-third lobectomy and amygdalohippocampectomy, Helmstaedter et al. [218, 219] found advantages for SAHE for material-specific memory in right-sided resections and one-third lobectomy with amygdalohippocampectomy in left-sided surgeries. Similarly, Loring et al. [233] found SAHE better for material-specific memory for right-sided but not for left-sided resections. Jones-Gotman et al. [168] comparing seizure-free cases after three resection types (ATL, SAHE, and ELE) found similar deficits in learning and retention tasks in all three groups. In the Freiburg series comprising 458 temporal patients, no differences in cognitive outcome regarding verbal or nonverbal learning or memory function as well as in selective attention after different resective procedures could be documented, whereas side of operation showed significant effects on measures of long-term verbal but not visual memory [39].

Overall, there is no consensus on the role of the temporal neocortex on cognitive functions.

Methodical issues of different studies, such as small subgroup sizes regarding approach and side of surgery or imperfect matching of subgroups concerning important clinical characteristics like IQ, age of seizure onset, or postoperative seizure outcome, may explain why the debate regarding cognitive outcomes of different surgical approaches is still open. Differences in neuropsychological outcome may rather depend on the preoperative performance status and postoperative seizure control than on the surgical approach [39]. Favorable postoperative seizure control has been discussed as an important factor for better cognitive outcome, which is induced by recovery or release of extratemporal functions [234, 235]. Helmstaedter et al. [210] demonstrated in a series of 161 adult patients stable cognitive performance 5–22 years after temporal resections and a positive course, if epilepsy was controlled and drug load reduced. Rehabilitation measures may support recovery of neuropsychological decline that is normally seen after temporal lobe resections [218, 219].

#### 6.3.2.5 Extent of Hippocampal Resection

As with the temporal neocortex, the influence of the extent of the hippocampus resection on neuropsychological outcome is discussed with controversy.

Early studies emphasized close relationship between postoperative memory deficits and the extent of hippocampal removal [236–238]. Thus, the operative concept aimed at minimalization of hippocampal resection [239, 240]. Katz et al. [221] analyzing 20 patients with a compartment model found a positive correlation of postoperative decrease of verbal material retention with the extent of mesial resection in left-sided procedures. Similarly, Skirrow et al. [241] found that verbal memory is better preserved with smaller left temporomesial resections, and Bonelli et al. [242] ascribed the posterior hippocampus a key role in preserving memory.

In a RCT, Wyler et al. [129] did not notice increased neuropsychological deficits with more extensive hippocampal resection. However, in this study, the extent of mesial resection was not controlled by MRI. The influence of MR-controlled short (2.5 cm) versus long (3.5 cm) hippocampal resections on cognitive functions was compared in a multicenter RCT [125, 126, 227, 228]. The trial did not show any statistically significant differences between both groups. However, cognitive outcomes negatively correlated with the volume of the resected hippocampus. In an observational study, Loring et al. [233] noted that a larger mesial resection was not associated with increased verbal memory deficit which is in line with others [168, 229]. Similarly, the Freiburg series [39] did not show a correlation between the length of hippocampal resection and neuropsychological performance irrespective of language dominance. In addition, it has been showed that postoperative short-term verbal memory deficits may be present even with minimal or no hippocampal resection [211, 243].

In sum, there is no evidence that shorter hippocampal resections correlate with a better cognitive outcome [227, 228]. However, the complete sparing of the hippocampus is associated with a benefit in verbal learning performance as compared to patients with hippocampus resection [98]. Yet, hippocampus-sparing temporal lobe resections within the language-dominant hemisphere can also be accompanied by a decline in verbal memory performance, since extrahippocampal temporal resections may alter verbal memory networks leading to hippocampal atrophy. However, the extent of decline in verbal memory performance after hippocampus-sparing procedures is not comparable to that observed in patients with hippocampus resection [98]. The postoperative left-sided hippocampal volume seems to be a significant predictor of postoperative verbal memory loss after left-sided hippocampus-sparing surgery [244].

#### 6.3.2.6 Multiple Hippocampal Transections (MHT)

Warsi et al. [172] analyzed 59 patients from 5 series who had left-sided MHT and completed pre- and postoperative neuropsychological evaluations for verbal memory at follow-up. Of them, 86.8% (range: 77.6–96%) showed complete preservation of verbal memory relative to preoperative functional baseline. Thus, MHT may be effective at preserving verbal memory in patients with a good baseline function [172].

#### 6.3.2.7 Prognostic Factors

The following predictors of a good cognitive outcome have been identified: (1) preoperatively evident dysfunction of the focus region, (2) lateralization to the nondominant hemisphere for language, (3) young age at the time of surgery, and (4) high general intelligence [205]. Conversely, factors indicating an increased risk of an unfavorable cognitive outcome include (1) unimpaired neuropsychological profile, (2) no MRI lesion, (3) very low presurgical performance corresponding to a limited reserve capacity, and (4) bilateral pathology such as bilateral hippocampal sclerosis [245].

These preoperative prognostic factors must be considered when selecting and advising potential surgical patients [246]. Other factors determining neuropsychological outcome that, however, cannot be sufficiently assessed preoperatively include the degree of age-dependent functional plasticity, postsurgical seizures, interictal epileptic discharges, and changes of anti-seizure medication [246, 247].

#### 6.3.2.8 Children/Adults

Comparing pre- and postsurgical neuropsychological performance after temporal resections in children and adults, Gleissner et al. [190] demonstrated that adults had lower presurgical scores for verbal memory, probably due to the longer epilepsy duration, and failed to recover after surgery. In this trial, children and adults were matched for pathology, epilepsy onset, and side and type of surgery. Additionally, children had better outcomes regarding attentional functions as compared to adults, with their vast majority improving 1 year after surgery. Recoveries following surgery that occurred exclusively in children and adolescents were attributed to the plasticity in the developing brain [190].

#### 6.3.2.9 Postoperative MRI Signal Alterations/Collateral Cortical Damage

Selective procedures in the temporal lobe are frequently accompanied by postoperative MRI signal intensity changes surrounding the approach. With respect to the limited access in selective procedures, these signal abnormalities within close proximity to the approach are thought to reflect collateral cortical damage, e.g., by surgical manipulation, impairing vascular supply or venous drainage, or by extensive tissue retraction. Helmstaedter et al. [205] evaluated collateral cortical damage in 34 patients who were randomly assigned to either transsylvian or transcortical SAHE. Losses in verbal learning and recognition memory positively correlated to signal intensity changes, independent of the side of the resection, the surgical approach, or the extent of the mesial resection. Losses in verbal memory were greater after left-sided surgery, while losses in figural learning were related to right-sided surgery. Thus, controlling for collateral damage as a measure of surgical quality may clarify controversial memory outcomes after SAHE reported [205].

### 6.3.3 Psychiatric Outcome

Postoperative psychiatric disorders may occur as either an exacerbation of a known psychiatric diagnosis, the re-emergence of a previous psychiatric disorder in remission, or the development of a de novo disorder [248].

#### 6.3.3.1 Pre/Postoperative Psychopathology

Earlier studies suggested that psychiatric disorders do not improve following surgery [249]. However, more actual studies have demonstrated that successful surgery with postoperative seizure control may improve psychiatric symptoms [246, 250–252].

Analyzing 360 patients, Devinsky et al. [253] noted preoperative rates of depression and anxiety of 22% and 25%, respectively, versus 11% and 13% at 24 months after surgery. Significant reduction in the prevalence of depression and anxiety in these patients was associated with improved seizure control [253]. Similarly, de Araujo Filho et al. [254] found in 115 patients undergoing ATL presurgical psychiatric disorders in 41% as compared to 27% postoperatively. In a prospective noncontrolled study, Spencer et al. [255] reported that 24% of temporal lobe patients had clinically elevated depression scores preoperatively as opposed to 13% at 24 months postoperatively. Macrodimitris et al. [256] reviewed psychiatric outcomes from 13 articles including 1322 patients who underwent resective surgery, most of them affecting the temporal lobe. All but two studies demonstrated either improved or unchanged psychiatric outcome after surgery. Only one study demonstrated deterioration of the psychiatric status, with a higher anxiety along with continued seizures, and another study reported an increased rate of psychosis after surgery [256].

Overall, there is consensus that preexistent psychopathology may improve with seizure control and therefore is not a contraindication for surgery [245].

#### 6.3.3.2 Risk Factors

The following risk factors for postoperative psychiatric problems have been identified: a presurgical affective disorder or a lifetime psychiatric diagnosis [241, 248, 251, 253, 257], persistent seizures [256], and a preoperative history of secondary generalized tonic-clonic seizures [251].

#### 6.3.3.3 De Novo Psychopathology

De novo psychopathology has been observed in 1–26% of patients after TLE surgery: depression (4–18%), anxiety (3–26%), and interictal psychosis (1–12%) [251]. Others found de novo psychopathology in 17% [258] and 10–16% [253, 254] of patients. Spencer et al. [259] reported postoperative psychosis in 1–5% and new affective disorders in 4–30% of cases. The incidence of new psychogenic non-epileptic seizures (PNES) following epilepsy surgery is estimated at 4%, but has been found as high as 8.5% in females with a psychiatric history [22, 246, 260].

Macrodimitris et al. [256] reported in their review including 1322 surgical patients a rate of 1.1–18.2% de novo psychiatric conditions, with milder psychiatric symptoms (e.g., adjustment disorders) being more common than more severe psychiatric problems (e.g., psychosis). In a meta-analysis comprising 2947 patients with temporal resections, Tebo et al. [261] found postoperative psychological and psychiatric problems in 1.3% of the patients. Brotis et al. [262] noted in another meta-analysis including 2842 patients de novo psychiatric disorders in 7% of patients.

#### 6.3.3.4 Burden of Normality

Experience shows that depression and anxiety may supervene when the handicap has been removed and seizure relief has been achieved [263]. Postsurgical seizure freedom can lead to adjustment issues, the so-called burden of normality [264]. Seizure relief decreases dependency and level of care by others and increases expectations towards the now "cured" patient. This may pose considerable pressure on the seizure-free patient [246]. Thus, in a subset of patients, despite an objective improvement in seizure control and cognitive indices, the quality of life as determined by the level of intrapersonal and intrapsychic adjustment may be adversely affected [263, 265].

## 6.4 Which Approach Should Be Preferred?

An extensive body of literature is available on different temporal approaches including modifications of lateral and mesial resection strategies all aiming at the ideal combination of maximal seizure freedom and minimal cognitive impairment. Starting with ATL in the 1950s, there is a tendency over the decades to reduce the extent of lateral resection in MTLE based on the hypothesis that smaller resections lead to the same favorable seizure outcome as ATL, but provide better cognitive function. Similarly, the extent of mesial resection has been modified hypothesizing that shorter mesial resections are advantageous with respect to the cognitive outcome while providing similar favorable seizure outcome as compared to larger mesial resections.

According to the data available, it seems that these hypotheses cannot be maintained longer. While smaller lateral and shorter mesial resections have been shown to provide the same favorable results in terms of seizure outcome as compared to larger resections, no significant differences in cognitive outcome between more extended and more restricted lateral and mesial resections have been proven [31, 39–41, 114, 125, 126, 130, 140, 166, 167, 227, 228].

It has been shown that SAHE may be accomplished with a minimal morbidity [225], and that the complication rate of different approaches may not show significant differences [39]. However, it is obvious that selective approaches providing only a limited overview on temporomesial structures, and, in particular transsylvian SAHE, requiring dissection of the Sylvian vessels, pose much higher challenges to surgical skills as compared to ATL. Since there is no evidence of any significant advantage of selective approaches from today's view, the surgeon should choose the approach according to his/her individual experience. Whether the preservation of the temporal neocortex may prove to be functionally advantageous in the long term over many decades with respect to cerebral comorbidities as may be expected remains an open question.

**Concluding Remarks**

- ***Outcome***. *Systematic reviews and meta-analyses consistently demonstrate seizure-free (Engel I) outcome in two-thirds of patients. Surgery-related neuropsychological deficits mainly referring to decline in verbal memory are observed in up to 40% of dominant temporal lobe procedures. No significant differences with respect to seizure outcome and neuropsychological performance have been found comparing different lateral and mesial resection strategies. Preexistent psychiatric disorders may improve with seizure control and therefore are not a contraindication for surgery.*
- ***Surgical approach***. *Neurosurgeons starting with epilepsy surgery are strongly advised to begin with ATL in order to became familiar with the topography of the temporomesial area. More circumscribed resections and, in particular SAHE, only provide a limited overview to temporomesial structures, and therefore are only advisable for surgeons with advanced technical skills who are very familiar with the temporomesial anatomy. With respect to selective approaches, the transsylvian route provides a good overview on the anterior circumference of the brainstem, while the subtemporal route focuses on its posterior aspects. Therefore, the transsylvian route is recommended for more anteriorly localized pathologies, while for lesions extending more posteriorly, the subtemporal route is advantageous.*
- ***Positioning of the patient***. *In principle, the smaller the extent of lateral resection, the less the head should be rotated, and the more the vertex should be lowered in order to provide sufficient overview on mesiotemporal structures without retracting the lateral temporal lobe. For subtemporal SAHE, the lateral position noticeably lowering the vertex is recommended facilitating the temporal base to sink back by gravity. It is advisable for all approaches to gradually lower the vertex the more mesial structures are reached.*
- ***Wernicke's language area***. *In order to preserve the sensory language area (Wernicke) localized at the dorsal aspect of the first temporal gyrus in the dominant hemisphere, some modifications of the classical ATL have been suggested. However, Wernicke's area does not begin before 6–7 cm, measured from the temporal pole. Keeping in mind this landmark, Wernicke's area is not endangered with ATL limiting the resection of the first temporal gyrus to 4.5 cm. Thus, the routine use of additional studies like fMRI is not necessary. Even more dorsal resection of the first temporal gyrus in the dominant hemisphere up to 6 cm from the pole is feasible without disadvantage. However, it is important in these cases to preserve arteries leaving the dorsal Sylvian fissure to the temporal lobe.*
- ***Vein of Labbé***. *In principle, it is advisable to preserve the vein of Labbé whenever possible.*

*However, with its anterior location, the vein of Labbé may be included in the resection area in classical ATL without any harm. With more limited lateral resections and in particular with selective procedures, the vein of Labbé must be preserved to prevent edema and hemorrhagic infarction.*

- ***Sylvian fissure***. *Dissection of the Sylvian fissure for transsylvian SAHE always starts at the frontal aspect of the superficial veins close to pars orbitalis of the inferior frontal gyrus, since superficial Sylvian veins are adherent to the temporal lobe by rough arachnoid layers. Exposing the temporal stem, it is advisable to cut minor temporal arteries rather at their superior-lateral, i.e., temporal, than inferior-mesial, i.e., basal ganglia aspect, and to push the vessels along with the arachnoid downward and mesially in order to avoid damage to perforating arteries.*
- ***Temporal base***. *With subtemporal SAHE, entry into the inferior horn mainly depends on the individual venous architecture. Major basal veins and in particular the vein of Labbé must be spared. Therefore, it is advisable to enter the inferior horn rather laterally than mesially, e.g., through the fusiform gyrus or—in critical cases—through the inferior temporal gyrus in order to avoid tension and damage to temporobasal veins.*
- ***Temporomesial arachnoid membrane***. *The arachnoid membrane surrounding the mesial temporal area protects important nervous and vascular structures. This membrane frequently shows gaps at its anterior aspects. Although additional opening of this membrane often is unavoidable during en bloc dissection of the hippocampus, it is important to preserve as much as possible of this protective layer using subtle microsurgical techniques. Using the ultrasound aspirator, it is advisable to limit its power to around 50% of the maximum, and to reduce suction strength to a value avoiding too strong aspiration of the arachnoid.*
- ***Inferior horn***. *With all approaches, it is important to enter the inferior horn of the lateral ventricle more basolaterally in order to avoid to bypass the ventricle at its superior and mesial aspect, thus erroneously entering the basal ganglia. The inferior horn is safely reached by continuously shifting dissection plane from laterally to mesially. Neuronavigation may be useful for selective approaches. With repect to Meyer's loop of the geniculocalcarine tract, the roof of the inferior horn should be spared to avoid visual field deficits as far as possible.*
- ***En bloc resection of the hippocampus***. *In order to facilitate histopathological analysis, the hippocampus should be removed en bloc. This is accomplished by blunt dissection. Vessels of the sulcus hippocampi should be cut close to the hippocampus not to endanger vascular structures of the crural and ambient cisterns. Moreover, these vessels should be cut at the last step of dissection, thus providing a vital specimen for scientific analysis.*
- ***Resection of the amygdala***. *While the bulging lateral parts of the amygdaloid body can be removed safely, it is not possible to completely remove its mesial part. The limit of mesial amygdala resection is ambiguous. The amygdaloid body can be safely removed to a plane of 3–4 mm (roughly corresponding to the external diameter of a sucker) mesial to the tip of the plexus of the inferior horn. Keeping this landmark in mind, damage to the optic tract and to vessels supplying basal ganglia is avoided.*
- ***Hemostasis***. *Electrocoagulation for hemostasis around the brainstem should be completely avoided. Usually, hemostasis is easily achieved applying some hemostatic agents such as oxidized cellulose gauze (Tabotamp R, Johnson and Johnson Medical, 22844 Norderstedt, Germany) or Surgicel (Johnson and Johnson, Brussels, Belgium). It is important to avoid coagulation-induced circulation disturbances or heat-induced vasospasms especially of the anterior choroid artery.*
- ***Suction drainage***. *It has been shown that extensive temporal lobe resections predispose to cerebellar foliar hemorrhage which is thought to result from a negative transtentorial pressure gradient caused by major loss of cerebrospinal fluid (CSF) due to forced suc-*

*tion drainage. Therefore, major suction should be avoided when a postoperative draining tube is used (see also Chap. 15).*

## References


1. Penfield W, Flanigin H. Surgical therapy of temporal lobe seizures. Arch Neurol Psychiatry. 1950;64(4):491–500.
2. Jasper HH. History of the early development of electroencephalography and clinical neurophysiology at the Montreal Neurological Institute: the first 25 years 1939–1964. Can J Neurol Sci. 1991;18(4 Suppl):533–48.
3. Jasper HH. Electrical potentials from the intact human brain. Science. 1935;81:51–3.
4. Jasper HH. Electroencephalography. In: Penfield WE, editor. Epilepsy and cerebral localization. Springfield, IL: Charles C Thomas; 1941. p. 380–454.
5. Bailey P, Gibbs FA. The surgical treatment of psychomotor epilepsy. JAMA. 1951;145(6):365–70.
6. Feindel W, Penfield W. Localization of discharge in temporal lobe automatism. Arch Neurol Psychiatry. 1954;72:605–30.
7. Penfield W, Paine K. Results of surgical therapy for focal epileptic seizures. Can Med Assoc J. 1955;73:515–30.
8. Falconer MA. Discussion on the surgery of temporal lobe epilepsy. Proc R Soc Med. 1953;46:971–5.
9. Falconer MA, Meyer A, Hill D, Mitchell W, Pond DA. Treatment of temporal lobe epilepsy by temporal lobectomy; a survey of findings and results. Lancet. 1955;268(6869):827–35.
10. Meyer A, Falconer MA, Beck C. Pathological findings in temporal lobe epilepsy. J Neurol Neurosurg Psychiatry. 1954;17:276–85.
11. Morris AA. Temporal lobectomy with removal of uncus, hippocampus and amygdala. Arch Neurol Psychiatry. 1956;76:479–96.
12. Bailey P. Surgical treatment of psychomotor epilepsy: five-year follow-up. South Med J. 1961;54:299–301.
13. Cahan LD, Engel J Jr. Surgery for epilepsy: a review. Acta Neurol Scand. 1986;73(6):551–60.
14. Coughlan A, Farrell M, Hardiman O, et al.. The results of removal of temporal lobe neocortex in the treatment of epilepsy in 40 patients. Meeting of the Association of British Neurologists with the American Neurological Association, London Hospital, November 1–2, 1985.
15. Polkey CE, Binnie CD, Janota I. Acute hippocampal recording and pathology at temporal lobe resection and amygdalohippocampectomy for epilepsy. J Neurol Neurosurg Psychiatry. 1989;52(9):1050–7.
16. Rasmussen TB. Surgical treatment of complex partial seizures: results, lessons, and problems. Epilepsia. 1980;24(Suppl 1):S65–76.
17. Scoville WB, Milner B. Loss of recent memory after bilateral hippocampal lesions. J Neurol Neurosurg Psychiatry. 1957;20(1):11–21.
18. Blakemore CB, Falconer MA. Long-term effects of anterior temporal lobectomy on certain cognitive functions. J Neurol Neurosurg Psychiatry. 1967;30(4):364–7.
19. Milner B. Amnesia following operation on the temporal lobes. In: Whitty CMW, Zangwill OL, editors. Amnesia. London: Butterworth; 1966. p. 109–33.
20. Milner B, Penfield W. The effect of hippocampal lesions on recent memory. Trans Am Neurol Assoc. 1955;80:42–8.
21. Serafetinides EA, Falconer MA. Some observations on memory impairment after temporal lobectomy for epilepsy. J Neurol Neurosurg Psychiatry. 1962;25:251–5.
22. Asadi-Pooya AA, Rostami C. History of surgery for temporal lobe epilepsy. Epilepsy Behav. 2017;70:57–60.
23. Loring DW. Neuropsychological evaluation in epilepsy surgery. Epilepsia. 1997;38(Suppl. 4):S18–23.
24. Serafetinides EA, Hoare RD, Driver M. Intracarotid sodium amylobarbitone test and cerebral dominance for speech and consciousness. Brain. 1965;88:107–30.
25. Silfvenius H, Christianson SA, Nilsson LG, Säisä J. Preoperative investigation of cerebral hemisphere speech and memory with the bilateral intracarotid Amytal test. Acta Neurol Scand Suppl. 1988;117:79–83.
26. Wieser HG, Engel JJ, Williamson PD. Surgical remediable temporal lobe syndromes. In: Engel Jr J, editor. Surgical treatment of the epilepsies. 2nd ed. New York: Raven Press; 1993. p. 49–63.
27. Engel J Jr. Multimodal approaches in the evaluation of epilepsy patients for surgery. Electroencephalogr Clin Neurophysiol Suppl. 1999;50:40–52.
28. Schmidt D, Elger C. Praktische Epilepsiebehandlung-Somatotope Einteilung fokaler Epilepsien. Stuttgart: Georg Thieme Verlag; 2002. p. 135.
29. Rolston JD, Englot DJ, Knowlton RC, Chang EF. Rate and complications of adult epilepsy surgery in North America: analysis of multiple databases. Epilepsy Res. 2016;124:55–62.
30. Binder DK, Schramm J. Resective surgical techniques: mesial temporal lobe epilepsy. In: Lüders HO, editor. Epilepsy surgery. London: Informa UK Ltd.; 2008. p. 1083–92.
31. Adada B. Selective amygdalohippocampectomy via the transsylvian approach. Neurosurg Focus. 2008;25(3):E5.
32. Chang EF, Englot DJ, Vadera S. Minimally invasive surgical approaches for temporal lobe epilepsy. Epilepsy Behav. 2015;47:24–33.
33. Cohen-Gadol AA, Wilhelmi BG, Collignon BSF, et al. Long-term outcome of epilepsy surgery among 399 patients with nonlesional seizure foci including mesial temporal lobe sclerosis. J Neurosurg. 2006;104:513–24.

34. Cossu M, Lo Russo G, Francione S, et al. Epilepsy surgery in children: results and predictors of outcome on seizures. Epilepsia. 2008;49(1):65–72.
35. Hemb M, Velasco TR, Parnes MS, et al. Improved outcomes in pediatric epilepsy surgery: the UCLA experience, 1986–2008. Neurology. 2010;74(22):1768–75.
36. Kim SK, Wang KC, Hwang YS, et al. Epilepsy surgery in children: outcomes and complications. J Neurosurg Pediatr. 2008;1(4):277–83.
37. Mathon B, Bédos Ulvin L, Adam C, Baulac M, Dupont S, Navarro V, et al. Surgical treatment for mesial temporal lobe epilepsy associated with hippocampal sclerosis. Rev Neurol (Paris). 2015;171(3):315–25.
38. Morino M, Uda T, Naito K, et al. Comparison of neuropsychological outcomes after selective amygdalohippocampectomy versus anterior temporal lobectomy. Epilepsy Behav. 2006;9(1):95–100.
39. Schmeiser B, Wagner K, Schulze-Bonhage A, Mader I, Wendling A-S, Steinhoff BJ, Prinz M, Scheiwe C, Weyerbrock A, Zentner J. Surgical treatment of mesiotemporal lobe epilepsy: which approach is favorable? Neurosurgery. 2017;81(6):992–1004. https://doi.org/10.1093/neuros/nyx138.
40. Wendling AS, Hirsch E, Wisniewski I, et al. Selective amygdalohippocampectomy versus standard temporal lobectomy in patients with mesial temporal lobe epilepsy and unilateral hippocampal sclerosis. Epilepsy Res. 2013;104(1-2):94–104.
41. Wieser HG, Ortega M, Friedman A, Yonekawa Y. Long-term seizure outcomes following amygdalohippocampectomy. J Neurosurg. 2003;98(4):751–63.
42. Yasargil MG. Microneurosurgery. Stuttgart, New York: Thieme; 1994.
43. Kiernan JA. Anatomy of the temporal lobe. Epilepsy Res Treat. 2012;2012:176157. https://doi.org/10.1155/2012/176157.
44. Wen HT, Rhoton AL, et al. Microsurgical anatomy of the temporal lobe: Part 2—Sylvian fissure region and its clinical application. Neurosurgery. 2009;65(ONS Suppl 1):ons1–ons36.
45. Seeger W. Atlas of Topographical Anatomy of the Brain and Surrounding Structures. Wien: Springer; 1978.
46. Seeger W. Microanatomical Aspects for Neurosurgeons and Neuroradiologists. Wien, New York: Springer; 2000.
47. Seeger W, Zentner J. Anatomical basis of cranial neurosurgery. Heidelberg: Springer; 2018.
48. Yasargil MG. Microneurosurgery. Vol I. Microsurgery Anatomy of the Basal Cisterns and Vessels of the Brain. Stuttgart, New York: Thieme; 1984.
49. Sindou M, Guenot M. Surgical anatomy of the temporal lobe. Adv Tech Stand Neurosurg. 2004;29:265–88.
50. Niewenhuys R, Voogd J, Van Huijzen C. The human cerebral nervous system: a synopsis and atlas. 3rd ed. Berlin, Heidelberg, New York, Tokyo: Springer; 1988.
51. Insausti R, Amaral DG. Hippocampal formation. In: Paxinos G, Mai JK, editors. The human nervous system. 2nd ed. Amsterdam, The Netherlands: Elsevier; 2004. p. 871–914.
52. Duvernoy HM. The human hippocampus. München: Bergmann; 1988.
53. Duvernoy HM. The human hippocampus: Functional anatomy, vascularization and serial sections with MRI. Berlin, Heidelberg, New York, Tokyo: Springer; 1998.
54. Zeidman P, Maguire EA. Anterior hippocampus: the anatomy of perception, imagination and episodic memory. Nat Rev. 2016;17:173–82.
55. Deng W, Aimone JB, Gage FH. New neurons and new memories: how does adult hippocampal neurogenesis affect learning and memory? Nat Rev Neurosci. 2010;11:339–50.
56. Babb TL, Wilson CL, Isokawa-Akesson M. Firing patterns of human limbic neurons during stereoencephalography (SEEG) and clinical temporal lobe seizures. Electroencephalogr Clin Neurophysiol. 1987;66(6):467–82.
57. Babb TL, Brown WJ, Pretorius J, Davenport C, Lieb JP, Crandall PH. Temporal lobe volumetric cell densities in temporal lobe epilepsy. Epilepsia. 1984;25(6):729–40.
58. Morimoto K, Fahnestock M, Racine RJ. Kindling and status epilepticus models of epilepsy. Prog Neurobiol. 2004;73(1):1–60.
59. Schmeiser B, Zentner J, Prinz M, et al. Extent of mossy fiber sprouting in patients with mesiotemporal lobe epilepsy correlates with neuronal cell loss and granule cell dispersion. Epilepsy Res. 2017d;129:51–8.
60. Schmeiser B, Li J, Brandt A, et al. Different mossy fiber sprouting patterns in ILAE hippocampal sclerosis types. Epilepsy Res. 2017e;136:115–22.
61. Borges K, Gearing M, McDermott DL, Smith AB, Almonte AG, Wainer BH, Dingledine R. Neuronal and glial pathological changes during epileptogenesis in the mouse pilocarpine model. Exp Neurol. 2003;182(1):21–34.
62. Rausch R, Babb TL. Hippocampal neuron loss and memory scores before and after temporal lobe surgery for epilepsy. Arch Neurol. 1993;50(8):812–7.
63. Vivash L, Tostevin A, Liu DS, Dalic L, Dedeurwaerdere S, Hicks RJ, Williams DA, Myers DE, O'Brien TJ. Changes in hippocampal GABAA/cBZR density during limbic epileptogenesis: relationship to cell loss and mossy fibre sprouting. Neurobiol Dis. 2011;41(2):227–36. https://doi.org/10.1016/j.nbd.2010.08.021.
64. Liu DS, O'Brien TJ, Williams DA, Hicks RJ, Myers DE. Lamina-specific changes in hippocampal GABA(A)/cBZR and mossy fibre sprouting during and following amygdala kindling in the rat. Neurobiol Dis. 2009;35:337–47.

65. Urbach H, Egger K, Nakagawa JM, et al. Bilateral cingulum fiber reductions in temporal lobe epilepsy with unilateral hippocampal sclerosis. Eur J Radiol. 2017;94:53–7.
66. Inman CS, Manns JR, Bijanki KR, Bass DI, Hamann S, Drane DL, Fasano RE, Kovach CK, Gross RE, Willie JT. Direct electrical stimulation of the amygdala enhances declarative memory in humans. Proc Natl Acad Sci. 2018;115(1):98–103.
67. Krolak-Salmon P, Guenot M, Tiliket C, et al. Anatomy of optic nerve radiations as assessed by static perimetry and MRI after tailored temporal lobectomy. Br J Ophthalmol. 2000;84:884–9.
68. Gonzales LF, Smith K. Meyer´s loop. Phoenix, AZ: Grand Rounds Publications and Media, Barrow Neurological Institute; 2002. p. 18.
69. Nowell M, Vos SB, Sidhu M, et al. Meyer's loop asymmetry and language lateralisation in epilepsy. J Neurol Neurosurg Psychiatry. 2016;87(8):836–42.
70. Dreessen de Gervai P, Sboto-Frankenstein UN, Bolster RB, et al. Tractography of Meyer's loop asymmetries. Epilepsy Res. 2014;108(5):872–82.
71. Jeelani NU, Jindahra P, Tamper MS, et al. Hemispherical asymmetry in the Meyer's loop: a prospective study of visual-field deficits in 105 cases undergoing anterior temporal lobe resection for epilepsy. J Neurol Neurosurg Psychiatry. 2010;81(9):985–91.
72. Winston GP. Epilepsy surgery, vision, and driving: What has surgery taught us and could modern imaging reduce the risk of visual deficits? Epilepsia. 2013;54(11):1877–88.
73. Winston GP, Daga P, White MJ, et al. Preventing visual field deficits from neurosurgery. Neurology. 2014;83(7):604–11.
74. Reisert M, Mader I, Anastasopoulos C, Weigel M, Schnell S, Kiselev V. Global fiber reconstruction becomes practical. Neuroimage. 2011;54(2):955–62.
75. Shattuck DW, Mirza M, Adisetiyo V, Hojatkashani C, Salamon G, Narr KL, Poldrack RA, Bilder RM, Toga AW. Construction of a 3D probabilistic atlas of human cortical structures. Neuroimage. 2008;39(3):1064–80. https://doi.org/10.1016/j.neuroimage.2007.09.03.
76. Ramantani G, Koessler L, Colnat-Coulbois S, et al. Intracranial evaluation of the epileptogenic zone in regional infrasylvian polymicrogyria. Epilepsia. 2013c;54(2):296–304.
77. San-juan D, Tapia CA, González-Aragón MF, et al. The prognostic role of electrocorticography in tailored temporal lobe surgery. Seizure. 2011;20(7):564–9.
78. Benifla M, Otsubo H, Ochi A, et al. Temporal lobe surgery for intractable epilepsy in children: an analysis of outcomes in 126 children. Neurosurgery. 2006;59(6):1203–14.
79. Li LM, Cendes F, Watson C, et al. Surgical treatment of patients with single and dual pathology: relevance of lesion and of hippocampal atrophy to seizure outcome. Neurology. 1997;48(2):437–44.
80. Mittal S, Montes JL, Farmer JP, et al. Long-term outcome after surgical treatment of temporal lobe epilepsy in children. J Neurosurg. 2005;103:401–142.
81. Ramantani G, Kadish NE, Anastasopoulos C, et al. Epilepsy surgery for glioneuronal tumors in childhood: avoid loss of time. Neurosurgery. 2014;74(6):648–57.
82. Salanova V, Markand O, Worth R. Temporal lobe epilepsy: analysis of patients with dual pathology. Acta Neurol Scand. 2004;109(2):126–31.
83. Falconer MA, Taylor DC. Surgical treatment of drug-resistant epilepsy due to mesial temporal sclerosis. Etiology and significance. Arch Neurol. 1968;19(4):353–61.
84. Penfield W, Baldwin M. Temporal lobe seizures and the technic of subtotal temporal lobectomy. Ann Surg. 1952;136(4):625–34.
85. Arruda F, Cendes F, Andermann F, et al. Mesial atrophy and outcome after amygdalohippocampectomy or temporal lobe removal. Ann Neurol. 1996;40(3):446–50.
86. McKhann GM 2nd, Schoenfeld-McNeill J, Born DE, Haglund MM, Ojemann GA. Intraoperative hippocampal electrocorticography to predict the extent of hippocampal resection in temporal lobe epilepsy surgery. J Neurosurg. 2000;93(1):44–52.
87. Radhakrishnan K, So EL, Silbert PL, et al. Predictors of outcome of anterior temporal lobectomy for intractable epilepsy: a multivariate study. Neurology. 1998;51(2):465–71.
88. Roberts DW. Technical advances in the surgical treatment of epilepsy. Adv Neurol. 2000;84:643–9.
89. Spencer SS. When should temporal-lobe epilepsy be treated surgically? Lancet Neurol. 2002;1(6):375–82.
90. Armon C, Radtke RA, Friedman AH, Dawson DV. Predictors of outcome of epilepsy surgery: multivariate analysis with validation. Epilepsia. 1996;37(9):814–21.
91. Bengzon AR, Rasmussen T, Gloor P, Dussault J, Stephens M. Prognostic factors in the surgical treatment of temporal lobe epileptics. Neurology. 1968;18(8):717–31.
92. Mansouri A, Fallah A, Valiante TA. Determining surgical candidacy in temporal lobe epilepsy. Epilepsy Res Treat. 2012;2012:706917.
93. Schulz R, Luders HO, Hoppe M, Tuxhorn I, May T, Ebner A. Interictal EEG and ictal scalp EEG propagation are highly predictive of surgical outcome in mesial temporal lobe epilepsy. Epilepsia. 2000;41(5):564–70.
94. Spencer DD, Spencer SS, Mattson RH, Williamson PD, Novelly RA. Access to the posterior medial temporal lobe structures in the surgical treatment of temporal lobe epilepsy. Neurosurgery. 1984;15(5):667–71.
95. Hori T, Tabuchi S, Kurosaki M, Kondo S, Takenobu A, Watanabe T. Subtemporal amygdalohippocampectomy for treating medically intractable temporal lobe epilepsy. Neurosurgery. 1993;33(1):50–6. discussion 56-57

96. Hori T, Yamane F, Ochiai T, et al. Selective subtemporal amygdalohippocampectomy for refractory temporal lobe epilepsy: operative and neuropsychological outcomes. J Neurosurg. 2007;106(1):134–41.
97. Niemeyer P. The transventricular amygdalohippocampectomy in temporal lobe epilepsy. In: Baldwin P, editor. Temporal lobe epilepsy. Springfield: Charles C Thomas; 1958. p. 461–82.
98. Wagner K, Uherek M, Horstmann S, et al. Memory outcome after hippocampus sparing resections in the temporal lobe. J Neurol Neurosurg Psychiatry. 2013;84(6):630–6.
99. Wieser HG, Yasargil MG. Selective amygdalohippocampectomy as a surgical treatment of mesiobasal limbic epilepsy. Surg Neurol. 1982;17(6):445–57.
100. Sindou M, Auque J, Jouanneau E. Neurosurgery and intracranial venous system. Acta Neurochir Suppl. 2005;94:167–75.
101. Sood S, Asano E, Chugani HT. Significance of preserving the vein of Labbé in epilepsy surgery involving temporal resection. J Neurosurg. 2006;105:210–3.
102. Walczak TS. Neocortical temporal lobe epilepsy: characterizing the syndrome. Epilepsia. 1995;36(7):633–5.
103. Cascino GD, Jack CR Jr, Parisi JE, et al. Operative strategy in patients with MRI-identified dual pathology and temporal lobe epilepsy. Epilepsy Res. 1993;14(2):175–82.
104. Lombardi D, Marsh R, de Tribolet N. Low grade glioma in intractable epilepsy: lesionectomy versus epilepsy surgery. Acta Neurochir Suppl. 1997;68:70–4.
105. Rougier A, Saint-Hilaire JC, Loiseau P, Bouvier G. Investigations et traitement chirurgical des epilepsies. Neurochirurgie. 1992;38:2–112.
106. Olivier A, Cukiert A, Andermann F. Transsulcal selective amygdalohippocampectomy: Surgical techniques and results in 50 cases. Book of abstracts of the XIth Meeting of WSSFN, Ixtapa, p 70. 1993
107. Olivier A. Transcortical selective amygdalohippocampectomy in temporal lobe epilepsy. Can J Neurol Sci. 2000;27(Suppl 1):S68–76; discussion S92-S66
108. Sarmento SA, Rabelo NN, Figueiredo EG. Minimally invasive technique (nummular craniotomy) for mesial temporal lobe epilepsy: a comparison of two approaches. World Neurosurg. 2020;134:e636–41. https://doi.org/10.1016/j.wneu.2019.10.160.
109. Shimizu H, Suzuki S, Ishijima B. Zygomatic approach for resection of mesial temporal epileptic focus. Neurosurgery. 1989;25:798–801.
110. Duckworth EA, Vale FL. Trephine epilepsy surgery: the inferior temporal gyrus approach. Neurosurgery. 2008;63(1 suppl 1):156–60. discussion 160-161
111. Yasargil MG, Teddy PJ, Roth P. Selective amygdalohippocampectomy. Operative anatomy and surgical technique. In: Symon L, et al., editors. Advances and technical standards in neurosurgery, vol. 12. Wien, New York: Springer; 1985. p. 93–123.
112. Mayanagi Y. Transsylvian unco-amygdalo-hippocampectomy: en-bloc resection. Proceedings of Second International Cleveland Clinic Epilepsy Symposium, Cleveland. Abstract T6; 1990. p 53
113. Liao C-H, Chen S-C, Yu H-Y, et al. Procedure-related temporal infarct after retractorless transsylvian selective amygdalohippocampectomy and impact on 2-year epilepsy outcome. Oper Neurosurg. 2020;18(4):430–7. https://doi.org/10.1093/ons/opz192.
114. Schmeiser B, Wagner K, Schulze-Bonhage A, Elger CE, Steinhoff BJ, Wendling A-S, Mader I, Prinz M, Scheiwe C, Zentner J. Transsylvian selective amygdalohippocampectomy for mesiotemporal epilepsy: Experience with 162 procedures. Neurosurgery. 2017a;80:454–64.
115. Beaton AE, Durnford A, Heffer-Rahn PE, Kirkham F, Griffin A, Gray WP. Transsylvian selective amygdalohippocampectomy in children with hippocampal sclerosis: seizure, intellectual and memory outcome. Seizure. 2012;21(9):699–705.
116. Kovanda TJ, Tubbs RS, Cohen-Gadol AA. Transsylvian selective amygdalohippocampectomy for treatment of medial temporal lobe epilepsy: surgical technique and operative nuances to avoid complications. Surg Neurol Int. 2014;5:133.
117. Morino M, Ichinose T, Uda T, Kondo K, Ohfuji S, Ohata K. Memory outcome following transsylvian selective amygdalohippocampectomy in 62 patients with hippocampal sclerosis. J Neurosurg. 2009;110(6):1164–9.
118. von Rhein B, Nelles M, Urbach H, Von Lehe M, Schramm J, Helmstaedter C. Neuropsychological outcome after selective amygdalohippocampectomy: subtemporal versus transsylvian approach. J Neurol Neurosurg Psychiatry. 2012;83(9):887–93.
119. Park TS, Bourgeois BF, Silbergeld DL, Dodson WE. Subtemporal transparahippocampal amygdalohippocampectomy for surgical treatment of mesial temporal lobe epilepsy. Technical note. J Neurosurg. 1996;85(6):1172–6.
120. Delev D, Schramm J, Clusmann H. How I do it—selective amygdalohippocampectomy via a navigated temporobasal approach, when veins forbid elevation of the temporal lobe. Acta Neurochir. 2018;160(3):597–601. https://doi.org/10.1007/s00701-017-3386-7.
121. Pitskhelauri D, Konovalov A, Kudieva E, et al. Burr hole microsurgery for intracranial tumors and mesial temporal lobe epilepsy: Results of 200 Consecutive Operations. World Neurosurg. 2019;126:e1257–67. https://doi.org/10.1016/j.wneu.2019.02.239.
122. Engel J Jr, McDermott MP, Wiebe S, Langfitt JT, Stern JM, Dewar S, et al. Early surgical therapy for drug-resistant temporal lobe epilepsy: a randomized trial. JAMA. 2012;307:922–30.
123. Hermann B, Davies K, Foley K, Kell B. Visual confrontation naming outcome after standard left anterior temporal lobectomy with sparing versus resection of the superior temporal gyrus: a randomized prospective clinical trial. Epilepsia. 1999;40:1070–6.

124. Lutz MT, Clusmann H, Elger CE, Schramm J, Helmstaedter C. Neuropsychological outcome after selective amygdalohippocampectomy with transsylvian versus transcortical approach: a randomized prospective clinical trial of surgery for temporal lobe epilepsy. Epilepsia. 2004;45:809–16.
125. Schramm J, Lehmann TN, Zentner J, et al. Randomized controlled trial of 2.5-cm versus 3.5-cm mesial temporal resection in temporal lobe epilepsy–Part 1: intent-to-treat analysis. Acta Neurochir. 2011a;153(2):209–19.
126. Schramm J, Lehmann TN, Zentner J, et al. Randomized controlled trial of 2.5-cm versus 3.5-cm mesial temporal resection–Part 2: volumetric resection extent and subgroup analyses. Acta Neurochir. 2011b;153(2):221–8.
127. Vogt VL, Delev D, Grote A, et al. Neuropsychological outcome after subtemporal versus transsylvian approach for selective amygdalohippocampectomy in patients with mesial temporal lobe epilepsy: a randomised prospective clinical trial. J Neurol Neurosurg Psychiatry. 2018;89(10):1057–63. https://doi.org/10.1136/jnnp-2017-316311.
128. Wiebe S, Blume WT, Girvin JP, Eliasziw M. Effectiveness, efficiency of surgery for temporal lobe epilepsy study G. A randomized, controlled trial of surgery for temporal-lobe epilepsy. N Engl J Med. 2001;345(5):311–8.
129. Wyler AR, Hermann BP, Somes G. Extent of medial temporal resection on outcome from anterior temporal lobectomy: a randomized prospective study. Neurosurgery. 1995;37(5):982–90. discussion 990-981
130. Engel JJ, Van Nes P, Rasmussen T, Ojemann L. Outcome with respect to epileptic seizures. In: Engel Jr J, editor. Surgical treatment of the epilepsies. 2nd ed. New York, NY: Raven Press; 1993. p. 609–21.
131. Téllez-Zenten JF, Dhar RJ, Wiebe S. Long-term seizure outcomes following epilepsy surgery: a systematic review and meta-analysis. Brain. 2005;128:1188–98.
132. Jobst BC, Cascino GD. Resective epilepsy surgery for drug-resistant focal epilepsy. A review. JAMA. 2015;313(3):285–93.
133. Clusmann H, Schramm J, Kral T, et al. Prognostic factors and outcome after different types of resection for temporal lobe epilepsy. J Neurosurg. 2002;97(5):1131–41.
134. Elliott RE, Bollo RJ, Berliner JL, et al. Anterior temporal lobectomy with amygdalohippocampectomy for mesial temporal sclerosis: predictors of long-term seizure control. J Neurosurg. 2013;119(2):261–72.
135. Foldvary N, Nashold B, Mascha E, et al. Seizure outcome after temporal lobectomy for temporal lobe epilepsy: a Kaplan-Meier survival analysis. Neurology. 2000;54(3):630–4.
136. Gleissner U, Helmstaedter C, Schramm J, Elger CE. Memory outcome after selective amygdalohippocampectomy in patients with temporal lobe epilepsy: one-year follow-up. Epilepsia. 2004;45(8):960–2.
137. Jutila L, Immonen A, Mervaala E, et al. Long term outcome of temporal lobe epilepsy surgery: analyses of 140 consecutive patients. J Neurol Neurosurg Psychiatry. 2002;73(5):486–94.
138. Mansouri A, Fallah A, McAndrews MP, et al. Neurocognitive and seizure outcomes of selective amygdalohippocampectomy versus anterior temporal lobectomy for mesial temporal lobe epilepsy. Epilepsy Res Treat. 2014;2014:306382.
139. Spencer SS, Berg AT, Vickrey BG, et al. Predicting long-term seizure outcome after resective epilepsy surgery: the multicenter study. Neurology. 2005;65(6):912–8.
140. Renowden SA, Matkovic Z, Adams CB, et al. Selective amygdalohippocampectomy for hippocampal sclerosis: postoperative MR appearance. AJNR. 1995;16(9):1855–61.
141. Josephson CB, Dykeman J, Fiest KM, et al. Systematic review and meta-analysis of standard vs. selective temporal lobe epilepsy surgery. Neurology. 2013;80(18):1669–76.
142. Hu WH, Zhang C, Zhang K, Meng FG, Chen N, Zhang JG. Selective amygdalohippocampectomy versus anterior temporal lobectomy in the management of mesial temporal lobe epilepsy: a meta-analysis of comparative studies. J Neurosurg. 2013;119(5):1089–97.
143. Kuang Y, Yang T, Gu J, Kong B, Cheng L. Comparison of therapeutic effects between selective amygdalohippocampectomy and anterior temporal lobectomy for the treatment of temporal lobe epilepsy: a meta-analysis. Br J Neurosurg. 2014;28(3):374–7.
144. Bate H, Eldridge P, Varma T, Wieshmann UC. The seizure outcome after amygdalohippocampectomy and temporal lobectomy. Eur J Neurol. 2007;14:90–4.
145. Clusmann H, Kral T, Fackeldey E, et al. Lesional mesial temporal lobe epilepsy and limited resections: prognostic factors and outcome. J Neurol Neurosurg Psychiatry. 2004a;75:1589–96.
146. Clusmann H, Kral T, Gleissner U, Sassen R, Urbach H, Blumcke I, Bogucki J, Schramm J. Analysis of different types of resection for pediatric patients with temporal lobe epilepsy. Neurosurgery. 2004b;54:847–59. discussion 859–860
147. Mackenzie RA, Matheson J, Ellis M, Klamus J. Selective versus non-selective temporal lobe surgery for epilepsy. J Clin Neurosci. 1997;4(2):152–4.
148. Hadar E, Bingaman W, Foldvary M, Chelune GJ, Comair YG. Prospective analysis of outcome after selective amygdalohippocampectomy and anterior temporal lobectomy for refractory epilepsy. San Diego, CA: Congress of Neurological Surgeons; 2001.
149. Paglioli E, Palmini A, Portuguez M, et al. Seizure and memory outcome following temporal lobe surgery: selective compared with nonselective

approaches for hippocampal sclerosis. J Neurosurg. 2006;104(1):70–8.
150. Pauli E, Pickel S, Schulemann H, Buchfelder M, Stefan H. Neuropsychologic findings depending on the type of the resection in temporal lobe epilepsy. Adv Neurol. 1999;81:371–7.
151. Tanriverdi T, Olivier A. Cognitive changes after unilateral corticoamygdalohippocampectomy unilateral selective-amygdalohippocampectomy mesial temporal lobe epilepsy. Turk Neurosurg. 2007;17(2):91–9.
152. Tanriverdi T, Dudley RWR, Hasan A, et al. Memory outcome after temporal lobe epilepsy surgery: corticoamygdalohippocampectomy versus selective amygdalohippocampectomy. J Neurosurg. 2010;113:1164–75.
153. Bujarski KA, Hirashima F, Roberts DW, et al. Long-term seizure, cognitive, and psychiatric outcome following trans-middle temporal gyrus amygdalohippocampectomy and standard temporal lobectomy. J Neurosurg. 2013;119(1):16–23.
154. Clusmann H. Predictors, procedures, and perspective for temporal lobe epilepsy surgery. Semin Ultrasound CT MRI. 2008;29:60–70.
155. Malikova H, Kramska L, Vojtech Z, et al. Different surgical approaches for mesial temporal epilepsy: resection extent, seizure, and neuropsychological outcomes. Stereotact Funct Nereuosurg. 2014;92(6):372–80.
156. Schmeiser B, Daniel M, Kogias E, et al. Visual field defects following different resective procedures for mesiotemporal lobe epilepsy. Epilepsy Behav. 2017c;EB 76:39–45.
157. Schmeiser B, Zentner J, Steinhoff BJ, et al. The role of presurgical EEG parameters and of reoperation for seizure outcome in temporal lobe epilepsy. Seizure. 2017f;51:174–9.
158. Staack AM, Wendling AS, Scholly J, et al. Quality control of elective surgery for drug-resistant epilepsy in a German reference centre – a long-term outcome study. Seizure. 2013;22(4):292–8.
159. Nayel MH, Awad IA, Luders H. Extent of mesiobasal resection determines outcome after temporal lobectomy for intractable complex partial seizures. Neurosurgery. 1991;29(1):55–60. discussion 60-51
160. Siegel AM, Wieser HG, Wichmann W, Yasargil GM. Relationships between MR-imaged total amount of tissue removed, resection scores of specific mediobasal limbic subcompartments and clinical outcome following selective amygdalohippocampectomy. Epilepsy Res. 1990;6(1):56–65.
161. Bonilha L, Kobayashi E, Mattos JP, Honorato DC, Li LM, Cendes F. Value of extent of hippocampal resection in the surgical treatment of temporal lobe epilepsy. Arq Neuropsiquiatr. 2004;62(1):15–20.
162. McIntosh AM, Wilson SJ, Berkovic SF. Seizure outcome after temporal lobectomy: current research practice and findings. Epilepsia. 2001;42:1288–307.
163. Tonini C, Beghi E, Berg AT, et al. Predictors of epilepsy surgery outcome: a meta-analysis. Epilepsy Res. 2004;62:75–87.
164. Bonilha L, Yaszda CL, Rorden C, et al. Does resection of the mesial temporal lobe improve the outcome of temporal lobe epilepsy surgery? Epilepsia. 2007;48(3):571–8.
165. Wolf RL, Ivnik RJ, Hirschorn KA, Sharbrough FW, Cascino GD, Marsh WR. Neurocognitive efficiency following left temporal lobectomy: standard versus limited resection. J Neurosurg. 1993;79:76–83.
166. Son EI, Howard MA, Ojemann GA, Lettich E. Comparing the extent of hippocampal removal to the outcome in terms of seizure control. Stereotact Funct Neurosurg. 1994;62(1-4):232–7.
167. Jack CR Jr, Sharbrough FW, Marsh WR. Use of MR imaging for quantitative evaluation of resection for temporal lobe epilepsy. Radiology. 1988;169(2):463–8.
168. Jones-Gotman M, Zatorre RJ, Olivier A, Andermann F, Cendes F, Staunton H, McMackin D, Siegel AM, Wieser HG. Learning and retention of words and designs following excision from medial or lateral temporal-lobe structures. Neuropsychologia. 1997;35:963–73.
169. Kanner AM, Kaydanova Y. deToledo-Morrell L, Morrell F, Smith MC, Bergen D, Pierre-Louis SJ, Ristanovic R. Tailored anterior temporal lobectomy. Relation between extent of resection of mesial structures and postsurgical seizure outcome. Arch Neurol. 1995;52:173–8.
170. Van Rijckevorsel K, Grandin C, de Tourtchaninoff M, Vaz G, Raftopoulos C. Selective amygdalohippocampectomy: seizure outcome in 26 consecutive cases compared to the amount of resection. Epilepsia. 2005;46:253–60.
171. Patil AA, Andrews R. Long term follow-up after multiple hippocampal transection (MHT). Seizure. 2013;22:731–4. https://doi.org/10.1016/j.seizure.2013.05.014.
172. Warsi N, Thiong'o GM, Zuccato J, et al. Multiple hippocampal transections: Post-operative memory outcomes and seizure control. Epilepsy Behav. 2019;100:106496. https://doi.org/10.1016/j.yebeh.2019.106496.
173. McIntosh AM, Kalnins RM, Mitchell A, et al. Temporal lobectomy: long-term seizure outcome, late recurrence and risks for seizure recurrence. Brain. 2004;127:2018–30.
174. Englot DJ, Rolston JD, Wang DD, et al. Seizure outcomes after temporal lobectomy in pediatric patients. J Neurosurg Pediatr. 2013;12(2):134–41.
175. Lopez-Gonzalez MA, Gonzalez-Martinez JA, Jehi L, Kotagal P, Warbel A, Bingaman W. Epilepsy surgery of the temporal lobe in pediatric population: a retrospective analysis. Neurosurgery. 2012;70(3):684–92.
176. Najim I, Jehi L, Palmini A, et al. Trempòral patterns and mechanisms of epilepsy surgery failure. Epilepsia. 2013;54:772–82.
177. Rowland NC, Englot DJ, Cage TA, et al. A meta-analysis of predictors of seizure freedom in the surgical management of focal cortical dysplasia. J Neurosurg. 2012;116:1035–41.

178. Schmeiser B, Hammen T, Steinhoff BJ, et al. Long-term outcome characteristics in mesial temporal lobe epilepsy with and without associated cortical dysplasia. Epilepsy Res. 2016;126:147–56.
179. Téllez-Zenteno JF, Hernández Ronquillo L, Moien-Afshari F, et al. Surgical outcomes in lesional and non-lesional epilepsy: a systematic review and meta-analysis. Epilepsy Res. 2010;89(2-3):310–8.
180. Barba C, Rheims S, Minotti L, et al. Temporal plus epilepsy is a major determinant of temporal lobe surgery failures. Brain. 2016;139(Pt 2):444–51. [Epub ahead of print] The first study to suggest that TPE represents the main reason for failed anterior temporal lobectomy
181. Bernasconi N, Bernasconi A, Caramanos Z, et al. Mesial temporal damage in temporal lobe epilepsy: a volumetric MRI study of the hippocampus, amygdala and parahippocampal region. Brain. 2003;126(Pt2):462–9.
182. Jeong SW, Lee SK, Hong KS, et al. Prognostic factors for the surgery for mesial temporal lobe epilepsy: longitudinal analysis. Epilepsia. 2005;46(8):1273–9.
183. Uijl SG, Leijten FSS, Arends JBAM, et al. Prognosis after temporal lobe epilepsy surgery: The value of combining predictors. Epilepsia. 2008;49(8):1317–23.
184. Bjellvi J, Olsson I, Malmgren K, et al. Epilepsy duration and seizure outcome in epilepsy surgery. Neurology. 2019;93:e159–66. https://doi.org/10.1212/WNL.0000000000007753.
185. Bialek F, Rydenhag B, Flink R, Malmgren K. Outcomes after resective epilepsy surgery in patients over 50 years of age in Sweden 1990–2009: a prospective longitudinal study. Seizure. 2014;23:641–5.
186. Dewar S, Eliashiv D, Walshaw PD, et al. Safety, efficacy, and life satisfaction & following epilepsy surgery in patients aged 60 years and older. J Neurosurg. 2016;124(4):945–51.
187. Murphy M, Smith PD, Wood M, et al. Surgery for temporal lobe epilepsy associated with mesial temporal sclerosis in the older patient: a longterm follow-up. Epilepsia. 2010;51:1024–9.
188. O'Dwyer R, Byrne R, Lynn F, et al. Age is but a number when considering epilepsy surgery in older adults. Epilepsy Behav. 2018;91:9–12. https://doi.org/10.1016/j.yebeh.2018.05.022.
189. Schmeiser B, Steinhoff BJ, Schulze-Bonhage A. Does early postoperative drug regimen impact seizure control in patients undergoing temporal lobe resections? J Neurol. 2018;265(3):500–9. https://doi.org/10.1007/s00415-017-8700-z.
190. Gleissner U, Sassen R, Schramm J, et al. Greater functional recovery after temporal lobe epilepsy surgery in children. Brain. 2005;128(Pt 12):2822–9.
191. Miserocchi A, Cascardo B, Piroddi C, et al. Surgery for temporal lobe epilepsy in children: relevance of presurgical evaluation and analysis of outcome. J Neurosurg Pediatr. 2013;11(3):256–67.
192. Mohamed A, Wyllie E, Ruggieri P, et al. Temporal lobe epilepsy due to hippocampal sclerosis in pediatric candidates for epilepsy surgery. Neurology. 2001;56(12):1643–9.
193. Smyth MD, Limbrick DD Jr, Ojemann JG, et al. Outcome following surgery for temporal lobe epilepsy with hippocampal involvement in preadolescent children: emphasis on mesial temporal sclerosis. J Neurosurg. 2007;106:205–10.
194. Terra-Bustamante VC, Inuzuca LM, Fernandes RM, et al. Temporal lobe epilepsy surgery in children and adolescents: clinical characteristics and post-surgical outcome. Seizure. 2005;14(4):274–81.
195. Blümcke I, Spreafico G, Haaker R, et al. Histopathological findings in brain tissue obtained during epilepsy surgery. N Engl J Med. 2017;377:1648–56.
196. Carrete H Jr, Abdala N, Lin K, Caboclo LO, Centeno RS, Sakamoto AC, Szjenfeld J, Nogueira RG, Yacubian EM. Temporal pole signal abnormality on MR imaging in temporal lobe epilepsy with hippocampal sclerosis: a fluid-attenuated inversion-recovery study. Arq Neuropsiquiatr. 2007;65(3A):553–60.
197. Choi D, Na DG, Byun HS, Suh YL, Kim SE, Ro DW, Chung IG, Hong SC, Hong SB. White-matter change in mesial temporal sclerosis: correlation of MRI with PET, pathology, and clinical features. Epilepsia. 1999;40(11):1634–41.
198. Mitchell LA, Harvey AS, Coleman LT, Mandelstam SA, Jackson GD. Anterior temporal changes on MR images of children with hippocampal sclerosis: an effect of seizures on the immature brain? AJNR Am J Neuroradiol. 2003;24(8):1670–7.
199. Naves PVF, Caboclo LOSF, Carrete H, et al. Temporopolar blurring in temporal lobe epilepsy with hippocampal sclerosis and long-term prognosis after epilepsy surgery. Epilepsy Res. 2015;112:76–83.
200. Schijns OEMG, Bien CG, Majores M, et al. Presence of temporal gray-white matter abnormalities does not influence epilepsy surgery outcome in temporal lobe epilepsy with hippocampal sclerosis. Neurosurgery. 2011;68:98–107.
201. Garbelli R, Milesi G, Medici V, Villani F, Didato G, Deleo F, D'Incerti L, Morbin M, Mazzoleni G, Giovagnoli AR, Parente A, Zucca I, Mastropietro A, Spreafico R. Blurring in patients with temporal lobe epilepsy: clinical, high-field imaging and ultrastructural study. Brain. 2012;135(Pt 8):2337–49.
202. Kuba R, Tyrlíková I, Paˇzourková M, Hermanová M, Horáková I, Brázdil M, Rektor I. Grey-white matter abnormalities in temporal lobe epilepsy associated with hippocampal sclerosis: inter-observer analysis, histopathological findings, and correlation with clinical variables. Epilepsy Res. 2012;102(1–2):78–85.
203. Mitchell LA, Jackson GD, Kalnins RM, Saling MM, Fitt GJ, Ashpole RD, Berkovic SF. Anterior temporal abnormality in temporal lobe epilepsy: a quantitative MRI and histopathologic study. Neurology. 1999;52(2):327–36.
204. Robinson S, Park TS, Blackburn LB, Bourgeois BF, Arnold ST, Dodson WE. Transparahippocampal selective amygdalohippocampectomy in children and adolescents: efficacy of the procedure and cognitive morbidity in patients. J Neurosurg. 2000;93(3):402–9.
205. Helmstaedter C, van Roost D, Clusmann H, et al. Collateral brain damage, a potential source of cogni-

tive impairment after selective surgery for control of mesial temporal lobe epilepsy. J Neurol Neurosurg Psychiatry. 2004;75(2):323–6.
206. Gollwitzer S, Scott CA, Farrell F, et al. The long-term course of temporal lobe epilepsy: From unilateral to bilateral interictal epileptiform discharges in repeated video-EEG monitorings. Epilepsy Behav. 2017;68:17–21.
207. King D, Spencer SS, McCarthy G, et al. Bilateral hippocampal atrophy in medial temporal lobe epilepsy. Epilepsia. 1995;36(9):905–10.
208. Jutila L, Aikia M, Immonen A, Mervaala E, Alafuzoff I, Kalviainen R. Long-term memory performance after surgical treatment of unilateral temporal lobe epilepsy (TLE). Epilepsy Res. 2014;108(7):1228–37.
209. Helmstaedter C, Reuber M, Elger CC. Interaction of cognitive aging and memory deficits related to epilepsy surgery. Ann Neurol. 2002;52:89–94.
210. Helmstaedter C, Elger CE, Vogt VL. Cognitive outcomes more than 5 years after temporal lobe epilepsy surgery: Remarkable functional recovery when seizures are controlled. Seizure. 2018;62:116–23. https://doi.org/10.1016/j.seizure.2018.09.023.
211. Ojemann G, Dodrill C. Verbal memory deficits after left temporal lobectomy for epilepsy. J Neurosurg. 1985;62:101–7.
212. Bauman K, Devinsky O, Liu AA. Temporal lobe surgery and memory: Lessons, risks, and opportunities. Epilepsy Behav. 2019:101, 106596. https://doi.org/10.1016/j.yebeh.2019.106596.
213. Sherman EM, Wiebe S, Fay-McClymont TB, et al. Neuropsychological outcomes after epilepsy surgery. Epilepsia. 2011;52(5):857–69.
214. Lee TM, Yip JT, Jones-Gotman M. Memory deficits after resection from left or right anterior temporal lobe in humans: a meta-analytic review. Epilepsia. 2002;43(3):283–91.
215. Helmstaedter C, Richter S, Roske S, et al. Differential effects of temporal pole resection with amygdalohippocampectomy versus selective amygdalohippocampectomy on material-specific memory in patients with mesial temporal lobe epilepsy. Epilepsia. 2008;49(1):88–97.
216. Acar G, Acar F, Miller J, Spencer DC, Burchiel KJ. Seizure outcome following transcortical selective amygdalohippocampectomy in mesial temporal lobe epilepsy. Stereotact Funct Neurosurg. 2008;86(5):314–9.
217. Bell ML, Rao S, So EL, et al. Epilepsy surgery outcomes in temporal lobe epilepsy with a normal MRI. Epilepsia. 2009;50(9):2053–60.
218. Helmstaedter C, Loer B, Wohlfart R, et al. The effects of cognitive rehabilitation on memory outcome after temporal lobe epilepsy surgery. Epilepsy Behav. 2008a;12:402–9.
219. Helmstaedter C, Richter S, Roske S, Oltmanns F, Schramm J, Lehmann TN. Differential effects of temporal pole resection with amygdalohippocampectomy versus selective amygdalohippocampectomy on material-specific memory in patients with mesial temporal lobe epilepsy. Epilepsia. 2008b;49:88–97.
220. Grivas A, Schramm J, Kral T, et al. Surgical treatment for refractory temporal lobe epilepsy in the elderly: seizure outcome and neuropsychological sequels compared with a younger cohort. Epilepsia. 2006;47(8):1364–72.
221. Katz A, Awad IA, Kong AK, et al. Extent of resection in temporal lobectomy for epilepsy. II. Memory changes and neurologic complications. Epilepsia. 1989;30(6):763–71.
222. Hori T, Yamane F, Ochiai T, Hayashi M, Taira T. Subtemporal amygdalohippocampectomy prevents verbal memory impairment in the language-dominant hemisphere. Stereotact Funct Neurosurg. 2003;80(1-4):18–21.
223. Goldstein LH, Polkey CE. Short-term cognitive changes after unilateral temporal lobectomy or unilateral amygdalohippocampectomy for the relief of temporal lobe epilepsy. J Neurol Neurosurg Psychiatry. 1993;56:135–40.
224. Helmstaedter C, Elger CE, Hufnagel A, Zentner J, Schramm J. Different effects of left anterior temporal lobectomy, selective amygdalohippocampectomy, and temporal cortical lesionectomy on verbal learning, memory, and recognition. J Epilepsy. 1996;9:39–45.
225. Yasargil MG, Krayenbuhl N, Roth P, Hsu SP, Yasargil DC. The selective amygdalohippocampectomy for intractable temporal limbic seizures. J Neurosurg. 2010;112(1):168–85.
226. Giovagnoli AR, Casazza M, Ciceri E, Avanzini G, Broggi G. Preserved memory in temporal lobe epilepsy patients after surgery for low-grade tumour. A pilot study. Neurol Sci. 2007;28(5):251–8.
227. Helmstaedter C, Roeske S, Kaaden S, Elger CE, Schramm J. Hippocampal resection length and memory outcome in selective epilepsy surgery. J Neurol Neurosurg Psychiatry. 2011a;82(12):1375–81.
228. Helmstaedter C, Roeske S, Kaaden S, et al. Hippocampal resection length and memory outcome in selective epilepsy surgery. J Neurol Neurosurg Psychiatry. 2011b;82(12):1375–81. https://doi.org/10.1136/jnnp.2010.240176.
229. Leonard G. Temporal lobe surgery for epilepsy: neuropsychological variables related to surgical outcome. Can J Neurol Sci. 1991;18:593–7.
230. Goldstein LH, Polkey CE. Behavioural memory after temporal lobectomy or amygdalohippocampectomy. Br J Clin Psychol. 1992;31(Pt 1):75–81.
231. Hader WJ, Pillay N, Myles ST, Partlo L, Wiebe S. The benefit of selective over standard surgical resections in the treatment of intractable temporal lobe epilepsy. Epilepsia. 2005;46:253–60.
232. Walton NH, Goodsman C, McCarter R, et al. An analysis of neuropsychological change scores following selective temporal resections of the non-dominant temporal lobe. Seizure. 1999;8(4):241–5.
233. Loring DW, Lee GP, Meador KJ, Smith JR, Martin RC, Ackell AB, Flanigin HF. Hippocampal contribution to verbal recent memory following dominant-hemisphere temporal lobectomy. J Clin Exp Neuropsychol. 1991;13:575–86.
234. Jain P, Tomlison G, Snead C, et al. Systematic review and network meta-analysis of resective surgery for

mesial temporal lobe epilepsy. Neurol Neurosurg Psychiatry. 2018;89:1138–44.
235. Helmstaedter C, Kurthen M, Lux S, et al. Chronic epilepsy and cognition. A longitudinal study in temporal lobe epilepsy. Ann Neruol. 2003;54:425–32.
236. Milner B. Psychological defects produced by temporal-lobe excision. Res Publ Assoc Res Nerv Ment Dis. 1958;36:244–57.
237. Milner B. Visually guided maze-learning in man: effects of bilateral hippocampal, bilateral frontal, and unilateral cerebral lesions. Neuropsychologia. 1965;3:317–38.
238. Milner B. Visual recognition and recall after right temporal-lobe excision in man. Neuropsychologia. 1968;6:191–209.
239. Blume WT, David RB, Gomez MR. Generalized sharp and slow wave complexes. Associated clinical features and long-term follow-up. Brain. 1973;96:289–306.
240. Blume WT, Parrent AG, Kaibara M. Stereotactic amygdalohippocampotomy and mesial temporal spikes. Epilepsia. 1997;38:930–6.
241. Skirrow C, Cross JH, Harrison S, et al. Temporal lobe surgery in childhood neuroanatomical predictors of long-term declarative memory outcome. Brain. 2015;138(Pt 1):80–93.
242. Bonelli SB, Thompson PJ, Yogarajah M, et al. Memory reorganization following anterior temporal lobe resection: a longitudinal functional MRI study. Brain. 2013;136(Pt 6):1889–900.
243. Ojemann G, Dodrill C. Intraoperative techniques for reducing language and memory deficits with left temporal lobectomy. Adv Epileptology. 1987;16:327–30.
244. Wagner K, Metternich B, Geiger M, et al. Effects of hippocampus-sparing resections in the temporal lobe: Hippocampal atrophy is associated with decline in memory performance. Epilepsia. 2020;61(4):725–34.
245. Hoppe C, Witt JA, Helmstaedter C. Depressed mood should not be regarded as a contraindication to epilepsy surgery. Epilepsy Behav. 2010;17(4):574. author reply 575-6
246. Vakharia VN, Duncan JS, Elger CE, Staba R. Getting the best outcomes from epilepsy surgery. Ann Neurol. 2018; https://doi.org/10.1002/ana.25205.
247. Busch RM, Love TE, Jehi LE, et al. Effect of invasive EEG monitoring on cognitive outcome after left temporal lobe epilepsy surgery. Neurology. 2015;85(17):1475–81.
248. Fasano RE, Kanner AM. Psychiatric complications after epilepsy surgery … but where are the psychiatrists? Epilepsy Behav. 2019;98:318–21.
249. Jensen I, Larsen JK. Mental aspects of temporal lobe epilepsy. Follow-up of 74 patients after resection of a temporal lobe. J Neurol Neurosurg Psychiatry. 1979;42:256–65.
250. Shahani L, Cervenka G. Impact of surgical intervention on seizure and psychiatric symptoms in patients with temporal lobe epilepsy. BMJ Case Rep. 2019;12:e229242. https://doi.org/10.1136/bcr-2019-229242.
251. Cleary RA, Baxendale SA, Thompson PJ, Foong J. Predicting and preventing psychopathology following temporal lobe epilepsy surgery. Epilepsy Behav. 2013;26(3):322–34.
252. Trebuchon A, Bartolomei F, McGonigal A, et al. Reversible antisocial behavior in ventromedial prefrontal lobe epilepsy. Epilepsy Behav. 2013;29(2):367–73.
253. Devinsky O, Barr WB, Vickrey BG, Berg AT, Bazil CW, Pacia SV, et al. Changes in depression and anxiety after respective surgery for epilepsy. Neurology. 2005;65:1744–9.
254. De Araujo Filho GM, Gomes FL, Mazetto L, Marinho MM, Tavares IM, Caboclo LO, et al. Major depressive disorder as a predictor of a worse seizure outcome one year after surgery in patients with temporal lobe epilepsy and mesial temporal sclerosis. Seizure. 2012;21(8):619–23. https://doi.org/10.1016/j.seizure.2012.07/002.
255. Spencer SS, Berg AT, Vickrey BG, Sperling MR, Bazil CW, Shinnar S, Langfitt JT, Walczak TS, Pacia SV, Ebrahimi N, Frobish D. Initial outcomes in the multicenter study of epilepsy surgery. Neurology. 2003;61:1680–5.
256. Macrodimitris S, Sherman EMS, Forde S, et al. Psychiatric outcomes of epilepsy surgery: A systematic review. Epilepsia. 2011;52(5):880–90.
257. Wrench JM, Wilson SJ, Bladin PF, Reuteins DC. Hippocampal volume and major depression: insights from epilepsy surgery. J Neurol Neurosurg Psychiatry. 2009;80:539–44.
258. Yang W, Chen C, Wu B, et al. Comprehensive analysis of presurgical factors predicting psychiatric disorders in patients with refractory temporal lobe epilepsy and mesial temporal sclerosis underwent corticoamygdalohippocampectomy. J Clin Lab Anal. 2018;33(3):e22724. https://doi.org/10.1002/jcla.22724.
259. Spencer S, Huh L. Outcomes of epilepsy surgery in adults and children. Lancet Neurol. 2008;7:525–37.
260. Markoula S, de Tisi J, Foong J, Duncan JS. De novo psychogenic nonepileptic attacks after adult epilepsy surgery: an underestimated entity. Epilepsia. 2013;54(12):e159–62.
261. Tebo CC, Evins AI, Christos PJ, Kwon J, Schwartz TH. Evolution of cranial epilepsy surgery complication rates: a 32-year systematic review and meta-analysis. J Neurosurg. 2014;120(6):1415–27.
262. Brotis AG, Giannis T, Kapsalaki E, Dardiotis E, Fountas KN. Complications after anterior temporal lobectomy for medically intractable epilepsy: a systematic review and meta-analysis. Stereotact Funct Neurosurg. 2019;2019 https://doi.org/10.1159/000500136.
263. Pilcher WH, Rusyniak WG. Complications of epilepsy surgery. Neurosurg Clin N Am. 1993;4(2):311–25.
264. Martin R. The burden of normality in the epilepsy postsurgery setting: out with the old and in with the new. Epilepsy Curr. 2016;16(6):375–7.
265. Ferguson SM, Rayport M. The adjustment to living without epilepsy. J Nerv Ment Dis. 1965;140:26–30.

# Extratemporal Resections 7

*There is no end to education. It is not that you read a book, pass an examination, and finish with education. The whole of life, from the moment you are born to the moment you die, is a process of learning.*

*Jiddu Krishnamurti*

## Contents





J. Zentner, *Surgical Treatment of Epilepsies*, https://doi.org/10.1007/978-3-030-48748-5_7

Extratemporal epilepsies (ETE) show a large variety of clinical syndromes. Variable seizure semiology can be attributed to the numerous neuronal systems connecting different structures. Limbic striae of the corpus callosum and in the basal cingulum (continuation of the hippocampus and of area dentata) connect all parts of the cortex. Frontomesial allocortical (limbic) and neocortical systems are connected by association pathways. Rapid propagation of ictal activity in a widespread network including projections to the contralateral side accounts to the complexity of extratemporal epileptic syndromes, thus rendering detection of respective seizure foci by clinical and electrophysiological assessment extremely difficult. Further problems restricting surgical treatment of ETE refer to the involvement of eloquent cortical areas including Broca's area, Rolandic cortex (pre- and postcentral gyrus), insula, and visual cortex [1–3]. Due to these obstacles, results of extratemporal resections reported in the past are not as favorable as in TLE [4–12].

Yet, advances in MR imaging facilitating detection of the structural basis of ETE and pointing to the epileptogenic zone have decisively changed this situation. In addition, PET and ictal SPECT [13–16], invasive diagnostic techniques based on the implantation of subdural and depth electrodes [17, 18], as well as intraoperative electrocorticography (ECoG) [19] may provide important information contributing to the definition of the epileptogenic zone. Overall, results of extratemporal resections have noticeably improved over time approximating or even exceeding now those obtained with temporal procedures. In fact, the success of epilepsy surgery over the last years has particularly become apparent in the treatment of extratemporal epilepsies [20–23], and this progress is reflected in the high variability of extratemporal outcome data comparing actual results with previous ones, while outcomes achieved with temporal procedures remained stable over the last decades [24, 25].

The first part of this chapter provides an overview on the functional anatomy of extratemporal areas. Epilepsy syndromes, resection strategies, overall seizure outcome, and prognostic factors are summarized in the second part, while the third part addresses specific aspects of frontal, Rolandic, posterior cortex, and insular epilepsies.

## 7.1 Functional Anatomy

### 7.1.1 Frontal Lobe

The frontal lobe can be divided into the *primary motor cortex*, *premotor cortex* including the *supplementary motor area (SMA)*, *frontal eye field*, and *Broca's area*, as well as *prefrontal cortex* (Fig. 7.1).

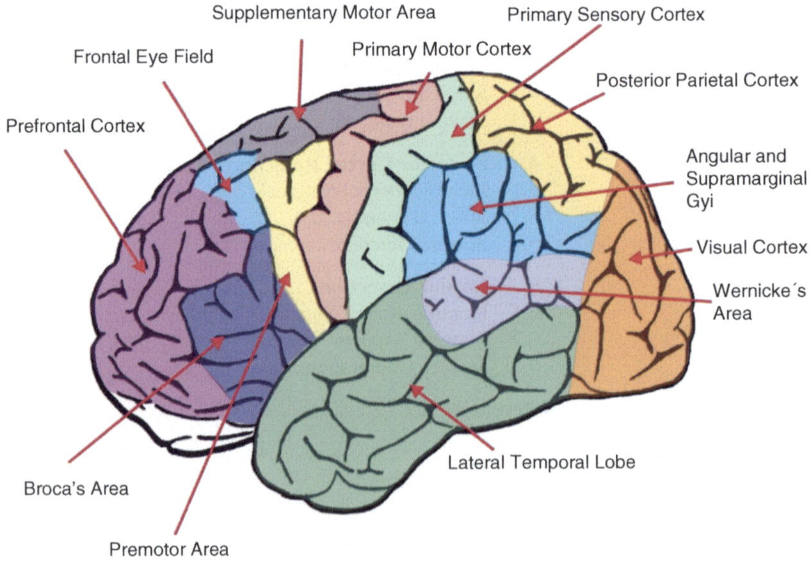


**Fig. 7.1** Schematic illustration of functional anatomy of the left (dominant) hemisphere in lateral view with particular attention to the frontal lobe and the posterior cortex

#### 7.1.1.1 Primary Motor Cortex

The primary motor cortex is located in the precentral gyrus and is topically organized as a "homunculus" as demonstrated by electrical stimulation studies [26]. The precentral "knob" corresponding to the hand area describes in axial view a consistent convolution that looks like an omega. However, 10% of individuals have an additional involution causing an epsilon sign. In sagittal view, the hand knob can be identified as a typical hook [27]. The mesial edge of the hand knob is 2–3 cm distant from the midline [27], and the distance of its lateral edge to the Sylvian fissure roughly measures 6 cm. The central sulcus can be identified by its anteriorly convex genu followed by a posteriorly convex genu and then another anteriorly convex genu. The precentral sulcus which reaches the midline in only roughly 10% of individuals is usually intersected in its inferior part by the inferior frontal sulcus and in its superior part by the superior frontal sulcus. The precentral knob is located opposite to the intersection of the superior frontal with the precentral sulcus [27]. It should be emphasized that the motor hand function frequently extends to the central sulcus and the anterior aspect of the postcentral gyrus [28].

#### 7.1.1.2 Premotor Cortex

The proper premotor cortex is located rostrally to the precentral gyrus and contains several areas, all of which are thought to control specific aspects of motor tasks via projection into primary motor cortex and to spinal cord neurons [29]. Similarly, the supplementary motor area (SMA), frontal eye field, and Broca's language area perform tasks within the scope of controlling motor functions, and thus can also be counted to the premotor cortex in the broader sense.

#### 7.1.1.3 Supplementary Motor Area (SMA)

The supplementary motor area (SMA) constitutes a complex anatomical and functional system for initiation and control of motor function and speech expression. It represents a segment of the premotor cortex located on the interhemispheric aspect of the frontal lobe anterior to the leg region of the primary motor cortex, mainly corresponding to the dorsal portion of the superior frontal gyrus. Boundaries of the SMA are the primary motor leg area dorsally, and the cingulate sulcus inferiorly. The anterior border of the SMA is not well defined and may correspond to a vertical line passing through the anterior commissure [30]. Stimulation studies suggest a somatotopic organization of the SMA with the lower extremity, upper extremity, and head representations extending from the posterior to the anterior borders [31]. However, this has been questioned by others [32, 33]. Anatomical studies revealed connections between the SMA and all components of the motor system, in particular to the contralateral SMA and bilaterally to the primary motor cortex, the cingulate gyri, the basal ganglia, the cerebellum, and the spinal cord, as well as the sensory system [34, 35]. In fact, the SMA is sensorimotor in representation, although predominantly motor in function [31]. It stands at an interface between limbic outflow and motor executive apparatus [36], and can be viewed as a paralimbic "protomotor" cortex [37] that functions in a "supramotor" fashion [38], participating earlier than the primary motor cortex in the translation of motive to intention to action, and exerting control over the primary motor cortex. Thus the SMA may play a key role in volitional processes [36, 39].

#### 7.1.1.4 Frontal Eye Field

The frontal eye field is located at between the proper premotor cortex, SMA, Broca's area, and prefrontal cortex. Its main function is the control of saccadic eye movements for visual field perception and awareness; thus it plays an important role in the control of visual attention as well as in voluntary eye movement. It communicates with extraocular muscles indirectly via the paramedian pontine reticular formation [4].

#### 7.1.1.5 Broca's Area

Broca's speech area is localized at the opercular and triangular parts of the inferior frontal gyrus in the dominant hemisphere. It is connected with Wernicke's temporal language area by the arcuate fasciculus and facilitates speech production as a premotor cortex. Broca's expressive aphasia is characterized by the loss of the ability to produce grammatically intact language, although the intended message may still be understood ("telegraphic speech"), while comprehension generally remains intact [4].

#### 7.1.1.6 Prefrontal Cortex

The prefrontal cortex receives projections from the mediodorsal nucleus of the thalamus. Its function is rather vaguely defined and includes executive control, monitoring in working memory, learning, temporal structuring of behavior, and control of behavior [40]. Some specific regions have been identified that are recruited by different demands indicating a prefrontal network involved in the solution of diverse cognitive tasks [4].

### 7.1.2 Posterior Cortex

The term posterior cortex comprises the parietal and the occipital lobes. It includes the *primary sensory cortex*, the *posterior parietal cortex*, the *angular and supramarginal gyri*, as well as the *visual cortex* (Fig. 7.1).

#### 7.1.2.1 Primary Sensory Cortex

The primary sensory cortex is located in the postcentral gyrus. As with the primary motor cortex, it is topically organized, and some body parts may be controlled by partially overlapping cortical areas. The area of the primary sensory cortex attributed to a body part reflects its relative density of cutaneous tactile receptors. Just posterior to the primary sensory cortex lies the sensory association cortex, which integrates sensory information from the primary sensory cortex (temperature, pressure, etc.) to construct an understanding of the object being felt.

#### 7.1.2.2 Angular and Supramarginal Gyri

The angular and supramarginal gyri constitute the transition area between the temporal, parietal, and occipital lobes. They include a network that is involved in several crucial functions such as language (Wernicke's area), writing, reading, calculation, and working memory in the dominant hemisphere, as well as musical memory, and face and object recognition in the nondominant hemisphere. The subcortical limits for performing safe resections within the temporo-parieto-occipital region have been described as follows: within the parietal region, the anterior horizontal part of the superior longitudinal fasciculus and, more deeply, the arcuate fasciculus, and dorsally, the vertical projective thalamocortical fibers [41].

#### 7.1.2.3 Posterior Parietal Cortex

The posterior parietal cortex is roughly synonymous with the precuneus or the quadrate lobule of Foville [42]. It has reciprocal cortical connections with the adjacent parietal cortex and the frontal cortex, as well as subcortical connections to the thalamus, striatum, claustrum, and brainstem [43]. Functional imaging studies suggest a key role of the posterior parietal cortex in a wide spectrum of highly integrated tasks including visuospatial recognition, episodic memory retrieval, symbol processing, and self-processing operations. Moreover, it has been suggested that the posterior parietal cortex is involved in the network of the neural correlates of self-consciousness [44].

#### 7.1.2.4 Visual Cortex

The occipital lobe is bordered anteriorly by the parieto-occipital sulcus which is located at the level of the lambdoid suture. While the lateral aspect of the occipital lobe does not consist of specific gyri or sulci, its internal aspect is of particular importance representing the end of visual pathways [45]. The optic radiation enfolding the temporal and occipital horn spreads out broadly to reach the area striata which represents the primary visual field. The fissura calcarina begins medially in the central polar region and lies in its transitional curvature between medial plane and base, rising forward. Despite variations, there is always a sharp bend forward and basally at its meeting with the sulcus cinguli [46].

### 7.1.3 Insula

The insular lobe or island of Reil, first described in 1809, constitutes a complex anatomical, functional, and physiological system [47]. It is formed by cortical layers covering the basal nuclei in the early embryological stages until the end of the fifth month of gestation [48, 49]. The apposition of the opercula is only completed with the end of gestation [48, 50]. In the adult human brain, the triangular shaped insular cortex lies in the depth of the Sylvian fissure, covered by the opercula of the surrounding frontal, parietal, and temporal lobes. It is separated from the overlying frontal and parietal opercula by the superior limiting sulcus and from the temporal opercula by the inferior limiting sulcus. Both sulci join at the caudal end and together form the circular sulcus, which surrounds the insula. The circular sulcus forms an oval ring that is open at its anterior pole, the limen insulae, which is located adjacent to the orbitofrontal cortex, but has no definite border.

#### 7.1.3.1 Anatomy

The central insular sulcus, which represents a direct continuation of the central sulcus separating the frontal and parietal lobes, divides the insula into two parts. The anterior part usually consists of three gyri termed the short gyri which ventrally unite at the limen. The posterior part consists of two long gyri. The posterior two short and the two long insular gyri are separated from each other by the pre- and postcentral insular sulci, respectively, which continue as the pre- and postcentral sulci of the frontal and parietal lobes [48, 49, 51] (Fig. 7.2). Arteries supplying the insula arise from M2 branches and are divided into three types: the short arteries that supply the insular cortex and extreme capsule, the medium-length arteries supplying the claustrum and external capsule, and the long arteries (perforating arteries amounting to 10% of insular arteries) that supply the corona radiata [53–55].

#### 7.1.3.2 Functional Aspects

The insular lobe is not a separate anatomical and functional entity but a part of the mesocortex connecting the allocortex with the neocortex. By cytoarchitectonic definition, the insula is part of the paralimbic system in which the agranular allocortex is transformed into the granular isocortex [48, 49]. Therefore, the insula cannot be separated from the limbic system and the neocortex. It represents an essential functional relay between

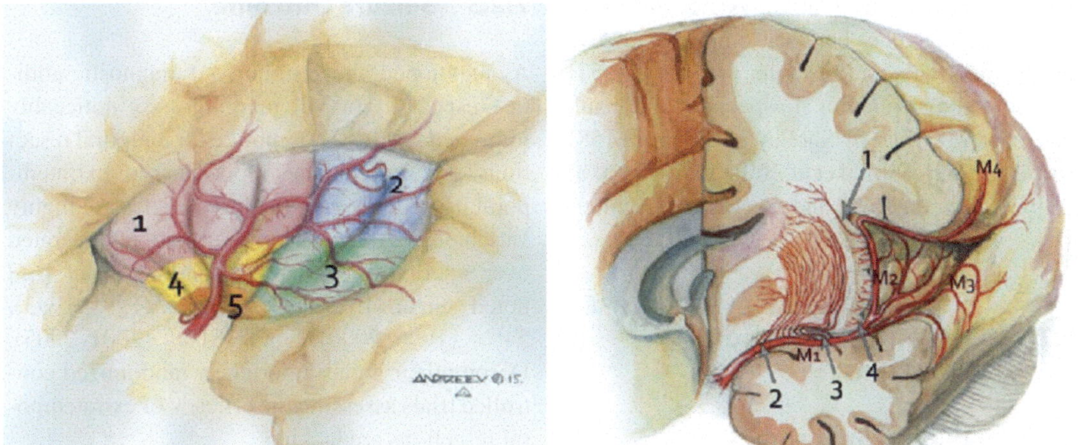


**Fig. 7.2** Artist's illustration of the insular cortex and arterial system of the insular region in sagittal (left) and coronal (right) views. Left: The insular cortex consists of five gyri. Parts of the insular cortex are shown in different colors: 1, anterior-superior; 2, posterior-superior; 3, posterior-inferior; 4, anterior-inferior; 5, limen insulae. The anterior part consists of three short gyri which unite at the limen. The posterior part consists of two long gyri. The central insular sulcus which continues as the central sulcus separating the frontal and parietal lobes is located between the short and long insular gyri. Right: The arteries supplying the insula arise from the M2 branch of the middle cerebral artery: 1, long perforating arteries; 2, medial lenticulostriate arteries (medium-length arteries); 3, lateral lenticulostriate arteries (medium-length arteries); 4, short perforating arteries (from [52], with permission)

those systems and is anatomically closely related and interconnected with them.

Multiple afferent and efferent connections of the insula have been identified to neocortical, limbic, thalamic, and various centers (such as the basal ganglia, capsula interna, and hypothalamus), which explain the complex functional spectrum of the insular lobe. In particular, the anterior part of the insula receives input from the basal part of the ventral medial nucleus of the thalamus and from the central nuclei of the amygdala. In addition, the anterior insula itself projects to the amygdala. The posterior part connects reciprocally with the secondary somatosensory cortex and receives input from ventral posterior inferior thalamic nuclei which convey homeostatic information such as pain, temperature, local oxygen status, and sensual touch [56]. The numerous behavioral affiliations of the insula seem to follow a topographical gradient in an anteroventral–dorsocaudal direction [49].

Overall, the most relevant functional aspects of the insula include (1) the insula as a primary visceral/autonomic sensory and motor area, (2) the insula as a supplementary motor area, (3) insular somatosensory and auditory functions, (4) complex language functions, and (5) connections with the limbic system, the insula as a balancing relay between empirical experiences, affectivity, and behavior [48, 49, 56, 57]. Anatomical and functional aspects of the insula have been reviewed by Shelley and Trimble [58], Türe et al. [59], Duffau et al. [60], Tanriover et al. [61], Wen et al. [62], and Seeger and Zentner [63].

## 7.2 Overall Extratemporal Resections

### 7.2.1 Epilepsy Syndromes

According to the location of the epileptogenic zone, frontal lobe epilepsy (FLE), parietal lobe epilepsy (PLE), occipital lobe epilepsy (OLE), and insular epilepsy can be distinguished. In addition, Rolandic epilepsy may be considered as a separate entity [4]. Gelastic epilepsy due to hypothalamic hamartomas is addressed in the chapter "Non-resective Epilepsy Surgery." Most studies refer to FLE, while data on other extratemporal locations are rather sparse.

### 7.2.2 Resection Strategies

With advanced diagnostics, lobectomy has declined in favor of lesionectomy (LE) and extended lesionectomy (ELE), the latter of which nowadays constitutes the most common extratemporal procedure. In the series of Delev et al. [20] comprising 383 extratemporal patients, ELE has been done in 66% of patients, and 48% of extratemporal procedures referred to the frontal lobe, 24% to the parietal, occipital, and insular cortex, while 28% included more than one lobe, thus referring to multilobectomy [20]. Elsharkawy et al. [64, 65] noted in a series of 154 adult patients frontal resections in 40%, posterior cortex procedures in 50%, and multilobectomies in 10%. In the literature, multilobectomies range between 12 and 22% [66].

### 7.2.3 Seizure Outcome

As mentioned above, improved diagnostic abilities, especially of MR imaging, have noticeably improved results. Thus, unlike for temporal resections, seizure outcomes reported from extratemporal procedures over the last decades are highly variable. In 208 extratemporal patients operated over a period of 15 years, Elsharkawy et al. [65] noted seizure-free rates of 45% (1991–1995), 54% (1996–2000), and 61% (2001–2005). Despite their great importance, randomized controlled trials assessing the efficacy of extratemporal resections are lacking.

#### 7.2.3.1 Mixed Follow-Up

Seizure freedom (Engel I) rates reported in ETE patients vary between 25 and 90% [13, 14, 22, 23, 25, 64, 65, 67–73]. In most studies, Engel I outcome ranges from 45 to 65% [6, 7, 67, 74–76]. Hanáková et al. [9] found 52.1% seizure-free patients (Engel I). In the series of Delev et al. [20] comprising 383 patients, 62.2% were seizure free (Engel I).

#### 7.2.3.2 Long-Term Follow-Up

Hanáková et al. [9] found decreasing seizure-free rates over years and only 37.5% seizure-free patients at the 5-year follow-up. Similarly, a meta-analysis reported by Tellez-Zenteno et al. [25] showed 34% seizure-free patients on long-term follow-up. McIntosh et al. [69] reported initial seizure freedom in 40.7% of their patients, which dropped to 14.7% at 5 years postoperatively. A study including 223 patients with ELE that focused on postoperative medication noted seizure freedom in 27% of the individuals with and without medication at a mean observation period of 84 months [77]. Contrarily, relatively stable Engel I outcome of approximately 50% has been reported in other series including adults and children [78–80].

#### 7.2.3.3 Histopathology

With cavernomas and glioneuronal tumors (gangliogliomas and DNET), seizure-free outcome (Engel I) rates of 89% and 85%, respectively, have been reported [20]. Analyzing 35 patients with focal cortical dysplasia (FCD) of the Cleveland Clinic, Edwards et al. [81] noted Engel I outcome in 49% of cases, while in the Bonn series including 53 patients, 72% seizure-free patients were documented [82]. The best outcome was reported in FCD type IIb lesions: With complete lesion resection, 92% of 50 patients were seizure free, but only 8%, when the lesion was incompletely resected [23]. In sum, seizure outcome depends to a major part on imaging quality to exactly delineate structural lesions facilitating their total removal.

#### 7.2.3.4 Preoperative Prognostic Factors

The following preoperative prognostic factors for favorable seizure outcome in ETE have been identified: MRI-visible lesion [6–8, 20, 23, 64, 65, 75, 83–85], younger age at surgery and short duration of epilepsy [8, 20, 64, 65], a larger distance of the epileptogenic zone to eloquent cortex [20], partial seizures [85], localizing EEG findings [8], and absence of generalized seizures [8]. In line, Bjellvi et al. [86] reported in a systematic review and meta-analysis that patients with shorter epilepsy duration are more likely to be seizure free at follow-up. Site of resection (frontal, parietal, occipital, insular, or multilobular) did not significantly influence seizure outcome [20].

#### 7.2.3.5 Postoperative Prognostic Factors

Postoperative factors indicating favorable seizure outcome include complete resection of the lesion [6, 7, 20, 23, 64, 65, 75, 85] and absence of epileptic activity [20, 87]. Rathore and Radhakrishnan [88] suggested that interictal epileptiform discharges in postoperative EEG may predict seizure outcome with only a fair degree of accuracy.

### 7.2.4 Neuropsychological Outcome

Only a few studies address cognitive and psychosocial outcome after extratemporal resections in adults, and most of them refer to the frontal lobe. The prospective study of Tanriverdi et al. [89, 90] including 23 patients demonstrated improvement of overall quality of life both at short-term (6 months) and at long-term (2 years) follow-up as compared with the preoperative condition regardless of the seizure status. El Hassani et al. [91] found in their series of 18 extratemporal resective cases improvement in the postoperative neuropsychological performance in 55%, while 17% of individuals had deteriorated. Overall stability of cognitive performance after frontal resections has been noted in other series [92, 93].

#### 7.2.4.1 Preoperative Prognostic Factors

The following preoperative positive predictors for neuropsychological outcome and quality of life after extratemporal resections have been identified: shorter duration of epilepsy [89, 90], resection outside eloquent cortex [92, 93], and posterior cortex resection [91]. Negative predictors for cognitive outcome were resection of the SMA [92, 93] and MST of the primary motor cortex [92]. Duration of epilepsy did not influence postoperative neuropsychological performance in the series of 126 patients reported by Holmes et al. [94] as well as in the series of El Hassani et al. [91], nor did resection site, gender, presence of neurological signs [94], and side of surgery [91].

#### 7.2.4.2 Postoperative Prognostic Factors

Seizure freedom has been identified as the most important postoperative positive prognostic factor for neuropsychological outcome [89–92]. Dulay et al. [95] found in a study of 64 cases depressive symptoms as a negative predictor for executive functions after frontal resections.

## 7.3 Frontal Lobe Resections

### 7.3.1 Identification of Surgical Candidates

#### 7.3.1.1 Epidemiology

Frontal lobe epilepsies (FLE) constitute the second most frequent partial epilepsy syndromes after temporal lobe epilepsies, and the most frequent ETE syndromes [25, 96, 97]. FLE account for 20–40% of all partial epilepsies [4]. However, incidence and prevalence of FLE may be overrated by the fact that motor signs are usually the most impressive features of epileptic seizures arising from extratemporal areas [4]. Frontal resections amount to around 25% of procedures in actual series [6, 7, 75]. As fewer patients with FLE were found to be good surgical candidates compared with TLE patients, FLE were underrepresented in earlier surgical series. In the MNI series of 2177 patients who underwent epilepsy surgery, 18% had frontal lobe epilepsies [98].

#### 7.3.1.2 Etiology

Malformations of cortical development, in particular focal cortical dysplasias (FCD), represent the most frequent etiology of FLE as observed in 20–80% of patients, followed by tumors (15–35%), gliosis including post-traumatic and ischemic lesions (10–30%), and vascular malformations (15%) [67, 76, 99–103].

#### 7.3.1.3 Seizure Semiology

Semiology of frontal lobe seizures is diverse and may be divided into three main subtypes: partial motor (see also below), supplementary motor, and complex-partial. However, there is considerable overlap among these seizure subtypes [6, 7, 75, 104, 105]. Complex partial seizures typically involve staring spells, vocalization, diminished responsiveness, and sometimes bizarre bimanual-bipedal movements [75, 104, 105]. Speech arrest, blinking, and asymmetrical tonic posturing suggest electrical spread to the SMA [102, 104].

### 7.3.2 Surgical Aspects

#### 7.3.2.1 Surgical Tools

In frontal lobe surgery, the primary motor cortex (see also below), supplementary motor cortex, and Broca's speech area are of particular importance. MRI- and fMRI-based neuronavigation is helpful to delineate the motor and language areas and to define resection borders. In addition, Broca's area can be localized by extraoperative mapping using a grid electrode. As an alternative to preoperative testing, awake craniotomy may be considered. Phase reversal of SEP [106, 107] facilitates delineation of the central area during general anesthesia, and MEP monitoring [57, 108] provides feedback for the surgeon on the functional integrity of the primary motor cortex.

#### 7.3.2.2 Surgical Techniques

Although en bloc resection of frontal lobe has become a rather unusual procedure, it shows some principles, application of which may also be useful for other extratemporal resection strategies. The main steps of frontal lobectomy are as follows:

- The patient is placed in supine position with the upper body slightly elevated and the head inclined avoiding compression of the jugular veins.
- A minimum 7 × 6 cm bone flap is created extending 4 cm before and 3 cm behind the bregma and 6 cm lateral from the midline.
- The precentral sulcus is exactly defined using neuronavigation and electrophysiological tools.
- Dissection starts at the mesial aspect of the frontal lobe and is continued along the arachnoid diagonal in frontal direction simulating the anterior bulging course of the corona radiata until the corpus callosum and the pericallosal artery are reached.
- As the level of the corpus callosum is reached, dissection is continued in lateral direction, thus creating a broad plane. Using this plane, dissection is continued following the pericallosal artery around the genu of the corpus callosum leaving the ventricle wall intact, and then downward along the A2 segment of the anterior cerebral artery (ACA) until its A1 segment is reached.
- Dissection is continued following the A1 segment of the ACA in lateral direction and visualizing the dorsal rim of the sphenoid and the optic nerves through the intact arachnoid until the carotid cistern is reached.
- Lateral disconnection is completed, and the major block of the frontal lobe is removed. Alternatively, the frontal lobe can be removed in several smaller blocks.
- In the nondominant hemisphere, frontal operculum is subpially removed until the Sylvian fissure is reached.

The main principles of frontal lobectomy are to consequently follow clearly visible guiding structures. These principles also apply to other extratemporal areas appreciating respective topographical landmarks. For most extratemporal procedures, positioning of the head in exact anterior-posterior direction is advantageous facilitating orientation in the midline with consistent landmarks.

Special attention has to be paid to circumscribed resections within highly vascularized areas, particularly if major vessels are traversing, such as in the frontal operculum and in the central area. In these locations, the technique of subpial gyral emptying preserving pial and arachnoidal banks including vessels is of particular importance. For resections in close vicinity to the motor cortex it seems to be advisable to completely expose the typically shaped motor hand area for better orientation.

#### 7.3.2.3 Broca's Area

Considerable interpersonal variability has been described in the location of frontal language area which may include not only the inferior but also the middle frontal gyrus. Damage to the proper motor language area is followed by long-lasting or even permanent severe deficits [109–111].

#### 7.3.2.4 SMA Deficiency Syndrome

Resection of the SMA (Figs. 7.3–7.6) is usually followed by reversible contralateral weakness and/or neglect and dysphasia without cognitive impairment that is termed the SMA deficiency syndrome [113]. Laplane et al. [114] reported a specific clinical evolution of the SMA deficiency syndrome in three stages: (1) immediately after surgery there is a global akinesia pronounced contralaterally with speech arrest in dominant hemisphere; (2) recovery begins within a few days, but reduction in spontaneous motor activity contralaterally, an emotional type of facial palsy, and a reduction in spontaneous speech may persist for weeks; (3) in the long run, only subtle deficits such as disturbance of the alternating movements of the hands may persist [114]. Akinesia is believed to be related to the function of the SMA in planning and initiating motor activity including speech output. Characteristically, the muscle tone of the "paralyzed" extremities is preserved. Most likely, reversibility of the SMA deficiency syndrome is based on the bilateral organization and representation of the SMA [115]. Indeed, bilat-

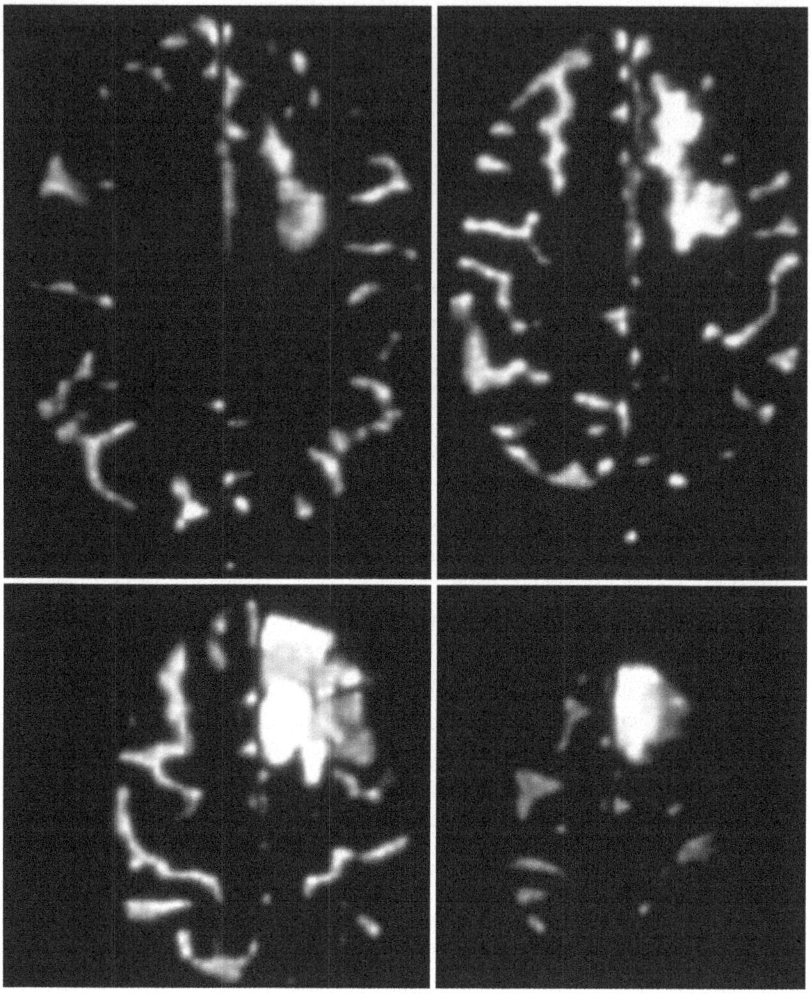

**Fig. 7.3** Astrocytoma (WHO grade II) of the left SMA. Axial T2-weighted MRI shows the residual tumor after previous partial resection. The patient suffered from a persistent medically intractable epilepsy. Thus, complete resection of the lesion including the SMA was planned (from [112], with permission)

eral extirpation of the SMA has been observed to be followed by a long-lasting akinesia and mutism [116].

The proportion of the SMA deficiency syndrome has been found to be related to the extent of SMA resection: deficits occur in almost all patients with complete removal of the SMA, while with incomplete resection partial or even no deficits may be observed [57]. Similar results have been found by Ibe et al. [117] emphasizing the risk of deficits with resection of the medial border of the SMA. However, others stated that deficits may occur independently of resected volume [30]. fMRI seems to be able to identify more clearly the area in the SMA at risk [30]. Nakajima et al. [118] felt that recovery time can be predicted with MR imaging at postoperative day 7.

### 7.3.3 Seizure Outcome

#### 7.3.3.1 Mixed Follow-Up

Earlier series of patients with FLE showed seizure freedom ranging from 13 to 41% after surgery [98]. Englot et al. [75] noted in a meta-

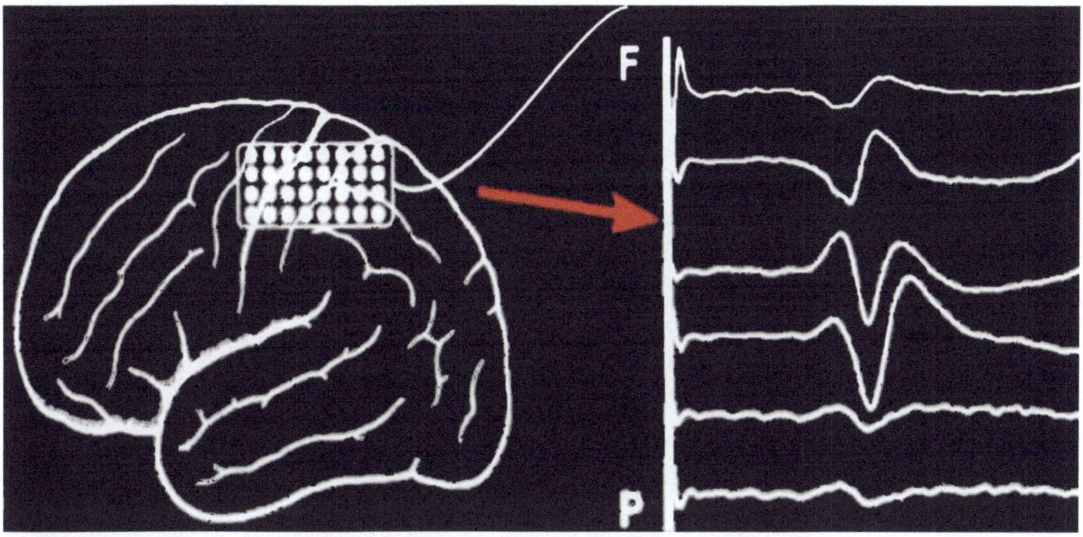


**Fig. 7.4** Illustration of phase reversal of SEP for localization of the central sulcus. Left: The grid electrode is placed over the area in question. Right: Recording of SEP after stimulation of the right median nerve. Phase reversal of SEP is demonstrated between lines 2 and 3 corresponding to the localization of the central sulcus. *F* frontal, *P* parietal

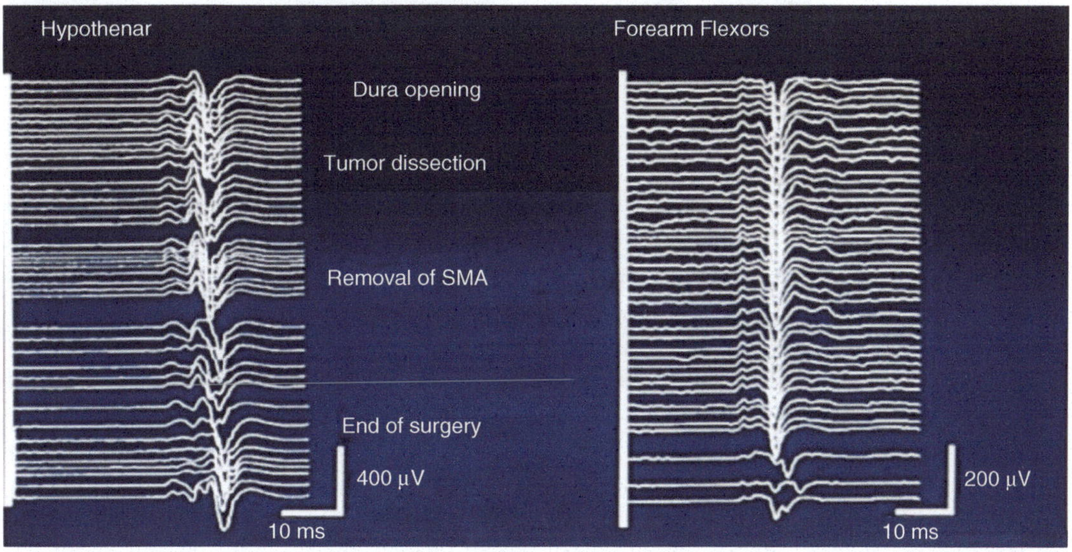


**Fig. 7.5** Intraoperative MEP monitoring during resection of the SMA in the case shown in Fig. 7.3. MEP were elicited by direct cortical stimulation and recorded from the right hypothenar and forearm flexors. Note that during resection of the SMA potentials remain stable. Postoperatively, a typical SMA deficiency syndrome lasting for 2 weeks was noted. There were no permanent deficits

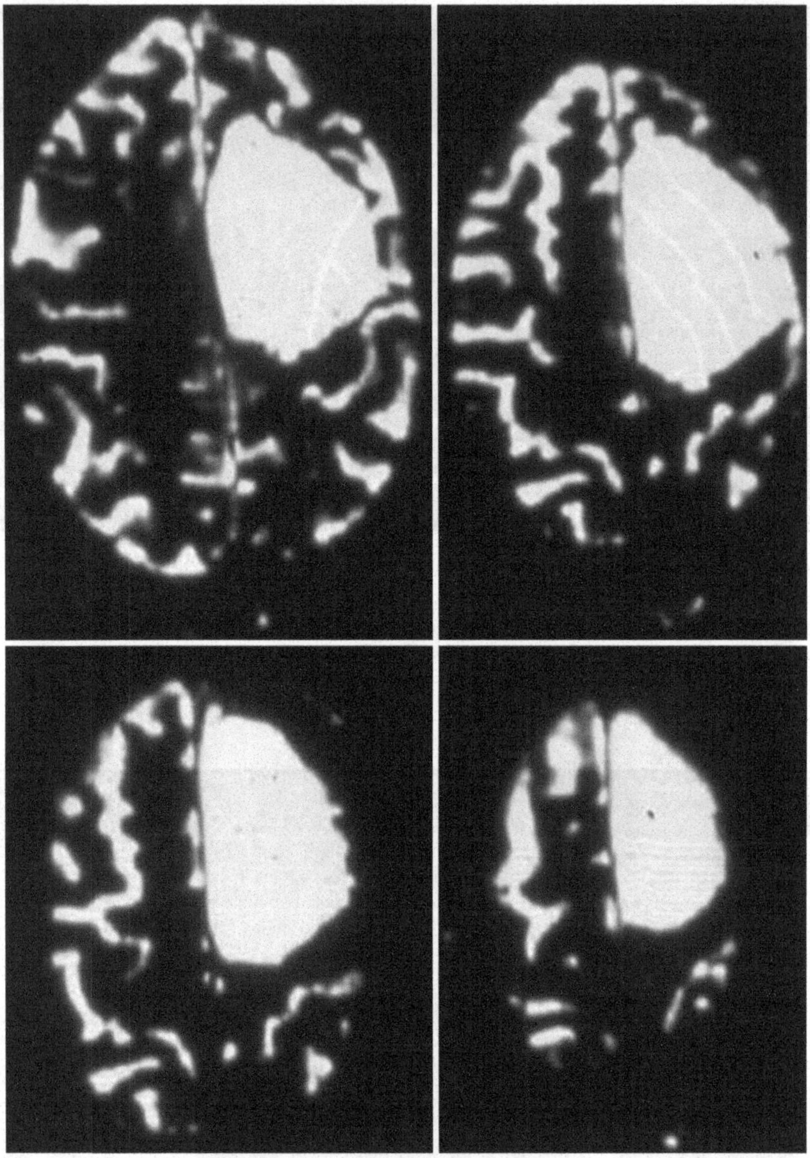

**Fig. 7.6** Postoperative T2-weighted MRI (axial view) of the case shown in Fig. 7.3. Tumor including SMA has been removed completely. Note that dorsal resection exactly borders to the precentral sulcus (from [112], with permission)

analysis comprising 1200 FLE patients seizure freedom (Engel I) in 45.1%. In other studies, seizure freedom or outcome with non-disabling or rare seizures was reported in 52–66% of patients [64, 65, 67, 76, 82, 102, 103]. A more actual series comprising 111 FLE patients demonstrated Engel I outcome in 65% [20]. Similarly, Morace et al. [21] noted seizure-free outcome (Engel I) in 68% of cases. Overall, most previous studies report Engel I outcome after frontal resections in the range between 45 and 60% [6, 7, 64, 65, 74–76, 103, 119, 120], while more actual studies show Engel I outcome between 60 and 70% of patients [20, 21].

#### 7.3.3.2 Long-Term Follow-Up

Long-term seizure-free outcome in the meta-analysis of Téllez-Zenteno et al. [25] comprising 7 studies and 486 FLE patients was 27%. Similarly, a meta-analysis summarizing data of 40 children with FLE documented long-term Engel I outcome in 27.5% [13]. In the Cleveland Clinic series [120], seizure-free outcome after frontal lobe resections dropped from 56% at 1-year follow-up to 30% at 5 years. Elsharkawy et al. [64] comprising 154 adult patients noted that seizure freedom rates decreased from 66 to 47% after 5 years but remained stable at 14-year follow-up with 51% seizure-free cases. In the series of Samuel et al. [121], seizure outcome was quite stable with seizure-free (Engel I) rates of 48% at 1 year, 41% at 2 years, 56% at 3 years, 57% at 4 years, and 53% at 5 years. In sum, long-term follow-up studies show seizure control rates after frontal resections mainly between 35 and 50% [75].

#### 7.3.3.3 Predictors for Seizure Control

The following predictors for seizure control have been identified: focal seizure onset, lesional epilepsy, complete resection of the lesion [6, 7, 64, 65, 75, 76, 82, 99, 103, 119, 122], type IIb FCD [6, 7, 23, 75, 123], and shorter epilepsy duration [121]. Of note, others did not observe a correlation between the presence of MRI-detectable lesions and a favorable seizure outcome [102, 124, 125].

## 7.4 Rolandic Resections

### 7.4.1 Identification of Surgical Candidates

#### 7.4.1.1 Epidemiology

While resections in the Rolandic cortex accounted to the most frequent procedures at the early beginning of epilepsy surgery [126–130], they amount nowadays to around 5–10% of all resective procedures performed for epilepsy [20]. In the MNI series of 2177 patients, 7% had resections in the Rolandic cortex, particularly affecting the precentral gyrus [98].

#### 7.4.1.2 Etiology

In the series of van Offen and van Rijen [131], the most frequent etiologies were dysembryoplastic neuroepithelial tumors (DNET), followed by focal cortical dysplasias (FCD) and gangliogliomas. Pondal-Sordo et al. [132] noted in descending order tumors, vascular malformations, FCD, and unspecific findings. Similarly, tumors were most frequently observed in other series [133, 134]. In the cohort of Delev et al. [5], FCD, followed by tumors, vascular malformations, and unspecific findings were observed, while Lehman et al. [135] found gliosis, cortical dysplasia, and microgyria in most cases.

#### 7.4.1.3 Seizure Semiology

Epilepsies arising from the precentral and postcentral gyri show motor and sensory symptoms, respectively. Partial motor seizures, sometimes demonstrating Jacksonian march with Todd's paralysis, are characterized by focal clonic activity, ranging from self-limiting forms to epilepsia partialis continua. Seizures originating from the interhemispheric motor area may show bilateral tonic posturing. Localization of the epileptic focus is facilitated by assessing initial seizure semiology pointing to its representation in the somatotopically organized homunculus [131].

### 7.4.2 Surgical Aspects

#### 7.4.2.1 Surgical Tools

As mentioned above, MRI- and fMRI-based neuronavigation is helpful to delineate the sensorimotor cortex. Functional topographic mapping and monitoring of the motor area can be accomplished during general anesthesia by recording motor evoked potentials (MEP) elicited by direct cortical stimulation. Similarly, cortical somatosensory evoked potentials (SEP) facilitate mapping and monitoring of the primary sensory cortex [57, 108]. In addition, phase reversal of SEP [106, 107] has proven to

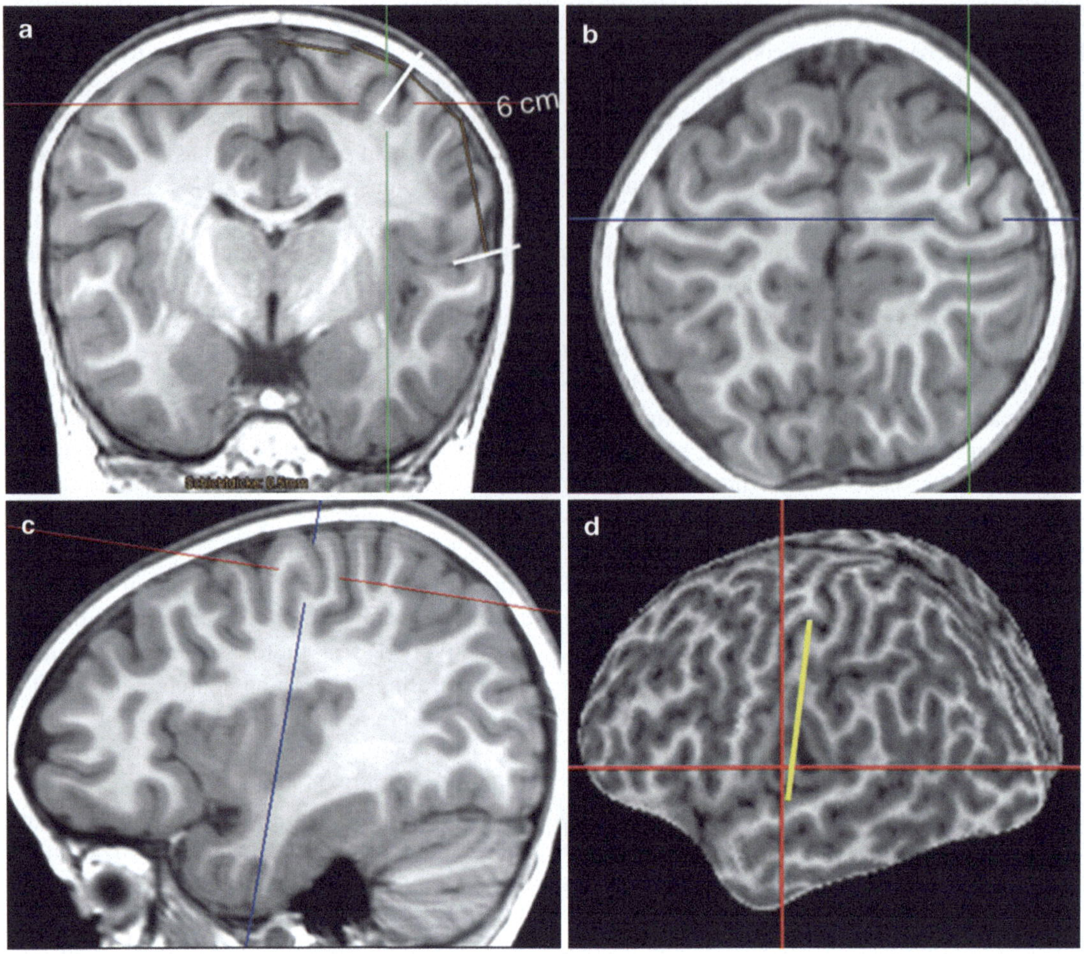


**Fig. 7.7** Coronal (**a**), axial (**b**), sagittal (**c**), and volume-rendering (**d**) MPRAGE slices with 1 mm³ voxels. Distance from the Sylvian fissure to the hand knob (hair cross in **a**–**c**) is shown. Measurement follows the axis of the precentral gyrus (yellow in **d**). Distance from the Sylvian fissure to the lateral edge of the hand knob along the convexity measures roughly 6 cm (with courtesy of H. Urbach, Dpt. of Neuroradiology, Freiburg)

be a useful tool for intraoperative localization of the central sulcus.

### 7.4.2.2 Primary Motor Cortex

Using the technique of subpial gyral emptying, the basal precentral Rolandic cortex can be resected from the Sylvian fissure up to the hand area (maximum roughly 6 cm) without permanent harm (Fig. 7.7). Resection of *the motor face and tongue area* is only followed by a temporary facial paresis and speech difficulties (on the dominant side) which usually resolve completely within 2–3 weeks due to their bilateral representation in the homunculus [111, 135, 136] (Fig. 7.8). Ostergard and Miller [28] noted moderate long-term facial weakness in 7 of 37 patients roughly corresponding to 20%, and dysphasia after resection of the motor face area on the dominant side in 8%. Figure 7.9 illustrates the resection of a circumscribed lesion in the primary motor hand area.

It should be noted that even after resection of major parts of *motor hand area*, functional recovery starts within 1–3 weeks in the proximal limb and proceeds distally over the next few months. Complete proximal recovery and restoration of functional grasp can be expected in the majority of individuals [135]. Similarly, gradual recov-

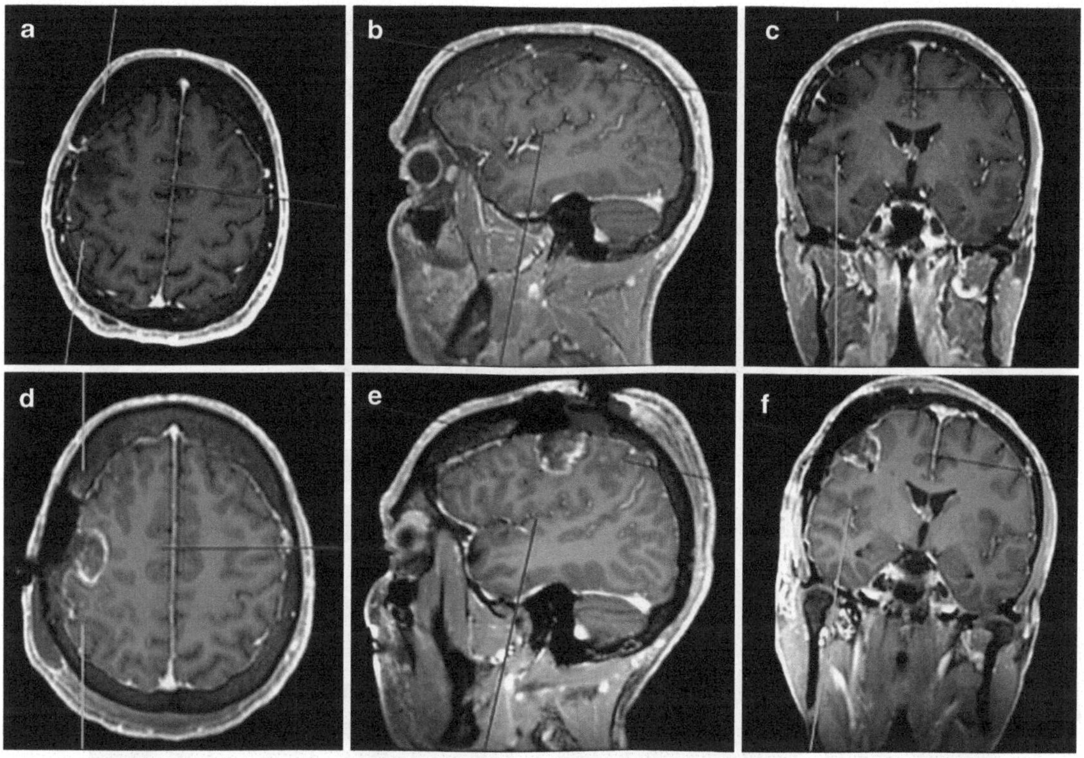


**Fig. 7.8** 45-year-old male patient with an oligodendroglioma (WHO grade II) of the right precentral suprasylvian area. Extended biopsy had been performed some months ago. Due to persistent seizures, tumor removal was indicated. Upper sequence shows the tumor with a small cystic defect after previous surgery on contrast-enhanced T1-weighted MRI in axial (**a**), sagittal (**b**), and coronal (**c**) views. Lower sequence (**d**–**f**) demonstrates complete removal of the MR-visible tumor. Note that the hand area (**d**) is still preserved. Postoperatively, the patient was seizure free. Facial paresis resolved completely within 3 weeks. Motor function of the left upper extremity remained intact

ery over months from proximal to distal can be expected after resection of the *motor leg area* [28, 111]. Lower extremity strength appears to recover better than upper extremity strength [28]. In a review of 280 cases, Ostergard and Miller [28] noted long-term weakness in 28% of cases. Functional recovery is thought to be related to networks facilitating recruitment of other cortical areas including the contralateral hemisphere. However, fine motor functions will remain lost [28]. It should be noted that deficits caused by cortical resection including the motor hand and leg areas have a much better prognosis than those caused by affection of the descending motor pathways, particularly of the tightly bundled pyramidal tract in the vicinity of the genu of the internal capsule, minimum injury of which is inevitably followed by major or complete permanent deficits [28].

Overall, limited resection of the motor cortex, particularly of the face area, is well tolerated in the long term, and well-delimitable lesions can be removed with favorable epileptological and functional results. Contrarily, more diffuse lesions requiring resection of larger parts of the motor hand and/or leg area will inevitably be followed by significant deficits. In these cases, multiple subpial transections (MST) may be considered as a stand-alone procedure or in addition to resection.

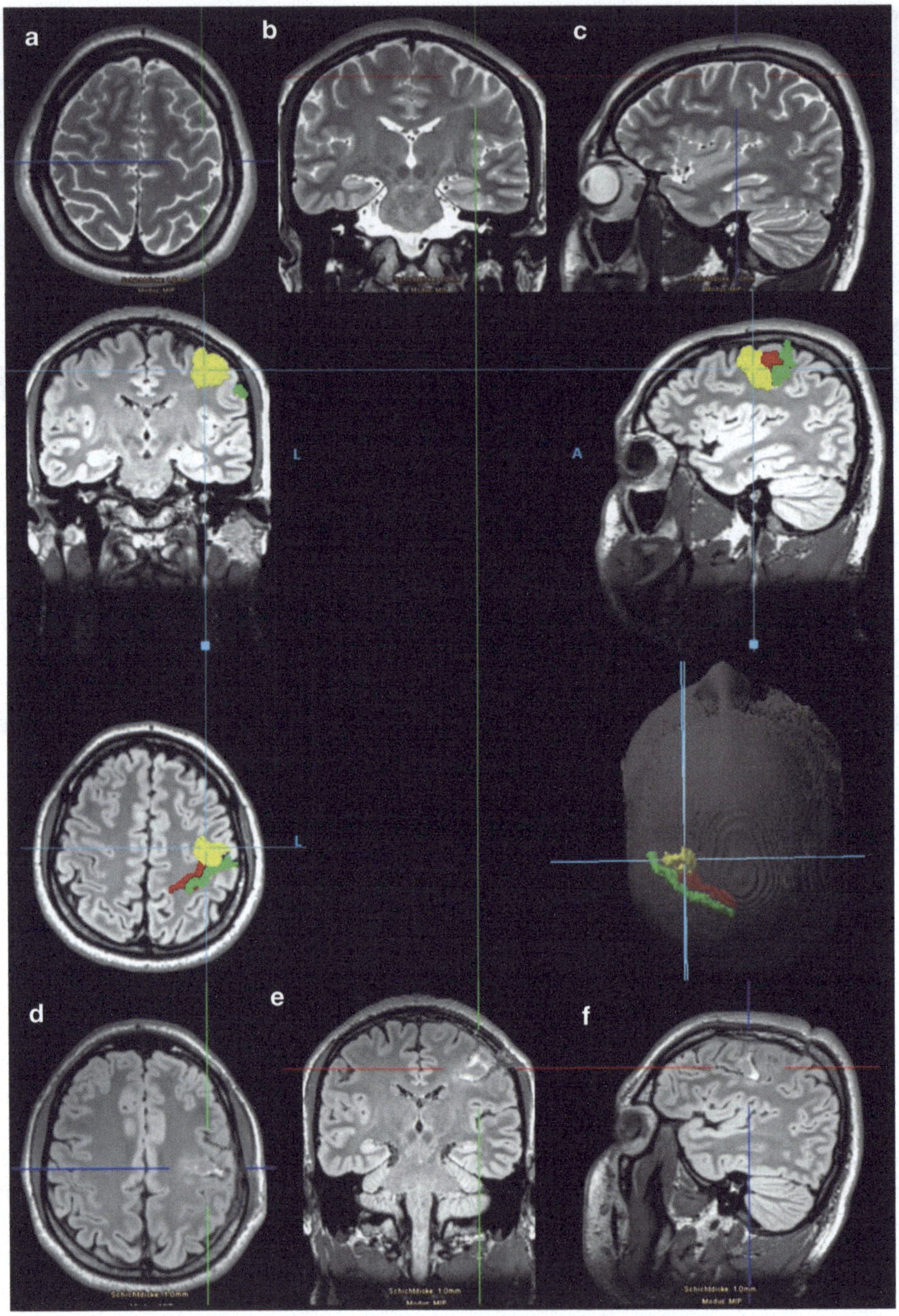


**Fig. 7.9** 23-year-old male patient with drug-resistant clonic seizures of right arm, in part followed by bilateral tonic-clonic seizures, since the age of 14 years (seizure frequency: 1–3/month). EEG showed a left fronto-central seizure onset. Upper sequence (**a–c**): Preoperative MRI revealed a signal abnormality resembling FCD in the left precentral gyrus. Middle sequences: fMRI and image fusion demonstrated the relationships between the lesion and the central area (yellow, lesion; red, primary motor cortex; green, primary sensory cortex). Lower sequence (**d–f**): Postoperative MRI shows result after lesionectomy performed with neuronavigation and electrophysiological mapping and monitoring (subcortical motor stimulation). Immediately after the operation, a marked paresis of the right arm, hand, and face, and dysarthria were noted. Up to postoperative day 6, hand and arm paresis recovered completely, with only a residual oral asymmetry persisting. At 3-month follow-up, the patient was completely seizure free (Engel Ia) (with courtesy of J. Beck, Dpt. of Neurosurgery, Freiburg)

#### 7.4.2.3 Primary Sensory Cortex

Similar to the primary motor cortex, resection of the *sensory face and tongue* area does not produce permanent deficits due to its bilateral representation [111, 135, 136]. In contrast to their motor counterparts, even partial resection of the primary sensory hand and leg area is usually not complicated by impairing deficits. However, complete resection of the *sensory hand area* is followed in around 70% of patients by significant clinical disabilities related to deficits in pressure sensitivity, two-point discrimination, point localization, position sense, and tactual object recognition [111, 137].

### 7.4.3 Seizure Outcome

In previous series, outcomes after Rolandic resections have been described summarizing Engel classes I and II as favorable outcome. More actual reports usually provide separate numbers for seizure-free (Engel I) patients.

#### 7.4.3.1 Previous Series

In the first series of Rolandic resections including 41 children and adults, favorable outcome (Engel I–II) at 6-year follow-up was achieved in 49% of the patients [138]. Similarly, Pondal-Sordo et al. [132] noted favorable outcome in 46% of patients, Devinsky et al. [139] in 54%, and Otsubo et al. [11] in 43% of cases. In two small cohorts including 4 [136] and 5 [140] patients, Engel I–II outcomes were 75% and 80%, respectively. Lehman et al. [135] summarizing 20 MNI cases found favorable outcome in 60%.

#### 7.4.3.2 More Actual Reports

In the Bonn series including 66 patients who underwent Rolandic and perirolandic resective surgery, which was in part combined with multiple subpial transections (MST), seizure freedom (Engel I) was achieved in 59% of the cases [5]. Independent predictors for excellent seizure outcome included specific histopathological findings, complete resection of the lesion, younger age at surgery, and absence of preoperative simple partial seizures [5]. Analyzing 9 studies including 280 patients, Ostergard and Miller [28] noted Engel I outcome in 50% of cases. Van Offen and van Rijen [131] reported complete seizure freedom (Engel Ia) in 59% of 22 individuals. Follow-up questionnaires revealed that most patients were satisfied with the results of surgery despite new deficits and impact on quality of life [131].

In sum, there is a broad range of outcomes after Rolandic resections reported in the literature ranging from 43% Engel I–II to 59% Engel Ia. Most previous studies noted favorable (Engel I–II) outcome in around 50% of cases, while more actual reports show seizure freedom (Engel I) in the same range (around 50%). Improved outcomes in more actual series reflect advances in diagnostics (high-resolution MRI) as well as better patient selection and more adequate surgical strategies including mapping and monitoring.

## 7.5 Posterior Cortex Resections

### 7.5.1 Identification of Surgical Candidates

#### 7.5.1.1 Epidemiology

Posterior cortex epilepsies (PCE) comprise seizure disorders originating from the parietal, occipital, or occipital border of the temporal lobe [141]. These epilepsies may be grouped together due to rather unspecific clinical and neurophysiological seizure patterns as well as difficulties in precise delineating the epileptogenic zone [142–145]. Seizures emanating from the posterior cortex are less common than those arising from the frontal lobe and account for 15–20% of extratemporal epilepsies [146–150], and for 5–10% of all epilepsy surgeries [68, 151].

#### 7.5.1.2 Etiology

Histopathologically, most series describe a predominance of malformations of cortical development which amount to around 40% of lesions in PCE [143, 148, 152, 153]. In accordance, Liava et al. [151] noted in their series of 208 PCE cases malformations of cortical development as the main etiologies with FCD identified in 43% of patients. Heo et al. [154] observed in a series of 42 occipital resections FCD (76%), tumors (19%), and encephalomalacia (5%). Others predominantly found scars, gliosis, and vascular malformations in PCE [142].

#### 7.5.1.3 Semiology of Parietal Seizures

Seizures arising from the parietal lobe frequently present with auras consisting of a variety of symptoms, such as somatosensory (paresthetic, painful, thermal, disturbances of body image), visual (amaurotic, elementary, and complex hallucinations, illusions), and other (anosognosia, apraxia, acalculia, alexia, aphemia, confusional states, gustatory, vertiginous, adversive, oculoclonic and eyelid flutter) phenomena [133, 145]. These symptoms can be contralateral or bilateral. The auras evolve typically into asymmetrical tonic posturing, unilateral clonic activity, or contralateral version when the ictal discharges activate the frontal region [155]. Propagation to the temporal lobe produces alteration of awareness and automatisms [155, 156].

#### 7.5.1.4 Semiology of Occipital Seizures

Symptoms of seizures arising from the occipital area can be divided into phenomena of occipital lobe origin and those induced by ictal spreading to adjacent areas. In contrast to children, the majority of adults with OLE report visual auras [144, 157–160]. Auras usually start in the contralateral visual field and propagate rapidly [161, 162]. Phenomena comprise elementary visual hallucinations, such as flashing colors or rotating lights or shapes, complex visual hallucinations, and ictal blindness. Other occipital phenomena include blinking, contralateral nystagmus, and contralateral eye pulling [144]. Due to fast ictal spread, as many as 50% of patients present with a frontal or temporal semiology [105, 144]. Infrasylvian seizure spread to the temporal lobe produces alteration of awareness and automatisms. Suprasylvian spread to the mesial frontal lobe induces asymmetrical tonic posturing, whereas lateral propagation results in focal motor or sensory seizures.

As with frontal epilepsies, accurate localization of the epileptogenic zone by clinical and electrophysiological tools in the posterior part of the brain is extremely difficult [163]. This holds particularly true, since there is no consistent seizure semiology due to wide propagation of the epileptic activity [164], scalp EEG is of poor lateralizing and localizing value [133, 159], and underlying pathologies frequently are ill defined [163]. However, actually available refined MRI techniques have improved visualization of those pathologies. In addition, information from invasive investigations is frequently required for planning resective surgery.

### 7.5.2 Surgical Aspects

#### 7.5.2.1 Interhemispheric Approaches

Interhemispheric approaches in PCE are frequently impaired by major bridging veins which have to be spared. These veins may partly run between the dural layers. Venous architecture should be appreciated on preoperative MRI studies. Moreover, attention should be paid to largely expose the fissura longitudinalis in order to have sufficient options to dissect the interhemispheric fissure between major veins.

#### 7.5.2.2 Parietal Operculum

Resection of the *parietal operculum* in the depth may cause contralateral lower quadrantic visual field defects which are much more disturbing than deficits of the superior visual field caused by temporal resections [111].

#### 7.5.2.3 Angular and Supramarginal Gyri, Visual Cortex

For resections around the angular and supramarginal gyri, the technique of subpial gyral emptying preserving pial and arachnoidal banks including vessels should be used. The same holds true for resections within the visual cortex to avoid complete homonymous hemianopia. As a result of the wide dispersion of the optic radiation, already superficial resections at the mesial aspects of the occipital lobe are frequently associated with visual field deficits [45, 46]. Upper and lower visual field defects should also be considered in planning parieto-occipital resections affecting white matter tracts or calcarine cortex [111].

#### 7.5.2.4 Occipital Lobe Landmarks

Important landmarks for anatomical resection of the occipital lobe include falx, tentorium, and ambient cistern. It is important to visualize the ventricular system. However, the distance from the cortical surface to the tip of the posterior horn is very variable. Limits of resection in the depth are defined by the thalamus which is covered by the plexus as well as the cisterna ambiens and quadrigemina which are covered at the edge of tentorium and falx by a tough arachnoidal layer. Figure 7.10 demonstrates a typical occipital lobe resection.

### 7.5.3 Seizure Outcome

#### 7.5.3.1 Mixed Follow-Up

Seizure-free outcome (Engel I) has been reported in most studies between 40 and 60% [6, 7, 57, 67, 74–76, 105, 141, 143, 144, 146, 152, 153, 160,

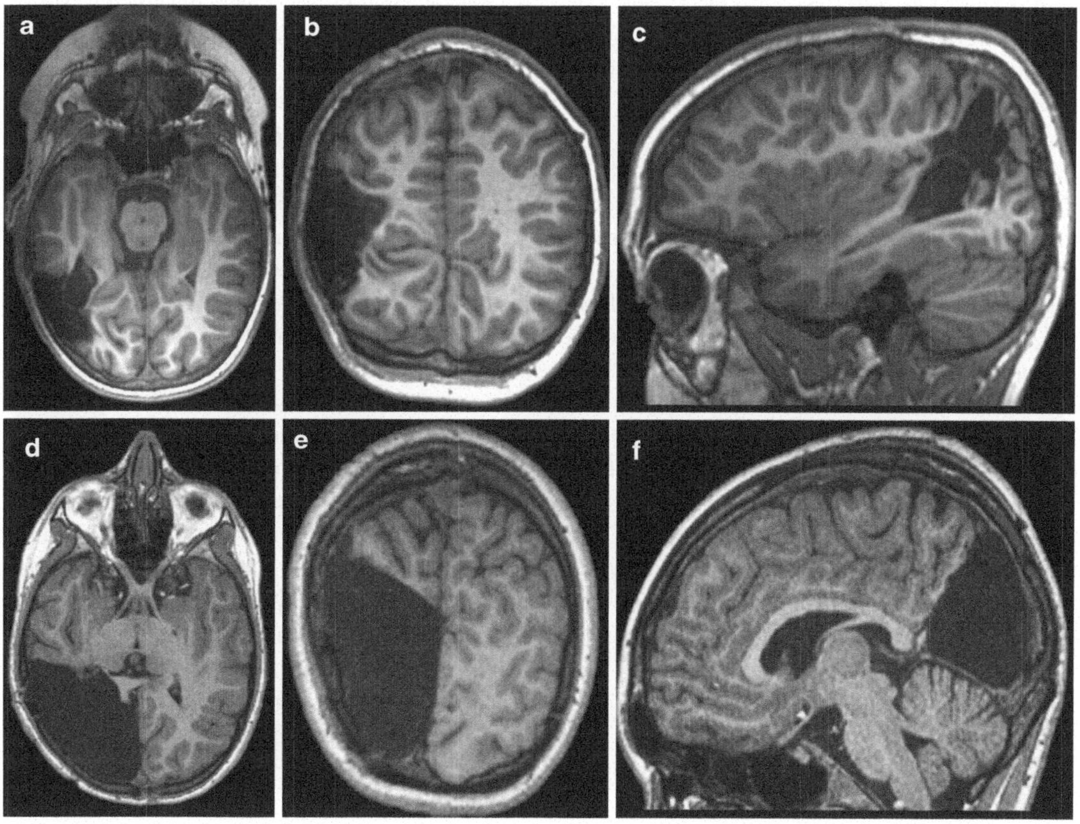


**Fig. 7.10** 10-year-old boy suffering from focal epilepsy after brain injury with impression fracture and hemorrhage of the right occipital lobe at the age of 6 months. There was an almost complete hemianopsia to the left side. Preoperative MRI (upper sequence) in axial (**a**), coronal (**b**), and sagittal (**c**) views shows an extensive cystic defect in the right temporo-parieto-occipital area. The EEG demonstrated epileptogenic activity predominantly in the right occipital lobe. Postoperative MRI (lower sequence, **d–f**) demonstrates resection of the occipital lobe and of the perilesional temporal and parietal cortex. Pathological evaluation of the operative specimen revealed a brain-dura scar. The child was seizure free except for some single questionable auras. Thus, outcome was classified as Engel Ib

165, 166]. Some centers report even better results with Engel I outcome between 60 and 70% [20, 142, 148, 167–169]. Jehi et al. [68] found seizure-free outcome in 89% of patients with occipital and in 93% of cases with parieto-occipital epilepsies. Daniel et al. [170] noted excellent seizure outcome in 92% of their 13 PCE patients.

#### 7.5.3.2 Long-Term Follow-Up

Meta-analyses demonstrated seizure-free (Engel I) outcome in 46% of 117 PCE patients [25] and in 65% of 584 occipital resections [171]. Liava et al. [151] analyzed a cohort of 208 patients (125 adults, 83 children) with PCE. At a mean follow-up of 9.6 years, seizure freedom (Engel I) was achieved in 70% [151]. Others noted seizure freedom (Engel I) in 46% [65], 64% [154], and 51% [172]. Overall, mean seizure freedom (Engel I) rates in posterior cortex resections range between 50 and 60%.

#### 7.5.3.3 Predictors for Seizure Control

The following prognostic factors indicating a favorable seizure outcome for resections in PCE have been identified: abnormal MRI findings [142, 143, 171], shorter duration of epilepsy [142, 143, 171, 173], complete removal of the lesion [69], presence of preoperative focal IED in scalp EEG [174], and pathologies other than FCD type I [69]. In the study of Liava et al. [151] comprising 208 PCE cases, short duration of epilepsy represented the most consistent positive predictor for seizure outcome. Contrarily, others found that the duration of epilepsy in PCE patients did not significantly influence seizure outcome [175, 176].

## 7.6 Insular Resections

### 7.6.1 Identification of Surgical Candidates

#### 7.6.1.1 Epidemiology

Seizures arising from the insula as a part of a complex epileptogenic network may only become evident after propagation of the ictal activity. Thus, insular cortex epilepsy seems to be an underrecognized syndrome, and reliable data on its frequency are lacking [177], since only intracranial EEG recordings using depth electrodes may prove insular seizure origin [178, 179]. Chevrier et al. [180] noted 6.4% insular and peri-insular epilepsies in their series of 920 patients.

#### 7.6.1.2 Etiology

Most frequent pathologies in the series of Chevrier [180] including 59 insular resections for epilepsy were neoplastic lesions (27%), followed by malformations of cortical development (21%), vascular malformations (19%), and atrophy/gliosis from an acquired insult (17%), whereas normal findings were observed in 8% of cases. Similar data have been reported by others [20, 57, 181].

#### 7.6.1.3 Seizure Semiology

According to the multiple connections of the insular cortex, semiology of insular seizures is variable [182–184]. Due to close relationships with temporomesial or fronto-orbital structures, insular seizures may resemble temporal [185] and frontal [186] origin. Nevertheless, there are some characteristics of insular seizures like vegetative, viscero-, and somatosensory symptoms [187–190]. Thus, insular epilepsy should be considered when a combination of somatosensory, visceral, and motor symptoms is observed early in a seizure [191]. Correlating insular-opercular seizure semiology with subregions based on connectional architecture, Wang et al. [192] identified four main subgroups following the anterior-inferior to posterior-superior axis: seizures involving the anterior insular region and mesial temporal lobe were characterized by epigastric sensations with or without feelings of fear or rage, seizures arising from the posterior temporal operculum showed auditory sensations and symmetric tonic signs, seizures involving the intermediate insulo-opercular region revealed orofacial and laryngeal signs, while seizures affecting the posterior insulo-opercular region with propagation to the mesial frontal lobe demonstrated somatosensory signs. Thus, anterior seizure origin predominantly showed limbic semiology, whereas posterior regions were associated with somatosensory semiology [192].

## 7.6.2 Surgical Aspects

### 7.6.2.1 History of Insular Resections

Guillaume and Mazars [193] were the first to attempt surgical treatment of epilepsies originating in the insular cortex. Others resected parts of the insula in addition to temporal lobectomy [194]. Silfvenius et al. [195] reviewing temporal cases at the MNI from 1946 to 1962 (106 patients, 58 of them had total or partial insulectomy, and 48 had no insular resection) found similar seizure-free outcome in both groups (45% in the insulectomy group compared to 42% in the non-insulectomy group). However, the rate of hemiparesis was increased from 3% in the non-insulectomy group to 21% in the insulectomy group. Thus, insular resections in addition to temporal lobectomy were abandoned, since they did not improve seizure outcome, but significantly increased surgical morbidity. In 1992, Yasargil reported a large series of 177 paralimbic tumors including 80 insular tumors. Surgical treatment mainly aiming at tumor control resulted in seizure freedom in 92.5% of the patients with minimal complications [196]. Stimulated by these favorable results demonstrating feasibility of insular resections, the interest at this area has renewed, and some larger series focused on insular tumors with or without pharmacoresistant epilepsy have been reported [57, 180, 181, 197].

### 7.6.2.2 Classification of Insular Tumors

Based on anatomical and functional characteristics of the insula, Yasargil [51] proposed a classification system for tumors of the insula as a part of paralimbic tumors. Tumors localized within the proper insular cortex, mainly at its middle and posterior parts, are categorized as Yasargil type 3A, while type 3B extends to adjacent opercula. At the anterior insula, the uncinate fasciculus connects the paralimbic areas with each other, and the paralimbic and limbic systems join at the piriform olfactory cortex. Therefore, tumor growth will always propagate along these two crossroads encompassing the entire paralimbic and/or limbic system and expanding into the corresponding neocortical areas, thus forming Yasargil types 5A (extending to orbitofrontal and/or temporo-polar structures) and 5B (extending to temporomesial structures) lesions [51, 196] (Fig. 7.11). Other classification systems for insular tumors proposed are based on tumor location with regard to a bisection plane through the foramen of Monro and a horizontal plane through the Sylvian fissure [199], as well as on tumor extension within the white matter tracts [200].

### 7.6.2.3 Surgical Approaches

Yasargil's classification of insular tumors provides a reasonable basis for planning approaches to different insular lesions. Most important approaches to the insula are the transsylvian and the transopercular route. Obviously, for pure insular lesions (corresponding to Yasargil's type 3A), the transsylvian approach preventing any damage to surrounding structures seems to be ideal. This approach is also suitable for lesions extending to the temporomesial area (corresponding to Yasargil's type 5B) [196, 201]. However, the transsylvian route requires dissection of the Sylvian vessels with the risk of direct or indirect (e.g., vasospastic reactions) damage [202, 203]. Yaşargil et al. [204] and others [201, 205] have emphasized the importance of wide splitting of the Sylvian fissure to avoid brain injury due to opercular retraction and to provide an overview on vascular architecture. In particular, the long arteries supplying the corona radiata must be preserved to avoid postoperative deficits [53, 55].

For lesions extending to the opercula (corresponding to Yasargil's type 3B), the transopercular approach is best suited, while lesions extending to the orbitofrontal and/or temporo-polar structures (corresponding to Yasargil's type 5A) may be removed using the transopercular, transfrontal, or transtemporal route [57, 168, 181, 206–208]. In principle, all insular tumors can be reached by the transoper-

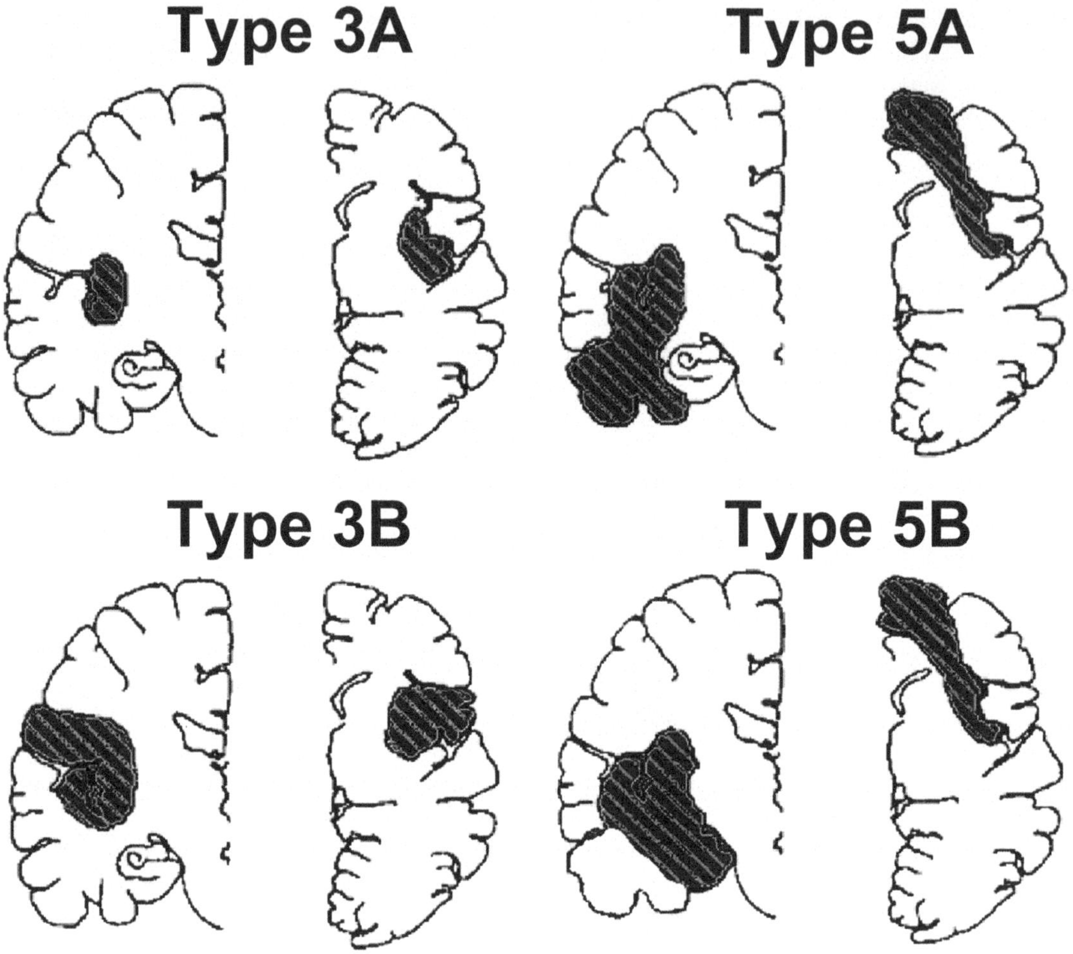


**Fig. 7.11** Schematic illustrations of Yasargil's classification of insular tumors in coronal (left side) and axial (right side) views. The gray areas represent patterns of tumors. Identical sections were used to display each type. Because type 5 lesions involve both frontal (shown in axial view) and temporal (shown in coronal view) areas, lesion may not appear to correspond when comparing the coronal and axial sections of each category (from [198], with permission)

cular route avoiding direct manipulation of the arteries within the Sylvian fissure [209, 210]. Different approaches to the insula are demonstrated in Fig. 7.12. The frontal and temporal approaches only serve to remove parts of the insula in addition to the respective lobar or intralobar resection.

#### 7.6.2.4 Resection Strategies

Insular resections are associated with a significant risk of temporary and permanent motor complications [57, 181] (see also Chap.15). These complications may be caused by direct and especially by indirect (i.e., ischemic) damage to the pyramidal tract. In particular, the long insular arteries, perforator-like arteries that are located in the posterior portion of the insula supplying parts of the corona radiata and the internal capsule, as well as the lenticulostriate arteries are endangered with resection of the posterior-superior aspect of the insula [196, 211, 212]. Therefore, it seems to be advisable to deliberately leave some tissue at that area and to confine resection to 80–90%.

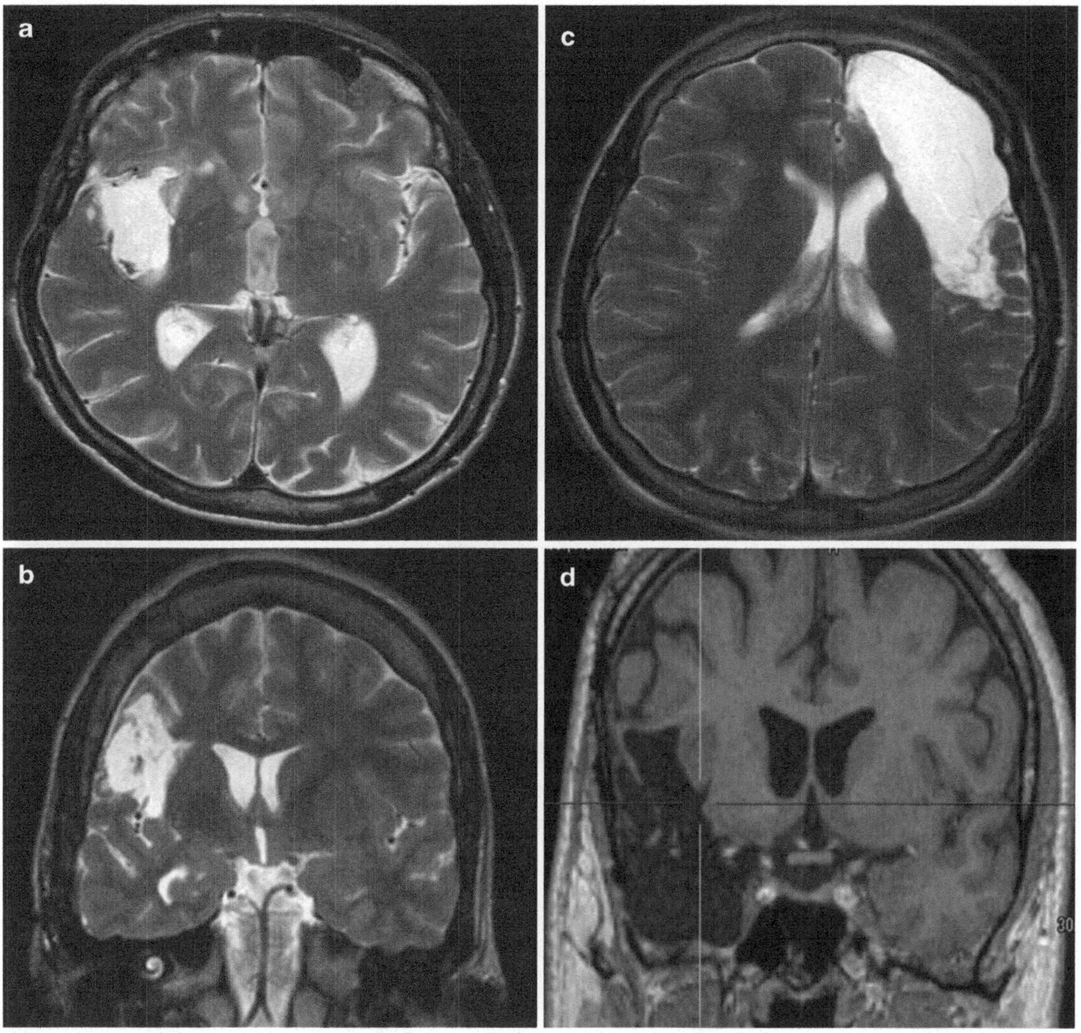


**Fig. 7.12** Different approaches to the insula demonstrated on postoperative MRI scans of single cases. (**a**) Transsylvian approach (axial view); (**b**) transopercular (frontal) approach (coronal view); (**c**) partial resection of the insula via the transfrontal route (axial view); (**d**) resection of parts of the insula via the transtemporal route (coronal view). Note that with the frontal and temporal approaches only parts of insula may be resected in addition to the proper lobar procedure

This strategy can be expected to noticeably reduce permanent morbidity [57]. Igekaya et al. [213] suggested to spare some tissue at the bottom of the peri-insular sulcus where the perforating arteries pass to the pyramidal tract in order to avoid neurological complications. Figures 7.13–7.16 show illustrative cases of insular resections. Figure 7.17 demonstrates the surgical steps of the transsylvian approach to the insula.

### 7.6.3 Seizure Outcome

Only a paucity of publications on the insula is available in the surgical literature. Most reports present single cases or small series, and only a few larger series have been published. Moreover, in most series, indications for surgery (epilepsy or tumor) are mixed, and different resection strategies (partial or complete insular resection, opercular-insular resection,

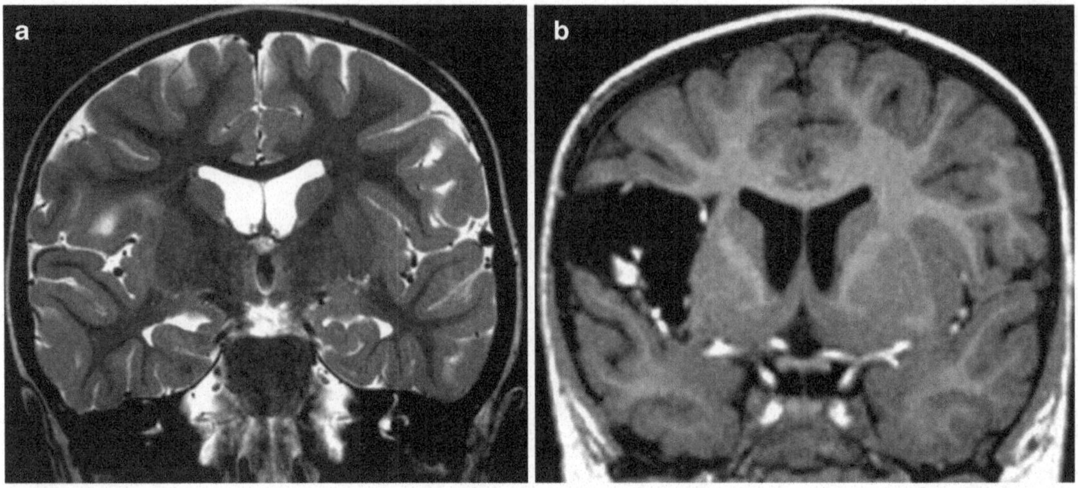

Fig. 7.13 Transopercular (frontal) approach to the insula. 3.5-year-old girl with epilepsy onset in the first days of life, multiple seizure types, pharmacoresistance, and poor response to the ketogenic diet. At the time of surgery, the girl had daily seizures and a developmental deficit as a result of the early epilepsy onset and very frequent seizures. (**a**) Preoperative MRI (coronal view) shows the lesion in the right frontal operculum and adjacent insula. (**b**) Postoperative MRI (coronal view) demonstrates complete removal of the MR-visible lesion by a frontal transopercular approach. Histopathological examination revealed FCD type IIa. The patient remained seizure free at long-term follow-up, even after antiepileptic drug withdrawal

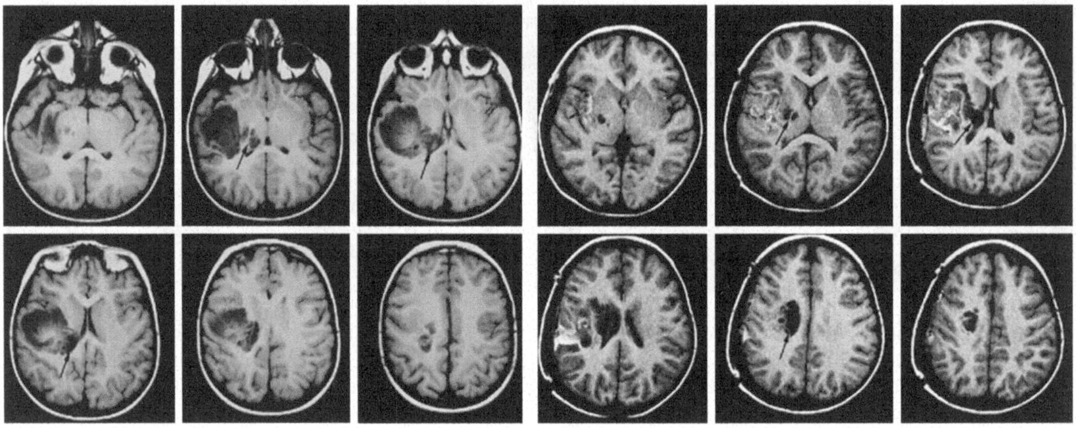

Fig. 7.14 Axial T1-weighted MRI of a 5-year-old girl who presented with a medically intractable epilepsy. Left: Preoperative MRI shows a right-sided tumor involving the insula and encroaching on the posterior part of the internal capsula and the thalamus (arrows). Tumor removal was accomplished using a transsylvian approach. Right: Early postoperative axial T1-weighted MRI shows residual tumor along the internal capsula and thalamus (arrows), which was left behind deliberately. The extent of resection was estimated to be more than 80%. Histopathological examination revealed a dysembryoplastic neuroepithelial tumor (WHO grade I). The postoperative course was uneventful. The patient remained completely seizure free (from [198], with permission)

etc.) have been applied. Thus, variable results in terms of seizure outcome have been reported, and data on long-term seizure outcome are largely lacking.

#### 7.6.3.1 Overall Results

In small series comprising 5–11 patients, seizure-free outcome (Engel I) has been reported in 81% [197], 83% [179], and 84% [191] of

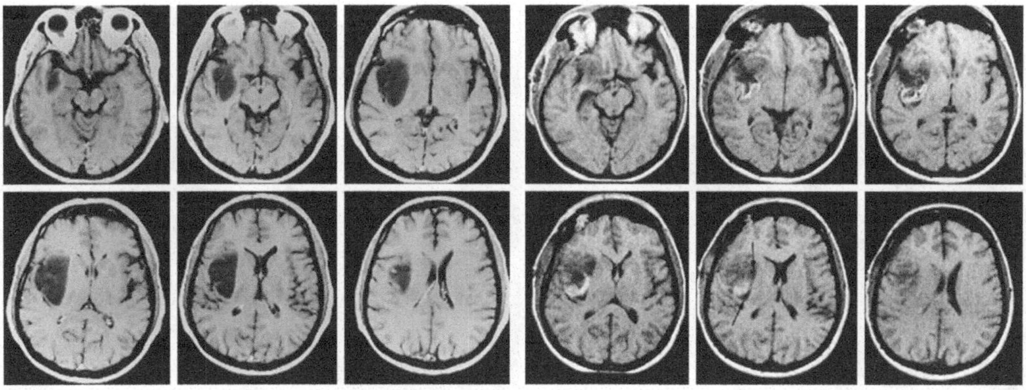

**Fig. 7.15** Axial T1-weighted MRI of a 48-year-old man with a 4-year history of partial seizures. Left: Contrast-enhanced MRI shows a well-demarcated tumor that is restricted to the right insula (Yasargil's type 3A). The tumor was removed via the transsylvian route. Right: Early postoperative MRI shows the defect after tumor removal. There are some small areas of residual tumor at the medial superior aspects of the tumor cavity (arrow). Tumor removal was estimated to be more than 80%. Histopathological examination revealed an astrocytoma (WHO grade II). The postoperative course was uneventful, and the patient became seizure free (from [198], with permission)

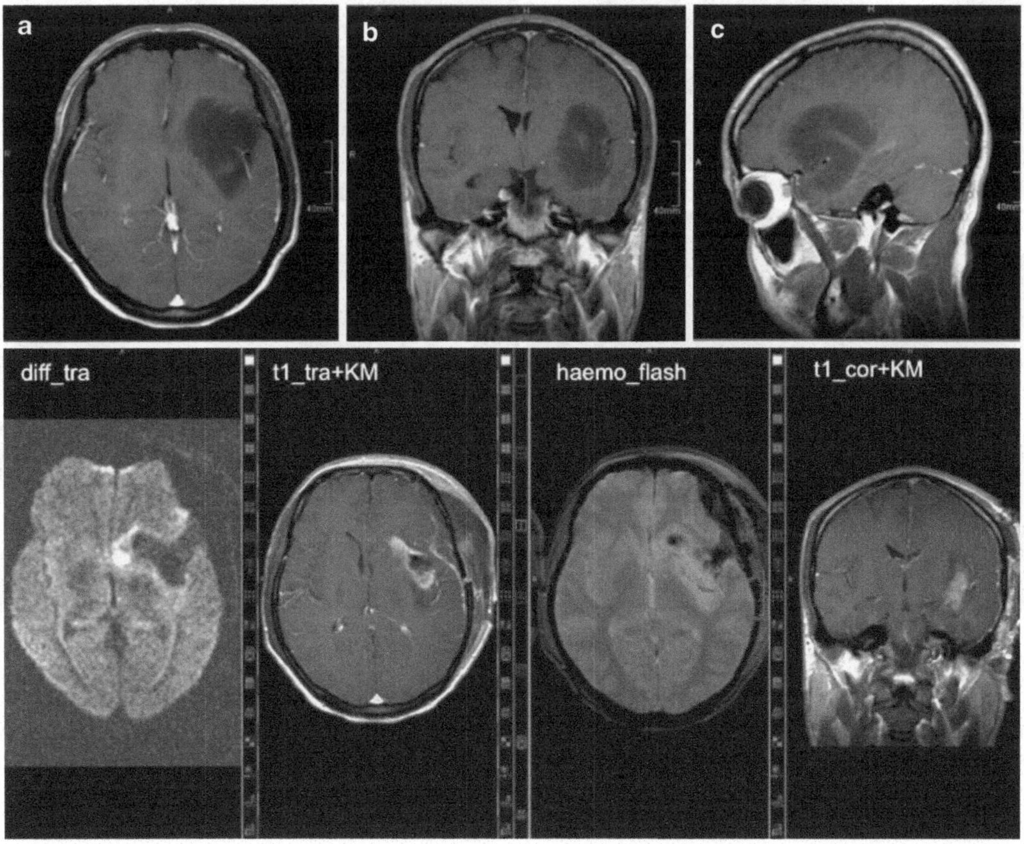


**Fig. 7.16** 29-year-old male patient with a pharmacoresistant epilepsy with focal and generalized tonic-clinic seizures. Upper sequence: Contrast-enhanced T1-weighted MRI in axial (**a**), coronal (**b**), and sagittal (**c**) views shows the tumor in the left insula (Yasargil type 3A). The tumor was removed using the transsylvian route. Lower sequence: Early postoperative MRI demonstrates about 80% tumor resection. Note some residual tumor in the superior-posterior aspect of the insula. Histopathological examination revealed an oligodendroglioma (WHO grade II). The postoperative course was uneventful, and the patient was seizure free

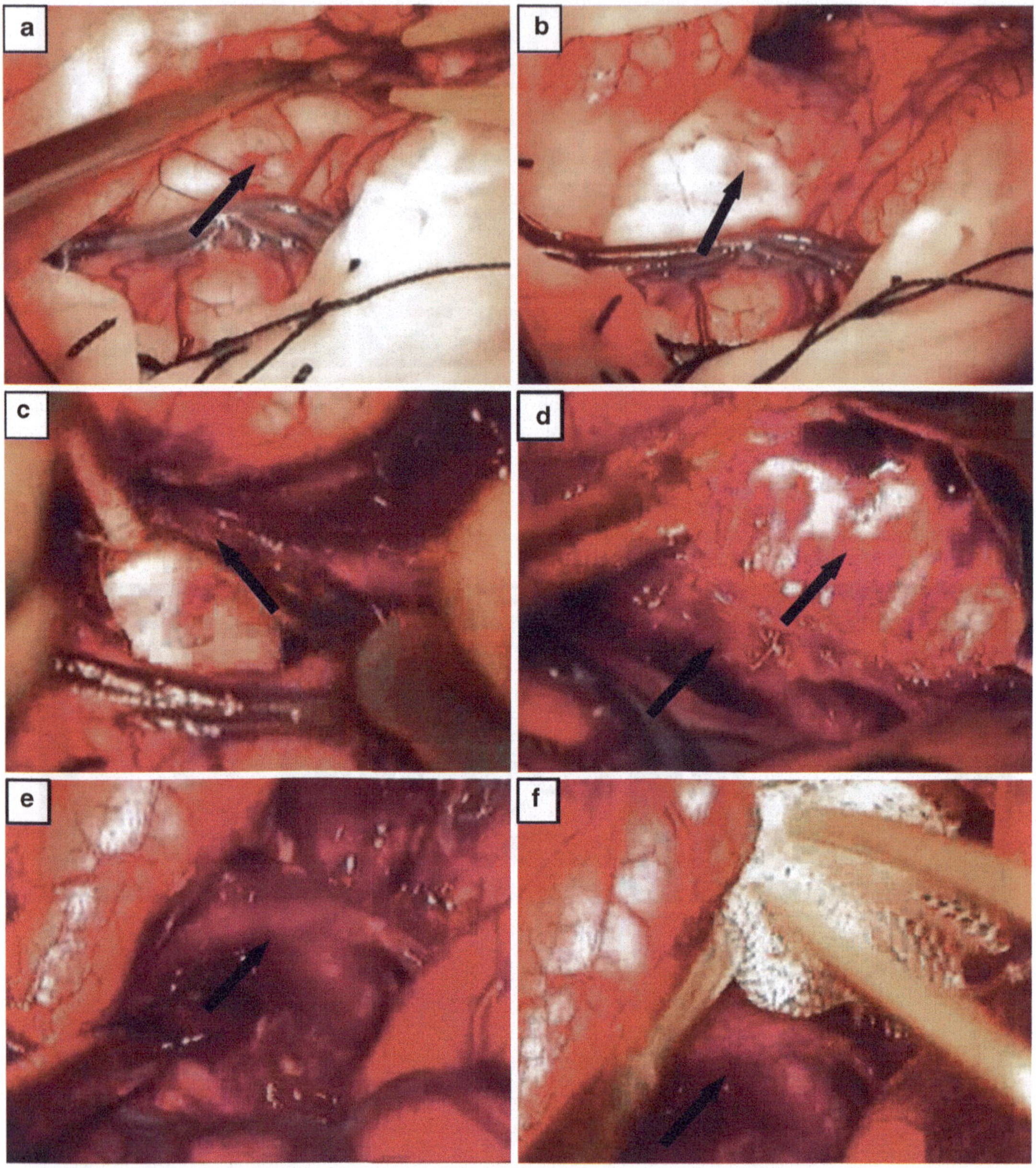


**Fig. 7.17** Surgical steps (intraoperative view) of removal of a left-sided insular tumor (case shown in Fig. 7.16): (**a**) The frontotemporal area is swollen by the underlying tumor (arrow: Sylvian fissure); (**b**) the Sylvian fissure is dissected, tumor of the insula is visualized (arrow: tumor between frontal and temporal lobes); (**c**) dissection of the tumor under the Sylvian vessels (arrow: MCA lifted by the sucker); (**d**) temporal dissection over Sylvian vessels (left arrow: MCA, right arrow: temporal tumor); (**e**) the Sylvian vessels are completely skeletonized (arrow; MCA); (**f**) hemostasis with Tabotamp (arrow: MCA). MCA: middle cerebral artery

cases. Von Lehe et al. [181] summarizing results of 24 patients found 62.5% seizure-free (ILAE I) cases, and Delev et al. [20] documented seizure freedom (Engel I) in 52% of patients. Favorable seizure outcome (Engel I–II) in between 50% and 70% of cases can be achieved with subtotal resection of the insula [53, 57, 181, 211]. With opercular-insular corticectomy, Bouthillier and

Nguyen [214] documented Engel class I outcome in 80% of their 25 patients. In sum, seizure-free outcome (Engel I) ranges between 50 and 60% in larger epilepsy surgical series [20, 53, 57, 181].

#### 7.6.3.2 Results in Children

In a pediatric series comprising 13 children undergoing opercular-insular corticectomy, seizure freedom (Engel I) has been noted in 69%, whereby 31% of children required a second procedure to complete resection and improve outcome [215]. These results compare favorably to the 28 reported pediatric cases of insular/perisylvian resections in whom seizure-free outcome (Engel I) was obtained in around 70% of cases [179, 181, 216–220].

**Concluding Remarks**

- ***Seizure outcome.*** *With availability of high-resolution MRI and postprocessing techniques facilitating delineation and complete resection of focal cortical dysplasias as the most frequent pathologies, results of extratemporal resections have noticeably improved and now approximate or even may exceed those achieved with temporal resections. Thus, the success of epilepsy surgery over the last decades has particularly become apparent in the treatment of extratemporal epilepsies.*
- ***Frontal operculum/Broca's area.*** *For resections in the frontal operculum, particularly around Broca's area, the technique of subpial gyral emptying should be used in order to prevent ischemic events in more distant areas.*
- ***Supplementary motor area (SMA).*** *The SMA can be removed completely without disadvantage in the long run. The SMA deficiency syndrome can be expected to recover almost completely over a period of around 3 weeks. Intraoperative mapping of the central area can easily be accomplished by phase reversal of SEP, and MEP monitoring provides reassurance with respect to the integrity of the primary motor cortex. Obviously, awake craniotomy would be misleading, since clinical testing cannot clearly differentiate between the SMA deficiency syndrome and motor deficits caused by injury to the primary motor cortex, while MEP do not change during resection of the SMA but immediately deteriorate if the primary motor cortex is affected.*
- ***Rolandic cortex.*** *The basal aspects of the precentral and postcentral gyri representing the motor and sensory face and tongue area can be resected up to the hand area (maximum roughly 6 cm above the Sylvian fissure) without permanent harm. Subsequent facial paresis/hypesthesia usually resolve completely within 2–3 weeks due to their bilateral representation. Well-delimitable lesions can be resected even in the motor hand and leg area with favorable epileptological and functional results. Limited removal of the upper primary sensory cortex is usually not complicated by significant permanent deficits.*
- ***Posterior cortex.*** *For resections dorsal to the central sulcus, the prone position should be preferred. By pronounced anteflexion of the head, the operation table can be brought in an inclined upward position, thus reducing brain swelling, while providing comfortable access to the operation field. Large exposure of the fissura longitudinalis is advantageous for interhemispheric approaches with respect to the individual venous anatomy.*
- ***Visual cortex.*** *As a result of the wide dispersion of the optic radiation, already superficial resections particularly at the mesial aspects of the occipital lobe are frequently associated with visual field deficits. Since Meyer's loop projects to the inferior bank of the calcarine sulcus, resection of the basal visual cortex mainly affects the superior visual fields, which much less impedes daily life activities than restriction of the inferior visual fields caused by resection of the upper bank of the calcarine sulcus.*
- ***Insula.*** *For pure insular lesions and pathologies extending to the temporomesial area, the transsylvian approach seems to be ideal. However, this approach should only be used by neurosurgeons who are familiar with the dissection of the Sylvian vessels, e.g., for*

*aneurysm surgery. For pathologies involving the opercula, the transopercular route offers itself. With this approach, the opercula can be removed by subpial dissection preserving pial banks and vessels, thus providing sufficient access to the proper insula. The transopercular route is much less dangerous compared to the transsylvian approach and can be used for all insular pathologies. Dissection of the superior-posterior aspect of the insula includes a high risk for damage to the pyramidal tract and internal capsule, either by direct injury or by occlusion of long insular or lenticulostriate arteries. It is therefore advisable to leave some tissue at the superior-posterior aspect of the insula in situ. Aiming at an 80–90% resection of the insula, favorable results in terms of seizure outcome are achieved similar to those with its complete resection, while neurological complications may be significantly reduced.*

## References

1. Behdad A, Limbrick DD Jr. Epilepsy surgery in children with seizures arising from the Rolandic cortex. Epilepsia. 2009;50(6):1450–61.
2. Chang EF, Clark A, Smith JS, et al. Functional mapping-guided resection of low-grade gliomas in eloquent areas of the brain: improvement of long-term survival. J Neurosurg. 2011;114(3):566–73.
3. Oliveira RS, Santos MV, Terra VC, Sakamoto AC, Machado HR. Tailored resections for intractable Rolandic cortex epilepsy in children: a single-center experience with 48 consecutive cases. Childs Nerv Syst. 2011;27(5):779–85.
4. Bauer S, Hamer HM. Extratemporal epilepsies. In: Stefan H, Theodore WH, editors. Epilepsy, part I, Handbook of Clinical Neurology, vol. vol 107. Edinburgh: Elsevier; 2012.
5. Delev D, Send K, Wagner J, et al. Epilepsy surgery of the Rolandic and immediate perirolandic cortex: surgical outcome and prognostic factors. Epilepsia. 2014;55(10):1585–93.
6. Englot DJ, Berger MS, Barbaro NM, Chang EF. Factors associated with seizure freedom in the surgical resection of glioneuronal tumors. Epilepsia. 2012a;53(1):51–7.
7. Englot DJ, Han SJ, Berger MS, Barbaro NM, Chang EF. Extent of surgical resection predicts seizure freedom in low-grade temporal lobe brain tumors. Neurosurgery. 2012b;70(4):921–8.
8. Englot DJ, Breshears JD, Sun PP, Chang EF, Auguste KI. Seizure outcomes after resective surgery for extra-temporal lobe epilepsy in pediatric patients. J Neurosurg Pediatr. 2013;12(2):126–33.
9. Hanáková P, Brázdil M, Novák Z, et al. Long-term outcome and predictors of resective surgery prognosis in patients with refractory extratemporal epilepsy. Seizure. 2014;23(4):266–73.
10. Hardy SG, Miller JW, Holmes MD, et al. Factors predicting outcome of surgery for intractable epilepsy with pathologically verified mesial temporal sclerosis. Epilepsia. 2003;44(4):565–8.
11. Otsubo H, Chitoku S, Ochi A, et al. Malignant rolandic-sylvian epilepsy in children: diagnosis, treatment, and outcomes. Neurology. 2001;57(4):590–6.
12. Roper SN. Surgical treatment of the extratemporal epilepsies. Epilepsia. 2009;50(suppl 8):69–74.
13. Ansari SF, Maher CO, Tubbs RS, et al. Surgery for extratemporal nonlesional epilepsy in children: a meta-analysis. Childs Nerv Syst. 2010a;26:945–51.
14. Ansari SF, Tubbs RS, Terry CL, Cohen-Gadol AA. Surgery for extratemporal nonlesional epilepsy in adults: an outcome meta-analysis. Acta Neurochir. 2010b;152(8):1299–305.
15. Kim S, Mountz JM. SPECT imaging of epilepsy: an overview and comparison with F-18 FDG PET. Int J Mol Imaging. 2011;2011(10):1–9.
16. Pardoe H, Kuzniecky R. Advanced imaging techniques in the diagnosis of nonlesional epilepsy: MRI, MRS, PET, and SPECT. Epilepsy Curr. 2014;14(3):121–4.
17. Cardinale F, Cossu M, Castana L, et al. Stereoelectroencephalography. Neurosurgery. 2013;72(3):353–66.
18. Shah A, Mittal S. Invasive electroencephalography monitoring: indications and presurgical planning. Ann Indian Acad Neurol. 2014;17(5):89.
19. Greiner HM, Horn PS, Tenney JR, et al. Preresection intraoperative electro-corticography (ECoG) abnormalities predict seizure-onset zone and outcome in pediatric epilepsy surgery. Epilepsia. 2016;57(4):582–9.
20. Delev D, Oehl B, Steinhoff BJ, Nakagawa J, Scheiwe C, Schulze-Bonhage A, Zentner J. Surgical treatment of extratemporal epilepsies. Neurosurgery. 2018;84:242. https://doi.org/10.1093/neuros/nyy099.
21. Morace RCasciato S, Quarato PP, et al. Long-term seizure outcome in frontal lobe epilepsy surgery. Epilepsy Behav. 2019;90:93–8.
22. Wagner J, Weber B, Urbach H, et al. Morphometric MRI analysis improves detection of focal cortical dysplasia type II. Brain. 2011a;134(10):2844–54.
23. Wagner J, Urbach H, Niehusmann P, et al. Focal cortical dysplasia type IIb: completeness of cortical, not subcortical, resection is necessary for seizure freedom. Epilepsia. 2011b;52(8):1418–24.
24. Engel JJ, Van Nes P, Rasmussen T, Ojemann L. Outcome with respect to epileptic seizures. In: Engel Jr J, editor. Surgical treatment of the epilepsies. 2nd ed. New York, NY: Raven Press; 1993. p. 609–21.

25. Tellez-Zenteno JF, Dhar R, Wiebe S. Long-term seizure outcomes following epilepsy surgery: a systematic review and meta-analysis. Brain. 2005;128:1188–98.
26. Penfield W, Boldrey E. Somatic motor and sensory representation in the cerebral cortex of man as studied by electrical stimulation. Brain. 1937;60:389–443.
27. Yousry TA, Schmid UD, Alkadhi H, Schmidt D, Peraud A, Buettner A, et al. Localization of the motor hand area to a knob on the precentral gyrus. A new landmark. Brain. 1997;120(Pt 1):141–57.
28. Ostergard TA, Miller JP. Surgery for epilepsy in the primary motor cortex: a critical review. Epilepsy Behav. 2018; https://doi.org/10.1016/j.yebeh.2018.06.036.
29. Dum RP, Strick PL. Motor areas in the frontal lobe of the primate. Physiol Behav. 2002;77:677–82.
30. Krainik A, Lehéricy S, Duffeau H, et al. Role of the supplementary motor area in motor deficit following medial frontal lobe surgery. Neurology. 2001;57:871–8.
31. Lim SH, Dinner DS, Pillay PK, et al. Functional anatomy of the human supplementary sensorimotor area: results of extraoperative electrical stimulation. Electroencephalo Clin Neurophysiol. 1994;91:179–93.
32. Talairach J, Bancaud J. The supplementary motor area in man (anatomo-functional findings by stereo-electroencephalography in epilepsy). Int J Neurol. 1966;5:330–47.
33. Van Buren JM, Fedio P. Functional representation on the medial aspect of the frontal lobes in man. J Neurosurg. 1976;44:275–89.
34. Hutchins KD, Martino AM, Strick PL. Corticospinal projections from the medial wall of the hemisphere. Exp Brain Res. 1988;71:667–72.
35. Jürgens U. The efferent and afferent connections of the supplementary motor area. Brain Res. 1984;300:63–81.
36. Goldberg G. Supplementary motor area structure and function: review and hypotheses. Behav Brain Sci. 1985;8:567–615.
37. Sanides F. The cyto-myeloarchitecture of the human frontal lobe and its relation to phylogenetic differentiation of the cerebral cortex. J Hirnforschung. 1984;6:269–82.
38. Orgogozo JM, Larsen B. Activation of the supplementary motor area during voluntary movement in man suggests it works as a supra-motor area. Science. 1979;206:847–50.
39. Fried I, Katz A, McCarthy G, Sass KJ, Williamson P, Spencer SS, Spencer DD. Functional organization of human supplementary motor cortex studied by electrical stimulation. J Neurosci. 1991;11:3656–66.
40. Duncan J, Owen AM. Common regions of the human frontal lobe recruited by diverse cognitive demands. Trends Neurosci. 2000;23:475–83.
41. De Benedictis A, Duffau H, Paradiso B, et al. Anatomo-functional study of the temporo-parieto-occipital: region: dissection, tractographic and brain mapping evidence from a neurosurgical perspective. J Anat. 2014;225:132–51.
42. Foville AL. Traite´ comple^t de l'anatomie, de la physiologie et de la pathologie du syste'me nerveux ce're'bro-spinal. Paris: Fortin, Masson; 1844.
43. Leichnetz GR. Connections of the medial posterior parietal cortex (area 7 m) in the monkey. Anat Rec. 2001;263:215–36.
44. Cavanna AE, Trimble MR. The precuneus: a review of its functional anatomy and behavioural correlates. Brain. 2006;129:564–83.
45. Campero A, Ajler P, Emmerich J, et al. Brain sulci and gyri: a practical anatomical review. J Clin Neurosci. 2014; https://doi.org/10.1016/j.jocn.2014.02.024.
46. Seeger W. Atlas of topographical anatomy of the brain and surrounding structures. Wien, New York: Springer; 1978.
47. Binder DK, Schaller K, Clusmann H. The seminal contributions of Johann Christian Reil to anatomy, physiology, and psychiatry. Neurosurgery. 2007;61:1091–6.
48. Augustine JR. The insular lobe in primates including humans. Neurol Res. 1985;7:2–10.
49. Mesulam MM, Mufson EJ. The insula of Reil in man and monkey. Architectonics, connectivity, and function. In: Peters A, Jones EG, editors. Cerebral cortex, Association and Auditory Cortices, vol. Vol 4. New York: Plenum Press; 1985. p. 179–226.
50. Jeanty P, Chervenak FA, Romero R, et al. The sylvian fissure: a commonly mislabeled cranial landmark. J Ultrasound Med. 1984;3:15–8.
51. Yasargil MG. Microneurosurgery, vol. Vol 4a. Stuttgart: Thieme; 1994.
52. Bykanov A, Piotskhelauri D, et al. Surgical anatomy of the insular cortex. Zhurnal voprosy neirokhirurgii imeni. 2015; https://doi.org/10.17116/neiro201579448-60.
53. Malak R, Bouthillier A, Carmant L, et al. Microsurgery of epileptic foci in the insular region. J Neurosurg. 2009;110:1153–63.
54. Pastor-Escartin F, Garcia-Catalán G, Holanda VM, et al. Microsurgical anatomy of the insular region and operculoinsular association fibers and its neurosurgical application. World Neurosurg. 2019;129:407–20.
55. Türe U, Yaşargil MG, Al-Mefty O, Yaşargil DC. Arteries of the insula. J Neurosurg. 2000;92:676–87.
56. Craig AD, Chen K, Bandy D, Reiman EM. Thermosensory activation of insular cortex. Nat Neurosci. 2000;3(2):184–90.
57. Zentner J, Hufnagel A, Ostertun B, Wolf HK, Behrens E, Campos MG, et al. Surgical treatment of extratemporal epilepsy: clinical, radiologic, and histopathologic findings in 60 patients. Epilepsia. 1996;37:1072–80.
58. Shelley BP, Trimble MR. The insular lobe of Reil—its anatamico-functional, behavioural and neuropsychiatric attributes in humans—a review. World J Biol Psychiatry. 2004;5:176–200.

59. Türe U, Yasargil DC, Al-Mefty O, Yasargil MG. Topographic anatomy of the insular region. J Neurosurg. 1999;90:720–33.
60. Duffau H, Capelle L, Lopes M, Faillot T, Sichez JP, Fohanno D. The insular lobe: physiopathological and surgical considerations. Neurosurgery. 2000;47:801–10; discussion 810–1
61. Tanriover N, Rhoton AL Jr, Kawashima M, Ulm AJ, Yasuda A. Microsurgical anatomy of the insula and the sylvian fissure. J Neurosurg. 2004;100:891–922.
62. Wen HT, Rhoton AL, de Oliveira E, et al. Microsurgical anatomy of the temporal lobe: Part 2–Sylvian fissure and its clinical application. Neurosurgery. 2009;65(ONS Suppl 1):1–36.
63. Seeger W, Zentner J. Anatomical basis of cranial neurosurgery. Heidelberg: Springer; 2018.
64. Elsharkawy AE, Alabbasi AH, Pannek H, et al. Outcome of frontal lobe epilepsy surgery in adults. Epilepsy Res. 2008a;81:97–106.
65. Elsharkawy AE, Pannek H, Schulz R, et al. Outcome after extratemporal epilepsy surgery. Experience of a single center. Neurosurgery. 2008b;63:516–26.
66. Sarkis RA, Jehi L, Najm IM, Kotagal P, Bingaman WE. Seizure outcomes following multilobar epilepsy surgery. Epilepsia. 2012;53(1):44–50.
67. Jehi LE, Najm I, Bingaman W, et al. Surgical outcome and prognostic factors of frontal lobe epilepsy surgery. Brain. 2007;130:574–84.
68. Jehi L, O'Dwyer R, Najm I, et al. A longitudinal study of surgical outcome and its determinants following posterior cortex epilepsy surgery. Epilepsia. 2009;50:2040–52.
69. McIntosh AM, Averill CA, Kalnins RM, et al. Long-term seizure outcome and risk factors for recurrence after extratemporal epilepsy surgery. Epilepsia. 2012;53(6):970–8.
70. Mulholland D, Ali Z, Delanty N, Shahwan A, O'Brien DF. An outcome of seventeen patients treated surgically for intractable extratemporal epilepsy. Ir Med J. 2010;103:211–3.
71. Spencer SS, Berg AT, Vickrey BG, et al. Initial outcomes in the Multicenter Study of Epilepsy Surgery. Neurology. 2003;61:1680–5.
72. Rossi GF. Evaluation of surgical treatment outcome in epilepsy. Crit Rev Neurosurg. 1998;8:282–9.
73. Siegel AM, Cascino GD, Meyer FB, McClelland RL, So EL, Marsh WR, Scheithauer BW, Sharbrough FW. Resective reoperation for failed epilepsy surgery: seizure outcome in 64 patients. Neurology. 2004;63:2298–302.
74. Binder DK, Podlogar M, Clusmann H, et al. Surgical treatment of parietal lobe epilepsy. J Neurosurg. 2009;110(6):1170–8.
75. Englot DJ, Wang DD, Rolston JD, Shih TT, Chang EF. Rates and predictors of long-term seizure freedom after frontal lobe epilepsy surgery: a systematic review and meta-analysis. J Neurosurg. 2012c;116(5):1042–8.
76. Schramm J, Kral T, Kurthen M, et al. Surgery to treat focal frontal lobe epilepsy in adults. Neurosurgery. 2002;51:644–54.
77. Park KI, Lee SK, Chu K, et al. Withdrawal of antiepileptic drugs after neocortical epilepsy surgery. Ann Neurol. 2010;67:230–8.
78. D'Argenzio L, Colonnelli MC, Harrison S, et al. Cognitive outcome after extratemporal epilepsy surgery in childhood. Epilepsia. 2011;52(11):1966–72.
79. Elsharkawy AE, Thorbecke R, Ebner A, May TW. Determinants of quality of life in patients with refractory focal epilepsy who were not eligible for surgery or who rejected surgery. Epilepsy Behav. 2012;24(2):249–55.
80. Engel J Jr, Wiebe S, French J, Sperling M, Williamson P, Spencer D, Gumnit R, Zahn C, Westbrook E, Enos B. Practice parameter: temporal lobe and localized neocortical resections for epilepsy. Epilepsia. 2003;44:741–51.
81. Edwards JC, Wyllie E, Ruggeri PM, et al. Seizure outcome after surgery for epilepsy due to malformation of cortical development. Neurology. 2000;55:1110–4.
82. Kral T, Kuczaty S, Blumcke I, et al. Postsurgical outcome of children and adolescents with medically refractory frontal lobe epilepsies. Childs Nerv Syst. 2001;17:595–601.
83. Tellez-Zenteno JF, Hernández Ronquillo L, Moien-Afshari F, Wiebe S. Surgical outcomes in lesional and non-lesional epilepsy: a systematic review and meta-analysis. Epilepsy Res. 2010;89(2–3):310–8.
84. Englot DJ, Berger MS, Barbaro NM, Chang EF. Predictors of seizure freedom after resection of supratentorial low-grade gliomas. J Neurosurg. 2011;115(2):240–4.
85. Rowland NC, Englot DJ, Cage TA, et al. A meta-analysis of predictors of seizure freedom in the surgical management of focal cortical dysplasia. J Neurosurg. 2012;116:1035–41.
86. Bjellvi J, Olsson I, Malmgren K, et al. Epilepsy duration and seizure outcome in epilepsy surgery. Neurology. 2019;93:e159–66. https://doi.org/10.1212/WNL.0000000000007753.
87. Di Gennaro G, De Risi M, Quarato PP, Sparano A, Mascia A, Grammaldo LG, Meldolesi GN, Esposito V, Picardi A. Prognostic significance of serial postoperative EEG in extratemporal lobe epilepsy surgery. Clin Neurophysiol. 2012;123:2346–51.
88. Rathore C, Radhakrishnan K. Prognostic significance of interictal epileptiform discharges after epilepsy surgery. J Clin Neurophysiol. 2010;27:255–62.
89. Tanriverdi T, Olivier NP, Olivier A, et al. Quality of life after extratemporal epilepsy surgery: a prospective clinical study. Clin Neurol Neurosurg. 2008a;110:30–7.
90. Tanriverdi T, Poulin N, Olivier A. Psychosocial outcome after extratemporal epilepsy surgery: a prospective clinical study. Turk Neurosurg. 2008b;18:114–24.
91. El Hassani Y, Fournet M, Momjian S, et al. Neuropsychological outcome after extra-temporal epilepsy surgery. Acta Neurochir. 2012;154:1337–42.
92. Helmstaedter C, Gleissner U, Zentner J, et al. Neuropsychological consequences of epilepsy sur-

gery in frontal lobe epilepsy. Neuropsychologia. 1998;36:681–9.
93. Ljunggren S, Andersson-Roswall L, Rydenhag B, Samuelsson H. Cognitive outcome two years after frontal lobe resection for epilepsy - a prospective longitudinal study. Seizure. 2015;30:50–6.
94. Holmes MD, Kutsy RL, Ojemann GA, Wilensky AJ, Ojemann LM. Interictal, unifocal spikes in refractory extratemporal epilepsy predict ictal origin and postsurgical outcome. Clin Neurophysiol. 2000;111:1802–8.
95. Dulay MF, Busch RM, Chapin JS. Executive functioning and depressed mood before and after unilateral frontal lobe resection for intractable epilepsy. Neuropsychologia. 2013;51:1370–6.
96. Kellinghaus C, Luders HO. Frontal lobe epilepsy. Epileptic Disord. 2004;6:223–39.
97. Salvanova V, Quesney LF, Rasmussen T, Andermann F, Olivier A. Reevaluation of surgical failures and the role of reoperation in 39 patients with frontal lobe epilepsy. Epilepsia. 1994;35:70–80.
98. Rasmussen T. Tailoring of cortical excisions for frontal lobe epilepsy. Can J Neurol Sci. 1991;18:606–10.
99. Ferrier CH, Engelsman J, Alarcon G, et al. Prognostic factors in presurgical assessment of frontal lobe epilepsy. J Neurol Neurosurg Psychiatry. 1999;66:350–6.
100. Frater JL, Prayson RA, Morris HH, 3rd. et al. Surgical pathologic findings of extratemporal-based intractable epilepsy: a study of 133 consecutive resections. Arch Pathol Lab Med 2000; 124: 545–549.
101. Janszky J, Fogarasi A, Jokeit H, et al. Are ictal vocalisations related to the lateralisation of frontal lobe epilepsy? J Neurol Neurosurg Psychiatry. 2000;69:244–7.
102. Jobst BC, Siegel AM, Thadani VM, et al. Intractable seizures of frontal lobe origin: clinical characteristics, localizing signs, and results of surgery. Epilepsia. 2000;41:1139–52.
103. Lee JJ, Lee SK, Lee SY, et al. Frontal lobe epilepsy: clinical characteristics, surgical outcomes and diagnostic modalities. Seizure. 2008;17:514–23.
104. Hosking PG. Surgery for frontal lobe epilepsy. Seizure. 2003;12:160–6.
105. Williamson PD, Thadani VM, Darcey TM, Spencer DD, Spencer SS, Mattson RH. Occipital lobe epilepsy: clinical characteristics, seizure spread patterns, and results of surgery. Ann Neurol. 1992;31:3–13.
106. Cedzich C, Taniguchi M, Schäfer S, Schramm J. Somatosensory evoked potential phase reversal and direct motor cortex stimulation during surgery in and around the central region. Neurosurgery. 1996;38:962–70.
107. Morris HH III, Lüders H, Hahn JF, et al. Neurophysiological techniques as an aid to surgical treatment of primary brain tumors. Ann Neurol. 1986;19:559–67.
108. Neuloh G, Pechstein U, Cedzich C, Schramm J. Motor evoked potential monitoring with supratentorial surgery. Neurosurgery. 2004;54:1061–72.
109. Lesser RP, Luders H, Klem G, et al. Cortical afterdischarge and functional response thresholds: results of extraoperative testing. Epilepsia. 1984;25:615–21.
110. Ojemann GA, Ojemann J, Lettich E, et al. Cortical language localization in left, dominant hemisphere. J Neurosurg. 1989;71:316–26.
111. Pilcher WH, Ojemann GA. Complications of epilepsy surgery. In: Post KD, Friedman E, McCormick P, editors. Postoperative complications in intracranial neurosurgery. Stuttgart: Thieme; 1993. p. 157–65.
112. Zentner J, Hufnagel A, Pechstein U, Wolf HK, Schramm J. Functional results after resective procedures involving the supplementary motor area. J Neurosurg. 1996a;85:542–9.
113. Rostomily RC, Berger MS, Ojemann GA, Lettich E. Postoperative deficits and functional recovery following removal of tumors involving the dominant hemisphere supplementary motor area. J Neurosurg. 1991;75:62–8.
114. Laplane D, Talairach J, Meininger V, Bancaud J, Orgogozo JM. Clinical consequences of corticectomies involving the supplementary motor area in man. J Neurol Sci. 1977;34:301–14.
115. Freund HJ. Premotor areas in man. Trends Neurosci. 1984;7:481–3.
116. Freund HJ. Premotor area and preparation of movement. Rev. Neurol. 1990;146:543–7.
117. Ibe Y, Tosaka M, Horiguchi K, et al. Resection extent of the supplementary motor area and postoperative neurological deficits in glioma surgery. Br. J Neurosurg. 2016; https://doi.org/10.3109/02688697.2015.1133803.
118. Nakajima R, Kinoshita M, Yahata T, Nakada M. Recovery time from supplementary motor area syndrome: relationship to postoperative day 7 paralysis and damage of the cingulum. J Neurosurg. 2019;8:1–10. https://doi.org/10.3171/2018.10.JNS182391. [Epub ahead of print]
119. Smith JR, Lee MR, King DW, Murro AM, et al. Results of lesional vs. nonlesional frontal lobe epilepsy surgery. Stereotact Funct Neurosurg. 1997;69:202–9.
120. Jeha LE, Najm I, Bingaman W, Dinner D, Widdess-Walsh P, Lüders H. Surgical outcome and prognostic factors of frontal lobe epilepsy surgery. Brain. 2007;130:574–84.
121. Samuel J, Menon RN, Chandran A, et al. Seizure outcome and its predictors after frontal lobe epilepsy surgery. Acta Neurol Scand. 2019;140(4):259–67.
122. Xu C, Zhang G, Wang Y, Li Y. Prognostic factors and longitudinal change in long-term outcome of frontal lobe epilepsy surgery. World Neurosurg. 2018; https://doi.org/10.1016/j.wneu.2018.08.192.
123. Bonini F, McGonigal A, Scavarda D, et al. Predictive factors of surgical outcome in frontal lobe epilepsy explored with stereoelectroencephalography. Neurosurgery. 2019;85:E790. https://doi.org/10.1093/neuros/nyz234.
124. Swartz BE, Gado-Escueta AV, Walsh GO, et al. Surgical outcomes in pure frontal lobe epilepsy and foci that mimic them. Epilepsy Res. 1998;29:97–108.

125. Zaatreh MM, Spencer DD, Thompson JL, et al. Frontal lobe tumoral epilepsy: clinical, neurophysiologic features and predictors of surgical outcome. Epilepsia. 2002;43:727–33.
126. Horsley V. Brain-surgery. Br Med J. 1886;2:670–5.
127. Keen WW. The successful cases of cerebral surgery. Am J Med Sci. 1888;96:452–65.
128. Nancrede CB. Two successful cases of brain surgery. Med News. 1888;53:584–8.
129. Lloyd JH, Deaver JB. A case of focal epilepsy successfully treated by trephining and excision of the motor centres. Am J Med Sci. 1888;96:477–87.
130. Sachs E. The subpial resection of the cortex in the treatment of Jacksonian Epilepsy (Horsley operation) with observations on areas 4 and 6. Brain. 1935;58:492–503.
131. Van Offen M, van Rijen PC, Leijten FS. Central lobe epilepsy surgery—(functional) results and how to evaluate them. Epilepsy Res. 2017;130:37–46.
132. Pondal-Sordo M, Diosy D, Téllez-Zenteno JF, et al. Epilepsy surgery involving the sensory-motor cortex. Brain. 2006;129:3307–14.
133. Kim DW, Lee SK, Yun CH, et al. Parietal lobe epilepsy: the semiology, yield of diagnostic workup, and surgical outcome. Epilepsia. 2004;45:641–9.
134. Sandok EK, Cascino GD. Surgical treatment for perirolandic lesional epilepsy. Epilepsia. 1998;39(Suppl 4):S42–8.
135. Lehman R, Andermann F, Olivier A, et al. Seizures with onset in the sensorimotor face area: clinical patterns and results of surgical treatment in 20 patients. Epilepsia. 1994;35:1117–24.
136. Cukiert A, Buratini JA, Machado E, et al. Seizure's outcome after cortical resections including the face and tongue Rolandic areas in patients with refractory epilepsy and normal. MRI submitted to subdural grids' implantation. Arq Neuropsiquiatr. 2001;59:717–21.
137. Corkin S, Milner B, Rasmussen T. Somatosensory thresholds: contrasting effects of postcentral gyrus and posterior parietal-lobe excisions. Arch Neurol. 1970;23:41–58.
138. Pilcher C, Meacham WR, Holbrook TJ. Partial excision of the motor cortex in treatment of Jacksonian convulsions. Results of forty cases. Arch Surg. 1947;54:633–43.
139. Devinsky O, Romanelli P, Orbach D, Pacia S, Doyle W. Surgical treatment of multifocal epilepsy involving eloquent cortex. Epilepsia. 2003;44:718–23.
140. Cohen-Gadol AA, Britton JW, Collignon FP, Bates LM, Cascino GD, Meyer FB. Nonlesional central lobule seizures: use of awake cortical mapping and subdural grid monitoring for resection of seizure focus. J Neurosurg. 2003;98:1255–62.
141. Blume WT, Whiting SE, Girvin JP. Epilepsy surgery in the posterior cortex. Ann. Neurol. 1991;29:638–45.
142. Binder DK, von Lehe M, Kral T, et al. Surgical treatment of occipital lobe epilepsy. J Neurosurg. 2008a;109(1):57–69.
143. Dalmagro CL, Bianchin MM, Velasco TR, Alexandre V Jr, Walz R, Terra-Bustamante VC, et al. Clinical features of patients with posterior cortex epilepsies and predictors of surgical outcome. Epilepsia. 2005;46:1442–9.
144. Salanova V, Andermann F, Olivier A, Rasmussen T, Quesney LF. Occipital lobe epilepsy: electroclinical manifestations, electrocorticography, cortical stimulation and outcome in 42 patients treated between 1930 and 1991. Surgery of occipital lobe epilepsy. Brain. 1992;115:1655–80.
145. Sveinbjornsdottir S, Duncan JS. Parietal and occipital lobe epilepsy: a review. Epilepsia. 1993;34:493–521.
146. Bidzinski J, Bacia T, Ruzikowski E. The results of the surgical treatment of occipital lobe epilepsy. Acta Neurochir. 1992;114:128–30.
147. Bien CG, Benninger FO, Urbach H, Schramm J, Kurthen M, Elger CE. Localizing value of epileptic visual auras. Brain. 2000;123:244–53.
148. Yu T, Wang Y, Zhang G, et al. Posterior cortex epilepsy: diagnostic considerations and surgical outcome. Seizure. 2009;18:288–92.
149. Yun CH, Lee SK, Lee SY, Kim KK, Jeong SW, Chung CK. Prognostic factors in neocortical epilepsy surgery: multivariate analysis. Epilepsia. 2006;47:574–9.
150. Kuzniecky R. Symptomatic occipital lobe epilepsy. Epilepsia. 1998;39(4 Suppl):S24–31.
151. Liava A, Mai R, Cardinale F, et al. Epilepsy surgery in the posterior part of the brain. Epilepsy Behav. 2016;64:273–82.
152. Aykut-Bingol C, Bronen RA, Kim JH, Spencer DD, Spencer SS. Surgical outcome in occipital lobe epilepsy: implications for pathophysiology. Ann Neurol. 1998;44:60–9.
153. Olivier A, Boling W Jr. Surgery of parietal and occipital lobe epilepsy. Adv Neurol. 2000;84:533–75.
154. Heo W, Kim JS, Chung CK, et al. Relationship between cortical resection and visual function after occipital lobe epilepsy surgery. J Neurosurg. 2017; https://doi.org/10.3171/2017.5.JNS162963.
155. Williamson PD, Boon PA, Thadani VM, et al. Parietal lobe epilepsy: diagnostic considerations and results of surgery. Ann Neurol. 1992a;31:193–201.
156. Salanova V, Andermann F, Rasmussen T, et al. Parietal lobe epilepsy. Clinical manifestations and outcome in 82 patients treated surgically between 1929 and 1988. Brain. 1995;118:607–27.
157. Blume WT, Wiebe S. Occipital lobe epilepsies. Adv Neurol. 2000;84:173–87.
158. Fogarasi A, Boesebeck F, Tuxhorn I, et al. A detailed analysis of symptomatic posterior cortex seizure semi- ology in children younger than seven years. Epilepsia. 2003;44:89–96.
159. Jobst BC, Williamson PD, Thadani VM, et al. Intractable occipital lobe epilepsy: clinical characteristics and surgical treatment. Epilepsia. 2010;51:2334–7.
160. Kun Lee S, Young Lee S, Kim DW, Soo Lee D, Chung CK. Occipital lobe epilepsy: clinical char-

acteristics, surgical outcome, and role of diagnostic modalities. Epilepsia. 2005;46:688–95.
161. Boesebeck F, Schulz R, May T. Lateralizing semiology predicts the seizure outcome after epilepsy surgery in the posterior cortex. Brain. 2002a;125:2320–31.
162. Boesebeck F, Schulz R, May T, Ebner A. Lateralizing semiology predicts the seizure outcome after epilepsy surgery in the posterior cortex. Brain. 2002b;125:2320–31.
163. Liava A, Mai R, Tassi L, et al. Paediatric epilepsy surgery in the posterior cortex: a study of 62 cases. Epileptic Disord. 2014;16:141–64.
164. Jayakar P, Duchowny M, Resnick TJ, et al. Localization of seizure foci: pitfalls and caveats. J Clin Neurophysiol. 1991;8:414–831.
165. Wyler AR, Hermann BP. Surgical treatment of occipital lobe epileptogenic foci. Epilepsia. 1990;31: 638.
166. Kuzniecki R, Gilliam F, Morawetz R, et al. Occipital lobe developmental malformations and epilepsy: clinical spectrum, treatment, and outcome. Epilepsia. 1997;38:175–81.
167. Caicoyaa AG, Macarrona J, Albısua J, Serratosa JM. Tailored resections in occipital lobe epilepsy surgery guided by monitoring with subdural electrodes: characteristics and outcome. Epilepsy Res. 2007;77:1–10.
168. Yang P-F, Jia Y-Z, Lin Q, et al. Intractable occipital lobe epilepsy: clinical characteristics, surgical treatment, and a systematic review of the literature. Acta Neurochir. 2015;157(1):63–75.
169. Asadollahi M, Sperling MR, Rabiei AH, Asadipooya AA. Drug-resistant parietal lobe epilepsy: clinical manifestations and surgery outcome. Epileptic Disord. 2017;19(1):35–9.
170. Daniel RT, Meagher-Villemure K, Farmer J-P. Posterior quadrantic epilepsy surgery: technical variants, surgical anatomy, and case series. Epilepsia. 2007;48(8):1429–37.
171. Harward SC, Chen WC, Rolston JD, et al. Seizure outcomes in occipital lobe and posterior quadrant epilepsy surgery: a systematic review and meta-analysis. Neurosurgery. 2018;82(3):350–8.
172. Davis KL, Murro AM, Park YD, et al. Posterior quadrant epilepsy surgery.: predictors of outcome. Seizure. 2012;21:722–8.
173. Simasathien T, Vadera S, Najm I, et al. Improved outcomes with earlier surgery for intractable frontal lobe epilepsy. Ann Neurol. 2013;73:646–54.
174. Noe K. Long-term outcomes after nonlesional extratemporal lobe epilepsy surgery. JAMA Neurol. 2013;70(8):1003–8. https://doi.org/10.1001/jamaneurol.2013.209.
175. Grivas A, Schramm J, Kral T, von Lehe M, Helmstaedter C, Elger CE, et al. Surgical treatment for refractory temporal lobe epilepsy in the elderly: seizure outcome and neuropsychological sequels compared with a younger cohort. Epilepsia. 2006;47: 1364–72.
176. Janszky J, Janszky I, Schulz R, Hoppe M, Behne F, Pannek HW, et al. Temporal lobe epilepsy with hippocampal sclerosis: predictors for long-term surgical outcome. Brain. 2005;128:395–404.
177. Sun T, Wang F, Cui J. Insular cortex and insular epilepsy. J Neurol Neurosci. 2015; https://doi.org/10.21767/2171-6625.10000.
178. Jobst BC, Gonzalez-Martinez J, Isnard J, et al. The insula and its epilepsies. Am Epil Soc. 2019; https://doi.org/10.1177/1535759718822847.
179. Park YS, Lee YH, Shim KW, Lee YJ, Kim HD, Lee JS, et al. Insular epilepsy surgery under neuronavigation guidance using depth electrode. Childs Nerv Syst. 2009;25:591–7.
180. Chevrier M-C, Bard C, Guilbert F, Nguyen DK. Structural abnormalities in patients with insular/peri-insular epilepsy: spectrum, frequency, and pharmacoresistance. Am J Neuroradiol. 2013; https://doi.org/10.3174/ajnr.A3636.
181. von Lehe M, Wellmer J, Urbach H, et al. Insular lesionectomy for refractory epilepsy: management and outcome. Brain. 2009;132:1048–56.
182. Bamiou DE, Musiek FE, Luxon LM. The insula (island of Reil) and its role in auditory processing. Literature review. Brain Res Brain Res Rev. 2003;42:143–54.
183. Frot M, Mauguiere F. Dual representation of pain in the operculo-insular cortex in humans. Brain. 2003;126:438–50.
184. Krolak-Salmon P, Henaff MA, Isnard J, Tallon-Baudry C, Guenot M, Vighetto A, et al. An attention modulated response to disgust in human ventral anterior insula. Ann Neurol. 2003;53:446–53.
185. Isnard J, Guenot M, Ostrowsky K, Sindou M, Mauguiere F. The role of the insular cortex in temporal lobe epilepsy. Ann Neurol. 2000;48:614–23.
186. Ryvlin P, Minotti L, Demarquay G, Hirsch E, Arzimanoglou A, Hoffman D, et al. Nocturnal hypermotor seizures, suggesting frontal lobe epilepsy, can originate in the insula. Epilepsia. 2006;47:755–65.
187. Isnard J, Guenot M, Sindou M, Mauguiere F. Clinical manifestations of insular lobe seizures: a stereo-electroencephalographic study. Epilepsia. 2004;45:1079–90.
188. Rossetti AO, Mortati KA, Black PM, Bromfield EB. Simple partial seizures with hemisensory phenomena and dysgeusia: an insular pattern. Epilepsia. 2005;46:590–1.
189. Catenoix H, Isnard J, Guenot M, Petit J, Remy C, Mauguiere F. The role of the anterior insular cortex in ictal vomiting: a stereotactic electroencephalography study. Epilepsy Behav. 2008;13:560–3.
190. Britton JW, Ghearing GR, Benarroch EE, et al. The ictal bradycardia syndrome: localization and lateralization. Epilepsia. 2006;47:737–44.
191. Laoprasert P, Ojemann JG, Handler MH. Insular epilepsy surgery. Epilepsia. 2017;58(Suppl. 1):35–45.
192. Wang H, McGonigal A, Zhang K, et al. Semiologic subgroups of insulo-opercular seizures based on connectional architecture atlas. Epilepsia. 2020; https://doi.org/10.1111/epi.16501.

193. Guillaume J, Mazars G. Technique de re'section de l'insula dans les e'pilepsies insulaires. Rev. Neurol (Paris). 1949;81:900–3.
194. Penfield W, Faulk ME Jr. The insula. Further observations on its function. Brain. 1955;78:445–70.
195. Silfvenius H, Gloor P, Rassmussen T. Evaluation of insular ablation in surgical treatment of temporal lobe epilepsy. Epilepsia. 1964;5:307–20.
196. Yasargil MG, von Ammon K, Cavazos E, et al. Tumors of the limbic and paralimbic systems. Acta Neurochir. 1992;118:40–52.
197. Duffau H, Capelle L, Lopes M, Bitar A, Sichez JP, van Effenterre R. Medically intractable epilepsy from insular low-grade gliomas: improvement after an extended lesionectomy. Acta Neurochir. 2002;144:563–72. discussion 572–3
198. Zentner J, Meyer B, Stangl A, Schramm J. Intrinsic tumors of the insula: a prospective surgical study of 30 patients. J Neurosurg. 1996b;85:263–71.
199. Sanai N, Polley MY, Berger MS. Insular glioma resection: assessment of patient morbidity, survival, and tumor progression. J Neurosurg. 2010;112:1–9.
200. Mandonnet E, Capelle L, Duffau H. Extension of paralimbic low grade glioma: toward an anatomical classification based on white matter invasion pattern. J Neurooncol. 2006;78:179–85.
201. Vanaclocha V, Saiz-Sapena N, Garcia-Casasola C. Surgical treatment of insular gliomas. Acta Neurochir (Wien). 1997;139:1126–35.
202. Schaller C, Zentner J. Vasospastic reactions in response to the transsylvian approach. Surg Neurol. 1998;49:170–5.
203. Finet P, Nguyen DK, Bouthillier A. Vascular consequences of operculoinsular corticectomy for refractory epilepsy. J Neurosurg. 2015;122(6):1293–8. https://doi.org/10.3171/2014.10.JNS141246.
204. Yaşargil MG, Krisht AF, Ture U, Al-Mefty O, Yaşargil DC. Microsurgery of insular gliomas part VI: surgical treatment and outcome. Contemp Neurosurg. 2002;24(14):1–8.
205. Wang L, Zhang MZ, Zhao JZ, Meng GL, Han XD. Clinical features and minimally invasive surgery of insular lesions: report of 42 cases. Chinese Med J (Engl). 2004;117:1104–8.
206. Hentschel SJ, Lang FF. Surgical resection of intrinsic insular tumors. Neurosurgery. 2005;57:176–83.
207. Lang FF, Olansen NE, DeMonte F, Gokaslan ZL, Holland EC, Kalhorn C, Sawaya R. Surgical resection of intrinsic insular tumors: complication avoidance. J Neurosurg. 2001;95:638–50.
208. Neuloh G, Pechstein U, Schramm J. Motor tract monitoring during insular glioma surgery. J Neurosurg. 2007;106:582–92.
209. Duffau H. A personal consecutive series of surgically treated 51 cases of insular WHO grade II glioma: advances and limitations. J Neurosurg. 2009;110:696–708.
210. Michaud K, Duffau H. Surgery of insular and paralimbic diffuse low-grade gliomas: technical considerations. J Neurooncol. 2016; https://doi.org/10.1007/s11060-016-2120-2.
211. Ikegaya N, Takahashi A, Kaido T, et al. Surgical strategy to avoid ischemic complications of the pyramidal tract in resective epilepsy surgery of the insula: technical case report. J Neurosurg. 2017; https://doi.org/10.3171/2017.1.JNS161278.
212. Tamura A, Kasai T, Akazawa K, et al. Long insular artery infarction: characteristics of a previously unrecognized entity. Am J Neuroradiol. 2014;35:466–71.
213. Igekaya N, Takahashi A, Kaido T, et al. Surgical strategy to avoid ischemic complications of the pyramidal tract in resective epilepsy surgery of the insula: technical case report. J Neurosurg. 2017; https://doi.org/10.3171/2017.1.JNS161278.
214. Bouthillier A, Nguyen DK. Epilepsy surgeries requiring an operculoinsular cortectomy: operative technique and results. Neurosurgery. 2017; https://doi.org/10.1093/neuros/nyx080.
215. Weil A, Minh N, Jayakar P, et al. Medically resistant pediatric insular opercular/perisylvian epilepsy. Part 2: outcome following resective surgery. J Neurosurg Pediatr. 2016; https://doi.org/10.3171/2016.4.PEDS15618.
216. Chiosa V, Granziera C, Spinelli L, Pollo C, Roulet-Perez E, Groppa S, Seeck M. Successful surgical resection in nonlesional operculo-insular epilepsy without intracranial monitoring. Epileptic Disord. 2013;15:148–57.
217. Dylgjeri S, Taussig D, Chipaux M, Lebas A, Fohlen M, Bulteau C, et al. Insular and insulo-opercular epilepsy in childhood: an SEEG study. Seizure. 2014;23:300–8.
218. Heffez DS. Stereotactic transsylvian, transinsular approach for deep-seated lesions. Surg Neurol. 1997;48:113–24.
219. Levitt MR, Ojemann JG, Kuratani J. Insular epilepsy masquerading as multifocal cortical epilepsy as proven by depth electrode. J Neurosurg Pediatr. 2010;5:365–7.
220. Roper SN, Levesque MF, Sutherling WW, Engel J Jr. Surgical treatment of partial epilepsy arising from the insular cortex. Report of two cases. J Neurosurg. 1993;79:266–9.

# Hemispherical Procedures: Hemispherectomy/ Hemispherotomy

# 8

*Do the difficult things while they are easy and do the great things while they are small. A journey of a thousand miles must begin with a single step.*

*Lao Tse*

## Contents





J. Zentner, *Surgical Treatment of Epilepsies*, https://doi.org/10.1007/978-3-030-48748-5_8

Hemispherectomy was primarily introduced for the treatment of malignant gliomas [1]. Early experience with this procedure showed beneficial effects on seizures [2]. Thus, already from the 1950s on, hemispherectomy has been recognized as a valuable tool for the surgical treatment of a subgroup of epileptic patients who show a diffuse pathology affecting one hemisphere which coincides with infantile hemiplegia [3–6]. Stimulated by excellent epileptological results, hemispherical procedures have been promoted and improved over decades, and even during the last years additional modifications have been introduced, all aiming at the best seizure control with the lowest morbidity. In fact, hemispherical procedures undoubtedly will continue to constitute an integral part of the epilepsy surgical program.

## 8.1 Selection of Surgical Candidates

When selecting candidates for hemispherical procedures, most important aspects are etiology, morphological (MRI) findings, and neurological as well as psychomotor performance, while seizure types and EEG findings are less relevant. Etiology as well as morphological and clinical findings provide important information with respect to the extent of hemispherical damage and to assess the functionality of the intact hemisphere [7]. In the case that the affected hemisphere is no longer functional but only produces seizures, thus negatively influencing the healthy and functional hemisphere, the indication for surgery seems to be clear. However, if partial functions are preserved in the affected hemisphere and additional neurological deficits are to be expected after its removal or disconnection, the decision to proceed with surgery becomes much more difficult [7]. A review on selection of surgical candidates has been given by Villemure et al. [7].

### 8.1.1 Etiology

Hemispherical procedures—hemispherectomy and hemispherotomy—are based on syndromes affecting major parts of the hemisphere. Respective pathologies can be divided into congenital and acquired disorders. Congenital or developmental syndromes may occur at various steps of the developing central nervous system during prenatal course. They include encephalomalacia, migrational disorders, multilobar cortical dysplasia, polymicrogyria, lissencephaly, hemimegalencephaly, and Sturge–Weber disease. Acquired syndromes arise during the perinatal or postnatal phase and can show an apoplectic or progressive course. They include perinatal infarction, hemorrhagic lesions, head trauma, vascular injury, and—most importantly—Rasmussen's encephalitis. Sturge–Weber syndrome and Rasmussen's encephalitis are characterized by progressive hemiparesis, hemispheric atrophy, and mental decline [8–10]. Analyzing 1237 hemispheric surgeries, Fallah et al. [11] found the following etiologies: porencephalic cyst/stroke (35.7%), cortical dysplasia (19.6%), hemimegalencephaly (14.4%), Rasmussen's encephalitis (12.5%), and Sturge–Weber syndrome (4·6%). A mix of other etiologies amounted to 13.2% [11].

MRI findings (Fig. 8.1) depend on the underlying pathology and include gray and white matter anomalies in migrational disorders, calcification in Sturge–Weber disease, and gyri-sulci malformations in hemimegalencephaly. A characteristic MRI feature of candidates for hemispherical procedures is unilateral atrophy which coincides with a smaller cerebral peduncle. The term porencephaly comprises several etiological categories such as stroke, infection, and trauma, all leading to cystic substance defects in an extensively damaged hemisphere [7]. Of particular importance is the question of whether the damage is strictly unilateral or whether both hemispheres are involved. With pathologies involving both hemispheres like diffuse infectious processes, prolonged hypoxia, and head injuries, restraint is called to consider hemispherical procedures [7].

### 8.1.2 Neurological and Psychomotor Status

#### 8.1.2.1 Neurological Status

Assessment of the preoperative neurological status is important to predict postoperative neurological condition. Typical candidates for hemispherical

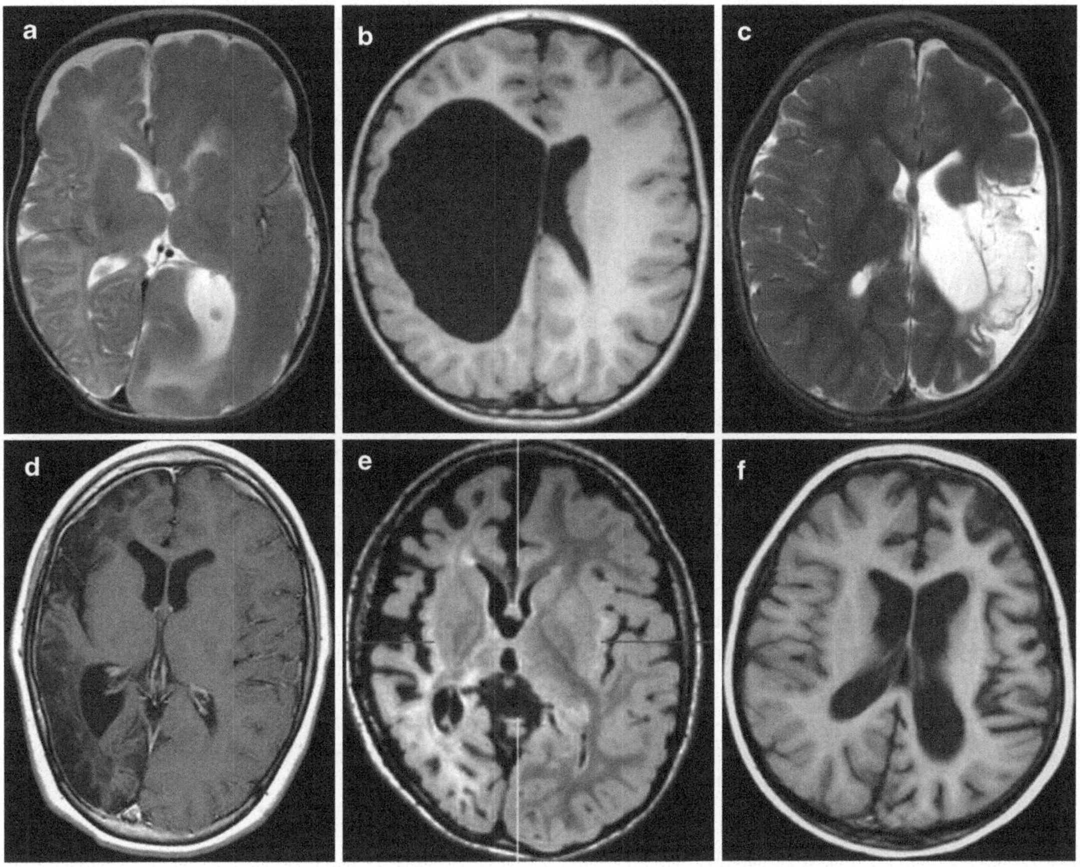


**Fig. 8.1** Hemispherical pathologies on MRI (axial view). (**a**) Hemimegalencephaly (left hemisphere); (**b**) hypoxic/ischemic lesion (right hemisphere); (**c**) perinatal middle cerebral artery infarct (left hemisphere); (**d**) meningoencephalitis (right hemisphere); (**e**) encephalitis of unknown origin (right hemisphere); (**f**) Rasmussen's encephalitis (left hemisphere) (with courtesy of H. Urbach, Dpt. of Neuroradiology, Freiburg)

procedures present with a contralateral spastic hemiparesis, but usually they are able to walk, and the arm is often more impaired than the leg. Frequently, fine motor control (pincer grasp) is absent, but gross motor control (e.g., handgrip) may be preserved. Although deficits may temporarily increase, hemispherical procedures usually do not aggravate such a motor performance in the long term, and patients can be expected to regain their preoperative abilities within a few weeks postoperatively [7]. Patients presenting with rather mild to moderate motor deficits are at risk of neurological deterioration postoperatively. In these cases, Wada testing [12] or—more recently used—DTI studies [13] may be helpful to estimate risks of surgery.

DTI studies have suggested that motor function in patients with hemispheric lesions may not only depend on the integrity of the pyramidal tract but also reflect functionality of alternative motor fibers such as the cortico-rubro-spinal and the cortico-reticulo-spinal pathways [14, 15]. Gaubatz et al. [13] characterized the roles of the pyramidal tract and alternative motor fibers in functional compensation by relating DTI parameters to measures of proximal and distal motor function in patients after hemispherotomy. Anisotropy of the pyramidal tract explained distal motor function, while that of alternative motor fibers originating in the contralateral cortex and crossing to the ipsilateral hemisphere related to the proximal motor function of the upper extremity. Thus, pyramidal tract and alternative motor fibers seem to have complementary roles in compensation of motor function that may be predicted by DTI. It is thought that surgical disconnection of the hemisphere interrupting the inhibitory influences via the transcallosal pathways facilitates neuroplastic reorganization of the intact hemisphere [16] with young age at surgery being a particular stimulus [13].

Postoperative sensory function is preserved or only moderately altered to all modalities in most patients, while stereognosis may be severely impaired. However, the sensory status does not have a significant impact on the decision to perform hemispherical procedures, since surgery leads to little if any change in the sensory system impairing daily life activities. Frequently, candidates for hemispherical procedures present with partial or complete hemianopia, while in some patients visual fields are intact or only minimally impaired. Absence of hemianopia should not prevent from an otherwise clearly indicated hemispherical procedure, since patients easily get used to hemianopia [7].

#### 8.1.2.2 Psychomotor Status

The degree of psychomotor retardation depends on severity and duration of epilepsy, the extent of hemispherical damage, and the social situation of the patient. In addition, the preoperative psychomotor status reflects the functionality of the intact hemisphere, and severe psychomotor retardation may point to bilateral cerebral damage predicting a less favorable outcome. In contrast, early and unilateral pathology usually coincides with the ability of the intact contralateral hemisphere for compensation. However, mental retardation is not considered a contraindication to surgery, and early surgery is thought to provide best chances for a favorable psychomotor development [7, 17].

### 8.1.3 Seizure Types and EEG Findings

Usually, patients exhibit a combination of seizure patterns including generalized seizures, drop attacks, and focal motor epilepsy, while complex partial seizures are rather rare. Over 80% of patients present a focal motor component affecting the contralateral side as their predominant seizure pattern. Most frequently, focal motor seizures are seen in epilepsia partialis continua, which is usually associated with Rasmussen's encephalitis. Seizure frequency varies considerably according to seizure types and underlying pathology, and some patients suffer as many as 200 seizures per day [7].

Electroencephalographic studies mainly demonstrate diffuse, but unilateral epileptic activity. Usually, low amplitude slow activity and multiple independent epileptic foci are observed. In about one half of candidates for hemispherical procedures, epileptic activity can be recorded from the intact hemisphere as well. This activity is either secondary or independent. However, seizure onset as assessed by both clinical and electroencephalographic studies must be restricted to the affected hemisphere. Independent interictal activity in the intact hemisphere does not mean a contraindication for surgery, since this activity may disappear after the hemispherical procedure [7, 18, 19]. Overall, detailed electrophysiological findings in hemispheric damage are not very meaningful. EEG mainly serves for the definition of the seizure onset side and to exclude psychogenic seizures.

## 8.2 Surgical Strategies

### 8.2.1 Goal

The goal of hemispherical procedures is to separate the central core of the hemisphere consisting of the basal ganglia, thalamus, internal, external and extreme capsules, and claustrum from the cortex [20]. The central core is covered by the insula and connects the frontal, temporal, and parietal lobes by the internal capsule and the corona radiata. From a lateral perspective, the superior, inferior, anterior, and posterior limits of the central core correspond to the same limits of the insula, namely its superior, inferior, and anterior limiting sulci [20].

### 8.2.2 Principles

Separation of the central core is achieved by resection and disconnection. Thus, all techniques for hemispherical procedures available follow common principles: disruption of the descending and ascending fibers through the corona radiata and internal capsule, removal of the mesial temporal structures, and callosotomy [21]. Main differences between variants of hemispherical procedures lie in different relationships of resection and disconnection, as well as in the different approaches to the lateral ventricle. Minor differences include the removal or preservation of the insula and the preservation of major vessels [20]. Important landmarks in hemispherical procedures include the tentorium cerebelli, the inferior rim of the falx, the corpus callosum, the pericallosal arteries, and the insula.

## 8.2.3 Techniques

The term hemispherectomy refers to the partial or total resection of the cerebral hemisphere. Hemispherotomy means that the hemisphere is made nonfunctional by disconnection interrupting all afferent and efferent fibers while sparing cortex and white matter. Starting with anatomical hemispherectomy, a variety of hemispherical procedures have evolved and noticeably changed over the decades. While some techniques are exclusively based on resective or disconnective strategies, the two surgical principles of resection and disconnection are combined in the most procedures actually used. Overall, there are three main technical modalities of hemispherical procedures.

### 8.2.3.1 Resective Procedures

Resective procedures include (1) anatomical hemispherectomy, which means complete removal of the hemisphere including white matter, and (2) hemidecortication/hemicorticectomy, which refers to complete removal of the cortex sparing white matter.

### 8.2.3.2 Disconnective Procedures

Disconnective procedures comprise (1) transsylvian hemispherotomy, which means complete disconnection of the hemisphere by the transsylvian-transventricular approach, and (2) vertical hemispherotomy aiming at the disconnection of the hemisphere using a parasagittal vertical approach.

### 8.2.3.3 Combined Resective/Disconnective Procedures

Combined resective/disconnective procedures include (1) Rasmussen's functional hemispherectomy consisting of removal of the temporal lobe and the central area, while the residual frontal and the parieto-occipital lobe are disconnected, and (2) its modifications: (a) hemispherical deafferentation, which means removal of the temporal lobe while disconnecting the rest of the hemisphere, and (b) periinsular hemispherotomy, which consists of removing the frontal and temporal opercula creating access to the ventricular system through which the complete hemisphere is disconnected.

## 8.2.4 Modifications

Modifications exist for all of these three main modalities. Thus, over the decades, the surgical techniques for hemispheric procedures have changed, in order to reduce surgical morbidity, while providing optimal epileptological results.

The following description of different surgical techniques reflects rather continuous development and improvement of procedures stimulated by complications with previous ones than the strict classification into resective and disconnective strategies. Comprehensive reviews on surgical anatomy, functional considerations, and hemispherical techniques have been given by Villemure [7], Schramm [22, 23], Morino et al. [21], Wen et al. [20], De Almeida et al. [24], and Seeger [25]. Uda et al. [26] demonstrated surgical steps of lateral approaches using cadaveric brain, 3-D reconstruction, and simulation models. Figure 8.2 provides a schematic illustration of different hemispherical techniques.

# 8.3 Procedures

## 8.3.1 Anatomical Hemispherectomy

The first anatomical hemispherectomy was done by Walter Dandy in 1923. Between 1923 and 1928, he carried out this procedure in five patients suffering from a diffusely infiltrating malignant glioma of the nondominant hemi-

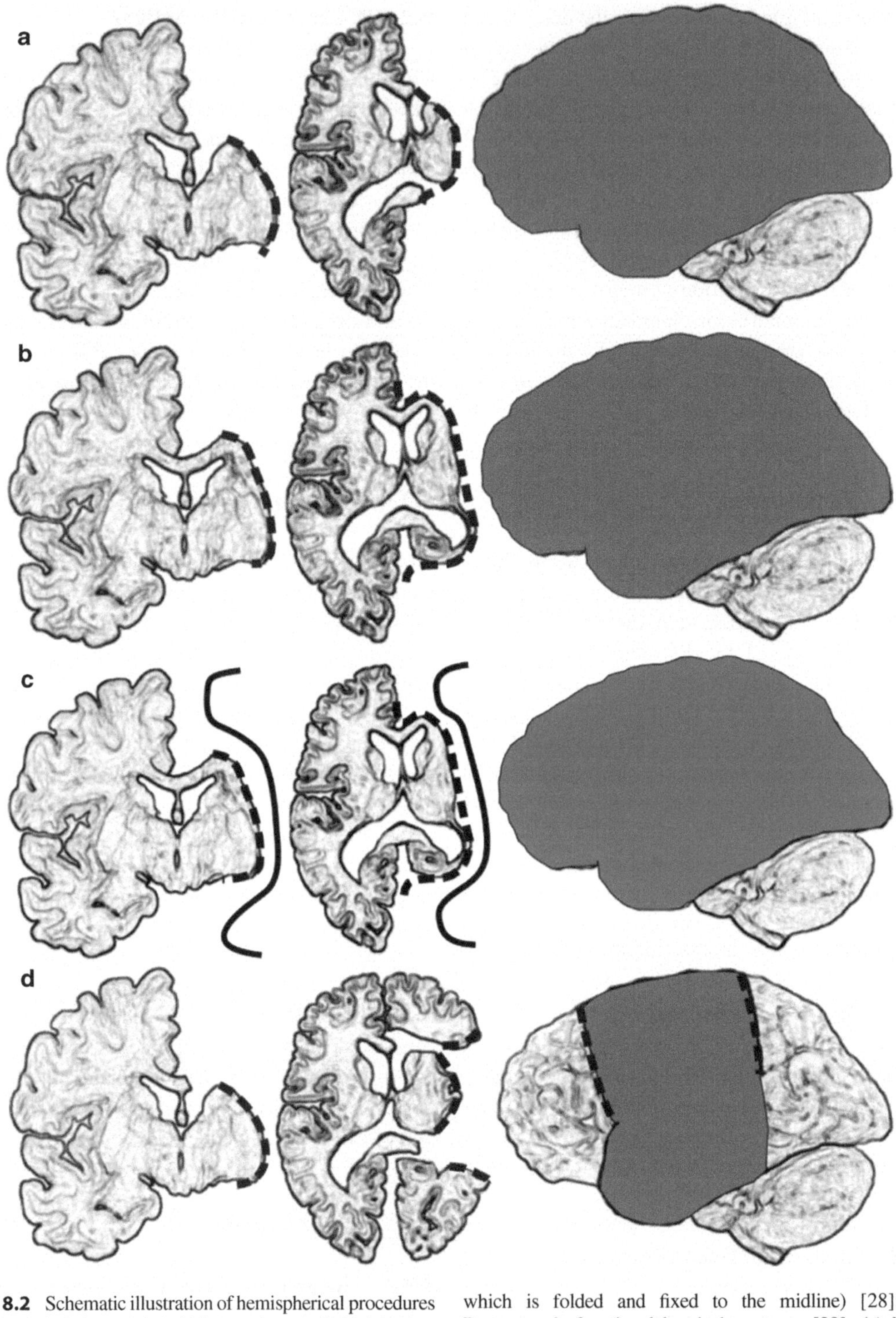


**Fig. 8.2** Schematic illustration of hemispherical procedures in coronal (left), axial (middle), and sagittal (right) view (except for j and k which show the right side in axial view). Dotted line: Resection line; Dark area: Resected area. (**a**) Anatomical hemispherectomy [1, 2], intraventricular approach; (**b**) anatomical hemispherectomy, extraventricular approach [27]; (**c**) Adam's modified hemispherectomy (Oxford modification) (continuous line represents the dura which is folded and fixed to the midline) [28]; (**d**) Rasmussen's functional hemispherectomy [29]; (**e**) hemispherical deafferentation [30]; (**f**) periinsular hemispherotomy [31]; (**g**) Japanese modified periinsular hemispherotomy [32]; (**h**) transsylvian keyhole functional hemispherectomy [33]; (**i**) hemidecortication [34]; (**j**) vertical hemispherotomy [35]; (**k**) modified vertical hemispherotomy [36] (modified from [24], with permission)

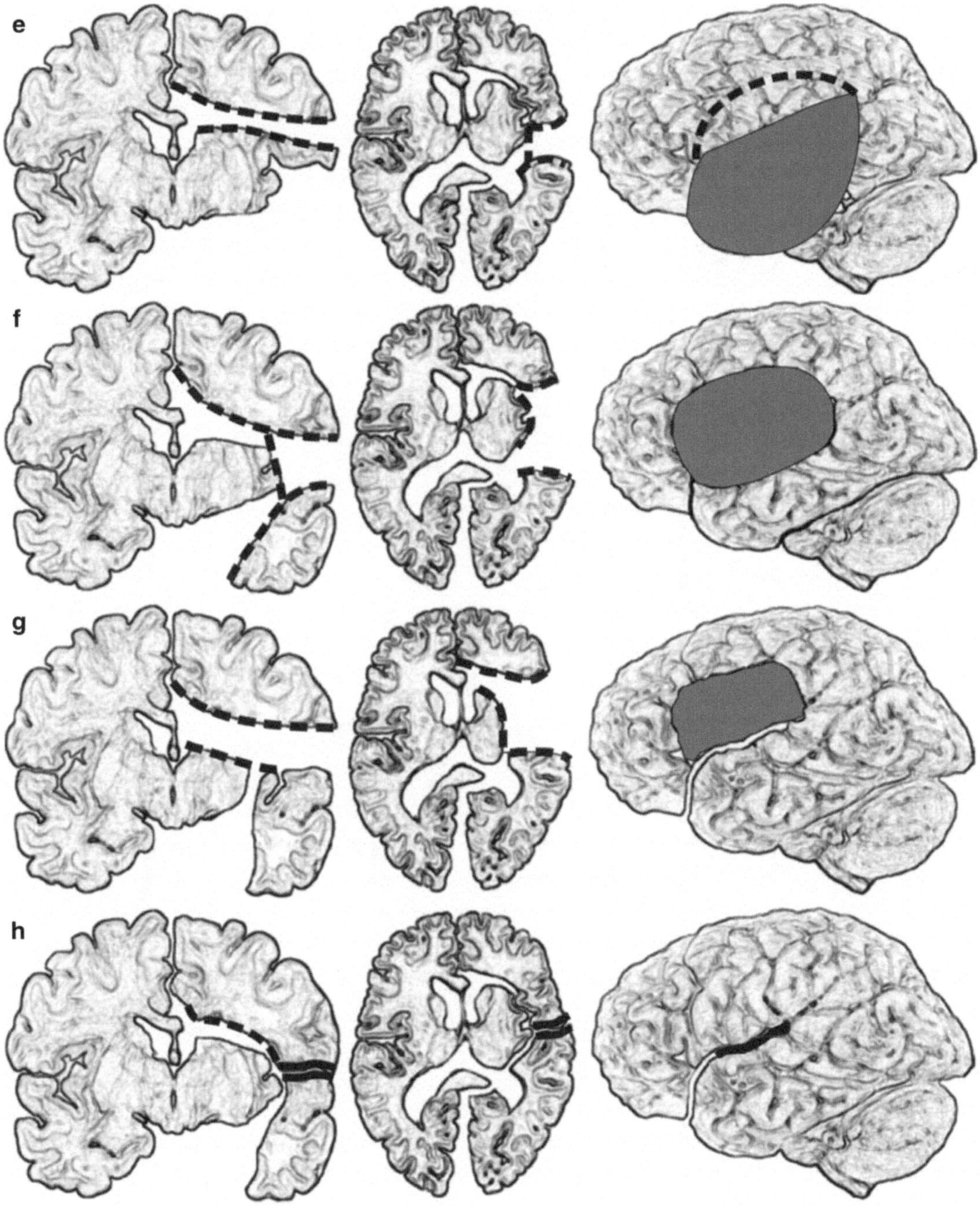


**Fig. 8.2** (continued)

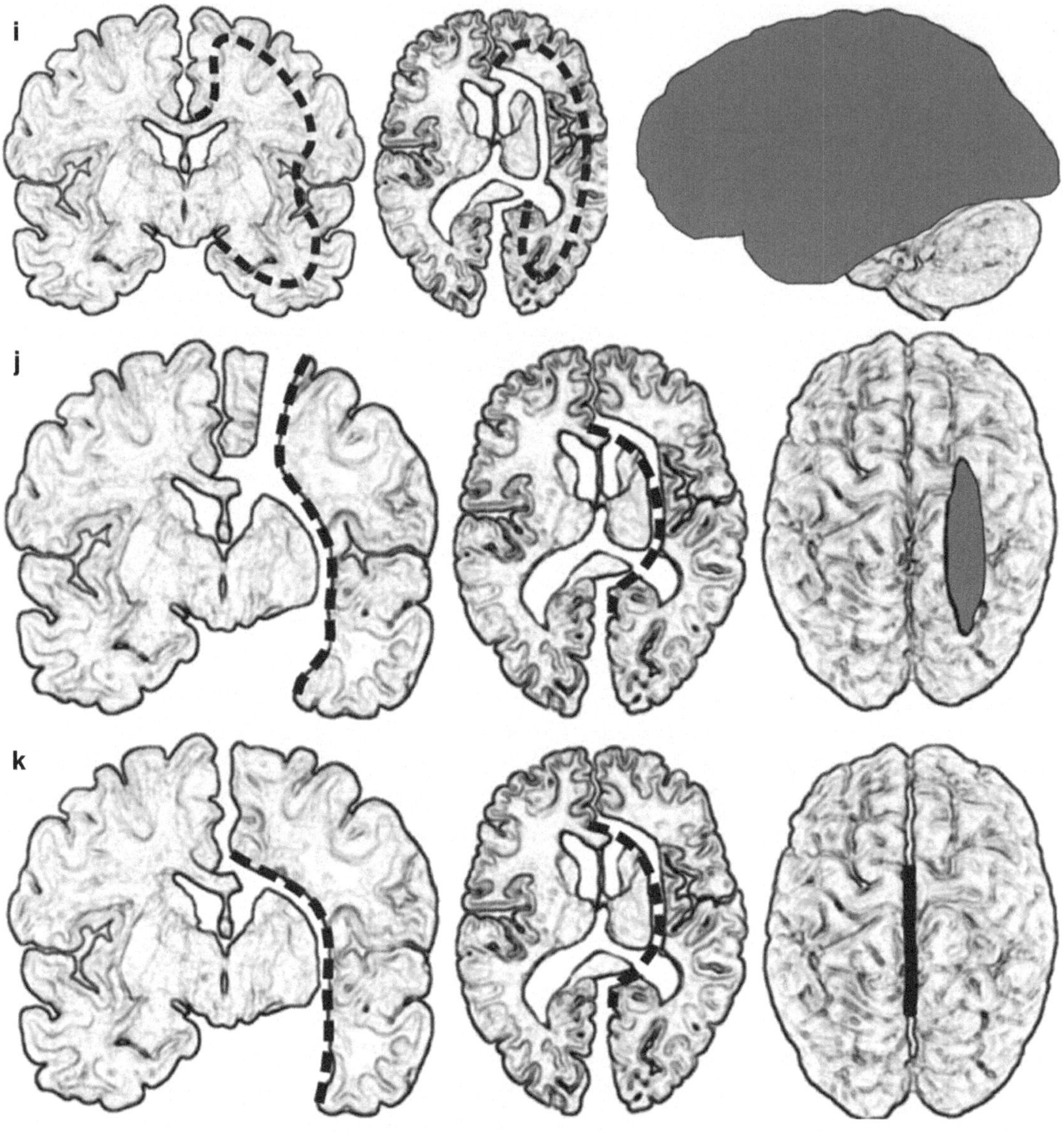


**Fig. 8.2** (continued)

sphere [1]. Anatomical hemispherectomy means complete removal of the hemisphere including gray and white matter, but preserving the thalamus. With this transventricular approach, the ventricles are largely opened. In his original paper, Dandy [1] described the procedure in the following matter:

- The patient is placed in a lateral park bench position. A large T-shaped fronto-occipital skin incision is made along the midline and then from the bregma down towards the temporal base in front of the ear. Large craniotomy reaching almost the midline and the frontal and occipital poles, respectively, is done.
- The anterior and middle cerebral arteries are divided at the carotid bifurcation.
- The parasagittal bridging veins are ligated at the sagittal sinus.
- The frontoparietal area is retracted, and adhesions of the hemisphere to the falx are cut. The interhemispheric fissure is dissected, thus exposing the corpus callosum.

- Frontal lobectomy is performed "requiring only a sweep of the scalpel."
- Connections to the anterior cerebral artery are divided, and "entering the anterior horn of the lateral ventricle with the index finger, to use it as a lever," sectioning of the corpus callosum is completed.
- The hemisphere is separated by transection underneath the insular cortex down to the mesial border of the temporal lobe. The posterior cerebral artery is divided at its P3-segment. Thus, the hemisphere can be removed en bloc.

Hemispherectomy for malignant gliomas has also been done by others [27, 37–42] speculating that removal of the hemisphere might be a curative treatment. However, the postoperative quality of life was very poor and far worse irrespective of the preoperative condition in these patients. More important was the fact that the gliomas were not cured. Thus, hemispherectomy that only prolonged very low quality of life of the patients was discarded for the treatment of malignant gliomas.

Kenneth McKenzie in Toronto did hemispherectomy in 1938 for the first time for the control of intractable epilepsy. His 16-year-old female patient with epilepsy and infantile hemiplegia was seizure free after the procedure [2]. Thus, others continued with this procedure [3–6]. Krynauw [43] reported on 12 children with infantile hemiplegia who underwent anatomical hemispherectomy with excellent seizure outcome. Following Krynauw's report, anatomical hemispherectomy obtained attention, and many reports were published during the next decade, that by 1961 there were already over 260 cases recorded in the literature [44]. Besides seizure relief, noticeable improvement of cognitive functions was observed [45, 46].

#### 8.3.1.1 Modifications

Dandy's original technique was modified using an extraventricular approach sparing basal ganglia. Gardner [27] proposed the preservation of the caudate nucleus, putamen, and globus pallidus, and modified the technique by ligating the anterior and middle cerebral arteries distal to the origin of the Heubner's and lenticulostriate arteries in order to preserve the vascularization of basal ganglia. Gardner assumed that preservation of the basal ganglia may provide better postoperative motor performance compared to Dandy's technique. This issue was addressed again in the 1950s by Laine in France [47] and French in the USA [48], who both performed anatomical hemispherectomy sparing basal ganglia and the caudate nucleus in one group of patients and excising them in the other. Lane and French concluded that the postoperative motor performance in the long-term was identical in both groups, although the initial postoperative performance was better when basal ganglia and the caudate nucleus had been preserved [7]. Similar observations have been reported by others [49–52].

Carson et al. [53] described a method by which the temporal, frontal, parietal, and occipital lobes are taken in sequence and the insular cortex was aspirated, while the ventricles largely remained intact. Similarly, removal of the hemisphere not en bloc but in smaller pieces has been recommended by others [43, 54]. Hoffman et al. [55] suggested to leave temporomesial structures intact if not involved in the epileptogenesis in order to keep the temporal horn closed.

#### 8.3.1.2 Complications

Anatomical hemispherectomy proved to be associated with early and late complications which finally led to a decline in its use despite excellent epileptological results. Early adverse events included severe intraoperative bleeding, the need for large transfusions, hypotension, and intraoperative cardiac arrest [53, 56, 57]. In order to prevent bleeding complications, Taha et al. [58] recommended two-staged surgery, while Schiff and Weinstein [59] advocated the use of preoperative erythropoietin. Another suggestion was to simply use a corpus callosotomy as a replacement for hemispherectomy [60]. In later series of anatomical hemispherectomies, those dramatic intraoperative events have rarely been described [53, 56, 57].

More important were late complications of anatomical hemispherectomy. Oppenheimer and Griffith [61] observed 3 of their 18 patients who a long time after an initially uneventful course continuously worsened and finally died. Autopsy revealed subdural formation of membranes lining the hemispherectomy cavity and the ventricular wall, subpial iron deposits in the brain and spinal cord, granular ependymitis, subependymal gliosis, and consequently hydrocephalus. Similar fatal courses along with the histopathological evidence of late hemorrhagic complications were observed in other series [28, 57, 62–71]. This hemorrhagic complication was eventually called superficial cerebral hemosiderosis [29, 72, 73]. Superficial cerebral hemosiderosis is a late complication that occurs at a median of 8 years following anatomical hemispherectomy (minimum 3–4 years, and up to 20 and more years). This late complication was observed in about 25–35% of patients and lead to death in up to 50% of individuals affected [74]. Rasmussen [72] reported superficial cerebral hemosiderosis in 9 out of 27 anatomical hemispherectomies with a 33% mortality. In fact, not hemosiderosis, but the subsequent hydrocephalus was the cause of death in the old series, since at the time before CT scans were available, hydrocephalus remained unrecognized [75].

It has been supposed that the bleeding complications of anatomical hemispherectomy leading to hemosiderosis and hydrocephalus were due to the large cavity left [72, 76]. Moreover, brain shift to the cavity has been reported which was thought to arise from gravity-induced dislocation [53]. This understanding gave rise to the suggestion to prevent hydrocephalus and dislocation of basal ganglia. In consequence, Di Rocco and Iannelli [64] sutured a band of lyophilized dura mater from the falx to the temporal fossa over the basal ganglia to retain the basal ganglia block in position and to prevent its dislocation as a result of head movement. To prevent hydrocephalus, McKissock [4] coagulated the choroid plexus. However, only Adams' and Rasmussen's modifications of anatomical hemispherectomy were able to abandon hemosiderosis and to significantly reduce the rate of hydrocephalus. In accordance with previous suggestions [72, 76], the common principle of both modifications was to reduce the subdural cavity. Adams [28] achieved this goal by tacking the dura to the midline, and Rasmussen [29] by disconnecting parts of the hemisphere which were left in place.

### 8.3.2 Adams' Modified Hemispherectomy (Oxford Modification)

The procedure completely corresponds to anatomical hemispherectomy. The essential new ideas were to reduce the size of hemispherectomy cavity and to interrupt the communication between the cavity and the ventricular system. These aspects as initially suggested by Wilson [70, 71] have been advocated by Adams [28]. The procedure is accomplished by the following steps:

- Anatomical hemispherectomy preserving basal ganglia is performed.
- At the end of anatomical hemispherectomy, the ipsilateral foramen of Monro is occluded with a muscle plug, eliminating the communication between the lateral ventricle and the hemispherectomy cavity.
- The dura is stripped off the bone and sutured to the falx, tentorium, and the floor of the middle fossa, thus reducing the hemispherectomy cavity and creating a large extradural space.

**Modifications**

In a report of 25 patients, Adams [28] noticed hydrocephalus in only one case. Thus, the rate of hydrocephalus was significantly reduced compared with anatomical hemispherectomy [69, 77]. With the same intention, Dunn et al. [78] used a duraplasty to isolate the hemispherectomy cavity. Other modifications refer to the use of omentum vascularized flaps [79], and the use of a silicone prosthesis to fill the hemispherectomy cavity [80]. Peacock et al. [57] kept an external drainage on a regular basis for a few postoperative days to drain blood products out of the subdural cavity, and inserted routinely a ventriculoperitoneal shunt thereafter.

### 8.3.3 Rasmussen's Functional Hemispherectomy

Rasmussen [72] reviewing the MNI results of anatomical hemispherectomy and multilobectomies found superficial cerebral hemosiderosis in about one-third of hemispherectomies, but none in multilobectomies. He attributed this syndrome to the lack of support of the remaining hemisphere and its consequent vulnerability to minimal repeated trauma or brief physiological increases in intracranial pressure, e.g., by coughing or sneezing, leading to repeated microhemorrhages into the cavity. Rasmussen began to leave epileptogenic brain (one-quarter to one-third) in place and called this procedure "subtotal hemispherectomy." While superficial cerebral hemosiderosis was not observed, seizure outcome was less efficacious, since only 70% of 48 patients became seizure free compared to 85% who underwent complete hemispherectomy [81].

Limited effectiveness of subtotal hemispherectomy led Rasmussen to further revise the operation by disconnecting the remaining part of the hemisphere resulting in a functional complete but anatomical subtotal hemispherectomy [29, 82]. He called this procedure "functional hemispherectomy." Already some years ago, Oppenheimer and Griffith [61] had suggested for the first time reduction of volume of the cavity by disconnection of a part of the hemisphere, but leaving it in place. Thus, functional hemispherectomy consists of a subtotal anatomical removal but complete disconnection of the hemisphere. The main principles of this procedure are as follows:

- As with the anatomical hemispherectomy technique, the patient is positioned in the lateral park-bench position, and the head is slightly tilted downward.
- A Large craniotomy is performed which is somewhat smaller than used for anatomical hemispherectomy.
- Two-thirds anterior temporal lobectomy is accomplished including temporomesial structures.
- The central area including the dorsal frontal lobe and the anterior parts of the parietal lobe is disconnected from the residual frontal and parietal lobes, respectively. Dissection starts at the base of the central area along the frontal and parietal opercula. Care has to be taken to preserve vessels to the frontal and parieto-occipital lobe which remain in place. Raising the disconnected flap, the lateral ventricle is entered. The arachnoidal granulations and veins of the parasagittal area are exposed and dissected from the sagittal sinus. The base of the central area is dissected along the inferior rim of the falx, and callosotomy is completed. Thus, the central area can be removed en bloc.
- The ventricular system is entered at the trigonum, and dissection is continued along the tentorium rim, thus disconnecting the residual parieto-occipital lobe. Care has to be taken to preserve the posterior cerebral artery.
- The residual frontal lobe is disconnected following the pericallosal artery around the genu of the corpus callosum and then downward to the floor of the anterior fossa. Finally, dissection follows the horizontal part of the anterior cerebral artery along the rim of the sphenoid wing continuously disconnecting the frontal lobe until the Sylvian fissure at the carotid cistern are reached.
- In a last step, frontal and temporal opercula are removed. Alternatively, opercula can be disconnected by undercutting.

Rasmussen demonstrated in his series of 54 functional hemispherectomies that seizure-free outcome rates after anatomical and functional hemispherectomies were very similar (83% and 85%, respectively), but the rate of complications from hydrocephalus was reduced from 35% to 7% [29]. Although Rasmussen's technique showed noticeable improvement in terms of hydrocephalus-associated morbidity and mortality, it remained still a large procedure, in particular for young children. One of the crucial points in this context was the resection of the central area, which is rather complex and time consuming. Therefore, further modifications aimed at diminishing parietal resection in order to reduce blood loss and the burden of the procedure for young children.

**Modifications**

Villemure et al. [7] modified Rasmussen's technique of functional hemispherectomy by removing only a narrow strip of the central area allowing to enter the lateral ventricle. The parasagittal tissue is removed, thus exposing the falx and the corpus callosum. Then, callosotomy is performed from within the ventricle anteriorly and posteriorly. Other steps are done according to the original technique [7]. A further modification refers to sparing of the upper central convexity. It has been shown that removal of the inferior central convexity is sufficient to get access to the lateral ventricle. This approach has been named the suprasylvian window technique [7]. It requires only the removal of the frontoparietal operculum to get access to the lateral ventricle through which the disconnection of the suprasylvian portion of the hemisphere is completed [7]. Callosotomy is performed from within the ventricle. Further disconnection can be accomplished according to the original technique [7].

### 8.3.4 Hemispherical Deafferentation

Schramm et al. [30, 75] described a modified Rasmussen's technique. This modification refers to complete preservation of the central area and its disconnection through the lateral ventricle (Figs. 8.3–8.4). Similar strategies have been used at MNI by Villemure and Rasmussen [83] and by Girvin and Baeesa [84]. Main steps are as follows:

- The patient is positioned in the lateral park-bench position, and the vertex is slightly lowered. The skin incision is a typical fronto-temporal question mark.
- Craniotomy is centered over the Sylvian fissure and should extend 3.5–4 cm below and 3.0–3.5 cm above the Sylvian fissure. The bone flap needs to be slightly longer than the corpus callosum.
- Two-thirds anterior temporal lobectomy is performed including amygdalohippocampectomy.
- Starting from the opened temporal horn, a transcortical incision along the outline of the lateral ventricular system in projection to its cortical surface down to the ventricle is per-

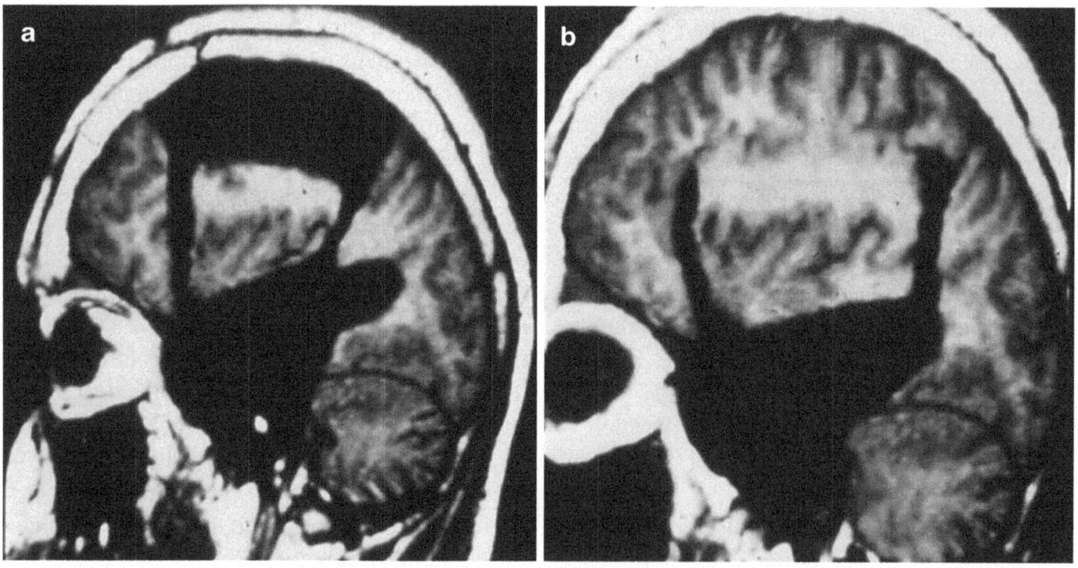


**Fig. 8.3** Differences between Rasmussen's functional hemispherectomy and Schramm's hemispherical deafferentation demonstrated on postoperative MRI scans of two single patients (sagittal view). With Rasmussen's technique (**a**), the temporal lobe and the central area are removed. With Schramm's hemispherical deafferentation (**b**), the central area is anatomically preserved, but disconnected

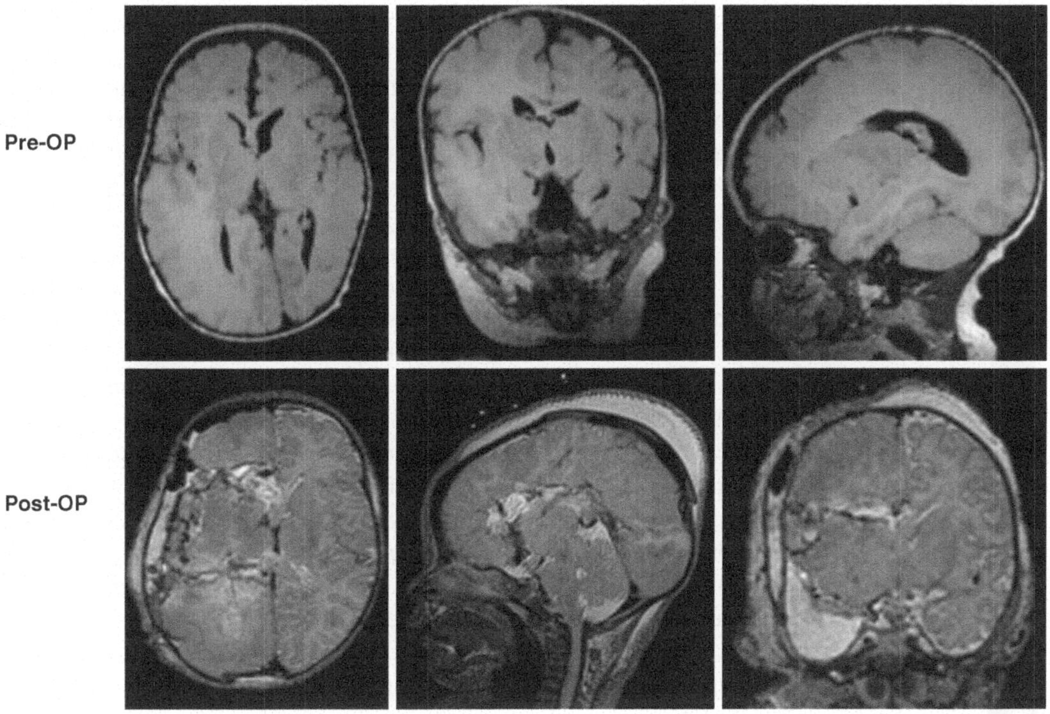


**Fig. 8.4** MRI scans of a 3-month-old child with hemimegalencephaly of the right hemisphere (upper line). Hemispherical deafferentation (modified Rasmussen's technique) has been applied with partial removal of the temporal lobe. The opercula have been undercut, while the proper insula is preserved (lower line). The postoperative course was uneventful

formed in a curve around the end of the Sylvian fissure and then anteriorly to the tip of the frontal horn. Care must be taken to preserve major branches of the middle cerebral artery as well as some of the major superficial veins.

- Dissection is continued through the white matter along the tentorial rim crossing the posterior cerebral artery, until the splenium of the corpus callosum is reached.
- From within the ventricle, posterior callosotomy is accomplished, running along the inferior margin of the falx to the posterior third of the cella media.
- Disconnection of the frontal lobe is performed dissecting from the anterior horn along the course of the anterior cerebral artery around the corpus callosum to the interhemispherical fissure and along the rim of the sphenoid wing.
- Disconnection of the central area and callosotomy are completed continuing dissection posteriorly until it joins the same line of dissection that has been prepared from the posterior aspect of the ventricular system. The arachnoid on the medial aspect of the hemisphere usually is not opened.

**Modifications**

Modifications of this technique refer to the extent of temporal resection. Schramm et al. [30] proposed to remove only the first 4 cm of the superior temporal gyrus instead of an anterior two-thirds temporal lobectomy. The inferior horn is opened and amygdalohippocampectomy is performed. This is followed by the procedure as described above.

During the last two decades, techniques have been developed which are rather based on disconnection than resection. For these techniques, the term hemispherotomy has been created. Hemispherotomy techniques require a small approach and offer the advantages of reduced operation time, reduced blood loss, and avoidance of exposure of large venous sinus [30, 31, 85]. Hemispherotomy benefits from the presence of enlarged ventricles. Currently two main approaches for hemispherotomy exist: the lateral approach advocated by Villemure [31, 83] and Schramm [30], and the vertical approach used by Delalande [85, 86].

### 8.3.5 Periinsular Hemispherotomy

The technique of periinsular hemispherotomy has been first mentioned in 1992 by Schramm [75], followed in 1993 by Villemure and Mascott [87]. In the mid-1990s, the first series of patients treated via the perisylvian approach have been reported [30, 31]. With the previously described technique, periinsular hemispherotomy shares the transventricular mesial disconnection. The key of this operation is the exposure of the lateral ventricle and the inferior horn which is accomplished by excising the operculum and transecting the white matter perpendicularly through the circular sulcus of the insula. From within the ventricle, callosotomy is accomplished, and the frontal lobe is disconnected reaching the edge of the sphenoid wing. Thereafter, the amygdala-hippocampal complex is removed, and the temporal and occipital lobes are disconnected [69]. Major features of the approach are as follows [7, 88]:

- A medium-sized craniotomy with the bone flap centered over the Sylvian fissure, about 3 cm above and below, is performed, thus exposing the frontal and temporal opercula in the whole length of the Sylvian fissure.
- A suprasylvian window is created by resection of the frontal and parietal operculum and underlying white matter, exposing the insular cortex. Major arteries and veins are preserved. An incision is made along the circular sulcus through the white matter, thus interrupting the fibers of the corona radiata and exposing the lateral ventricle from the frontal horn to the trigone.
- A vertical incision through the ependyma and the parasagittal tissue is made until the inferior rim of the falx, the pericallosal arteries, and the callosum are reached. The corpus callosum is identified in its midportion. Once the level of the callosum has been recognized, callosotomy is completed from within the lateral ventricle.
- To complete the suprasylvian step, a coronal section is carried out from the anterior portion of the opercular region, reaching the inferior frontal region at the level of the sphenoid wing. This incision transects the head of the caudate nucleus and reaches the frontal horn as well as the rostral extent of callosotomy, thus disconnecting the frontal lobe.
- An infrasylvian window is created by resection of the first temporal gyrus, and the insular cortex below the Sylvian fissure is exposed. The temporal stem is transected to enter the inferior horn from front to back, reaching posteriorly the suprasylvian window, thus disconnecting the temporal and the occipital lobe. Uncus, amygdala, and hippocampus are removed.
- Finally, the insular cortex is removed by subpial aspiration above and below the Sylvian fissure preserving large vessels. Alternatively, the insular cortex may be undercut.

### 8.3.6 Japanese Modified Periinsular Hemispherotomy

This technique proposed by Shimizu and Maehara [32] constitutes a further modification of Rasmussen's hemispherectomy. It combines elements of the periinsular window technique with subcortical access to the mesial temporal lobe as described by Delalande et al. [85]. Pursuing a wider view to the ventricular system, Shimizu and Maehara advocated a window in the superior part of the insula along with the inferior frontal gyrus. Through this space, the authors coagulate the middle cerebral artery and its branches, remove the mesial structures of the temporal lobe, and disconnect the rest of the hemisphere. They named it "modified periinsular hemispherectomy." The following main steps are included:

- The patient is placed in supine position with the head horizontal. A medium-sized rectangular bone flap is created extending from the tip of the anterior horn to the trigone, and from the middle temporal gyrus to the roof of the corpus callosum.

- The upper half of the insula is exposed by dissecting between the lower margin of the frontal operculum and the Sylvian veins. All ascending insular arteries running over the insular surface are coagulated and divided.
- The frontal and parietal operculum and the upper half of the insular cortex are resected, thus creating a rectangular cavity along the superior margin of the Sylvian fissure. From the opercular cavity, the lateral ventricle is exposed from the anterior horn to the trigone. With this procedure, the transitional zone from the corona radiata to the internal capsule is sectioned.
- The dissection line from the opercular cavity to the trigone is extended to the inferior horn, and the amygdalohippocampal complex is removed.
- The pericallosal cistern is opened, and the pericallosal artery is exposed. Following this artery, callosal section is completed.
- As the last step, the frontal horizontal fibers which are composed of the internal and external sagittal layers running lateral to the anterior horn are sectioned.

Compared with periinsular hemispherotomy as described by Villemure and Mascott [31], the upper half of the insula is resected, and the temporal horn is accessed behind the insula. Thus, the insula is disconnected during access from the frontal opercular cavity to the temporal horn. Moreover, the upper extent of the frontoparietal operculum is determined on the basis of the level of the corpus callosum, which facilitates access from the resection cavity to the ventricle when there is no ventricular dilation. Therefore, this technique can be called a "transopercular hemispherotomy."

**Modifications**

A similar procedure was used by Comair and named "transsylvian functional hemispherectomy" [89]. Also looking for a better exposure, Cook et al. [90] routinely excised the thalamus, basal ganglia, and deeper structures of the hemisphere. Others limited the suprasylvian window and extended the temporal resection [91]. In cases where there is a porencephalic cyst around the middle cerebral artery, Smith et al. [92] suggested removing the gliotic lesion en bloc. Finally, Kanev et al. [93] described a procedure guided by ultrasound, by which the hemisphere is disconnected while preserving the ventricular integrity.

### 8.3.7 Transsylvian Keyhole Hemispherotomy

This approach has been described by Schramm et al. [33] as a refined version of the perisylvian technique (Figs. 8.5–8.7). Key features are:

- The patient is placed in a lateral park-bench position with the head slightly tilted downward. A small bone flap between 4 × 4 cm and 5 × 6 cm is created through a linear slightly anteriorly curved fronto-temporal incision. The anterior border of the trephination which is located approximately 80% above and 20% below the Sylvian fissure should correspond to the limen insulae.
- The Sylvian fissure is opened, and the frontal and temporal opercula are retracted to expose the superior and inferior insular sulcus (circular sulcus). The temporal horn is opened through the anterior limb of the insular sulcus, and the uncus and the amygdalohippocampal complex are removed.
- Following the outline of the circular sulcus and sparing major branches of the middle cerebral artery, the ventricular system is opened around the trigone and the pulvinar thalami to the tip of the frontal horn.
- Disconnection of the frontobasal cortex and white matter is performed along a line drawn from the ascending middle cerebral artery (MCA) through the bulk of lateral frontal lobe to the tip of the frontal horn. The disconnection continues by following the M1 segment and then the anterior cerebral artery (ACA),

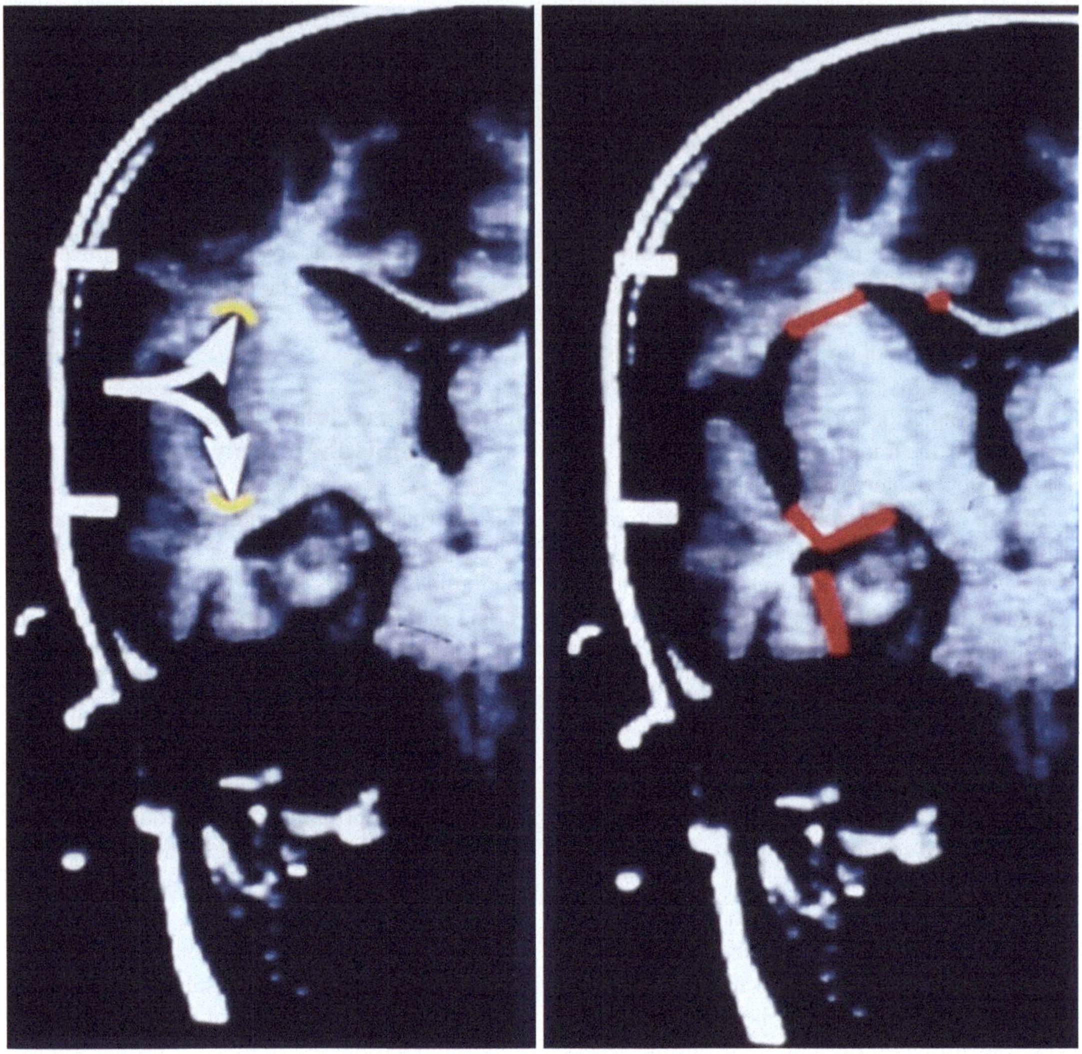

**Fig. 8.5** Schematic illustration of the principles of the transsylvian keyhole hemispherotomy on MRI (coronal view). After exposure of the Sylvian fissure (left), dissection is continued to the inferior horn and then to the lateral ventricle (right), thus the hemisphere can be disconnected from within the ventricles

**Fig. 8.6** Transsylvian keyhole hemispherotomy; left hemisphere (intraoperative view; author's modification of steps are shown, see also "*Concluding remarks*"). (**a**): Dissection of the Sylvian fissure; (**b**): removal of the uncus; (**c**) blunt dissection of the hippocampus (arrow); (**d**) disconnection of the temporo-occipital area dissecting along the tentorial rim (arrow); (**e**): continued occipital disconnection leaving major vessels intact (arrow); (**f**): parietal disconnection and callosotomy as well as disconnection of the frontal lobe following the pericallosal artery (arrow) around the genu of the corpus callosum and then down to and along the sphenoid wing until the Sylvian fissure is reached; (**g**): overview: temporal disconnection is completed (arrow); (**h**): overview: frontoparietal disconnection is completed (arrow pointing to the pericallosal artery)

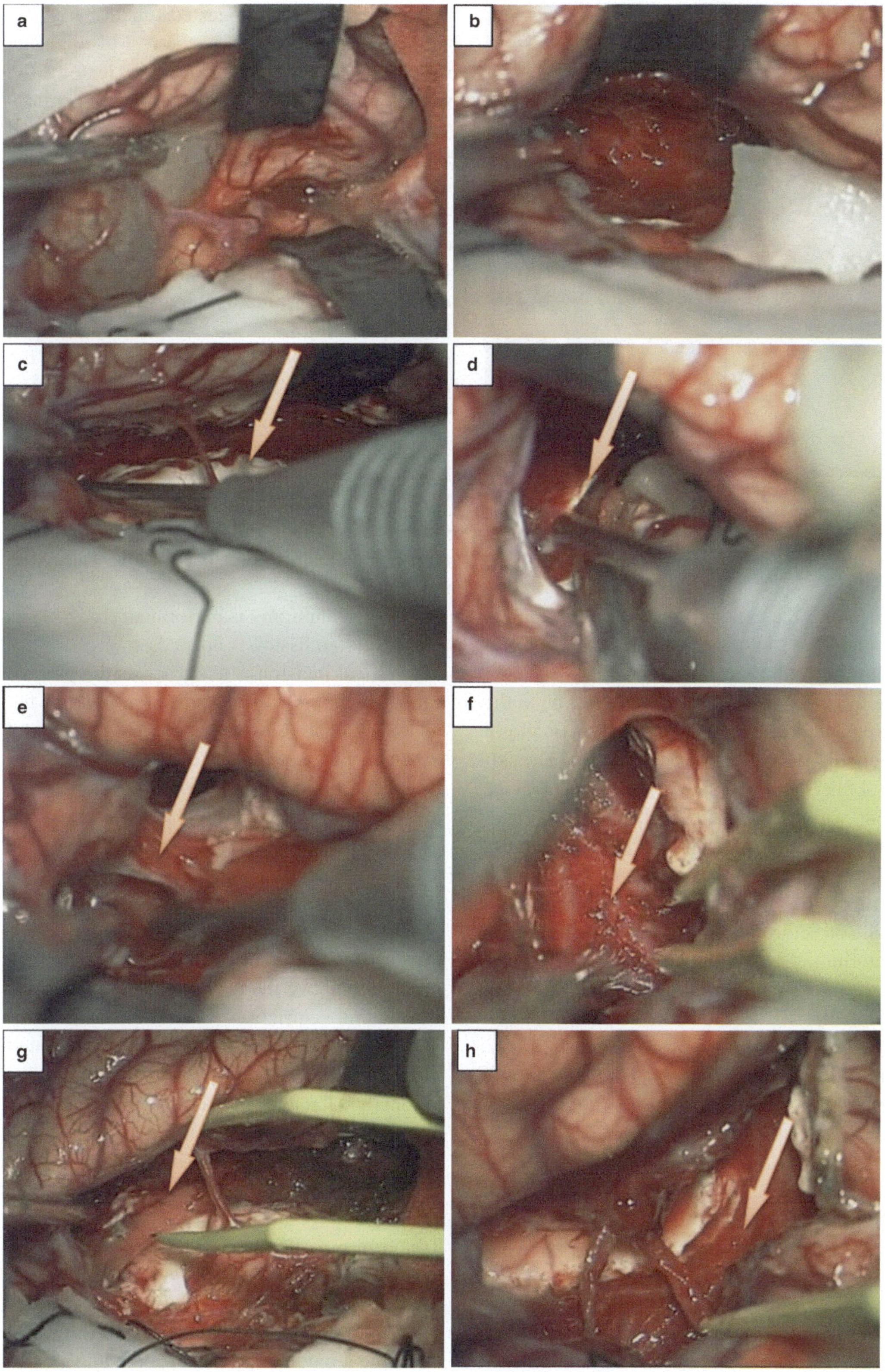
a
b
c
d
e
f
g
h

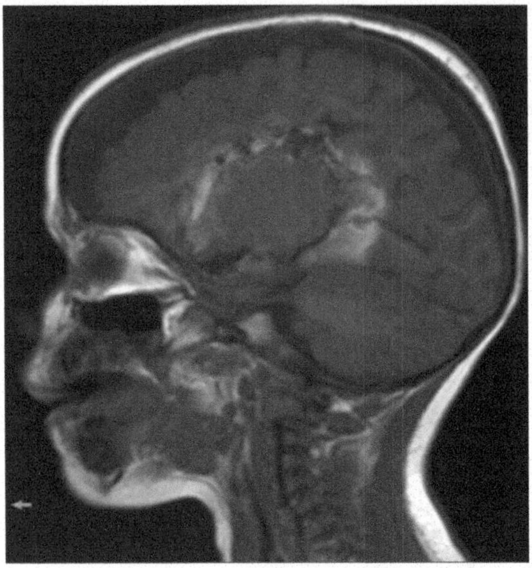

**Fig. 8.7** Transsylvian keyhole approach. Disconnection of the hemisphere is demonstrated on early postoperative MRI (sagittal view)

first along the A1 and later the A2 segment around the anterior knee of the corpus callosum.

- Medial disconnection is continued around the corpus callosum following the pericallosal artery disconnecting the parietal lobe. The callosal fibers are sectioned in a paramesial plane from within the ventricle back to the splenium. As the pericallosal artery becomes smaller and runs upward to supply its cortical territory, the inferior rim of the falx serves as a guide structure and turns into the rim of the tentorium.
- Posterior disconnection follows the anterior falcotentorial rim. The calcar avis is crossed sparing the posterior cerebral artery. Dissection is continued crossing the hippocampal tail, until the temporomesial resection cavity is reached.

### 8.3.8 Hemidecortication/Hemicorticectomy

The procedure is based on the principle that only the ictogenic cortex needs to be removed sparing white matter, thus avoiding a large cavity. Laine et al. [68] suggested functionally disconnecting the cortex from the rest of the brain by a series of stereotactic lesions, leaving the brain in place. The proper procedure of hemidecortication has been described by Ignelzi and Bucy in 1968 [34] as an alternative to anatomical hemispherectomy. With this procedure, the entire cortex of one hemisphere is removed in a piecemeal dissection, while leaving a layer of white matter surrounding ventricular ependyma intact except for some openings, particularly in the temporal horn.

Winston et al. [52] reported on a variant of the hemidecortication technique that they termed "hemicorticectomy." In this technique, the principles of hemidecortication are respected, but the cortex is removed in slabs of tissue rather than piecemeal. The procedure is best conceptualized as a "degloving" dissection around the lateral ventricle. It consists of the following main steps:

- A large craniotomy is performed.
- The Sylvian fissure is opened.
- A vertical incision is made across the parietal lobe, beginning in the posterior Sylvian fissure and continuing upward across the parietal lobe to the vertex. Subsequently, a plane of dissection is developed from the edges of the insula below the cortex and around the ventricles to the falx above the corpus callosum.
- A fanlike incision is made into the frontal opercular cortex and the underlying white matter. This incision undermines the cortex anteriorly and superiorly and is extended medially above the body and anterior horn of the lateral ventricle.
- Bridging veins along the vertex are coagulated and divided. The hemisphere is retracted away from the falx, and the pia of the medial surface is entered. This incision is extended laterally into the white matter to meet the fanlike incision as mentioned in the previous step. The anterior cerebral artery is interrupted. Thus, the fronto-parietal cortex except for the cortex in the posterior inferior part of the frontal region is disconnected and removed.
- A plane of dissection is developed inferiorly into the temporal operculum and white matter,

and around the inferior horn facilitating removal of the temporal cortex.
- Dissection is continued around the occipital horn allowing removal of the remaining parietal and occipital cortex. Remaining portions of mesial occipital area and above the corpus callosum are removed in a piecemeal fashion.

With this technique, the lateral ventricle remains largely closed. However, removal of the hippocampus makes opening of the temporal horn unavoidable. This approach requires a large exposure similar to that necessary for anatomical hemispherectomy. Moreover, resorption of cerebrospinal fluid through the granulations at the midline is blocked. In cases of hemimegalencephaly, where dysplastic epileptogenic tissue may be located deeper inside the white matter, orientation can be difficult. In addition, hemimegalencephaly requires extensive dissection, which may induce the same intraoperative problems as seen with anatomical hemispherectomy [56, 57, 67]. Moreover, there is a certain risk of incomplete deafferentation in these cases [22, 67].

### 8.3.9 Vertical Hemispherotomy

The term hemispherotomy was created by Delalande et al. [85] who described in an abstract a functional hemispherectomy through a small vertex approach. Once the lateral ventricle is entered, the parasagittal callosotomy is accomplished, and the hemisphere is disconnected by an incision through the basal ganglia, from the trigone reaching the medial frontal region. Later, this procedure has been described in more detail [35]. It includes the following features:

- The patient is placed in supine with the head in neutral position, but slightly elevated in the horizontal plane. A small parasagittal craniotomy (approximately 3 × 5 cm, 1–2 cm from the midline, one-third anterior and two-thirds posterior to the coronal suture) is performed.
- A high parietal corticectomy of about 3 × 2 cm is performed. The mesial border is about 2 cm from the sagittal sinus. Major bridging veins should be preserved. The resection extends down to the roof of the lateral ventricle, which is entered by a parasagittal opening through the parenchyma, avoiding manipulation of the anterior cerebral artery and its branches.
- Following the roof of the lateral ventricle mesially, the corpus callosum is identified. The callosal section is first performed posteriorly towards the splenium. Resection of the splenium is continued until the roof of the third ventricle and the arachnoid of the cisterna ambiens are exposed.
- The hippocampal commissure curving downward is cut behind the pulvinar thalami, and the white matter is dissected around the trigone. Incision through the corona radiata lateral to the thalamus is performed using the posterior part of the choroid plexus of the temporal horn as a guide. This incision is performed strictly vertically and extends from the trigone to the most anterior part of the temporal horn while unroofing the temporal horn entirely. Dissection has to remain within the white matter as laterally as possible to avoid damage to the lateral aspect of the thalamus.
- Completion of callosotomy is achieved anteriorly, resecting the genu until just above the anterior commissure. As for the posterior part of the corpus callosum, the section is performed intracallosally to the interhemispheric cistern.
- The most posterior part of the gyrus rectus is resected allowing visualization of the first segment of the anterior cerebral artery, and providing space for the next step.
- Starting from the anterior end of the opened roof of the inferior horn, a straight incision oriented anterolaterally through the caudate nucleus towards the exposure in the prechiasmatic gyrus rectus is performed. This last dissection will cut all the connections from the anterior temporal lobe, the amygdala, and the frontal lobe, and thus the hemispherotomy is complete.

Using a similar technique, Danielpour et al. [36] reached the lateral ventricle through an interhemispheric approach and then disconnected the hemisphere. A new variant of disconnective vertical hemispherotomy termed vertical extraventricular parasagittal hemispherotomy has been described by Giordano et al. [94]. This procedure aims to further reduce the rate of postoperative hydrocephalus

### 8.3.10 Endoscopic Hemispherotomy

Chandra and Tripathi [95] described a novel technique of hemispherical disconnection using an interhemispheric transcallosal approach. This technique is based on cadaveric studies by Bahuleyan et al. [96], and they named it "interhemispheric endoscope-assisted hemispherotomy." It combines the standard vertical hemispherotomy approach with endoscopic technique. The procedure includes the following main steps:

- The patient is placed in the supine with the head slightly flexed in neutral position. A transverse skin incision is made on the coronal suture, and a 4 × 3 cm bone flap is created with the mesial border just over the lateral part of the sagittal sinus.
- After microsurgical dissection of the mesial aspect of the hemisphere and exposure of the callosum, the endoscope is placed in, and endoscope-assisted dissection is continued beginning with corpus callosotomy.
- Anterior disconnection starts at the genu of the corpus callosum and passes down to the anterior skull base at the level of the sphenoid wing, thus disconnecting the frontal lobe. At this stage, the anterior cerebral artery is visualized.
- Middle disconnection starts from the sphenoid ridge and divides the hemisphere lateral to the thalamus and the choroidal fissure, until the atrium is reached. Dissection is completed disconnecting the anterior temporal lobe including the amygdalohippocampal complex.
- Posterior disconnection includes division of limbic structures around the plexus of the atrium and the posterior temporal and occipital lobes.

Similar to the approach proposed by Danielpour et al. [36], endoscope-assisted interhemispheric transcallosal hemispherotomy provides a "cisternal to ventricular" access unlike the "parenchymal to ventricular" access of Delalande's technique [85]. In his 2018 report on 32 patients, Chandra et al. used a robotic device both as a holder for the endoscope and as a neuronavigation system. Based on a 10 mm thick and 310 mm long endoscope, they described a hybrid technique facilitating both visualization of the target and dissection with the working instruments being far distal to the telescopic lens [97]. Comparing endoscope-assisted hemispherotomy with conventional (interhemispheric and periinsular) approaches, Chandra et al. [97] found the endoscopic technique as affective as the other procedures with similar seizure and behavioral outcomes. Mean operation time was 302 min with the endoscopic technique and 351 min with other procedures, while mean blood loss was significantly reduced with the endoscopic approach (210 ml versus 720 ml) as was the mean postoperative hospital stay (15 days versus 19 days).

## 8.4 Special Surgical Aspects

### 8.4.1 Insular Cortex

Whether the removal of the insular cortex is necessary for complete seizure relief is open for discussion. In Holhausen's series of 323 patients from 13 centers, the outcome was not worse if the insular cortex had not been removed [8]. Villemure et al. [98, 99] reviewed 55 cases of hemispherectomies (functional and anatomical) in which 27 patients had the insular cortex excised, while 28 had the insula preserved. There were more seizure-free patients in the group where the insula was preserved, suggesting that the removal of the insular cortex seems not to be essential for an excellent seizure outcome. Contrarily, Cats et al. [100] found that the preservation of the insular cortex was associated with a lower rate of seizure freedom in 28 patients. This is in line with others reporting individual cases of persisting seizures arising from the insula [98, 99, 101]. Overall, the value of insular resection is unproved [52, 102].

### 8.4.2 Which Approach Should Be Preferred?

Development of different techniques for hemispherical procedures has been stimulated by the intention to provide patients with the best seizure outcome, while lowering the risks involved with the procedure. Variations of techniques mainly refer to the approach (lateral versus vertical), and proportions of the two main principles of hemispherical procedures, resection and disconnection, and thus the extent of exposure necessary which depends on the proportion of resection. In fact, there is a clear trend towards less resection in favor of disconnection [30, 31, 36, 103–105]. Variations described may influence duration of operation, blood loss, and rate of infection. Choosing the most appropriate approach for the individual patient, the underlying pathology coinciding with different volumes of the affected hemisphere as well as the age of patients have to be taken into account. This is particularly true, since hemimegalencephaly in a small baby poses quite different challenges to the surgical and the anesthesiological team than hemiatrophy in older children or adolescents [22, 88].

#### 8.4.2.1 Resective Procedures

For anatomical hemispherectomy as well as for hemidecortication/hemicorticectomy, a wide access to the whole extent of the hemisphere is necessary requiring a large exposure. Although more actual series of anatomical hemispherectomy rarely describe dramatic intraoperative events due to extensive blood loss [53, 56, 57], the mortality is still around 4–6%. Infection rate is higher compared to modified procedures, possibly as a result of the large bone flap sizes and long operation times. Moreover, anatomical hemispherectomy frequently requires a shunt [28, 57, 62, 64, 67, 69].

Essential weaknesses of hemidecortication/hemicorticectomy include the large exposure, removal of granulations in the midline, thus limiting resorption of cerebrospinal fluid, and extensive dissection with limited orientation in cases of hemimegalencephaly. On the other hand, hemidecortication sparing the white matter may be difficult in the presence of a noticeable atrophy, too [31].

Overall, both anatomical hemispherectomy and hemidecortication/hemicorticectomy representing pure resective techniques have been largely abandoned. Most recent approaches refer to pure disconnective procedures and to combined resective/disconnective strategies. Sood et al. [106], however, re-advocated anatomical hemispherectomy to minimize seizure recurrence due to incomplete disconnection following hemispherotomy. Reporting 77 procedures, mortality was 1.3% and serious morbidity 3.8%. Shunting was required in 21% of patients without previous surgery but in 50% with previous surgery (invasive monitoring or resection) [106].

#### 8.4.2.2 Disconnective Procedures

Pure disconnective procedures have proven to further reduce extent of exposure, operative time, blood loss, as well as the rate of hydrocephalus. The transsylvian-transventricular keyhole approach [22, 30] seems to be ideal for atrophic hemispheres with enlarged ventricles, especially for cases with perinatal infarction, encephalomalacia, and large porencephalic cysts [22, 32, 67, 90]. However, it is not recommended in hemimegalencephaly. Although vertical hemispherotomy has proven to be best suitable for atrophic hemispheres, this approach can also be applied in cases of hemimegalencephaly [7, 85]. The place of endoscopic hemispherotomy among disconnective techniques remains to be awaited.

#### 8.4.2.3 Combined Resective/ Disconnective Procedures

Combining the principles of resection and disconnection, Rasmussen's technique represented great progress to reduce surgical morbidity compared to pure resective procedures, and modified Rasmussen's approaches sparing the central area constitute further major achievements with respect to surgical feasibility. Comparing the size of craniotomy, duration of surgery, and blood loss, some advantageous effects of these modifications are apparent, as, for example, in small children for whom the positive effects of a shorter operation time and less blood loss certainly add up to a less stressful situation [22]. In fact, all modified Rasmussen's approaches combining elements of resection and disconnection including hemispherical deafferentation, periinsular hemispherotomy, and its Japanese modification can be used for cases with normal as well as enlarged hemispheres and hemimegalencephaly.

## 8.4.3 Postoperative Care

### 8.4.3.1 Postoperative Course

Postoperatively, patients are observed in the intensive care unit. The classic parameters are monitored, including wakefulness, motor reaction, pupillary function, and verbal response. Especially in young children, coagulation parameters must be controlled, and some blood replacement may be necessary. Early postoperative MRI (within 72 h) in which the blood-tinged Surgicel[R] outlines the disconnection line may prove complete disconnection [22]. Typically, patients run a mild to moderate increase of temperature for 7–12 days due to contamination of the cerebrospinal fluid (CSF) with detritus and blood. Therefore, it is advisable to place an external drain into the resection cave to avoid repeated lumbar puncture. This is especially important in young children for whom lumbar puncture is stressful and time consuming. The external drain should be kept at normal level (about 10 cm above the lateral ventricle), and drainage should be continued until CSF is clear, usually for 1 week. Thereafter, the external drain is removed.

### 8.4.3.2 Persistent Seizures

In case of persistent seizures, it has to be clarified whether seizures originate from the operated hemisphere or from the contralateral side. Incomplete disconnection is the main reason for persistent seizures, and has been described for all types of surgery [7–9, 32, 64, 107–110]. Persistent seizures due to incomplete disconnection have been found for Rasmussen's functional hemispherectomy in 19% [111] and 21% [57], with the perisylvian hemispherotomy technique in 8.1% [112], using different techniques in 17% [113], and for hemidecortication/hemicorticectomy in 4.5% [8, 9] of the procedures. Persistent seizures may also arise from the opercula or the insula if left in place. So far disconnection is considered to be incomplete or seizures are thought to come from residual epileptogenic tissue according to MRI, reoperation may be indicated. Di Rocco and Iannelli [64] described second surgeries in 8 of 15 hemimegalencephaly patients. Another reason for persistent seizures may be dysplastic features and/or electroencephalographic abnormalities in the intact hemisphere [7, 57, 110].

## 8.4.4 Timing of Surgery

Timing of surgery depends to a great extent on the severity of the epilepsy, the efficacy of therapeutic trials with anticonvulsant medication, and particularly on the natural history of the disease. Although some recommendations can be given, each clinical situation should be individualized.

### 8.4.4.1 Infancy and Early childhood

Before the age of 5, the two hemispheres appear to be largely equipotential for language, and children will acquire this function with either hemisphere alone, provided that this remaining hemisphere is intact. Therefore, with respect to the plasticity of the developing brain, it is advisable in hemispheric epilepsy syndromes that are progressive and in whom the natural course of disease can be expected to lead to maximum deficits within a few years (e.g., Rasmussen's encephalitis or Sturge–Weber syndrome) to consider hemispherectomy/hemispherotomy at an early stage accepting neurological deterioration, which anyway is temporary with respect to the progressive nature of the underlying disease in order to seize the chance for an improved psychosocial development with seizure control [7, 105, 114]. Hemispherical procedures, especially for hemimegalencephaly, should preferably be performed after the age of 5–6 months. In certain conditions, e.g., catastrophic infantile epilepsy, very early surgery even at 3–4 months of age depending on the body weight may be considered [115–117].

#### 8.4.4.2 Later Childhood and Adolescence

In cases with later onset of epilepsy, timing of surgery is controversial. By the age of more than 5 years, hemispherical dominance evolves, such that injury to the respective hemisphere inevitably will produce persisting deficits [118]. Complete postoperative transfer of language and motor function to the healthy hemisphere cannot be expected in these children. The motor status to be expected postoperatively, however, may be predicted by DTI [13]. Nevertheless, surgery may be required due to neuropsychological deterioration caused by intractable epilepsy. This is particularly true, since seizures themselves as opposed to the pathologic substrate may significantly delay cognitive development [119]. Overall, the sooner drug-resistant seizures are abolished by surgery, the more favorable the cognitive developmental outcome, including the outcome for speech and language [118].

#### 8.4.4.3 Adult Age

While young children can better compensate potential new deficits, some concern has been voiced about risking new deficits in adults [120, 121]. Only sparse data with few patients addressing hemispherical procedures in adults are available [122–127]. While some authors report excellent results with more than 75% seizure-free patients and improvement of quality of life [126, 128, 129], others found seizure control in only 55% after 2 years and 38% in the long-term follow-up [121].

In a meta-analysis comprising 90 cases of adult hemispherectomy, Schusse et al. [130] found seizure-free outcome in 80% at a follow-up ranging from 9 to 456 months. No patient lost ambulatory or significant functional abilities, and two patients had objective ambulatory improvement. Among the 41 patients who underwent postoperative neuropsychological testing, overall stability or improvement was seen [130]. McGovern et al. [126] noted that postoperative ambulatory status and hand function were unchanged in most cases. Patients who could walk unaided preoperatively and had no cerebral peduncle atrophy on MRI were more likely to experience worsening of motor function postoperatively. Of the 19 patients who completed neuropsychological testing, 17 demonstrated stable or improved postoperative outcomes [126]. Similarly, others reported that despite possible motor deterioration and hemianopia, quality of life had improved in nearly all cases after surgery [128, 129].

Althausen et al. [122] analyzed the epileptological, cognitive-behavioral, and psychosocial long-term outcome in 61 hemispherectomies performed at early age (<7 years), intermediate age (7–16 years), and late age (>16 years). Although younger patients showed a minimally better seizure outcome (90% seizure-free patients versus 74% in the total group), high-functioning older patients have proven to be excellent candidates. It has been concluded that the overall cognitive and psychosocial long-term outcome is mainly determined by the presurgical intelligence and cognitive status representing an indicator of the functional integrity of the contralateral hemisphere [122]. In fact, the data available show that favorable seizure and cognitive outcome can be achieved in older patients with moderate risks. Therefore, the adult age should not be considered to be an argument against hemispherical procedures [122, 130, 131].

### 8.4.5 Special Considerations in Infancy and Childhood

#### 8.4.5.1 Physiological Profile

Procedures in the pediatric age require special precautions related to physiological profile of children because of the differences in body fat, body surface-to-body volume ratio, metabolism, and, most importantly, blood volume. Since the first report by King et al. [132], hemimegalencephaly increasingly has become an indication for surgery in early childhood. Besides the large volume, hamartomatous structures around the ventricle and ectopic gray matter can make orientation difficult. The midline and sagittal sinus may be displaced to the intact side. Higher blood loss may result not only from the larger volume but also from increased vascularization in hemimegalencephaly [64, 133, 134].

#### 8.4.5.2 Surgical/Anesthesiological Team

In the few reports on neuroanesthesia for children with hemimegalencephaly, dangerous situations have been mentioned, including episodes of severe hypotension, hemodynamic instability, metabolic acidosis, hypothermia, and even episodes of cardiac arrest [53, 56, 67, 110, 135]. Special care needs to be taken to prevent hypothermia, to start blood replacement early, and to correct disturbed serum parameters quickly [56, 135]. It cannot be overemphasized that close collaboration and communication between the surgical and the anesthesiological team is necessary to successfully manage the problems involved with hemispherical procedures in infancy.

#### 8.4.5.3 Surgical Approach

It should be emphasized that minimalistic procedures such as transsylvian hemispherotomy cannot be recommended for young children with enlarged hemisphere volumes and small ventricles or hemimegalencephaly. Besides technical and anesthesiological challenges, the large volume predisposes to postoperative swelling in the absence of reserve space. In these cases, it is strongly recommended to create more space, e.g., by performing temporal lobectomy or a larger perisylvian window. Alternatively, the vertical approach (vertical hemispherotomy) may be used [133].

## 8.5 Seizure Outcome

### 8.5.1 Overall Results

Hemispherectomy was the type of epilepsy surgery with the highest rate of seizure control (77.3%) in the survey of the First Palm Desert Conference [136]. In the 1993 survey of the Second Palm Desert Conference, 67.4% of patients were seizure free after hemispherical procedures [137]. In a systematic review of 29 reports including 1161 patients, the overall seizure freedom rate for hemispherotomy was 76.0% [138]. In line, a meta-analysis performed by Hu et al. [139] including 1528 patients pooled across 56 studies demonstrated seizure freedom in 73% of patients. Similarly, a multicenter study comprising 333 hemispherectomies showed seizure freedom in 70.4% of the patients [8]. Tellez-Zenteno et al. [140] noted in a meta-analysis comprising 2 studies and 169 patients seizure freedom in 61%. In a series of 170 hemispherectomy procedures in children, approximately two-thirds of patients remained seizure free at a mean of 5 years after surgery [141]. A 73% seizure freedom rate has been reported in an Italian study [142]. In sum, seizure-free outcome is achieved in around 70% of patients after hemispherical procedures [8, 9, 139, 141, 142].

### 8.5.2 Predictors

Fallah et al. [11] analyzed 1237 hemispheric surgeries performed in pediatric patients across 31 centers and 12 countries to identify predictors for seizure outcome. Overall, 1050/1237 patients (85%) were seizure free at 12 months after surgery and 817/1237 (66%) at a median follow-up of 24 months. Children with early seizure onset, presence of generalized seizures, contralateral interictal FDG-PET hypometabolism, non-stroke etiology, and a history of previous resective surgery were more likely to experience seizure recurrence. Based on the estimated regression coefficients in the logistic model, a Hemispheric Surgery Outcome Prediction Scale (HOPS) was developed, with scores of 0–2, 3–4, and 5–6 predicting "excellent," "good," and "moderate" chance for seizure freedom, respectively. According to this model, a patient with perinatal infarction, seizure onset at 5 years of age, no contralateral interictal FDG-PET hypometabolism, no generalized seizure semiology, and no previous resective epilepsy surgery would calculate a HOPS score of 0, indicating excellent outcome with >95% likelihood of seizure freedom at 12 months following surgery, while a patient with cortical dysplasia, seizure onset at 5 months of age, contralateral interictal FDG-PET hypometabolism, generalized seizure semiology, and a prior non-hemispheric resective epilepsy surgery would result in a HOPS score of 5, indicating a moderate prognosis with 65% likelihood of seizure freedom [11].

Generalized seizure semiology, developmental etiologies, non-lateralizing EEG, and contralateral MRI abnormalities were predictors of seizure recurrence in the meta-analysis of Hu et al. [139] including 1528 patients. In line, comparing different hemispherotomy techniques, de Palma et al. [142] found that presurgical focal to bilateral tonic-clonic seizures were the strongest predictor of seizure recurrence after surgery, independently from the type of hemispherotomy.

### 8.5.3 Surgical Technique

In theory, all different surgical techniques should have identical results with respect to seizure control for a given indication. Removing the whole hemisphere, removing the whole cortex, or disconnecting the hemisphere rendering it nonfunctional can be expected to similarly abolish seizures arising from the affected hemisphere [128]. Differences between lateral and vertical approaches may, if at all, most likely be related to the opercular-insular cortex, which frequently remains connected in part with lateral approaches. Griessenauer et al. [138] found in a review of 29 reports including 1161 patients similar outcomes with different techniques. In the multicenter study of Holthausen et al. [8], a better seizure outcome with functional hemispherectomy as compared to hemidecortication/hemicorticectomy was observed. With vertical hemispherotomy, Delalande et al. [103] noticed in their series of 83 children seizure freedom in 77%. Schramm et al. [133] documented in his pediatric series of 92 patients mainly treated using the transsylvian keyhole technique Engel I outcome in 85%.

Overall, similar excellent results have been reported for lateral and vertical approaches: With lateral approaches, seizure freedom rates range between 68 and 90% [31, 128, 133, 143] and with vertical approaches between 77 and 91% [103, 104].

### 8.5.4 Etiology

While the influence of the surgical technique on seizure outcome remains unclear and may reflect the volume of the affected hemisphere and the question whether the epileptic cortex has been resected/disconnected completely or incompletely, the underlying disease definitively constitutes an important factor determining results.

#### 8.5.4.1 Acquired Pathologies/ Sturge–Weber Syndrome

The best results are achieved with acquired pathologies mainly causing hemiatrophy such as perinatal infarction, hemorrhage, and Rasmussen's encephalitis, as well as with Sturge–Weber syndrome. With Rasmussen's encephalitis, seizure-free outcome of 65% [144], 77% [8], 88% [145], and 90% [146] has been reported. For Sturge–Weber syndrome, seizure freedom was found in 81% [144], 82% [8], and 100% [128, 133, 147] of patients. In a multicenter study including 1237 pediatric cases, Fallah et al. [11] noted the following seizure freedom rates at 1 year follow-up: 89.9% (282/314) with stroke, 82·4% (26/31) with Sturge–Weber syndrome, and 76·6% (74/96) with Rasmussen's encephalitis. De Palma et al. [142] observed seizure-free outcome in 77% of patients with different acquired pathologies.

#### 8.5.4.2 Congenital or Developmental Pathologies

Developmental pathologies such as hemimegalencephaly, migrational disorders, multilobar cortical dysplasia, and polymicrogyria show a lower rate of seizure control. Devlin et al. [91] found only 31% seizure-free patients for developmental pathologies versus 82% for acquired pathologies. In contrast, De Palma et al. [142] noted seizure-free outcome in 68% of patients with developmental pathologies. For hemimegalencephaly, Kossoff et al. [148] reported seizure-free outcome in 40% of the patients. Similarly, Shimizu and Maehara [32] noted 31% seizure-free patients with hemimegalencephaly as opposed to 66% in the total group. In the series of Schramm et al. [128, 133], patients with hemimegalencephaly showed seizure control in 60% compared to 81% in the total group.

Patients with developmental pathologies other than hemimegalencephaly seem to achieve somewhat better seizure outcomes than those with hemimegalencephaly. For cortical dysplasia, complete seizure control was achieved in 57% in the series of Kossoff et al. [144]. With hemispheric polymicrogyria, seizure freedom was noted in 11 of 12 cases (92%) by Jalin et al. [149] and in 16 of 18 patients (89%) by Fohlen et al. [150]. Holthausen et al. [8] reported complete seizure control in 56.6% of patients with cortical dysplasia, and in 53.2% with hemimegalencephaly. In the study of Fallah et al. [11], 142 of 175 patients (81·3%) with non-hemimegalencephaly malformations of cortical development and 73 of 101 patients (72·4%) with hemimegalencephaly were seizure free at 1 year follow-up.

**Concluding Remarks**

- ***Outcome.*** *Systematic reviews and meta-analyses consistently demonstrate seizure-free (Engel I) outcome in around 70% of patients. Whereas the surgical technique* per se *may not influence seizure outcome, the underlying disease constitutes an important factor determining outcome with best results achieved with acquired pathologies and Sturge–Weber syndrome mainly causing hemiatrophy, while seizure outcome with developmental pathologies, in particular hemimegalencephaly, is less favorable. Given the compensatory abilities of young children, hemispherical procedures are advocated in the early age. However, favorable seizure and cognitive outcome can also be achieved in older patients and adults with moderate risks.*
- ***Surgical approach.*** *All hemispherical procedures require high surgical skills. Modified Rasmussen's techniques are suitable for patients with atrophic, normal, and enlarged hemispheres. The transsylvian-transventricular key-hole approach is ideal for atrophic hemispheres and enlarged ventricles and can also be applied in normal hemispheric volumes, but should not be used for hemimegalencephaly. Vertical hemispherotomy constitutes a good alternative to combined resective and disconnective strategies that works well in almost all conditions, in particular with normal and enlarged hemispheres. It should be emphasized that the choice of the surgical approach within the limits given by different techniques and the patient's situation depends to major parts on the individual training and experience of the surgeon.*
- ***Modified steps for deafferentation and key-hole approach.*** *As an alternative to the original description of hemispherical deafferentation (modified Rasmussen's technique) and transsylvian key-hole hemispherotomy, the following modified steps may be considered: After removal of the amygdalo-hippocampal complex, dissection is continued following the rim of the tentorium to the inferior rim of the falx, thus disconnecting the occipital lobe, then following the pericallosal artery disconnecting the parietal lobe and sectioning the callosum. Finally, dissection is proceeded around the genu of the callosum down to the sphenoid wing following the descending and then the horizontal part of the anterior cerebral artery, until the Sylvian fissure is reached, thus disconnecting the frontal lobe. This sequence facilitates continuous dissection from the temporo-occipital over the parietal to the frontobasal area in a circular fashion avoiding change the preparation site.*

- ***Landmarks.*** *Orientation constitutes a major problem with all hemispherical techniques. Important landmarks include the rim of tentorium cerebelli, the inferior rim of the falx, the corpus callosum, the pericallosal artery, the sphenoid wing, and the anterior cerebral artery. These landmarks are either directly visible (corpus callosum, pericallosal and anterior cerebral arteries) or can be made visible through the intact arachnoid by gentle suction with a cotton pad (rim of tentorium cerebelli, inferior rim of falx, and sphenoid wing). Navigation may be helpful in critical cases with enlarged hemispheres.*
- ***Infancy.*** *Hemispherical procedures in infancy pose major challenges regarding preservation of hemodynamic and metabolic stability. Especially in hemimegalencephaly, surgery should preferably be performed after the age of 5–6 months and not before the age of 3–4 months, depending on the body weight. It is advisable to start with some blood replacement just at skin incision. In critical situations of hemodynamic or metabolic instability, it may be reasonable to intraoperatively decide for a staged procedure, and to proceed with the second operation a few weeks later when the patient has recovered.*
- ***Opercula/insula.*** *The value of resection of the insula is still unproven. Thus, with lateral approaches, the insula and parts of the opercula are not infrequently left behind. However, cases with persistent seizures after hemispherical procedures arising from the insula or the adjacent opercula are well known. Therefore, it seems to be advisable to remove or undercut the opercula completely, and to remove major parts of the insular cortex.*
- ***External drainage.*** *Opening of the ventricles -at least of the inferior horn- is associated with all hemispherical procedures, thus causing aseptic meningitis which leads to mild temperatures and headaches during the first postoperative week. It is advisable to place an external drain into the resection cavity to avoid repeated lumbar puncture. This is especially important in young children for whom lumbar puncture is stressful. External drainage should be continued,* e.g., *for 7–10 days, until the CSF becomes more clear, and cell counts as well as CSF protein levels noticeably drop.*

## References


1. Dandy W. Removal of the right cerebral hemisphere for certain tumors with hemiplegia. JAMA. 1928;90:823–5.
2. Mc Kenzie KC. The present status of a patient who had the right cerebral hemisphere removed. JAMA. 1938;111:168.
3. Cairns H. Hemispherectomy in the treatment of infantile hemiplegia. Lancet. 1951;2:411–5.
4. McKissock W. The operative technique for cerebral hemispherectomy in the treatment of infantile hemiplegia. Zentralbl Neurochir. 1954;14:42–8.
5. Meyers R. Recent advances in the neurosurgery of cerebral palsy. In: Illingworth RS, editor. Recent advances in cerebral palsy. London: Churchill; 1958. p. 330–86.
6. Polani PE. Encephalo-trigeminal angiomatosis (Sturge-weber syndrome) treated by removal of the affected cerebral hemisphere. Proc R Soc Med. 1952;45:860–2.
7. Villemure JG, Vernet O, Delalande O. Hemispheric disconnection: callosotomy and hemispherectomy. Adv Tech Stand Neurosurg. 2000;26:25–78.
8. Holthausen H, May TW, Adams CTB, Andermann F, Comair Y, Delalande O, Duchowny M, Freeman JM, Hoffman HJ, et al. Seizures post hemispherectomy. In: Tuxhorn I, Holthausen H, Boenigk H, editors. Paediatric epilepsy syndromes and their surgical treatment. London: John Libbey; 1997a. p. 749–73.
9. Holthausen H, Strobl K, Pieper T, Teixeira VA, Oppel F. Prediction of motor functions post hemispherectomy. In: Tuxhorn I, Holthausen H, Boenigk H, editors. Paediatric epilepsy syndromes and their surgical treatment. London: John Libbey; 1997b. p. 785–98.
10. Meagher-Villemure K. Neuropathological findings in paediatric functional hemispherectomies. In: Tuxhorn I, Holthausen H, Boenigk H, editors. Paediatric epilepsy syndromes and their surgical treatment. London: John Libbey; 1997. p. 799–811.
11. Fallah A, Weil AG, Lewis EC, et al. Hemispheric surgery outcome prediction scale: development and validation of a seizure freedom prediction tool 2020. (submitted).
12. Wada J, Rasmussen T. Intracarotid injection of sodium amytal for the lateralization of cerebral speech dominance: experimental and clinical observations. J Neurosurg. 1960;17:266–82.
13. Gaubatz J, Ernst L, Prillwitz CC, et al. Pyramidal tract and alternate motor fibers complementarily mediate motor compensation in patients after hemi-

spherotomy. Nature Sci Rep. 2020;1(10):1010. https://doi.org/10.1038/s41598-020-57504-x.
14. Koch P, Schulz R, Hummel FC. Structural connectivity analyses in motor recovery research after stroke. Ann Clin Transl Neurol. 2016;3:233–44.
15. Nelles M, et al. Functional hemispherectomy: postoperative motor state and correlation to preoperative DTI. Neuroradiology. 2015;57:1093–102.
16. Benecke R, Meyer BU, Freund HJ. Reorganisation of descending motor pathways in patients after hemispherectomy and severe hemispheric lesions demonstrated by magnetic brain stimulation. Exp Brain Res. 1991;83:419–26.
17. Lindsay J, Ounsted C, Richards P. Hemispherectomy for childhood. Epilepsy: a 36 years study. Dev Med Child Neurol. 1987;29:592–600.
18. Smith SJM, Andermann F, Villemure JG, Rasmussen TR, Quesney LF. Functional hemispherectomy: EEG findings, spiking form isolated brain postoperatively, and prediction of outcome. Neurology. 1991;41:1790–4.
19. Weenberg RA, Quesney LF, Villemure JG. Epileptiform and non-epileptiform paroxysmal activity from isolated cortex after functional hemispherectomy. Clin Neurophysiol. 1997;102:437–42.
20. Wen HT, Rhoton AL, Marino J. Anatomical landmarks for hemispheotomy and their clinical application. J Neurosurg. 2004;101:747–55.
21. Morino M, Shimizu H, Ohata K, Tanaka K, Hara M. Anatomical analysis of different hemispherotomy procedures based on dissection of cadaveric brains. J Neurosurg. 2002;97:423–31.
22. Schramm J. Hemispherectomy techniques. Neurosurgery. 2002;37:113–34.
23. Schramm J. Hemispheric disconnection procedures (chapter 77). In: Youmans and Winn (HR Winn, ed). Neurological surgery, 7th edition, Vol 1, Elsevier, Philadelphia, 2017, pp. 515–524.
24. De Almeida AN, Marino R, Aguiar PH, Teixeira MJ. Hemispherectomy: a schematic review of the current techniques. Neurosurg Rev. 2006;29:97–102.
25. Seeger W, Zentner J. Anatomical basis of cranial neurosurgery. Heidelberg: Springer; 2018.
26. Uda T, Kunihiro N, Koh S, et al. Anatomic understanding of subtotal hemispherotomy using cadaveric brain, 3-dimensional simulation models, and intraoperative photographs. Oper Neurosurg. 2019; https://doi.org/10.1093/ons/opz354.
27. Gardner WJ. Removal of the right cerebral hemisphere for infiltrating gliomas. JAMA. 1933;12:154–64.
28. Adams CBT. Hemispherectomy: a modification. J Neurol Neurosurg Psychiatry. 1983;46:617–9.
29. Rasmussen TB. Surgical treatment of complex partial seizures: results, lessons, and problems. Epilepsia. 1983;24(Suppl. 1):S65–76.
30. Schramm J, Behrens E, Entzian W. Hemispherical deafferentation: an alternative to functional hemispherectomy. Neurosurgery. 1995;36:509–16.
31. Villemure JG, Mascott CR. Peri-insular hemispherectomy: surgical principles and anatomy. Neurosurgery. 1995;37:975–81.
32. Shimizu H, Maehara T. Modification of peri-insular hemispherectomy and surgical results. Neurosurgery. 2000;47:367–72.
33. Schramm J, Kral T, Clusmann H. Transsylvian keyhole functional hemispherectomy. Neurosurgery. 2001;49:891–901.
34. Ignezli RJ, Bucy PC. Cerebral hemidecortication in the treatment of infantile cerebral hemiatrophy. J Nerv Ment Dis. 1968;147:14–30.
35. Delalande O, Fohlen M, Jalin C, Pinard JM. From hemispherectomy to hemispherotomy. In: Lüders H, Comair YG, editors. Epilepsy surgery. 2nd ed. Philadelphia: Lippincott Williams and Wilkins; 2001. p. 741–6.
36. Danielpour M, von Koch CS, Ojemann SG, Peacock WJ. Disconnective hemispherectomy. Pediatr Neurosurg. 2001;35:169–72.
37. Austin GM, Grant FC. Physiologic observations following total hemispherectomy in man. Surgery. 1955;38:239–58.
38. Bell E, Karnosh LJ. Cerebral hemispherectomy. Report of a case ten years after operation. J Neurosurg. 1949;6:285–93.
39. Gardner WJ. Removal of cerebral hemisphere for glioma. Proceedings of the fifth international conference on neurology, Lisbon 1953, vol 4. p. 307–313.
40. Hillier WF. Total left cerebral hemispherectomy for malignant glioma. Neurology. 1954;4:718–21.
41. L'Hermitte J. L'ablation complete de l'hémisphère droit dans les cas de rumeur cérébrale localisée compliquée d'hemiplégie: la decerebration suprathalamique unilateréale chez l'homme. L'Encéphale. 1928;23:314–23.
42. Zollinger R. Removal of left cerebral hemisphere. Report of a case. Arch Neurol Psychiatr. 1935;34:48–63.
43. Krynauw RA. Infantile hemiplegia treated by removing one cerebral hemisphere. J Neurol Neurosurg Psychiatry. 1950;13:243–67.
44. White HH. Cerebral hemispherectomy in the treatment of infantile hemiplegia. Review of the literature and report of two cases. Confin Neurol. 1961;21:1–50.
45. McFie J. The effects of hemispherectomy on intellectual functioning in cases of infantile hemiplegia. J Neurol Neurosurg Psychiatry. 1961;24:240–9.
46. Smith A, Sugar O. Development of above normal language and intelligence 21 years after left hemispherectomy. Neurology. 1975;25:813–8.
47. Laine E, Pruvot P, Osson D. Résultats éloignés de l´hémisphérectomie dans les cas d´hémiatrophie cérébrale inantile génératrice d´épilepsie. Neurochirurgie. 1964;10:507–22.
48. French LA, Johnson DR, Brown IA, Van Bergen FB. Cerebral hemispherectomy for control of intractable convulsive seizures. J Neurosurg. 1955;12:154–64.
49. Chugani HT, Jacobs B. Metabolic recovery in caudate nucleus of children following cerebra hemispherectomy. Ann Neurol. 1994;36:794–7.
50. Machado AGG, Shoji A, Ballester G, Marino R. Motor area after hemispherectomy: the hemi-

spheres as potentially independent motor brains. Epilepsia. 2003;44:500–6.
51. Marino R, Machado AGG, Timo-Iaria C. Functional recovery after combined cerebral and cerebellar hemispherectomy in the rat. Stereotact Funct Neurosurg. 2001;76:83–93.
52. Winston KR, Welch K, Adler JR, Erba G. Cerebral hemicorticectomy for epilepsy. J Neurosurg. 1992;77:889–95.
53. Carson BS, Javedan SP, Freeman JM, Vining EP, Zuckerberg AL, Lauer JA, Guarnieri M. Hemispherectomy: a hemidecortication approach and review of 52 cases. J Neurosurg. 1996;84:903–11.
54. Gros C, Vlahovitch B. Hemispherectomies: neurophysiological considerations. Rev Neurol. 1951;85:482–8.
55. Hoffman HJ, Hendrick EB, Dennis M, Armstrong D. Hemispherectomy for Sturge-weber syndrome. Childs Brain. 1979;5:233–48.
56. Brian JE, Deshpande JK, McPherson RW. Management of cerebral hemispherectomy in children. J Clin Anesth. 1990;2:91–5.
57. Peacock WJ, Wehby-Grant MC, Shields WD, Shewmon DA, Chugani HT, Sankar R, Vinters HV. Hemispherectomy for intractable seizures in children: a report of 58 cases. Childs Nerv Syst. 1996;12:376–84.
58. Taha JM, Crone KR, Berger TS. The role of hemispherectomy in the treatment of of holohemispheric hemimegalencephaly. J Neurosurg. 1994;81:37–42.
59. Schiff SJ, Weinstein SL. Use of recombinant human erythropoietin to avoid blood transfusion in a Jehova's witness requiring hemispherectomy. Case report. J Neurosurg. 1993;79:600–2.
60. Wilson DH, Culver C, Waddington M, Gazzaniga M. Disconnection of the cerebral hemispheres: an alternative to hemispherectomy for the control of intractable seizures. Neurology. 1975;25:1149–53.
61. Oppenheimer DR, Griffith HB. Persistent intracranial bleeding as a complication of hermispherectomy. J Neurol Neurosurg Psychiatry. 1966;9:229–40.
62. Beardsworth ED, Adams CB. Modified hemispherectomy for epilepsy: early results in 10 cases. Br J Neurosurg. 1988;2:73–84.
63. Cabieses F, Jeri R, Landa R. Fatal brain-stem shift following hemispherectomy. J Neurosurg. 1957;14:74–91.
64. Di Rocco C, Iannelli A. Hemimegalencephaly and intractable epilepsy: complications of hemispherectomy and their correlations with the surgical technique. A report on 15 cases. Pediatr Neurosurg. 2000;33:198–207.
65. Falconer MA, Wilson PJE. Complications related to delayed hemorrhage after hemispherectomy. J Neurosurg. 1969;30:413–26.
66. Griffith HB. Certebral hemispherectomy for infantile hemiplegia in the light of the late results. Ann R Coll Surg. 1967;41:183–201.
67. Kestle J, Connolly M, Cochrane D. Pediatric peri-insular hemispherotomy. Pediatr Neurosurg. 2000;32:44–7.
68. Laine E, Pruvot P, Osson D. Resultats eloignes de l'hemispherectomie dans les cas d'hemiatrophie cerebrale infantile generatrice dépilepsie. Neurochirurgie. 1964;10:507–22.
69. Villemure J-G. Hemispherectomy techniques. In: Tuxhorn I, Holthausen H, Boenigk H, editors. Paediatric epilepsy syndromes and their surgical treatment. London: John Libbey; 1997. p. 729–38.
70. Wilson PJE. Cerebral hemispherectomy for infantile hemiplegia. A report of 50 cases. Brain. 1970a;93:147–80.
71. Wilson PJE. More "second thoughts" on hemispherectomy in infantile hemiplegia. Dev Med Child. 1970b;12:799–800.
72. Rasmussen T. Postoperative superficial cerebral hemosiderosis of the brain, its diagnosis, treatment and prevention. Am Neurol Assoc. 1973;98:133–7.
73. Rasmussen T, Andermann F. Hemispherectomy for seizures revisited. Can J Neurol Sci. 1983;10:71–8.
74. Wilson PJE. More "second thoughts" on hemispherectomy in infantile hemiplegia. Dev Med Child Neurol. 1980;12:799–800. (letter)
75. Schramm J, Behrens E, Entzian W. Hemispherical deafferentation: a modified functional hemispherectomy technique (abstract). Epilepsia. 1992;33:71.
76. Ransohoff J, Hess W. Discussion in: Rasmussen T. Post-operative superficial cerebral hemosiderosis of the brain, its diagnosis, treatment and prevention. Am Neurol Assoc. 1973;98:133–7.
77. Adams CTB. Periinsular Hemispherotomy—comment. Neurosurgery. 1995;37:981.
78. Dunn LT, Miles JB, May PL. Hemispherectomy for intractable seizures: a further modification and early experience. Br J Neurosurg. 1995;9:775–83.
79. Matheson JM, Truskett P, Davies MA, Vonau M. Hemispherectomy: a further modification using omentum vascularized free flaps. Aust NZ J Surg. 1993;63:646–50.
80. Sorano V, Esposito S. Hemispherectomy complications in the light of craniocerebral disproportion: review of the literature and rationale for a filling-reduction cranioplasty. Childs Nerv Syst. 1998;14:440–7.
81. Rasmussen T. Surgery for epilepsy arising in regions other than the temporal and frontal lobes. In: Purpura DP, Penry JK, Walter RD, editors. Advances in neurology, vol. 8. New York: Raven Press; 1975. p. 206–26.
82. Tinuper P, Andermann F, Villemure JG, Rasmussen TB, Quesney LF. Functional hemispherectomy for the treatment of epilepsy associated with hemiplegia: rationale, indications, results, and comparison with callosotomy. Ann Neurol. 1988;24:27–34.
83. Villemure JG, Rasmussen TB. Functional hemispherectomy: methodology. J Epilepsy. 1990;(Suppl 3):177–82.
84. Girvin JP, Baeesa SS. Functional hemispherectomy for the treatment of intractable seizures. Neurosciences. 2006;11:72–7.
85. Delalande O, Pinard JM, Basdevant C, Gauthe M, Plouin P, Dulac O. Hemispherotomy: a new

procedure for central disconnection. Epilepsia. 1992;33(Suppl 3):99–100.
86. Delalande O. Chirurgie de l`épilepsie chez l`lenfant. Techniques chirurgicales. Soins Chirurgie. 1996;178:18–21.
87. Villemure JG, Mascott CR. Hemispherotomy: the peri-insular approach—technical aspects. Epilepsia. 1993;34(Suppl 6):48.
88. Villemure JG. Functional hemispherectomy: evolution of techniques and results in 65 cases. In: Lüders H, Comair YG, editors. Epilepsy surgery. 2nd ed. Philadelphia: Lippincott Williams and Wilkins; 2001. p. 733–9.
89. Comair YG. The Transsylvian functional hemispherectomy: patient selection and results. In: Lüders H, Comair YG (eds). Epilepsy surgery, 2nd edn, 2001. Lippincott Williams and Wilkins, Philadelphia 699–704.
90. Cook SW, Nguyen ST, Hu B, Yudovin S, Shields WD, Vinters HV, Van de Wiele BM, Harrisoin RE, Mathern GW. Cerebral hemispherectomy in pediatric patients with epilepsy: comparison of three techniques by pathological substrate in 115 patients. J Neurosurg Ped. 2004;100:125–41.
91. Devlin AM, Cross JH, Harkness W, Chong WK, Harding B, Vargha-Khadem F, Neville BGR. Clinical outcomes of hemispherectomy for epilepsy in childhood and adolescence. Brain. 2003;126:556–66.
92. Smith JR, Fountas KN, Lee MR. Hemispherectomy: description of surgical technique. Childs Nerv Syst. 2005;21:466–72.
93. Kanev PM, Foley CM, Miles D. Ultrasound-tailored functional hemispherectomy for surgical control of seizures in children. J Neurosurg. 1997;86:762–7.
94. Giordano F, Spacca B, Barba C, Mari F, Pisano T, Guerrini R, et al. Vertical extraventricular functional hemispherotomy: a new variant for hemispheric disconnection. Technical notes and results in three patients. Childs Nerv Syst. 2015;31:2151–60. https://doi.org/10.1007/s00381-015-2788-1.
95. Chandra SP, Tripathi M. Endoscopic epilepsy surgery: emergence of a new procedure. Neurology India. 2015; https://doi.org/10.4103/0028-3886.162056.
96. Bahuleyan B, Manjila S, Robinson S, Cohen AR. Minimally invasive endoscopic transventricular hemispherotomy for medically intractable epilepsy: a new approach and cadaveric demonstration. J Neurosurg Pediatr. 2010;6:536–40.
97. Chandra PS, Subianto H, Bajaj J, Girishan S, Doddamani R, Ramanujam B, Chouhan MS, Garg A, Tripathi M, Bal CS, Sarkar C, Dwivedi R, Sapra S, Tripathi M. Endoscope-assisted (with robotic guidance and using a hybrid technique) interhemispheric transcallosal hemispherotomy: a comparative study with open hemispherotomy to evaluate efficacy, complications, and outcome. J Neurosurg Pediatr. 2018;23(2):187–97.
98. Villemure JG, Mascott C, Andermann F, Rasmussen T. Hemispherectomy and the insula. Epilepsia. 1989a;30:5.
99. Villemure JG, Mascott C, Andermann F, Rasmussen T. Is removal of the insular cortex in hemispherectomy necessary? Epilepsia. 1989b;30(Suppl):728.
100. Cats EA, Kho KH, Van Nieuwenhuizen O, Van Veelen CW, Gosselaar PH, Van Rijen PC. Seizure freedom after functional hemispherectomy and a possible role for the insular cortex: the Duch experience. J Neurosurg. 2007;107:275–80.
101. Freeman JM, Arroyo S, Vining EPG, Breiter SN, Barker PB, Pardo CA, Carson BS, Zuckerberg AL. Insular seizures: a study in Sutton's law. Epilepsia. 1994;35(Suppl 8):49.
102. Cosgrove GR, Villemure JG. Cerebral hemicorticectomy for epilepsy. J Neurosurg. 1993;79:473–4.
103. Delalande O, Bulteau C, Dellatolas G, Fohlen M, Jalin C, Buret V, Viguier D, Dorfmuller G, Jambaque I. Vertical parasagittal hemispherectomy: surgical procedures and clinical long-term outcomes in a population of 83 children. Neurosurgery. 2007;60:19–32.
104. Dorfer C, Czech T, Dressler A, et al. Vertical perithalamic hemispherotomy: a single-center experience in 40 pediatric patients with epilepsy. Epilepsia. 2013;54:1905–12.
105. Villemure JG. Anatomical to functional hemispherectomy: from Krynauw to Rasmussen. Epilepsy Res. 1992;5:209–15.
106. Sood S, Ilyas M, Marapudi NI, et al. Anatomical hemispherectomy revisited—outcome, blood loss, hydrocephalus, and absence of chronic hemosiderosis. Childs Nerv Syst. 2019;35:1341–9.
107. Gonzalez-Martinez JA, Gupta A, Kotagal P, Lachhwani D, Wyllie E, Luders HO, Bingaman WE. Hemispherectomy for catastrophic epilepsy in infants. Epilepsia. 2005;46:1518–25.
108. Kawai KS. Clinical outcome and comparison of surgical procedures in hemispherectomy for children with malformation of cortical development. Epilepsia. 2004;(Suppl 3):168.
109. Shimizu H. Our experience with pediatric epilepsy surgery focusing on corpus callosotomy and hemispherectomy. Epilepsia. 2005;46(Suppl 1):30–1.
110. Peacock WJ. Hemispherectomy for the treatment of intractable seizures in childhood. Neurosurg Clin North Am. 1995;6:549–63.
111. Pinto A, Takeoka M, Bergin AM, Bourgeois BF, Duffy FH, Sarco D, Black P, Poduri A. Surgery for intractable epilepsy due to unilateral cortical disease: comparison between anatomical and functional hemispherectomy. Epilepsia. 2009;50(Suppl 4): 148.
112. Limbrick DD, Narayan P, Powers AK, Ojeman JG, Park TS, Bertrand M, Smyth MD. Hemispherectomy: efficacy and analysis of seizure recurrence. J Neurosurg Pediatr. 2009;4:323–32.
113. Kwan A, Ng WH, Otsubo H, Ochi A, Snead OC, Tamber MS, Rutka JT. Hemispherectomy for the control of intractable epilepsy in childhood: comparison of 2 surgical techniques in a single institution. Neurosurgery. 2010;67:429–36.

114. Vining EP, Freeman JM, Brandt J, et al. Progressive unilateral encephalopathy of childhood (Rasmussen's syndrome): a reappraisal. Epilepsia. 1993;34:639–50.
115. Ballantyne AQ, Spilkin AM, Hesselink J, Trauner DA. Plasticity in the developing brain: intellectual, language and academic functions in children with ischaemic perinatal stroke. Brain. 2008;131:2975–85.
116. Ramantani G, Kadish NE, Strobl K, Brandt A, Stathi A, Mayer H, et al. Seizure and cognitive outcomes of epilepsy surgery in infancy and early childhood. Eur J Paediatr Neurol. 2013;17(5):498–506.
117. Villemure JG, Daniel T. Functional hemispherectomy and periinsular hemispherectomy. In: Baltuch GH, Villemure JG, editors. Operative techniques in epilepsy surgery. New Delhi: Thieme; 2012. p. 138–45.
118. Vargha-Khadem F, Mishkin M. Speech and language outcome after hemispherectomy in childhood. In: Tuxhorn I, Holthausen H, Boenigk H, editors. Paediatric epilepsy syndromes and their surgical treatment. London: John Libbey; 1997. p. 774–84.
119. Jonas R, Nguyen S, Hu B, Asarnow RF, LoPresti C, Curtis S, de Bode S, Yudovin S, Shields WD, Vinters HV, Mathern GW. Cerebral hemispherectomy: hospital course, seizure, developmental, language, and motor outcomes. Neurology. 2004;62:1712–21.
120. Benabis S, Vale F, Dubeau F, Duchowny M. Huh? Hemispherectomy in adults? An exercise in risk-benefit analysis. Epileptic Disord. 2009;11:258–9.
121. Verdinelli C, Olsson I, Edelvik A, et al. A long-term patient perspective after hemispherotomy—A population based study. Seizure. 2015;30:76–82.
122. Althausen A, Gleissner U, Hoppe C, et al. Long-term outcome of hemispheric surgery at different ages in 61 epilepsy patients. J Neurol Neurosurg Psychiatry. 2013;84(5):529–36.
123. Cukiert A, Cukiert CM, Argentoni M, Baise-Zung C, Forster CR, Mello VA, Burattini JA, Mariani PP. Outcome after hemispherectomy in hemiplegic adult patients with refractory epilepsy associated with early middle cerebral artery infarcts. Epilepsia. 2009;50:1381–4.
124. De Francisco J, Fernandez S, Carreno M, Rumia J, Donaire A, Maestro I, Bargallo N, Candela S, Pintor L, Boget T, Setoain X. Successful functional hemispherectomy in adult patients with refractory epilepsy. Neurologia. 2009;24:9–14.
125. McClelland S, Maxwell RE. Hemispherectomy for intractable epilepsy in adults: the first reported series. Ann Neurol. 2007;61:372–6.
126. McGovern RA, Moosa ANV, Jehi L, et al. Hemispherectomy in adults and adolescents: seizure and functional outcomes in 47 patients. Epilepsia. 2019;60:2416. https://doi.org/10.1111/epi.16378.
127. Steinhoff BJ, Staack AM, Bilic S, Kraus U, Schulze-Bonhage A, Zentner J. Functional hemispherectomy in adults with intractable epilepsy syndromes: a report of 4 cases. Epileptic Disord. 2009;11:251–7.
128. Schramm J, Delev D, Wagner J, Elger CE, von Lehe M. Seizure outcome, functional outcome, and quality of life after hemispherectomy in adults. Acta Neurochir. 2012a;154:1603–12.
129. Steinhoff BJ, Schulze-Bonhage A, Zentner J, Staack AM. Funktionelle Hemisphärektomien, Langzeitverlauf bei erwachsenen Patienten. Z Epileptol. 2016;29:144–50.
130. Schusse CM, Smith K, Drees C. Outcomes after hemispherectomy in adult patients with intractable epilepsy: institutional experience and systematic review of the literature. J Neurosurg. 2018;3:657–9.
131. Schmeiser B, Zentner J, Steinhoff BJ, Schulze-Bonhage A, Kogias E, Wendling A-S Hammen T. Functional hemispherectomy is safe and effective in adult patients. Epilepsy Behav. 2017;77:19–25.
132. King M, Stephanson JBP, Ziervogel M, Doyle D, Galbraith S. Hemimegalencephaly —a case for hemispherectomy? Neuropediatrics. 1985;16:46–55.
133. Schramm J, Kuczaty S, Sassen R, Elger CE, von Lehe M. Pediatric functional hemispherectomy: outcome in 92 patients. Acta Neurochir. 2012b;154:2017–28.
134. Andermann F, Villemure JG. Hemispherectomy: results for control of seizures in patients with hemiparesis. In: Lüders H, editor. Epilepsy surgery. Raven Press: New York; 1991. p. 625–32.
135. Eldredge EA, Soriano SG, Rockoff MA. Neuroanesthesia. Neurosurg Clin North Am. 1995;6:505–20.
136. Engel J. Outcome with respect to epileptic seizures. In: Engel J, editor. Surgical treatment of the epilepsies. New York: Raven Press; 1987. p. 553–71.
137. Engel J, Van Ness PC, Rasmussen TB, Ojeman LM. Outcome with respect to epileptic seizures. In: Engel J, editor. Surgical treatment of the epilepsies. New York: Raven Press; 1993. p. 609–21.
138. Griessenauer CJ, Salam S, Hendrix P, Patel DM, Tubbs RS, Blount JP, et al. Hemispherectomy for treatment of refractory epilepsy in the pediatric age group: a systematic. review. J Neurosurg Pediatr. 2015;15:34–44.
139. Hu WH, Zhang C, Zhang K, Shao XQ, Zhang JG. Hemispheric surgery for refractory epilepsy: a systematic review and meta-analysis with emphasis on seizure predictors and outcomes. J Neurosurg. 2016;124:952–61.
140. Tellez-Zenteno JF, Dhar R, Wiebe S. Long-term seizure outcomes following epilepsy surgery: a systematic review and meta-analysis. Brain. 2005;128:1188–98.
141. Moosa AN, Gupta A, Jehi L, Marashly A, Cosmo G, Lachhwani D, et al. Longitudinal seizure outcome and prognostic predictors after hemispherectomy in 170 children. Neurology. 2013;80:253–60.
142. De Palma L, Pietrafusa N, Gozzo F, et al. Outcome after hemispherotomy in patients with intractable epilepsy: comparison of techniques in the Italian experience. Epilepsy Behav. 2019;93:22–8.
143. Villemure JG, Daniel RT. Peri-insular hemispherotomy in paediatric epilepsy. Childs Nerv Syst. 2006;22:967–81. https://doi.org/10.1007/s00381-006-0134-3.

144. Kossoff EH, Vining EP, Pillas DJ, Pyzik PL, Avellino AM, Carson BS, Freeman JM. Hemispherectomy for intractable unihemispheric epilepsy. Etiology versus outcome. Neurology. 2003;61:887–90.
145. Lam S, Mathern GW. Functional hemsispherectomy at UCLA. In: Cataltepe O, Jallo GI, editors. Pediatric epilepsy. New York: Thieme; 2010. p. 230–40.
146. Ramesha KN, Rajesh B, Ashalatha R, Kesavadas C, Abraham M, Radhakrishnan VV, Sarma PS, Radhakrishnan K. Rasmusse's encephalitis: experience from a developing country based opn a group of medically and surgically treated patients. Seizure. 2009;18:567–72.
147. Burgeois M, Crimmins DW, de Oliveira RS, Arzimanoglou A, Garnett M, Roujeau T, DiRocco F, Sainte-Rose C. Surgical treatment of epilepsy in Sturge-weber syndrome ion children. J Neurosurg. 2007;106:20–8.
148. Kossoff EH, Vining EP, Pillas DJ, et al. Hemispherectomy for intractable unihemispheric epilepsy: etiology versus outcome. Neurology. 2003;61:887–90.
149. Jalin C, Fohlen M, Dorfmueller G, et al. Polymicrogyria: electro-clinical and anatomical aspects. A study of 12 children with unilateral polymicrogyria associated with epilepsy with continuous spikes and waves syndrome treated by hemispherectomy. Epilepsia. 2009;21:17–33.
150. Fohlen M, Dorfmüller G, Ferrand-Sorberts S, et al. Parasagittal hemispherotomy in hemispheric polymicrogyria with electrical status epilepticus during slow sleep: indications, results and follow-up. Eur J Epilepsy. 2019;71:190–200.

# Long-Term Epilepsy-Associated Tumors (LEATs)

# 9

*Tell me and I forget. Teach me and I remember.*
*Involve me and I learn.*

*Benjamin Franklin*

## Contents





J. Zentner, *Surgical Treatment of Epilepsies*, https://doi.org/10.1007/978-3-030-48748-5_9

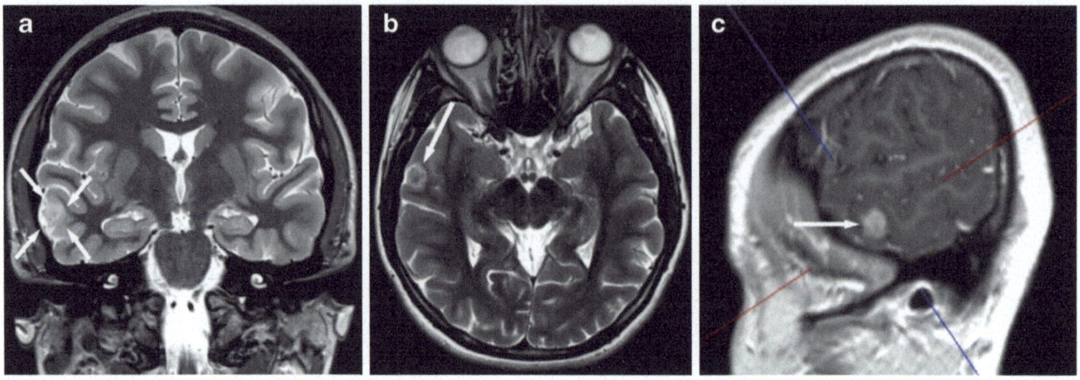


**Fig. 9.1** Ganglioglioma WHO°I of the right middle temporal gyrus. (**a**) Coronal T2-weighted fast spin echo; (**b**) axial T2-weighted fast spin echo; (**c**) sagittal contrast-enhanced MPRAGE images. Note the cortical location of the tumor (**a**, **b**: arrow) which is the most important clue for considering a ganglioglioma. Around 1/3 of gangliogliomas show contrast enhancement (**c**: arrow) (with courtesy of H. Urbach, Dpt. of Neuroradiology, Freiburg)

Epileptic seizures are the initial symptom or occur during the course of the disease in around 50–60% of patients with brain tumors [1, 2]. Incidence and frequency of seizures depend on the type and localization of the tumor. While in higher-grade and subcortically localized tumors of the middle to higher adult age focal neurological deficits are the main symptoms, benign and cortically localized tumors especially of the younger age are more associated with epilepsy. For these benign tumors which present with severe intractable epilepsy as the leading symptom and for which the oncologic burden is usually indolent, the name "long-term epilepsy-associated tumors, LEATs" has been proposed by Luyken et al. [3], whereby long-term means causing drug-resistant seizures lasting for more than 2 years (see also Chap. 13). There is now growing consensus that the adjective "long-term" in this sense has become obsolete [4–8], and it has been proposed to maintain the name LEATs, changing its meaning to "low-grade epilepsy-associated neuroepithelial tumors" [4].

## 9.1 Histopathological Features

LEATs are generally slow-growing, low-grade, and cortically localized tumors that often arise in younger patients and, in many cases, show both neuronal and glial differentiation [3, 9–11]. These glioneuronal tumor types include gangliogliomas (GG) and dysembryoplastic neuroepithelial tumors (DNET) (Figs. 9.1 and 9.2). Other less frequent LEATs are angiocentric gliomas, papillary glioneuronal tumors (PGNT), pleomorphic xanthoastrocytomas (PXA), pilocytic astrocytomas, and extraventricular neurocytomas. These tumors are mainly of WHO grade I. Less frequently, refractory epilepsy may be caused by more aggressive LEATs of WHO grade II such as diffuse astrocytomas and oligodendrogliomas [8, 12–15]. There is ongoing debate on consensus for histopathological diagnosis, since correct histopathological and molecular diagnosis is important for both epileptological and oncological reasons [4, 8, 11–13, 16, 17].

Although LEATs account only for around 1.5% of all brain tumors, they have been found in epilepsy surgical series in 10–15% of cases [18, 19]. In the European Epilepsy Brain Bank (EEBB) comprising 9606 specimens, tumors as the cause of epilepsy were found in 2190 patients (22.8%). GG as observed in 1046 cases (10.9%) formed the largest group, followed by DNET (6%). In a summary of different series, the incidence of DNET among LEATs ranged between 7 and 80% [15]. Evaluating 207 LEATs [20], found 75 GG (36.2%) and 25 DNET (12.1%). Pasquier et al. [21] observed among 94 WHO grade I and grade II tumors 61 DNET (64.9%) and 29 GG (30.9%). LEATs may have mixed features (GG

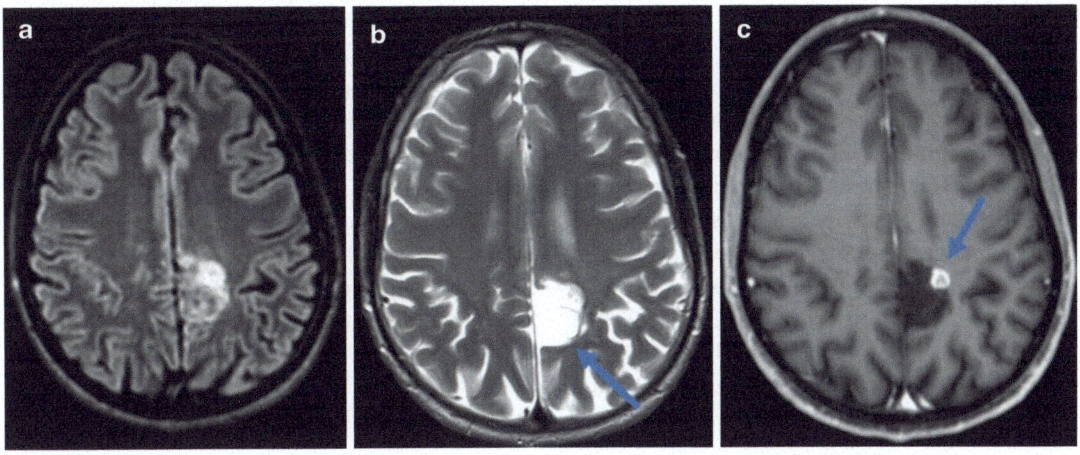


**Fig. 9.2** Dysembryoplastic neuroepithelial tumor (DNET) of the left paracentral/postcentral gyrus. (**a**) Axial FLAIR fast spin echo, (**b**) axial T2-weighted fast spin echo, (**c**) reformatted axial T1-weighted contrast-enhanced gradient echo images. The DNT has a multicystic appearance, which is best appreciated on T2-weighted images (**b**: arrow). Ring-like contrast-enhancement (**c**: arrow) may appear and even disappear (with courtesy of H. Urbach, Dpt. of Neuroradiology, Freiburg)

and DNET; PXA and GG; PXA and DNET) [5, 11, 15, 22]. Location of LEATs is temporal in most cases, followed by the frontal and parietal areas. In temporal location, most tumors are temporomesially extending to limbic and/or paralimbic areas [8, 15, 23–28].

It has been noted that especially in glioneuronal tumors (GG and DNET), the region surrounding the neoplasm is characterized by cortical disorganization in 80% of cases [29, 30]. In particular, a strong association of LEATs with focal cortical dysplasia (FCD) has been found in most series between 40 and 80%. This raises the question as to the pathophysiologic processes underlying the development of these distinct entities and which of the two coexisting lesions carries the leading role in seizure generation. In contrast, the coincidence of LEATs with hippocampal sclerosis is more rare (2–25%) [3, 5, 9–11, 15, 16, 21, 25, 27, 31–41].

## 9.2 Clinical Aspects

Gangliogliomas (GG) and dysembryoplastic neuroepithelial tumors (DNET) representing WHO grade I tumors are in 90–100% of patients associated with pharmacoresistant epilepsy [14, 41]. Other WHO grade I gliomas which predominantly occur in children and adolescents like pilocytic astrocytomas, pleomorphic xanthoastrocytomas (PXA), and angiocentric gliomas are frequently associated with epilepsy as well [14]. With diffuse WHO grade II gliomas, epilepsy is observed in between 60 and 90% of patients [24, 42]. These diffuse gliomas mainly constitute cortically localized protoplasmatic astrocytomas, but also oligodendrogliomas and oligoastrocytomas [41]. In addition, among WHO grade II astrocytomas, a subtype named isomorphic astrocytoma has been described which coincides with a particular long duration of epilepsy and a low tendency of recurrence. This tumor is characterized by a low cellular density, absence of mitotic activity, and special molecular features [43].

The most frequent seizure pattern as seen in 30–50% of patients with LEATs is complex partial seizure with or without secondary generalization [18, 44–46]. About 10–15% of patients present with generalized seizures only, and a small number (5%) have simple partial seizures [45, 47]. However, up to 30% of patients present with more than one seizure type. The mean duration of seizures in patients with LEATs until surgery ranges from 6 to 12 years, but may be as long as up to 20 or 30 years [1, 18, 46, 48].

## 9.3 Pathophysiological Considerations

Pathogenesis of LEATs-associated seizures seems to be multifactorial depending on the type, growth characteristics, and localization of the tumor. Epileptogenic mechanisms include cellular components with hyperexcitable neurons, different neurochemical characteristics, and neurotransmitter disturbances [3, 15, 28, 42, 49]. Overviews on mechanisms have been provided by Rudà et al. [41, 50], Pallud and MCKhann [51], and Samudra et al. [42].

### 9.3.1 Cellular Components

Invasive EEG studies have demonstrated that in cases of glioneuronal tumors, more abundant epileptiform activity may be recorded in patients with a coexisting FCD [36]. Other data, however, have shown that glioneuronal tumors can be intrinsically epileptogenic, even when associated with FCD [49]. These tumor cells can overregulate transmitters and neuropeptides, which may cause a dysbalance between excitatory and inhibitory activities. Rosati et al. [52] found a relationship between seizures and downregulation of glutamine synthetase. Impaired activity of potassium chloride cotransporter (KCC2) affects inhibitory gamma-aminobutyric acid (GABA) related chloride channels [53]. Moreover, inflammatory reactions with accumulation of microglial cells may contribute to epileptogenesis [36]. However, the specific role of each of them in epileptogenesis is still ill defined [16, 23, 25, 27, 38].

### 9.3.2 Peritumoral Milieu

By partial deafferentation of cortical areas, LEATs can produce a hypersensitive peritumoral environment [54]. Changes in connectivity and in formation of networks could be proven by means of MEG. MR-spectrographic studies showed decreased levels of *N*-acetylaspartate which is a marker of neuronal cell function in the epileptogenic cortex. Moreover, the space-occupying effect of the tumor may cause increased excitability by hypoxia and acidosis coinciding with changes of concentration of ions and disturbances of the blood–brain barrier in the surrounding tissue. In addition, tumor and perilesional tissue can cause changes in expression of neurotransmitters as well as of their receptors, thus inducing imbalance in favor of the excitatory effect of glutamate and reducing the inhibitory effect of GABA at the same time [47, 51, 55].

### 9.3.3 Persisting Neurons

Morphologic studies in LEATs showed aberrant migrations with persisting neurons in the white matter which develop to a lesser extent inhibitory, but to a larger extent excitatory synapses [55]. By means of immunohistochemistry, changed expression profiles of connexins have been proven in the perilesional cortex of low-grade gliomas [9, 10].

### 9.3.4 Molecular Profiles

Molecular genetic studies in glioneuronal tumors demonstrated changed profiles of gene expression, which may influence tumor-associated epilepsy as well as tumor growth [56]. B1 (BRAF) mutations have been found in a large percentage of cases [4, 57–61]. Mutant BRAF V600E protein in gangliogliomas is expressed predominantly by neuronal tumor cells [58]. Characterizing molecular signatures could be very helpful, allowing a more precise pathological definition and a better comprehension of both oncologic behavior [4, 16, 57, 59] and the epileptogenic mechanisms [62].

### 9.3.5 Secondary Epileptogenesis

Long-standing tumoral epilepsy may lead to secondary epileptogenicity with far distant seizure foci or mirror foci, especially in young patients. Theses secondary epileptogenic foci have been found to disappear in many instances after resection of the primary focus, but may also persist [63–65].

## 9.4 Surgical Strategies

### 9.4.1 Surgical Goals

For surgical treatment of LEATs, both oncological and epileptological aspects have to be considered. From an oncological point of view, it is the main goal to achieve a long-term tumor control. At the same time, epilepsy predominantly impairing the patients should be completely cured. Seizure control, however, can only be achieved per definition by removing the epileptogenic area. Pursuing both aims—tumor control and seizure freedom—can be rendered difficult, since the relationships between the tumor and the epileptogenic area can be variable.

### 9.4.2 Conceptual Considerations

Controversies exist about the site of ictal onset and the concept of an epileptogenic area in the presence of a LEAT. As mentioned above, dysplastic foci within GG, DNET, and low-grade gliomas have been demonstrated. These benign tumors may behave like dysplasia and be inherently epileptogenic [47, 49]. However, most authors agree that the seizure generator is not entirely within the tumor itself, but more often involves the brain immediately adjacent to it, and that the irritative interictal area is in close proximity to the lesion [66–68]. In some cases, even more distant areas have been shown to be epileptogenic and capable of triggering seizures. These distant areas may refer to limbic and/or paralimbic structures in extrahippocampal temporal tumors. Thus, relationships between LEATs and the epileptogenic area are variable.

### 9.4.3 Surgical Options

Depending on the relationships between tumor and epileptogenic focus as hypothesized by presurgical workup, different surgical options are available: (1) removal of the tumor only (lesionectomy), (2) removal of the tumor including an intact margin (extended lesionectomy), and (3) tailored resection of the epileptogenic area. Lesionectomy and extended lesionectomy represent morphologically-guided approaches and follow results of MR imaging. Contrarily, tailored resection of the epileptogenic area is based on extensive functional presurgical workup. Optimal surgical strategy with respect to different pathologies remains controversial, since reliable data based on prospective controlled studies are lacking [8, 25, 27, 31, 37, 38, 69–71]. Thus, only some arbitrary recommendations for proceedings can be given that have proven to be useful in clinical practice.

#### 9.4.3.1 Lesionectomy

In principle, a morphologically (MRI) based procedure in the sense of lesionectomy can be sufficient both for tumor control and for the treatment of epilepsy. However, lesionectomy for control of epilepsy is only efficient in the minority of cases, i.e., in very well delimitable tumors in neocortical location that are at a great distance from limbic structures. In these cases, epilepsy may be caused by the tumor itself [8, 72, 73].

#### 9.4.3.2 Extended Lesionectomy

In the majority of cases, a circumscribed involvement of the perilesional area into the epileptogenic zone can be assumed. In this situation, seizure control can be achieved by a morphologically-guided approach in the sense of an extended lesionectomy. Removing an intact margin of about 0.5–1 cm around the tumor seems to be sufficient to provide more reliability in terms of seizure control and can be recommended whenever possible with respect to the functionality of the surrounding brain. The situation with more diffusely growing gliomas or tumors involving limbic and/or paralimbic areas is much more difficult. Here, lesionectomy and extended lesionectomy frequently provide unsatisfactory results.

#### 9.4.3.3 Functional Approach

The association of a more diffusely growing temporal tumor in close relationship to a sclerotic hippocampus known as a dual pathology should encourage to remove both the tumor and the hippocampal area, since a sclerotic hippocampus rarely has a significant role in memory function. If the hippocampal formation seems to be morphologically intact as assessed by MRI, a functional approach with extensive presurgical workup to define the epileptogenic area and to facilitate tailored resection is recommended, which can be expected to provide optimal results in terms of seizure control and preservation of function. Similarly, in more diffusely growing tumors in extratemporal location a functional strategy may be required to achieve satisfying epileptological results [3, 9, 10, 28, 70, 74–80].

## 9.5 Seizure Outcome

### 9.5.1 Overall Results

In a meta-analysis comprising 39 studies with a total of 910 patients [69] considering both pediatric and adult cohorts with glioneuronal tumors (GG and DNET), seizure freedom (Engel I) was reported in 80% of the patients. A previous systematic overview comprising 737 patients demonstrated seizure freedom in 71% of the patients after complete removal of the tumor [81]. No significant differences in terms of seizure outcome were observed between temporal and extratemporal tumor location, between adults and children, and between patients operated with and without intraoperative ECoG [81]. In a nationwide Italian study, Giulioni et al. [12] reported on 339 patients with LEATs. Tumor location was temporal in 70.2%, and complete seizure control was achieved in 89.7% of patients [12].

### 9.5.2 Prognostic Factors

The following significant prognostic factors indicating favorable seizure outcome have been identified: complete tumor removal [12, 69, 81], shorter duration of epilepsy [12, 69], preoperatively medicamentous well controlled epilepsy [69], and absence of secondary generalized seizures before surgery [69, 71]. Giulioni et al. [12] noted in their series of 339 LEAT cases 98.2% seizure-free patients after surgery in the drug-responsive group, compared to 88.0% in the drug-refractory cohort. Longer duration of epilepsy indicated a less favorable outcome, with the probability of unfavorable outcome increasing by 4% for every year waiting for surgery. Moreover, longer duration of epilepsy was significantly associated with preoperative neuropsychological deficits [12].

### 9.5.3 Surgical Strategy

All studies available agree that complete removal of the tumor is the most important prognostic factor providing seizure freedom in 70–90% of patients. This is true for both temporal and extratemporal tumor localization [3, 5, 8, 23, 26, 27, 33, 37, 38, 69, 71, 76, 82]. However, most studies do not differentiate between lesionectomy alone and extended lesionectomy. In more diffuse temporal gliomas showing close relationships to temporomesial structures, several studies have demonstrated more favorable epileptological results with tailored resection of the epileptogenic zone as opposed to lesionectomy alone [69, 81]. In the series of Giuloni et al. [37], only 43% of patients were seizure free after lesionectomy as opposed to 93% when a tailored resection has been performed.

### 9.5.4 Tumor Type

It has been shown that the type of tumor correlates with seizure outcome. More favorable epileptological results have been found in patients with glioneuronal tumors (GG and DNET) with seizure freedom of 94% as opposed to patients with diffuse gliomas showing seizure freedom in 79% [83]. Luyken et al. [3] observed seizure freedom in more than 90% of patients with GG and oligodendrogliomas compared to 66% in patients with WHO grade II astrocytomas, and 61% in patients with pilocytic astrocytomas. Garcia-Fernández [84] noted seizure-free outcome in 95.2% of patients with GG and

DNET. Similar results were observed by Ozlen et al. [85] with seizure freedom in 92.8% of patients with DNET and 87.5% with GG. In a Swedish cohort comprising 67 patients with GG and DNET, Rydenhag et al. [86] documented seizure freedom in 79% of patients. Chassoux et al. [75] noted seizure freedom in 83% of patients with DNET.

#### 9.5.4.1 DNET and Dysplastic Cortex

Seizure-free outcome with DNET has been reported to range between 70 and 90% of cases [3, 34, 74, 77, 78, 87–93]. Among other factors, surgical failure with DNET has been attributed to the presence of dysplastic cortex adjacent to the tumor that is not clearly visible on MRI. Removing such dysplastic epileptogenic areas that may be detected by intraoperative ECoG has been found to be necessary to achieve seizure freedom [34, 40, 87, 92, 94, 95]. Dependent on the presence or absence of neighboring dysplastic cortex, Chassoux et al. [75] defined three main structural MRI types in a series of 78 patients operated for DNET, and they found that the epileptogenic zone differed significantly according to these types. The epileptogenic zone was found to be co-localized with the tumor in MRI type 1 (absence of dysplastic cortex), to include perilesional cortex in MRI type 2 (small dysplastic area), and to involve extensive areas in MRI type 3 (large dysplastic areas) [75]. Thus, Chassoux et al. [75] concluded that in MRI type 1, restricting the resection to the MRI lesion may be adequate, in MRI type 2 it may be advisable to include the perilesional cortex, while in MRI type 3 more extended resection strategies are recommended.

#### 9.5.4.2 DNET and HS

Hippocampal sclerosis (HS) associated with DNET has been rarely found by Li et al. [96]. Contrarily, Thom et al. [15] observed HS associated with DNET in 40% of cases and emphasized the predominance of atypical DNET patterns. Chassoux et al. [75] noted hippocampal atrophy in 15% in their DNET series, especially in MRI type 3 DNET. Accordingly, they recommended for these cases anterior temporal lobectomy as the best surgical strategy.

#### 9.5.4.3 LEATs and FCD

Cossu et al. [25] evaluated clinical characteristics and postoperative seizure outcome of patients with LEATs associated with FCD. Particular attention has been paid to FCD type IIIb which is defined by the association of FCD type I with a glial or glioneuronal tumor. Clinical variables and postoperative seizure outcome of patients with coexisting tumor and FCD (FCD IIIb and tumor-associated FCD II) were similar to those of patients with a solitary tumor and solitary FCD II, but differed significantly from patients with solitary FCD I. Seizure freedom was 81% in patients with solitary tumors, 83% with FCD IIIb, 76% in patients with tumor and FCD II, 84% with FCD II, but only 47% in patients with FCD I. The authors supposed that FCD I is likely to represent a more widespread structural abnormality compared to the dysplastic component of FCD IIIb [25]. Similar seizure outcomes of patients with LEATs alone and tumor-associated FCD have been observed in another study [12].

## 9.6 Tumor Control

### 9.6.1 Survival Rate/Tumor Recurrence

Patients with LEATs show a high survival rate and a low tendency to tumor recurrence. A 10-year survival rate of 90% to almost 100% has been found in many studies [37, 76, 82]. Luyken et al. [3] reported a 10-year survival rate of 90% and a 10-year recurrence rate of 25% in epilepsy-associated supratentorial WHO grade II and WHO grade III astrocytomas. Among 144 patients with GG, DNET, and pilocytic astrocytomas, Luyken et al. [3] observed tumor recurrence in only one case of a ganglioglioma WHO grade I which showed malignant transformation at a mean observation time of 8 years.

### 9.6.2 Prognostic Factors

The following factors were associated with a longer survival and low recurrence rate: (1) temporal localization of the tumor, (2) age below 30 years at

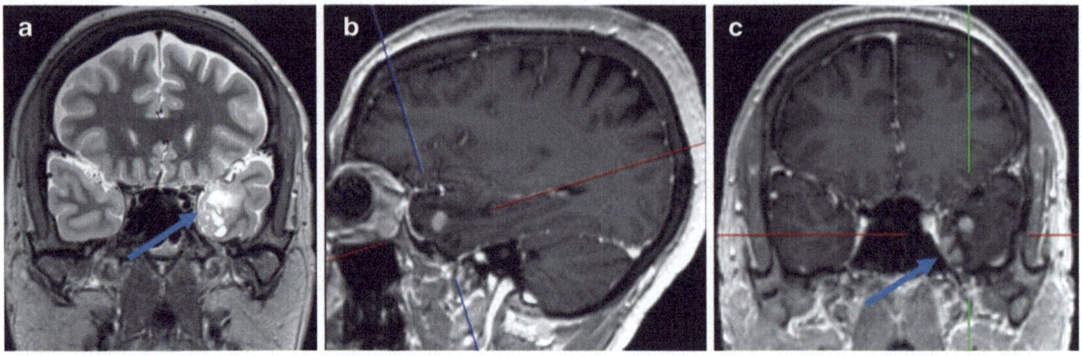


**Fig. 9.3** Tumor of the left temporal pole. (**a**) Coronal T2-weighted fast spin echo, (**b**) sagittal T1-weighed contrast-enhanced gradient echo, (**c**) reformatted coronal T1-weighed contrast-enhanced gradient echo image. Note the cortical and subcortical location (**a**: arrow) and the meningo-cerebral contrast enhancement (**c**: arrow). The latter one is suggestive for a pleomorphic xanthoastrocytoma; however a clear differentiation to a ganglioglioma is not possible. Pathological analysis revealed a pleomorphic xanthoastrocytoma (WHO grade III) with mutation of BRAF-V600E and TP53 (with courtesy of H. Urbach, Dpt. of Neuroradiology, Freiburg)

operation, (3) insignificant gemistocytic fraction of the tumor, (4) complete removal of the tumor, and (5) long history of epilepsy [3]. Schramm et al. [97] observed a 10-year survival rate of 80% in patients with astrocytomas and a long history of epilepsy as opposed to 49% in cases without long duration of epilepsy. Correspondingly, tumor recurrence rate after 10 years was 25% in patients with a long history of epilepsy versus 89% without a long duration of epilepsy [97]. Overall, the most important prognostic factor to achieve long-term tumor control is complete tumor removal. The idea of supratotal resection of these tumors based on functional boundaries has been thought to further improve long-term survival [98].

### 9.6.3 Malignant Transformation

Despite the benign course as usually observed, several reports have demonstrated that GG, glial tumors such as PXA, and even DNET can show malignant transformation in rare cases [3, 13, 15, 27, 33, 99, 100] (Fig. 9.3). Therefore, strict reluctance towards surgical treatment and concentration to observation only seems not to be adequate. Weighing up benefits and risks, complete tumor removal to achieve long-term tumor control and to avoid malignant transformation should at least be considered [97].

## 9.7 Special Considerations in Children and Adolescents

Besides focal cortical dysplasias (FCD) as observed in between 40 and 60% of cases, tumors account with 20–30% for the most frequent etiologies of focal epilepsy in children and adolescents. Glioneuronal tumors (GG and DNET) amounting to 40% of pathologies constitute the largest group in pediatric patients undergoing temporal resections [101].

### 9.7.1 Seizure Control

A number of studies have analyzed surgical treatment and epileptological outcome of children and adolescents with LEATs. These studies demonstrate excellent results with seizure control rates around 90% [25, 39, 87, 102–105]. Ramantani et al. [70] found seizure freedom in children and adolescents operated for glioneuronal tumors in 86% of patients at 12 months after surgery. Seizure recurrence was mainly caused by incomplete resection of the tumor as it has been confirmed by others [69]. Ko et al. [106] noted seizure-free outcome in 51 of 58 cases (88%). Pelliccia et al. [8] compared the outcome of patients with LEATs operated before and after the age of 18 years (pediatric group versus adult group). In the pediatric group, 93.3% were in Engel I and 80% in Engel Ia as opposed to 77% Engel I and 53.3% Engel Ia in the adult group.

### 9.7.2 Prognostic Factors

Short history of epilepsy and complete removal of the tumor have proven to be essential positive prognostic factors regarding seizure control in the pediatric age [106, 107]. Thus, data available strongly support early presurgical evaluation in children and adolescents with LEATs. Early surgical intervention provides excellent chances for seizure control and prevents adverse effects of seizures and anticonvulsant medication on the developing brain. Moreover, it may also prevent the possibility of long-term malignant transformation [3, 8–10, 105, 106].

**Concluding Remarks**

- ***Definition.*** *Long-term epilepsy-associated tumors (LEATs) constitute a special clinicopathological group of benign brain tumors mainly in temporal and frontal location, which characteristically occur in young age, show a stable course over years, and become symptomatic by a pharmacoresistant epilepsy. Therapeutic goals include both tumor and seizure control.*
- ***Tumor control.*** *With respect to color and consistency of tumor tissue, most LEATs are well recognized under the operation microscope, while definition of tumor borders is rendered difficult. With complete removal of the MRI visible tumor as the most important prognostic factor, 10-year survival rates of 90% to almost 100% can be achieved.*
- ***Seizure control.*** *The optimal surgical strategy to achieve seizure control remains controversial. In the absence of robust data from controlled studies only arbitrary recommendations can be given that have proven to be useful in clinical practice. In well delimitable tumors, extended lesionectomy additionally removing an intact margin of 0.5–1.0 cm around the tumor can be recommended providing seizure control in between 70 and 90% of patients. In more diffusely growing tumors infiltrating limbic and/or paralimbic structures, extensive presurgical workup is necessary in order to define the epileptogenic area as well as its functionality and to facilitate an adequate tailored resection.*

## References


1. Blume WT, Girvin JP, Kaufmann JC. Childhood brain tumors presenting as chronic uncontrolled focal cerebral discharges. Ann Neurol. 1989;12:538–41.
2. Lynam LM, Lyons MK, Drazkowski JF, et al. Frequency of seizures in patients with newly diagnosed brain tumors: a retrospective review. Clin Neurol Neurosurg. 2007;109:634–8.
3. Luyken C, Blümcke I, Fimmers R, Urbach H, Elger CE, Wiestler OD, Schramm J. The spectrum of long-term epilepsy-associated tumors: long-term seizure and tumor outcome and neurosurgical aspects. Epilepsia. 2003;44:822–30.
4. Blümcke I, Aronica E, Becker A, et al. Low-grade epilepsy-associated neuroepithelial tumours—the 2016 WHO classification. Nat Rev Neurol. 2016;12:732–40.
5. Giulioni M, Marucci G, Martinoni M, et al. Epilepsy associated tumors: review article. World J Clin Cases. 2014;2:623–41.
6. Giulioni M, Martinoni M, Marucci G. Observations on epilepsy associated low-grade tumors and focal cortical dysplasias. Childs Nerv Syst. 2015;31:507–9.
7. Giulioni M, Martinoni M, Marucci G. Challenges in epilepsy associated tumors. J Neuro-Oncol. 2016;130:239–40.
8. Pelliccia V, Deleo F, Gozzo F, et al. Early and late epilepsy surgery in focal epilepsies associated with long-term epilepsy-associated tumors. J Neurosurg. 2017;127(5):1147–52.
9. Aronica E, Gorter JA, Jansen GH, et al. Expression of connexin 43 and connexin 32 gap-junction proteins in epilepsy-associated brain tumors and in the perilesional epileptic cortex. Acta Neuropathol. 2001a;101:449–59.
10. Aronica E, Leenstra S, van Veelen CW, van Rijen PC, Hulsebos TJ, Tersmette AC, et al. Glioneuronal tumors and medically intractable epilepsy: a clinical study with long-term follow-up of seizure outcome after surgery. Epilepsy Res. 2001b;43:179–91.
11. Blümcke I, Aronica E, Urbach H, Alexopoulos A, Gonzalez-Martinez JA. A neuropathology-based approach to epilepsy surgery in brain tumors and proposal for a new terminology use for long-term epilepsy-associated brain tumors. Acta Neuropathol. 2014;128:39–54.

12. Giulioni M, Marucci G, Pelliccia V, Gozzo F, Barba C, et al. Epilepsy surgery of "low grade epilepsy associated neuroepithelial tumors": a retrospective nationwide Italian study. Epilepsia. 2017;58:1832. https://doi.org/10.1111/epi.13866.
13. Louis DN, Ohgaki H, Wiestler OD, et al. WHO classification of tumours of the central nervous system. Lyon: IARC; 2016.
14. Prayson R, Fong J, Najm I. Coexistent pathology in chronic epilepsy patients with neoplasms. Mod Pathol. 2010;23:1097–103.
15. Thom M, Blümcke I, Aronica E. Long-term epilepsy-associated tumors. Brain Pathol. 2012;22:350–79.
16. Holthausen H, Blümcke I. Epilepsy-associated tumours: what epileptologists should know about neuropathology, terminology, and classification systems. Epileptic Disord. 2016;18:240–51.
17. Marucci G, Giulioni M. Pathological assessment of epilepsy surgery brain tissue. Pathologica. 2016; 108:80–6.
18. Boon PA, Williamson PD, Fried I, et al. Intracranial, intraaxial, space-occupying lesions in patients with intractable partial seizures: an anatomicoclinical, neuro-psychological and surgical correlation. Epilepsia. 1991;32:467–76.
19. De Tisi J, Bell GS, Peacock JL, McEvoy AW, Harkness WF, Sander JW, Duncan JS. The long-term outcome of adult epilepsy surgery, patterns of seizure remission, and relapse: a cohort study. Lancet. 2011;378:1388–95.
20. Luyken C, Blümcke I, Fimmers R, et al.: Supratentorial gangliogliomas: Histopathological grading and tumor recurrence during a median of eight years in 184 patients. Cancer. 2004; 101, 146–55.
21. Pasquier B, Péoc'H M, Fabre-Bocquentin B, et al. Surgical pathology of drug-resistant partial epilepsy. A 10-year-experience with a series of 327 consecutive resections. Epileptic Disord. 2002;4:99–119.
22. Prayson RA, Napekoski KM. Composite ganglioglioma/dysembryoplastic neuroepithelial tumor: a clinicopathologic study of 8 cases. Hum Pathol. 2012;43:1113–8.
23. Bonney PA, Boettcher LB, Conner AK, et al. Review of seizure outcomes after surgical resection of dysembryoplastic neuroepithelial tumors. J Neuro-Oncol. 2016;126:1–10.
24. Brogna C, Gil Robles S, Duffau H. Brain tumors and epilepsy. Expert Rev Neurother. 2010;8:941–55.
25. Cossu M, Fuschillo D, Bramerio M, et al. Epilepsy surgery of focal cortical dysplasia-associated tumors. Epilepsia. 2013;54(Suppl. 9):115–22.
26. Radhakrishnan A, Abraham M, Vilanilam G, et al. Surgery for "long-term epilepsy associated tumors (LEATs)": seizure outcome and its predictors. Clin Neurol Neurosurg. 2016;141:98–105.
27. Tomita T, Volk JM, Shen W, et al. Glioneuronal tumors of cerebral hemisphere in children: correlation of surgical resection with seizure outcomes and tumor recurrences. Childs Nerv Syst. 2016;32:1839–48.
28. Zaghloul KA, Schramm J. Surgical management of glioneural tumors with drug-resistant epilepsy. Acta Neurochir. 2011;153:1551–9.
29. Kleihues P, Cavanee WK. World Health Organization classification of tumors. Pathology and genetics of tumors of the nervous system. Lyon, France: IARC Press; 2000.
30. Morris HH, Matkovic Z, Estes ML, Prayson RA, Comair YG, Turnbull J, Najm I, Kotagal P, Wyllie E. Ganglioglioma and intractable epilepsy: clinical and neurophysiologic features and predictors of outcome after surgery. Epilepsia. 1998;39:307–13.
31. Babini M, Giulioni M, Galassi E, et al. Seizure outcome of surgical treatment of focal epilepsy associated with low-grade tumors in children. J Neurosurg Pediatr. 2013;11:214–23.
32. Blümcke I, Wiestler OD. Gangliogliomas: an intriguing tumor entity associated with focal epilepsies. J Neuropathol Exp Neurol. 2002;61:575–84.
33. Bonney PA, Glenn CA, Ebeling PA, et al. Literature review seizure freedom rates and prognostic indicators after resection of gangliogliomas: a review. World Neurosurg. 2015;84:1988–96.
34. Chang EF, Christie C, Sullivan JE, Garcia PA, Tihan T, Gupta N, et al. Seizure control outcomes after resection of dysembryoplastic neuroepithelial tumor in 50 patients. J Neurosurg Pediatr. 2010;5:123–30.
35. Chang EF, Wang DD, Barkovich AJ, Tihan T, Auguste KI, Sullivan JE, et al. Predictors of seizure freedom after surgery for malformations of cortical development. Ann Neurol. 2011;70:151–62.
36. Ferrier CH, Aronica E, Leijten FSS, Spliet WGM, Van Huffelen AC, Van Rijen PC, Binnie CD. Electrocorticographic discharge patterns in glioneuronal tumors and focal cortical dysplasia. Epilepsia. 2006;47:1477–86.
37. Giulioni M, Rubboli G, Marucci G, et al. Seizure outcome of epilepsy surgery in focal epilepsies associated with temporomesial glioneural tumors: lesionectomy compared with tailored resection. J Neuosurg. 2009;111:1275–82.
38. Giulioni M, Marucci G, Martinoni M, et al. Seizure outcome in surgically treated drug-resistant mesial temporal lobe epilepsy based on the recent histopathological classifications. J Neurosurg. 2013;119:37–47.
39. Nolan MA, Sakuta R, Chuang N, Otsubo H, Rutka JT, Snead OC III, et al. Dysembryoplastic neuroepithelial tumors in childhood: long-term outcome and prognostic features. Neurology. 2004;62:2270–6.
40. Sakuta R, Otsubo H, Nolan MA, Weiss SK, Hawkins C, Rutka JT, et al. Recurrent intractable seizures in children with cortical dysplasia adjacent to dysembryoplastic neuroepithelial tumor. J Child Neurol. 2005;20:377–84.
41. Rudà R, Trevisan E, Soffietti R. Epilepsy and brain tumors. Curr Opin Oncol. 2010;22:611–20.

42. Samudra N, Zacharias T, Plitt A, et al. Seizures in glioma patients: an overview of incidence, etiology, and therapies. J Neurol Sci. 2019;404:80–5.
43. Blumcke I, Luyken C, Urbach H, Schramm J, Wiestler OD. An isomorphic subtype of long-term epilepsy-associated astrocytomas associated with benign prognosis. Acta Neuropathol. 2004;107:381–8.
44. Berger MS, Ghatan S, Haglund MM, Dobbins J, Ojemann GA. Low-grade gliomas associated with intractable epilepsy: seizure outcome utilizing electrocorticography during tumor resection. J Neurosurg. 1993;79:62–9.
45. Hirsch JF, Sainte-Rose C, Kahn PA, et al. Benign astrocytic and oligodendrocytic tumors of the cerebral hemispheres in children. J Neurosurg. 1989;70:568–72.
46. Spencer DD, Spencer SS, Mattson RH, et al. Intracerebral masses in patients with intractable partial epilepsy. Neurology. 1984;34:432–6.
47. Olivier A, Boling WW, Tanriverdi T. Epilepsy and brain tumors. In: Olivier A, Boling WW, Tanriverdi T, editors. Techniques in epilepsy surgery. The MNI approach. Cambridge: University Press; 2012. p. 216–33.
48. Goldring S, Gregory GM. Experience with gliomas and lesions which mimic them in patients presenting with chronic seizure disorders. Part II. Clin Neurosurg. 1986;33:43–70.
49. Barba C, Coras R, Giordano F, Buccoliero AM, Genitori L, Blümcke I, Guerrini R. Intrinsic epileptogenicity of gangliogliomas may be independent from co-occurring focal cortical dysplasia. Epilepsy Res. 2011;97:208–13.
50. Rudà R, Bello L, Duffau H, Soffietti R. Seizures in low-grade gliomas: natural history, pathogenesis, and outcome after treatments. Neuro-Oncology. 2012;14:iv55. https://doi.org/10.1093/neuonc/nos199.
51. Pallud J, McKhann GM. Diffuse low-grade glioma-related epilepsy. Neurosurg Clin N Am. 2019;30(1):43–54.
52. Rosati A, Tomassini A, Pollo B, et al. Epilepsy in cerebral glioma: timing of appearance and histological correlations. J Neuro-Oncol. 2009;93: 395–400.
53. Campbell SL, Robel S, Cuddapah VA, et al. GABAergic disinhibition and impaired KCC2 cotransporter activity underlie tumor-associated epilepsy. Glia. 2015;63:23–36.
54. Van Breemen MS, Wilms EB, Vecht CJ. Epilepsy in patients with brain tumours: epidemiology, mechanisms, and management. Lancet Neurol. 2007;6:421–30.
55. Shamij MF, Fric-Shamij EC, Benoit BG. Brain tumors and epilepsy: pathophysiology of peritumoral changes. Neurosurg Rev. 2009;32:275–84.
56. Berntsson SG, Malmer B, Bondy ML, et al. Tumor-associated epilepsy and glioma: are there common genetic pathways? Acta Oncol. 2009;48:955–63.
57. Marucci G, Giulioni M. Pathological assessment of epilepsy surgery brain tissue. Pathologica. 2016;108:80–6.
58. Koelsche C, Wöhrer A, Jeibmann A, et al. Mutant BRAF V600E protein in ganglioglioma is predominantly expressed by neuronal tumor cells. Acta Neuropathol. 2013;125:891–900.
59. Lassaletta A, Zapotocky M, Bouffet E, et al. An integrative molecular and genomic analysis of pediatric hemispheric low-grade gliomas: an update. Childs Nerv Syst. 2016;32:1789–97.
60. Marucci G, de Biase D, Visani M, et al. Mutant BRAF in low-grade epilepsy-associated tumors and focal cortical dysplasia. Ann Clin Transl Neurol. 2014;1:130–4.
61. Chappé C, Padovani L, Scavarda D, et al. Dysembryoplastic neuroepithelial tumors share with pleomorphic xanthoastrocytomas and gangliogliomas BRAF V600E mutation and expresssion. Brain Pathol. 2013;23:574-83.
62. Liubinas SV, D'Abaco GM, Moffat BM, et al. IDH1 mutation is associated with seizures and protoplasmic subtype in patients with low-grade gliomas. Epilepsia. 2014;55:1438–43.
63. Montes JL, Rosenblatt B, Farmer J-P, et al. Lesionectomy of MRI detected lesions in children with epilepsy. Pediatr Neurosurg. 1995;22:167–73.
64. Morell F. Secondary epileptogenesis in man. Arch Neurol. 1985;42:318–35.
65. Rosenow F, Menzler K. Invasive EEG-studies in tumor-related epilepsy: when are they indicated and with what kind of electrodes? Epilepsia. 2013;54(Suppl.9):60–4.
66. Awad IA, Rosenfeld J, Ahl J, et al. Intractable epilepsy and structural lesions of the brain: mapping, resection strategies, and seizure outcome. Epilepsia. 1991;32:179–86.
67. Berger MS, Ojemann GA, Lettich E. Neurophysiological monitoring during astrocytoma surgery. Neurosurg Clin North Am. 1990;1:65–80.
68. Goldring S, Rich KM, Picker S. Experience with gliomas in patients presenting with a chronic seizure disorder. Clin Neurosurg. 1984;33:15.
69. Englot DJ, Berger MS, Barbaro NM, Chang EF. Factors associated with seizure freedom in the surgical resection of glioneuronal tumors. Epilepsia. 2012;53:51–7.
70. Ramantani G, Kadish NE, Anastasopoulos C, Brandt A, Wagner K, Strobl K, Mayer H, Schubert-Bast S, Stathi A, Korinthenberg R, Feuerstein TJ, Mader I, van Velthoven V, Zentner J, Schulze-Bonhage A. Epilepsy surgery for glioneuronal tumors in childhood: avoid loss of time. Neurosurgery. 2014;74:648–57.
71. Yang I, Chang EF, Han SJ, et al. Early surgical intervention in adult patients with ganglioglioma in associated with improved clinical seizure outcomes. J Clin Neurosci. 2011;18:29–33.
72. Bourgeois M, Sainte-Rose C, Lellouch-Tubiana A, et al. Surgery of epilepsy associated with focal lesions in childhood. J Neurosurg. 1999;90:833–42.

73. Cascino GD, Kelly PJ, Sharbrough FW, Hulihan JF, Hirschorn KA, Trenerry MR. Long-term follow-up of stereotactic lesionectomy in partial epilepsy: predictive factors and electroencephalographic results. Epilepsia. 1992;33:639–44.
74. Campos AR, Clusmann H, von Lehe M, et al. Simple and complex dysembryoplastic neuroepithelial tumors (DNT) variants: clinical profile, MRI, and histopathology. Neuroradiology. 2009;51:433–43.
75. Chassoux F, Rodrigo S, Mellerio C, Landré E, Miquel C, Turak B, Laschet J, Meder J-F, Roux F-X, Daumas-Duport C, Devaux B. Dysembryoplastic neuroepithelial tumors. An MRI-based scheme for epilepsy surgery. Neurology. 2012;79:1699–707.
76. Clusmann H, Kral T, Gleissner U, et al. Analysis of different types of resection for pediatric patients with temporal lobe epilepsy. Neurosurgery. 2004;54:847–60.
77. Hennessy MJ, Elwes RD, Honavar M, Rabe-Hesketh S, Binnie CD, Polkey CE. Predictors of outcome and pathological considerations in the surgical treatment of intractable epilepsy associated with temporal lobe lesions. J Neurol Neurosurg Psychiatry. 2001;70:450–8.
78. Raymond AA, Halpin SF, Alsanjari N, et al. Dysembryoplastic neuroepithelial tumor: features in 16 patients. Brain. 1994;117:461–75.
79. Schulze-Bonhage A, Zentner J. The preoperative investigation and surgical treatment of epilepsy. Deutsch Ärztebl Int. 2014;111:313–9.
80. Weyerbrock A, Zentner J. Epilepsiechirurgie bei Gliomen. In: Simon M, editor. Glomchirurgie. Heidelberg: Springer; 2018. p. 169–80.
81. Englot DJ, Berger MS, Barbaro NM, Chang EF. Predictors of seizure freedom after resection of supratentorial low-grade gliomas. J Neurosurg. 2011;115:240–4.
82. Giulioni M, Gardella E, Rubboli G, et al. Lesionectomy in epileptogenic gangliogliomas: seizure outcome and surgical results. J Clin Neurosci. 2006;13:529–35.
83. Clusmann H, Schramm J, Kral T, et al. Prognostic factors and outcome after different types of resection for temporal lobe epilepsy. J Neurosurg. 2002;97:1131–41.
84. Garcia-Fernández M, Fournier-Del CC, Ugalde-Canitrot A, et al. Epilepsy surgery in children with developmental tumors. Seizure. 2011;20;616–27.
85. Ozlen F, Gunduz A, Asan Z, et al. Dysembryoplastic neuroepithelial tumors and gangliogliomas: clinical results of 52 patients. Acta Neurochir. 2010;152:1661–71.
86. Rydenhag B, Flink R, Malmgren K. Surgical outcomes in patients with epileptogenic tumours and cavernomas in Sweden: good seizure control but late referrals. J Neurol Neurosurg Psychiatry. 2013;84(1):49–53.
87. Bilginer B, Yalnizoglu D, Soylemezoglu F, et al. Surgery for epilepsy in children with dysembryoplastic neuroepithelial tumor: clinical spectrum, seizure outcome, neuroradiology, and pathology. Childs Nerv Syst. 2009;25:485–91.
88. Burneo JG, Tellez-Zenteno J, Steven DA, et al. Adult-onset epilepsy associated with dysembryoplastic neuroepithelial tumors. Seizure. 2008;17:498–504.
89. Daumas-Duport C, Scheithauer BW, Chodkiewicz JP, Laws ER, Vedrenne C. Dysembryoplastic neuroepithelial tumor: a surgically curable tumor of young patients with intractable partial seizures. Neurosurgery. 1988;23:545–56.
90. Daumas-Duport C, Varlet P, Bacha S, Beuvon F, Cervera-Pierot P, Chodkiewicz JP. Dysembryoplastic neuroepithelial tumors: nonspecific histological forms: a study of 40 cases. J Neuro-Oncol. 1999;41:267–80.
91. Devaux B, Chassoux F, Guenot M, et al. Epilepsy surgery in France: evaluation of activity. Neurochirurgie. 2008;54:453–65.
92. Lee J, Lee BL, Joo EY, et al. Dysembryoplastic neuroepithelial tumors in pediatric patients. Brain and Development. 2009;31:671–81.
93. Sharma MC, Jain D, Gupta A, et al. Dysembryoplastic neuroepithelial tumor: a clinicopathological study of 32 cases. Neurosurg Rev. 2009;32:161–70.
94. Prayson RA. Diagnostic challenges in the evaluation of chronic epilepsy-related surgical neuropathology. Am J Surg Pathol. 2010;34:e1. https://doi.org/10.1097/PAS.0b013e3181d9ba38.
95. Takahashi A, Hong SC, Seo DW, Hong SB, Lee M, Suh YL. Frequent association of cortical dysplasia in dysembryoplastic neuroepithelial tumor treated by epilepsy surgery. Surg Neurol. 2005;64:419–27.
96. Li LM, Cendes F, Andermann F, et al. Surgical outcome in patients with epilepsy and dual pathology. Brain. 1999;122:799–805.
97. Schramm A, Luyken C, Urbach H, et al. Evidence for a clinically distinct new subtype of grade II astrocytomas in patients with long-term epilepsy. Neurosurgery. 2004;55:340–8.
98. Duffau H. Brain mapping in tumors: intraoperative or extra-operative? Epilepsia. 2013;54(Suppl. 9):78–82.
99. Hirsch M, Coenen VA, Heiland DH, Lützen N, Straszewski O, Schulze-Bonhage A. Epilepsieassoziierte Tumoren des Zentralnervensystems. Nervenarzt. 2015;87:402. https://doi.org/10.1007/s00115-015-0031-7.
100. Majores M, von Lehe M, Fassunke J, et al. Tumor recurrence and malignant progression of gangliogliomas. Cancer. 2008;113:3355–63.
101. Harvey AS, Cross JH, Shinnar S, et al. Pediatric epilepsy task force: defining the spectrum of international practice in pediatric epilepsy surgery patients. Epilepsia. 2008;49:146–55.
102. Cataltepe O, Turanli G, Yalnizoglu D, Topçu M, Akalan N. Surgical management of temporal lobe tumor-related epilepsy in children. J Neurosurg. 2005;102(Suppl 3):280–7.
103. Gaggero R, Consales A, Fazzini F, Mancardi MM, Baglietto MG, Nozza P, et al. Epilepsy associated

with supratentorial brain tumors under 3 years of life. Epilepsy Res. 2009;87:184–9.
104. Gilliam F, Wyllie E, Kashden J, Faught E, Kotagal P, Bebin M, et al. Epilepsy surgery outcome: comprehensive assessment in children. Neurology. 1997;48:1368–74.
105. Kim NR, Wang KC, Bang JS, Choe G, Park Y, Kim SK, et al. Glioblastomatous transformation of ganglioglioma: case re- port with reference to molecular genetic and flow cytometric analysis. Pathol Int. 2003;53:874–82.
106. Ko A, Kim SH, Kim SH, et al. Epilepsy surgery for children with low-grade epilepsy-associated tumors (LEATs): factors associated with seizure recurrence and cognitive function. Pediatr Neurol. 2019;91:50–6.
107. Ramantani G, Kadish NE, Strobl K, et al. Seizure and cognitive outcomes of epilepsy surgery in infancy and early childhood. Eur J Paediatr Neurol. 2013;17:498–506.

# MRI-Negative Epilepsies

# 10

*Nothing in life is to be feared, it is only to be understood. Now is the time to understand more, so that we may fear less.*

*Marie Curie*

## Contents



The presence or absence of a lesion can be based on MRI or on histopathological analysis [1]. In the proper sense, the term non-lesional implies the absence of a lesion not only on MRI, but also in histopathology [2], while the term MRI-negative refers to patients in whom presurgical MRI fails to demonstrate a potentially epileptogenic structural abnormality [3]. Since preoperative decision-making processes are based on MRI as the most precise imaging modality, most studies refer to MRI findings when distinguishing between lesional and non-lesional epilepsies, and in clinical praxis, the terms "non-lesional" and "MRI-negative" are used synonymously [4, 5] In principle, however, the definition of which epilepsies may be called MRI-negative remains dynamic and depends on the technology used and the interpretation of images.

Due to advancements in MRI technology and post-processing algorithms, the rate of MRI-negative epilepsies has significantly decreased. Subtle signal deviations and poorly visible lesions are now more clearly identified [6, 7, 8]. The rate of formerly overlooked FCD is likely around 30% [9–11], but rates as high as 41% [12] and 79% [13] have been reported. Automated volumetry and relaxometry analysis have been found to reveal signs of hippocampal sclerosis in 99% of patients with visually detected hippocampal sclerosis, and in 28% with visually normal



J. Zentner, *Surgical Treatment of Epilepsies*, https://doi.org/10.1007/978-3-030-48748-5_10

MRI findings [14]. Multi-parametric MRI in adequate angulation using volumetry, FLAIR and T2-weighted fast spin-echo sequences can detect neuronal loss in hippocampal sclerosis with an accuracy approximating histopathological analysis [15, 16]. Furthermore, temporal lobe epilepsy (TLE) coinciding with enlargement of the amygdala has been thought to represent a subtype of TLE that so far is classified as MRI-negative [17]. Therefore, from today's view, the synonymous use of the terms "MRI-negative" and "non-lesional" seems to be justified, while previous data on the frequency of MRI-negative epilepsies based on uncontrolled imaging quality do not allow this de facto equation.

## 10.1 Prevalence

In a systematic review and meta-analysis, Téllez-Zenteno et al. [2] comprised 40 articles including 697 patients with non-lesional and 2860 patients with lesional epilepsies. The overall prevalence of patients with non-lesional epilepsy in all surgical studies was 26%. It was significantly higher in extratemporal (45%) than in temporal (24%) location as well as in children (31%) compared to adults (21%). According to the above-mentioned limitations, the prevalence strongly depended on the method used to define non-lesional epilepsy: It was much higher in cases defined by MRI (44%) than by histopathology (16%) [2]. Overall, 20–40% of patients with drug-resistant focal epilepsy (dependent on quality of MRI), roughly 25% of patients with temporal epilepsy and 35% of those with extratemporal epilepsy, evaluated for surgery have been defined as MRI-negative [2, 3, 18–24]. Most reports on MRI-negative epilepsies refer to the temporal lobe [25–34].

## 10.2 Diagnostics

While a distinct MRI-lesion represents the most important feature pointing to the epileptogenic zone, its absence constitutes an obstacle against surgical candidacy and may lead to exclusion from presurgical evaluation and surgical treatment [35, 36]. Localization of seizure origin is even more challenging in children with MRI-negative epilepsy in whom widespread extratemporal epileptogenesis caused by malformations of cortical development is common. Thus, the lack of an MRI-detectable lesion calls for a more extensive and multimodal presurgical evaluation [35]. Assessment of MRI-negative epilepsies has been reviewed by So and Lee [6] and So and Ryvlin [3].

### 10.2.1 Diagnostic Tools

MRI-negative epilepsy is more easily localized and more successfully treated in temporal than in extratemporal location [37], and typical auras are of high localizing value [17]. Yet, with improved localization techniques, also MRI-negative extratemporal cases more frequently become amenable to surgical resection [17]. Advanced 3T-MRI techniques including voxel-based morphometric analysis and DTI, fMRI, MRS, MEG, FDG-PET coregistered with MRI, SPECT, and subtraction ictal SPECT coregistered to MRI (SISCOM) may demonstrate abnormalities pointing to the epileptogenic zone [17, 22, 38–43]. The localizing value of scalp EEG may be further enhanced by the use of electrical source imaging (ESI) [17, 44–46] and EEG-fMRI [47–49]. Frequently, intracranial EEG recordings using strip, grid, or depth electrodes (SEEG) [30, 32, 35] and/or ECoG [50] are required to localize the epileptogenic zone [6, 51, 52] (Figs. 10.1, 10.2, and 10.3).

### 10.2.2 Diagnostic Significance

Sensitivity of FDG-PET in MRI-negative temporal lobe epilepsy (TLE) was 84% [53], but only 19% in MRI-negative extratemporal epilepsy (ETE) [54]. However, correct localization of the epileptigenic area in ETE by focal or regional FDG-PET hypometabolism has been noted in 68% of patients by Rubí et al. [55] and in 84% by Chassoux et al. [56]. Coregistration of PET and MRI (PET-MRI) demonstrating relationships between the abnormal PET focus and the topographical anatomy was positive in 40% of FCD

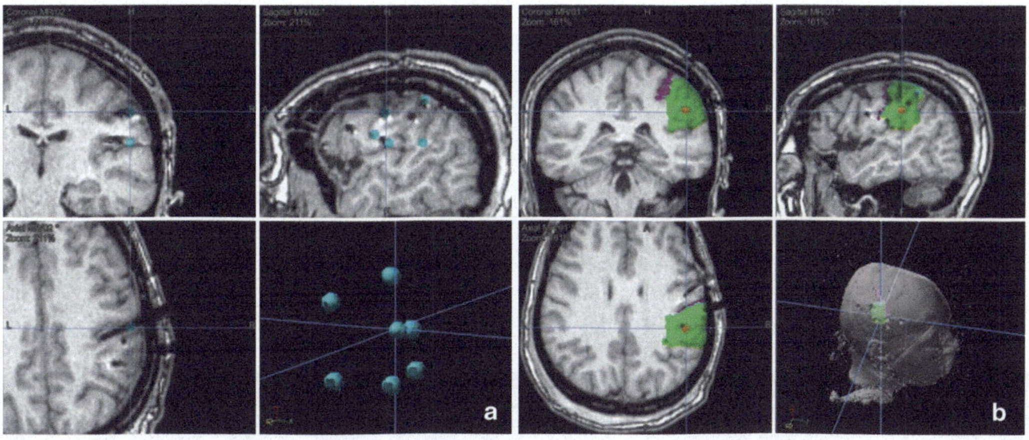


**Fig. 10.1** (**a**) Resection plan for MRI-negative epilepsy after intracranial EEG recordings with nine intracerebral depth electrodes. The relevant electrode contacts defining the epileptogenic zone haven been marked with blue dots. (**b**) The resection scheme is manually interpolated (green volume). The biopsy site is marked orange. The central sulcus is marked purple. (From Kogias et al. [51], with permission)

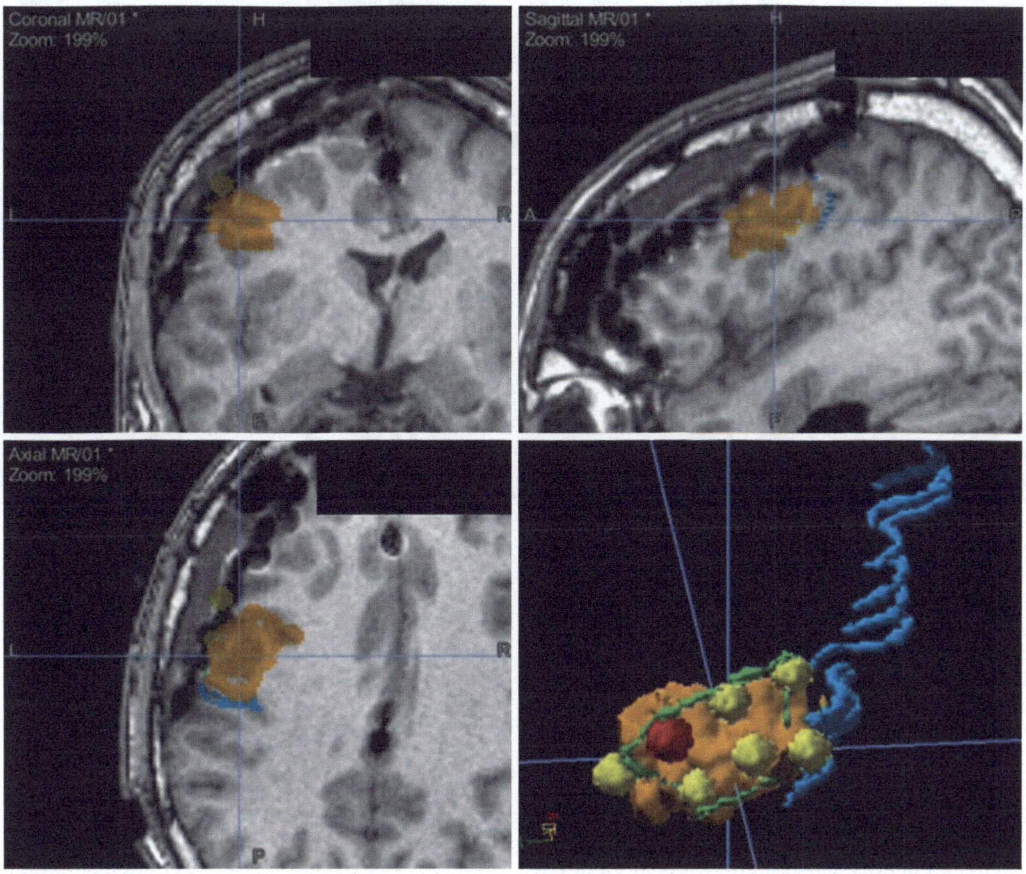


**Fig. 10.2** Resection plan for MRI-negative frontal lobe epilepsy after intracranial EEG recordings with subdural electrodes. The relevant electrode contacts defining the epileptogenic zone are marked yellow. The resection scheme is manually interpolated as an orange volume. The biopsy site is marked red. The precentral sulcus is marked light blue. (From Kogias et al. [51], with permission)

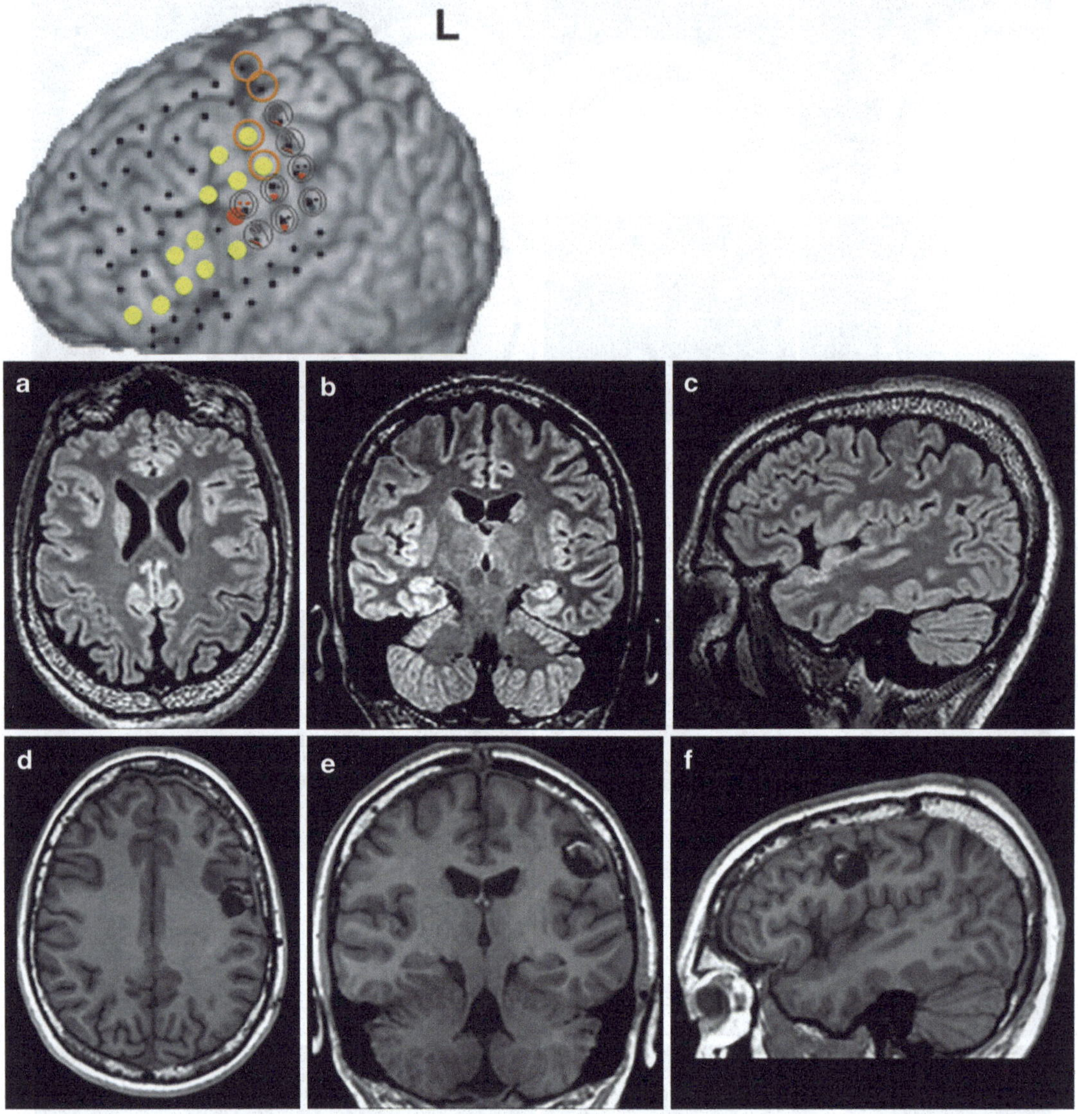


**Fig. 10.3** 20-year-old female patient with an MRI-negative left frontal lobe epilepsy suffering from versive and bilateral tonic-clonic seizures. Above: An 8 × 8 cm grid electrode was implanted for electrocorticography and extraoperative functional-topographic mapping. Yellow: language; orange: negative motor response; red dot: provocation of a habitual seizure corresponding to the epileptogenic area. Below: preoperative MRI in axial (**a**), coronal (**b**), and sagittal (**c**) view does not show any lesion. Corresponding postoperative MRI (**d–f**) demonstrate resection left frontolateral. Pathological evaluation of the operative specimen revealed a focal cortical dysplasia (Palmini type IIa). Postoperatively, the patient was completely seizure-free (Engel class Ia) without any neurological deficit

patients in whom optimized MRI studies were normal, and in 86% when there was a subtle focal MRI abnormality [57, 58]. Subtraction ictal SPECT coregistered to MRI (SISCOM) has been shown to have a sensitivity of 82% to localize an abnormal focus in MRI-negative temporal [25] and 77% in extratemporal [59] epilepsy patients.

Lee et al. [60] studied 89 temporal and extratemporal epilepsy patients with normal MRI. Diagnostic sensitivities of interictal EEG, ictal scalp EEG, FDG-PET, and SISCOM were 37.1%, 70.8%, 44.3%, and 41.1%, respectively. Jung et al. [61] reported 21 MRI-negative patients who had been investigated with MEG and intracranial EEG. They found that MEG modeling of spikes is a promising tool and that selection of patients for localization of the seizure focus by SEEG can be optimized by this technique. Smith et al. [62] noted that seizure freedom was achieved in 80% of cases when the MEG focus was resected, but only in 10% when it was not. Similarly, Oishi et al. [63] concluded that MEG may be useful to define the epileptogenic area.

Doelken et al. [54] investigated the contribution of morphometric MRI analysis in comparison to MEG, SPECT, and PET in 51 patients with MRI-negative epilepsy to a focus hypothesis based on seizure semiology and video-EEG monitoring. Sensitivity and specificity of voxel-based MR analysis were 24% and 96%, respectively. MEG sensitivity was 62%, and sensitivity of interictal and ictal SPECT were 20% and 50%, respectively. PET sensitivity was 19% in extratemporal and 82% in temporal location. The best concordance of morphometric analysis was noted with PET (88%) and MEG (80%), followed by interictal (63%) and ictal (60%) SPECT [54].

## 10.3 Surgical Treatment

A limited number of MRI-negative series mainly with small numbers of patients have been published so far. Despite the extensive and time-consuming presurgical work-up, surgical treatment of MRI-negative focal epilepsies carries significantly lower chances of postsurgical seizure freedom than lesional cohorts [2, 64]. A meta-analysis including 2860 lesional and 697 non-lesional patients reported a 2.5-times higher likelihood of a seizure-free outcome in the presence of a lesion on MRI or histopathology than when there was no structural abnormality to be resected [2]. Most studies summarize temporal and extratemporal MRI-negative epilepsies, as well as children and adults [4, 18, 22, 61, 65–67].

### 10.3.1 Overall Seizure Outcome

Seizure-free outcome (Engel I) in MRI-negative epilepsies has been reported in between 36% and 70% of cases [4, 66–71], and favorable outcome (Engel I–II) in between 41% and 83% [4, 18, 22, 25, 28, 33, 35, 37, 61, 65–67, 72–75]. Wang et al. [76] analyzing data of 90 MRI-negative patients, observed seizure freedom in 70% and 63% at 6 and 12 months follow-up, respectively. Evidence of a positive histopathology was significantly associated with seizure-free outcome at 6 months, but not at 12 months follow-up [76]. In the series of 89 non-lesional patients reported by Lee et al. [60], 47% were seizure-free, and 80% had a favorable outcome. Jayakar et al. [35] analyzed 102 MRI-negative patients, most of them being children. Resections were unilobar in 66 cases, and multilobar in 36. At 1-year follow-up, 43.6% of patients, at 5 years 46%, and at 10 years 37.2% were seizure-free [35]. A pediatric series comprising 22 patients [77] reported seizure freedom in 36%. Overall, seizure-free outcome in MRI-negative epilepsies mainly ranges between 30% and 50% [61, 78–80].

### 10.3.2 Temporal Lobe Epilepsies (TLE)

#### 10.3.2.1 Clinical Features

Clinical features of MRI-negative TLE include older age at seizure onset, and a lower rate of initial precipitating events, i.e., febrile seizures and infections [81]. Similar findings have been reported by others [17]. Kim et al. [82] found in MRI-negative temporal epilepsies a lower prevalence of auras, automatisms, and secondarily generalized seizures compared to lesional cases. These features have been associated with a milder course of the disease and better drug response compared to mesiotemporal lobe epilepsies (MTLE) based on hippocampal sclerosis (HS) [81]. While TLE in general has a high tendency to develop drug-resistance (up to 71%) [83], a longitudinal study on MRI-negative TLE showed that 43 of 73 patients (59%) had a mild course and were seizure-free or had ≤2 seizures per year for at least 3 years on medical treatment [84].

Similarly, favorable response on just 1 or 2 drugs with a mean seizure-free period of 4.3 years has been shown in 55% of MRI-negative TLE cases by others [83]. In these studies, familial cases of TLE which also tend to be associated with a late seizure onset and demonstrate a benign course along with a non-lesional MRI in a high percentage, have been excluded [85]. In sum, MRI-negative TLE seems to constitute a distinct syndrome running a milder course with better drug response as compared with classical MTLE caused by HS.

#### 10.3.2.2 Pathophysiological Aspects

In MRI-negative TLE, multifocal seizure onset and the presence of subcortical seizure generators have been suspected [86–88]. Muhlhofer et al. [17] found a greater tendency for secondary generalization of seizures which has been suggested to reflect an epileptogenic network more efficiently spreading ictal activity, or to indicate a lower epileptogenic threshold of the brain in MRI-negative TLE as compared to classical MTLE. The greater tendency for secondary generalization of seizures has been found to be associated with an up to 10.8-fold increased risk for seizure recurrence following surgical resection in the MRI-negative TLE cohort [28]. Immonen et al. [37] stated that primary involvement of lateral temporal neocortical rather than mesial structures constitutes the main pathophysiological basis of MRI-negative TLE, a view that has also been supported by others [17, 19].

#### 10.3.2.3 Seizure Outcome

In a systematic review and *meta-analysis*, Téllez-Zenteno et al. [2] comprising 20 articles including 398 patients found in non-lesional TLE 45% seizure-free patients as compared to 69% in lesional TLE. Based on MRI, seizure freedom was 51% in non-lesional, and 75% in lesional epilepsies. Evaluating histopathology, seizure freedom was 36% in non-lesional and 65% in lesional cases. Outcomes were similar in children and adults [2].

*Observational studies* report seizure-free outcome rates in MRI-negative patients varying between 18% and 80% [4, 18, 19, 25, 33, 37, 65, 67, 72, 78, 80, 89–91]. Fong et al. [28] found seizure freedom in 66% of cases at 2 years and in 47% at 7 or more years follow-up. In a series of 127 MRI-negative TLE patients, Grewal et al. [92] noted seizure freedom in 60% of cases. Alarcón et al. [65] found no significant differences in seizure control between individuals with normal and those with abnormal imaging: 92% with normal MRI, and 80% with abnormal imaging had a favorable outcome [65].

Overall, seizure-free outcome in MRI-negative temporal epilepsies is achieved in between 40% and 50% of patients [25, 33, 37, 69, 78, 79, 93, 94].

#### 10.3.2.4 FDG-PET and Seizure Outcome

Willmann et al. [95] assessed the predictive diagnostic value of PET on seizure outcome in a meta-analysis of 46 TLE studies. Ipsilateral PET hypometabolism showed a predictive value of 80% for a favorable outcome in patients with normal MRI, but did not appear to add value in MRI-positive cases. In line, focal temporal hypometabolism on FDG-PET ipsilateral to the EEG side of seizure onset has been found to be associated with Engel class I postoperative outcomes in 75–80% of MRI-negative TLE patients in other studies [19, 29, 53, 79, 96, 97]. Capraz et al. [98] compared in a series of 24 cases with unilateral temporal hypometabolism on FDG-PET patients with HS on MRI to those without. Seizure freedom was similar in both groups (79.2% in MRI-negative and 82% in HS patients). Similar results have been reported by others [19, 53, 65]. In addition, it has been shown that FDG-PET hypometabolism is not correlated with the degree of hippocampal cell loss [99]. In sum, data available clearly indicate that unilateral FDG-PET hypometabolism correlates with a favorable seizure outcome [37, 95].

#### 10.3.2.5 Prognostic Factors

The following preoperative prognostic factors indicating favorable seizure outcome have been identified for patients with MRI-negative temporal resections: History of febrile seizures [17, 100], short duration of epilepsy [17, 101], subtle non-specific MRI findings [17, 25, 28], absence of contralateral or extratemporal interictal epileptiform discharges [17, 25, 26, 33, 89, 101], absence of secondary generalized seizures [102–104], hypometabolism on FDG-PET [19, 29, 53, 79, 95–97], and concordance of a subtraction ictal SPECT coregistered to MRI (SISCOM) hyperperfusion focus to the resection site [17, 25, 28]. Conversely, a higher baseline seizure frequency and the presence of generalized tonic-clonic seizures have been identified as negative prognostic factors [17, 102–104]. Evaluating the role of intraoperative ECoG in 127 MRI-negative TLE patients who underwent ATL, Grewal et al. [92] showed that incomplete resection of tissue generating interictal epileptiform discharges (IED) was associated with an increased risk of seizure recurrence.

#### 10.3.2.6 Neuropsychological Outcome

The neuropsychological outcome of patients with non-lesional TLE strongly depends on the lateralization of seizures and surgery and is consistent with reports on lesional cases [105–107]. The most significant clinical finding is decline in verbal memory in patients undergoing resections in the dominant temporal lobe.

### 10.3.3 Extratemporal Epilepsies (ETE)

#### 10.3.3.1 Seizure Outcome

In a systematic review and *meta-analysis*, Téllez-Zenteno et al. [2] comprising 13 articles and 156 patients found in non-lesional ETE 34% seizure-free patients as opposed to 66% in lesional cases. Using MRI, seizure freedom was 35% in non-lesional and 60% lesional ETE cases. Based on histopathology, seizure freedom was 32% in non-lesional and 74% in lesional patients. There were no differences between children and adults [2]. Contrarily, the meta-analysis of Shaheryar et al. evaluating children and adults [108, 109] did not reveal significant differences in seizure outcome between patients with normal versus abnormal MRI findings. Ansari et al. [110] reported in his meta-analysis including 131 patients with non-lesional ETE seizure freedom (Engel I) in 45.8% of cases.

Seizure-free outcome in MRI-negative ETE has been reported in *observational studies* to range between 23% and 81% [65, 67, 68, 73, 111–120]. Analyzing 36 MRI-negative extratemporal patients, Delev et al. [13] noted Engel I outcome in 44%. Long-term seizure control rates of 42% at 2 years [121] and 38% at 10 years [122] follow-up have been reported. Favorable seizure outcomes have been shown in single cases of MRI-negative insular epilepsies [123–125]. In small 3T MRI-negative series, seizure-free outcomes between 50% and 65% have been reported [61, 79, 126]. Bauman et al. [113] favored resection of non-lesional epileptic foci in multiple stages in order to improve outcome. Overall, seizure-free outcome in MRI-negative ETE mainly ranges between 30% and 40% [2, 4, 127].

#### 10.3.3.2 Prognostic Factors

The following preoperative factors indicating favorable seizure outcome have been identified for MRI-negative ETE: Unspecific MRI abnormalities [21, 110], shorter duration of epilepsy [102], localizing ictal EEG findings [102], absence of generalized seizures [102, 110], FDG-PET hypometabolism [55, 56, 79, 128], and concordance of an SISCOM hyperperfusion focus to the resection site [128]. Age at surgery, age at seizure onset, duration of epilepsy, and seizure semiology did not significantly correlate with seizure outcome in the meta-analysis of Ansari et al. [110].

### 10.3.4 Multilobar Epilepsies

Patients with MRI-negative epilepsies requiring multilobar resection constitute a particularly challenging subgroup. This subgroup accounts for up to one-third of MRI-negative procedures [35, 129]. While most studies include single multilobar cases, only a few reports focus on MRI-negative multilobar epilepsy surgery presenting patient series. Long-term seizure freedom has been achieved in 25–52% of the cases [130–132]. Jayakar et al. [35] reported 102 patients with non-lesional epilepsy, and most of them were children. Thirty-six resections were multilobar, and 66 unilobar. Overall seizure-free outcome was 43.6% at 2-years follow-up, 46% at 5-years, and 37.2% at 10-years follow-up.

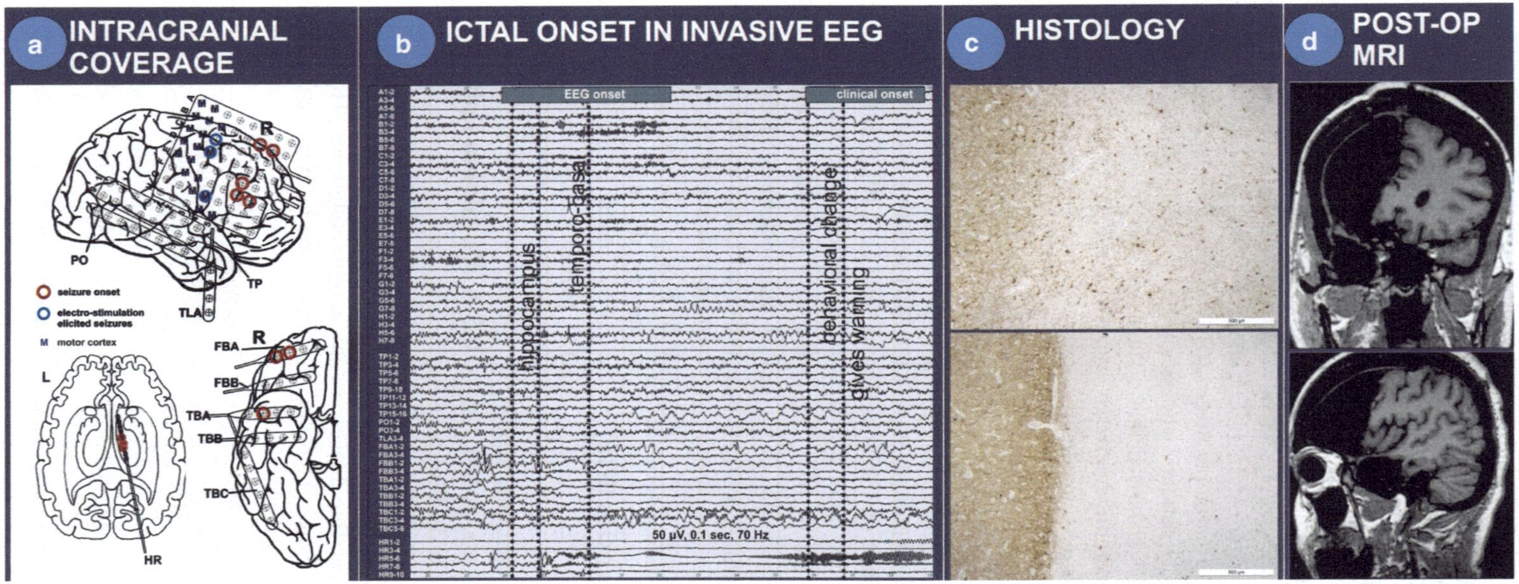


**Fig. 10.4** Thirty-five-year-old female patient with an MRI-negative right frontotemporal epilepsy. (**a**) Illustration of the subdural electrode coverage; (**b**) Temporomesial and temporobasal seizure onset shown on an intracranial EEG; (**c**) Histological slides (microtubule-associated protein 2 immunohistochemistry) show blurring of the gray-white matter boundaries with many ectopic white matter neurons in the epilepsy patient (Top) compared with relatively sharp gray-white matter boundaries with only isolated white matter neurons in a control patient (Bottom). Histopathological diagnosis was mMCD; (**d**) Postoperative MRI scans demonstrate frontal and temporal resection cavities including AHE in coronal (Top) and sagittal (Bottom) view. In addition, MST of the motor cortex have been performed. There were no postoperative deficits. During follow-up of 11 years, the patient remained completely seizure-free (Engel Ia). (From Kogias et al. [36], with permission)

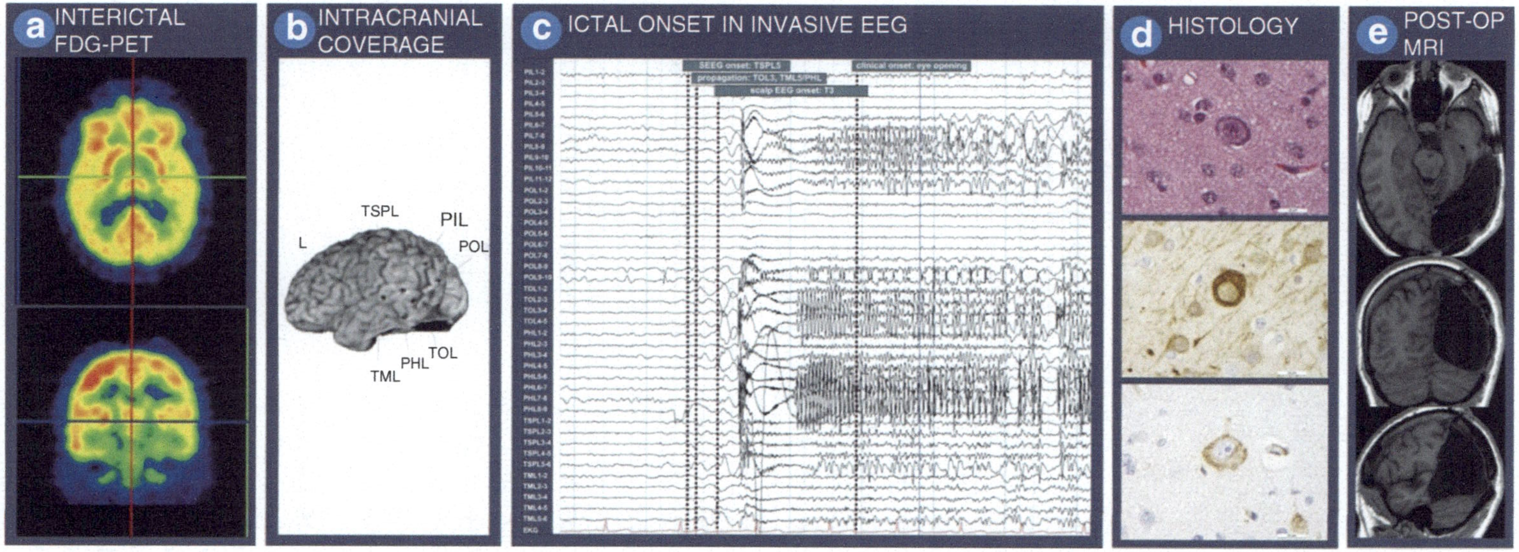


**Fig. 10.5** Fourteen-year-old female patient with an MRI-negative left temporo-parieto-occipital epilepsy. (**a**) Interictal FDG-PET shows left temporo-parieto-occipital hypometabolism; (**b**) Illustration of depth electrodes placed for SEEG; (**c**) Seizure onset shown on invasive EEG; (**d**) Histological slides demonstrate dysmorphic neurons with pathological accumulation of Nissl substance (hematoxylin and eosin stain) (Top), pathological accumulation of neurofilament protein (Middle), and immunoreactivity for phosphorylated S6 (Bottom). Histopathological diagnosis was FCD type IIa; (**e**) Postoperative MRI scans demonstrate the temporo-parieto-occipital resection cavity in the axial (Top), coronal (Middle), and sagittal (Bottom) planes. Wernicke's area has been spared. Postoperatively, the patient had a complete right hemianopia as expected, but no additional deficits. During follow-up of 2.2 years, she was almost seizure-free (Engel Ic). (From Kogias et al. [36], with permission)

There were no differences in outcome with respect to temporal versus extratemporal cases, one-stage versus two-stage procedures, and unilobar versus multilobar resections [35]. Kogias et al. [36] noted seizure freedom (Engel I) in 3 of the 4 patients with 3T MRI-negative drug-resistant focal epilepsy who had undergone multilobar resection (Figs. 10.4 and 10.5). In sum, seizure-free outcome rates after MRI-negative multilobar resections mainly range between 30% and 40% [35].

### Concluding Remarks

- ***Definition.*** *"MRI-negative" means the absence of an MRI-detectable lesion, while the term "non-lesional" refers to the absence of a specific abnormality on pathological evaluation. During the last years, the quality of MRI has enormously improved facilitating detection of subtle lesions to the range of 1 mm$^3$, that is to an accuracy approximating histopathological analysis. Therefore, from today's view, the synonymously use of the terms "MRI-negative" and "non-lesional" seems to be justified.*
- ***Characteristics.*** *MRI-negative epilepsies constitute a heterogeneous group of focal epilepsies amounting to 20–40% (dependent on quality of MRI) of surgical candidates in epilepsy centers. MRI-negative TLE seems to represent* a distinct syndrome *associated with a milder course of the disease and better drug response as compared to classical MTLE caused by HS and has been thought to primarily involve neocortical rather than mesiotemporal structures. Thus, classical ATL may be the treatment of choice.*
- ***Outcome.*** *Surgical results in MRI-negative epilepsies are less favorable as compared with lesional cases. However, careful selection of appropriate candidates using noninvasive and invasive EEG recordings and radionuclide imaging including FDG-PET and subtraction ictal SPECT coregistered to MRI (SISCOM) facilitates seizure-free outcome mainly ranging between 40% and 50% in temporal and between 30% and 40% in extratemporal and multilobar procedures.*

## References

1. Sinclair DB, Wheatley M, Aronyk K, Hao C, Snyder T, Colmers W, McKean JD. Pathology and neuroimaging in pediatric temporal lobectomy for intractable epilepsy. Pediatr Neurosurg. 2001;35:239–46.
2. Téllez-Zenteno JF, Hernández Ronquillo L, Moien-Afshari F, Wiebe S. Surgical outcomes in lesional and non-lesional epilepsy: a systematic review and meta-analysis. Epilepsy Res. 2010;89:310–8. https://doi.org/10.1016/j.eplepsyres.2010.02.007.
3. So EL, Ryvlin P. MRI-negative epilepsy. Cambridge: Cambridge University Press; 2015.
4. Siegel AM, Jobst BC, Thadani VM, Rhodes CH, Lewis PJ, Roberts DW, et al. Medically intractable, localization-related epilepsy with normal MRI: presurgical evaluation and surgical outcome in 43 patients. Epilepsia. 2001;42:883–8.
5. Pardoe H, Kuzniecky R. Advanced Imaging Techniques in the Diagnosis of Nonlesional Epilepsy: MRI, MRS, PET, and SPECT. Epilepsy Currents. 2014; 14 (3): 121–4.
6. So EL, Lee RW. Epilepsy surgery in MRI-negative epilepsies. Curr Opin Neurol. 2014;27:206–12.
7. Toledano R, Jimenez-Huete A, Campo P, et al. Small temporal pole encephalocele: a hidden cause of "normal" MRI temporal lobe epilepsy. Epilepsia. 2016;57:841–51.
8. Winston GP. Epilepsy surgery, vision, and driving: What has surgery taught us and could modern imaging reduce the risk of visual deficits? Epilepsia. 2013;54(11):1877–88.
9. Jin B, Krishnan B, Adler S, et al. Automated detection of focal cortical dysplasia type II with surface-based magnetic resonance imaging postprocessing and machine learning. Epilepsia. 2018;59:982–92.
10. Wagner J, Weber B, Urbach H, et al. Morphometric MRI analysis improves detection of focal cortical dysplasia type II. Brain. 2011a;134(10):2844–54.
11. Wagner J, Urbach H, Niehusmann P, et al. Focal cortical dysplasia type IIb: completeness of cortical, not subcortical, resection is necessary for seizure freedom. Epilepsia. 2011b;52 (8):1418–24.
12. Wang ZI, Jones SE, Jaisani Z, et al. Voxel-based morphometric magnetic resonance imaging (MRI) postprocessing in MRI-negative epilepsies. Ann Neurol. 2015;77(6):1060–75.
13. Delev D, Quesada CM, Grote A. A multimodal concept for invasive diagnostics and surgery based on neuronavigated voxel-based morphometric MRI postprocessing data in previously nonlesional epilepsy. J Neurosurg. 2018;128(4):1178–86.
14. Coan AC, Kubota B, Bergo FPG, et al. 3T MRI quantification of hippocampal volume and signal in mesial temporal lobe epilepsy improves detection of hippocampal sclerosis. AJNR Am J Neuroradiol. 2014;35:77–83.
15. Goubran M, Bernhardt BC, Cantor-Rivera D, et al. In vivo MRI signatures of hippocampal subfield

pathology in intractable epilepsy. Hum Brain Mapp. 2016;37:1103–19.
16. Urbach H, Mast H, Egger K, Mader I. Presurgical MR imaging in epilepsy. Clin Neuroradiol. 2015;25(Suppl 2):151–5.
17. Muhlhofer W, Tan Y-L, Mueller S, Knowlton R. MRI-negative temporal lobe epilepsy—what do we know? Epilepsia. 2017; https://doi.org/10.1111/epi.13699.
18. Bien CG, Szinay M, Wagner J, et al. Characteristics and surgical outcomes of patients with refractory magnetic resonance imaging-negative epilepsies. Arch Neurol. 2009;66:1491–9. https://doi.org/10.1001/archneurol.2009.283.
19. Carne RP, O'Brien TJ, Kilpatrick CJ, MacGregor LR, Hicks RJ, Murphy MA, Bowden SC, Kaye AH, Cook MJ. MRI-negative PET-positive temporal lobe epilepsy: a distinct surgically remediable syndrome. Brain. 2004;127:2276–85.
20. Cascino GD, Jack CRJ, Parisi JE, et al. Magnetic resonance imaging based volume studies in temporal lobe epilepsy: pathological correlations. Ann Neurol. 1991;30:31–6.
21. Englot DJ, Ouyang D, Garcia PA, et al. Epilepsy surgery trends in the United States, 1990–2008. Neurology. 2012;78:1200–6. https://doi.org/10.1212/WNL.0b013e318250d7ea.
22. Hong KS, Lee SK, Kim JY, Lee DS, Chung CK. Presurgical evaluation and surgical outcome of 41 patients with nonlesional neocortical epilepsy. Seizure. 2002;11:184–92.
23. Kutsy RL. Focal extratemporal epilepsy: clinical features, EEG patterns, and surgical approach. J Neurol Sci. 1999;166:1–15.
24. Semah F, Picot MC, Adam C, et al. Is the underlying cause of epilepsy a major prognostic factor for recurrence? Neurology. 1998;51:1256–62.
25. Bell ML, Rao S, So EL, et al. Epilepsy surgery outcomes in temporal lobe epilepsy with a normal MRI. Epilepsia. 2009;50:2053–60.
26. Burkholder DB, Sulc V, Hoffman EM, et al. Interictal scalp electroencephalography and intraoperative electrocorticography in magnetic resonance imaging-negative temporal lobe epilepsy surgery. JAMA Neurol. 2014;71:702–9.
27. Cukiert A, Burattini JA, Mariani PP, et al. Outcome after corticoamygdalohippocampectomy in patients with temporal lobe epilepsy and normal MRI. Seizure. 2010;19:319–23.
28. Fong JS, Lehi L, Najm I, et al. Seizure outcome and its predictors after temporal lobe epilepsy surgery in patients with normal MRI. Epilepsia. 2011;52:1393–401. https://doi.org/10.1111/j.1528-1167.2011.03091.x.
29. Kuba R, Tyrlikova I, Chrastina J, et al. "MRI-negative PET-positive" temporal lobe epilepsy: invasive EEG findings, histopathology, and postoperative outcomes. Epilepsy Behav. 2011;22:537–41.
30. Lee RW, Hoogs MM, Burkholder DB, et al. Outcome of intracranial electroencephalography monitoring and surgery in magnetic resonance imaging-negative temporal lobe epilepsy. Epilepsy Res. 2014;108:937–44.
31. Smith AP, Sani S, Kanner AM, et al. Medically intractable temporal lobe epilepsy in patients with normal MRI: surgical outcome in twenty-one consecutive patients. Seizure. 2011;20:475–9.
32. Suresh S, Sweet J, Fastenau PS, et al. Temporal lobe epilepsy in patients with nonlesional MRI and normal memory: an SEEG study. J Neurosurg. 2015;23:1368–74.
33. Sylaja PN, Radhakrishnan K, Kesavadas C, Sarma PS. Seizure outcome after anterior temporal lobectomy and its predictors in patients with apparent temporal lobe epilepsy and normal MRI. Epilepsia. 2004;45(7):803–8.
34. Vale FL, Effio E, Arredondo N, et al. Efficacy of temporal lobe surgery for epilepsy in patients with negative MRI for mesial temporal lobe sclerosis. J Clin Neurosci. 2012;19:101–6.
35. Jayakar P, Dunoyer C, Dean P, et al. Epilepsy surgery in patients with normal or nonfocal MRI scans: Integrative strategies offer long-term seizure relief. Epilepsia. 2008;49(5):758–64.
36. Kogias E, Schmeiser B, Dooskamp S, et al. Multilobar resections for 3T MRI-negative epilepsy: worth the trouble? World Neurosurg. 2019; https://doi.org/10.1016/j.wneu.2018.11.170.
37. Immonen L, Jutila A, Muraja-Murro E, Mervaala M, Äikiä S. Lamusuo, et al., Long-term epilepsy surgery outcomes in patients with MRI-negative temporal lobe epilepsy. Epilepsia. 2010;51:2260–9. https://doi.org/10.1111/j.1528-1167.2010.02720.x.
38. Bast T, Ramantani G, Boppel T, et al. Source analysis of interictal spikes in polymicrogyria: loss of relevant cortical fissures requires simultaneous EEG to avoid MEG misinterpretation. NeuroImage. 2005;25:1232–41.
39. Chassoux F, Rodrigo S, Semah F, et al. FDG-PET improves surgical outcome in negative MRI Taylor-type focal cortical dysplasias. Neurology. 2010;75:2168–75.
40. Davis KA, Nanga RPR, Das S, et al. Glutamate imaging (GluCEST) lateralizes epileptic foci in nonlesional temporal lobe epilepsy. Sci Transl Med. 2015;7:309ra161. https://doi.org/10.1126/scitranslmed.aaa7095.
41. Krsek P, Kudr M, Jahodova A, et al. Localizing value of ictal SPECT is comparable to MRI and EEG in children with focal cortical dysplasia. Epilepsia. 2013;54:351–8.
42. O'Brien TJ, So EL, Cascino GD, et al. Subtraction SPECT coregistered to MRI in focal malformations of cortical development: localization of the epileptogenic zone in epilepsy surgery candidates. Epilepsia. 2004;45:367–76.
43. Ramantani G, Boor R, Paetau R, et al. MEG versus EEG: influence of background activity on interictal spike detection. J Clin Neurophysiol. 2006;23:498–508.

44. Brodbeck V, Spinelli L, Lascano AM, et al. Electrical source imaging for presurgical focus localization in epilepsy patients with normal MRI. Epilepsia. 2010;51:583–91.
45. Ramantani G, Dümpelmann M, Koessler L, et al. Simultaneous subdural and scalp EEG correlates of frontal lobe epileptic sources. Epilepsia. 2014;55:278–88.
46. Rikir E, Koessler L, Gavaret M, et al. Electrical source imaging in cortical malformation-related epilepsy: a prospective EEG-SEEG concordance study. Epilepsia. 2014;55:918–32.
47. Jacobs J, Menzel A, Ramantani G, et al. Negative BOLD in default-mode structures measured with EEG-MREG is larger in temporal than extratemporal epileptic spikes. Front Neurosci. 2014;8:335.
48. Jacobs J, Stich J, Zahneisen B, et al. Fast fMRI provides high statistical power in the analysis of epileptic networks. NeuroImage. 2014;88:282–94.
49. Jäger V, Dümpelmann M, LeVan P, et al. Concordance of epileptic networks associated with epileptic spikes measured by high-density EEG and fast fMRI. PLoS One. 2015;10:e0140537.
50. Luther N, Rubens E, Sethi N, et al. The value of intraoperative electrocorticography in surgical decision making for temporal lobe epilepsy with normal MRI. Epilepsia. 2011;52:941–8.
51. Kogias E, Evangelou P, Schmeiser B, et al. The oxymoron of image-guided resection in 3 T MRI-negative extratemporal epilepsy: technique and postoperative results. Clin Neurol Neurosurg. 2018;166:16–22.
52. Kogias E, Altenmüller D-M, Klingler J-J, et al. Histopathology of 3 Tesla MRI-negative temporal lobe epilepsies. J Clin Neurosci. 2018;47:273–7.
53. Gok B, Jallo G, Hayeri R, et al. The evaluation of FDG-PET imaging for epileptogenic focus localization in patients with MRI positive and MRI negative temporal lobe epilepsy. Neuroradiology. 2013;55:541–50.
54. Doelken MT, Mennecke A, Huppertz HJ, et al. Multimodality approach in cryptogenic epilepsy with focus on morphometric 3T MRI. J Neuroradiol. 2012;39:87–96.
55. Rubí S, Setoain X, Donaire A, et al. Validation of FDG-PET/MRI coregistration in nonlesional refractory childhood epilepsy. Epilepsia. 2011;52:2216–24.
56. Chassoux F, Devaux B, Landré E, et al. Stereoelectroencephalography in focal cortical dysplasia: a 3D approach to delineating the dysplastic cortex. Brain. 2000;123:1733–51.
57. Salamon N, Kung J, Shaw SJ, et al. FDG-PET/MRI coregistration improves detection of cortical dysplasia in patients with epilepsy. Neurology. 2008;71:1594–601.
58. Colombo N, Salamon N, Raybaud C, et al. Imaging of malformations of cortical development. Epileptic Disord. 2009;11:194–205.
59. O'Brien T, So E, Mullan P, et al. Subtraction periictal SPECT is predictive of extratemporal epilepsy surgery outcome. Neurology. 2000;55:1668–76.
60. Lee SK, Lee SY, Kim KK, Hong KS, Lee DS, Chung CK. Surgical outcome and prognostic factors of cryptogenic neocortical epilepsy. Ann Neurol. 2005;58:525–32.
61. Jung J, Bouet R, Delpuech C, et al. The value of magnetoencephalography for seizure-onset zone localization in magnetic resonance imaging-negative partial epilepsy. Brain. 2013;136:3176–86.
62. Smith JR, King DW, Park YD, et al. A 10-year experience with magnetic source imaging in the guidance of epilepsy surgery. Stereotact Funct Neurosurg. 2003;80:14–7.
63. Oishi M, Kameyama S, Masuda H, et al. Single and multiple clusters of magnetoencephalographic dipoles in neocortical epilepsy: significance in characterizing the epileptogenic zone. Epilepsia. 2006;47:355–64.
64. Liava A, Francione S, Tassi L, Lo Russo G, Cossu M, Mai R, et al. Individually tailored extratemporal epilepsy surgery in children: anatomo-electro-clinical features and outcome predictors in a population of 53 cases. Epilepsy Behav. 2012; 25(1):68–80.
65. Alarcón G, Valentin A, Watt C, Selway RP, Lacruz ME, Elwes RD, Jarosz JM, Honavar M, Brunhuber F, Mullatti N, Bodi I, Salinas M, Binnie CD, Polkey CE. Is it worth pursuing surgery for epilepsy in patients with normal neuroimaging? J Neurol Neurosurg Psychiatry. 2006;77:474–80.
66. Blume W, Ganapathy GR, Munoz D, Lee DH. Indices of resective surgery effectiveness for intractable nonlesional focal epilepsy. Epilepsia. 2004;45(1):46–53.
67. Chapman K, Wyllie E, Najm I, Ruggieri P, Bingaman W, Luders J, Kotagal P, Lachhwani D, Dinner D, Luders HO. Seizure outcome after epilepsy surgery in patients with normal preoperative MRI. J Neurol Neurosurg Psychiatry. 2005;76:710–3.
68. Ferrier CH, Engelsman J, Alarcon G, et al. Prognostic factors in presurgical assessment of frontal lobe epilepsy. J Neurol Neurosurg Psychiatry. 1999;66:350–6.
69. Jeha LE, Najm IM, Bingaman WE, Khandwala F, Widdess-Walsh P, Morris HH, Dinner DS, Nair D, Foldvary-Schaeffer N, Prayson RA, Comair Y, O'Brien R, Bulacio J, Gupta A, Luders HO. Predictors of outcome after temporal lobectomy for the treatment of intractable epilepsy. Neurology. 2006;66:1938–40.
70. Stavem K, Bjornaes H, Langmoen IA. Predictors of seizure outcome after temporal lobectomy for intractable epilepsy. Acta Neurol Scand. 2004; 109:244–9.
71. Wieshmann UC, Larkin D, Varma T, Eldridge P. Predictors of outcome after temporal lobectomy for refractory temporal lobe epilepsy. Acta Neurol Scand. 2008;118:306–12.
72. Feng R, Hu J, Pan L, et al. Surgical treatment of MRI negative temporal lobe epilepsy based on PET: a retrospective cohort study. Stereotact Funct Neurosurg. 2014;92:354–9. https://doi.org/10.1159/000365575.
73. Cukiert A, Buratini JA, Machado E, et al. Results of surgery in patients with refractory extratempo-

ral epilepsy with normal or nonlocalizing magnetic resonance findings investigated with subdural grids. Epilepsia. 2001a;42:889–94.
74. Kim S, Mountz JM. SPECT imaging of epilepsy: an overview and comparison with F-18 FDG PET. Int J Mol Imaging. 2011;2011(10):1–9.
75. Cohen-Gadol AA, Bradley CC, Williamson A, Kim JH, Westerveld M, Duckrow RB, Spencer DD. Normal magnetic resonance imaging and medial temporal lobe epilepsy: the clinical syndrome of paradoxical temporal lobe epilepsy. J Neurosurg. 2005;102:902–9.
76. Wang ZI, Alexopouzlos AV, Jones SE, et al. The pathology of magnetic-resonance imaging-negative epilepsy. Mod Pathol. 2013;26:1051–8.
77. Ramachandran Nair R, Otsubo H, Shroff MM, Ochi A, Weiss SK, Rutka JT, Snead OC 3rd. MEG predicts outcome following surgery for intractable epilepsy in children with normal or nonfocal MRI findings. Epilepsia. 2007;48:149–57.
78. Berkovic SF, McIntosh AM, Kalnins RM, Jackson GD, Fabinyi GC, Brazenor GA, Bladin PF, Hopper JL. Preoperative MRI predicts outcome of temporal lobectomy: an actuarial analysis. Neurology. 1995;45:1358–63.
79. Kogias E, Klingler J-H, Urbach H, et al. 3 Tesla MRI-negative focal epilepsies: presurgical evaluation, postoperative outcome and predictive factors. Clin Neurol Neurosurg. 2017;163:116–20.
80. Scott CA, Fish DR, Smith SJM, et al. Presurgical evaluation of patients with epilepsy and normal MRI: role of scalp video-EEG telemetry. J Neurol Neurosurg Psychiatry. 1999;66:69–71.
81. Labate A, Aguglia U, Tripepi G, et al. Long-term outcome of mild mesial temporal lobe epilepsy: the National General Practice Study of Epilepsy. The syndromic classification of the International League Against Epilepsy applied to epilepsy in a general population. A prospective longitudinal cohort study. Neurology. 2016;86:1904–10.
82. Kim J, Kim SH, Lim SC, et al. Clinical characteristics of patients with benign nonlesional temporal lobe epilepsy. Neuropsychiatr Dis Treat. 2016;12:1887–91.
83. Hernandez-Ronquillo L, Buckley S, Ladino LD, et al. How many adults with temporal epilepsy have a mild course and do not require epilepsy surgery? Epileptic Disord. 2016;18:137–47.
84. Aguglia U, Gambardella A, Le Piane E, et al. Mild non-lesional temporal lobe epilepsy. A common, unrecognized disorder with onset in adulthood. Can J Neurol Sci. 1998;25:282–6.
85. Kobayashi E, Lopes-Cendes I, Guerreiro CA, et al. Seizure outcome and hippocampal atrophy in familial mesial temporal lobe epilepsy. Neurology. 2001;56:166–72.
86. Salanova V, Markand O, Worth R. Temporal lobe epilepsy: analysis of failures and the role of reoperation. Acta Neurol Scand. 2005;111:126–33.
87. Siegel AM, Cascino GD, Meyer FB, McClelland RL, So EL, Marsh WR, Scheithauer BW, Sharbrough FW. Resective reoperation for failed epilepsy surgery: seizure outcome in 64 patients. Neurology. 2004;63:2298–302.
88. Wyler AR, Hermann BP, Richey ET. Results of reoperation for failed epilepsy surgery. J Neurosurg. 1989;71:815–9.
89. Holmes MD, Born DE, Kutsy RL, Wilensky AJ, Ojemann GA, Ojemann LM. Outcome after surgery in patients with refractory temporal lobe epilepsy and normal MRI. Seizure. 2000;9:407–11.
90. McIntosh AM, Wilson SJ, Berkovic SF. Seizure outcome after temporal lobectomy: current research practice and findings. Epilepsia. 2001;42:1288–307.
91. Radhakrishnan K, So EL, Silbert PL, Jack CR Jr, Cascino GD, Sharbrough FW, O'Brien PC. Predictors of outcome of anterior temporal lobectomy for intractable epilepsy: a multivariate study. Neurology. 1998;51:465–71.
92. Grewal SS, Alvi MA, Perkins WJ, et al. Reassessing the impact of intraoperative electrocorticography on postoperative outcome of patients undergoing standard temporal lobectomy for MRI-negative temporal lobe epilepsy. J Neurosurg. 2019; https://doi.org/10.3171/2018.11.JNS182124.
93. Cohen-Gadol AA, Bradley CC, Williamson A, Kim JH, Westerveld M, Duckrow RB, Spencer DD. Normal magnetic resonance imaging and medial temporal lobe epilepsy: the clinical syndrome of paradoxical temporal lobe epilepsy. J Neurosurg. 2005;102:902–9.
94. Ivanovic J, Larsson PG, Ostbury Y, et al. Seizure outcomes of temporal lobe epilepsy surgery in patients with normal MRI and without specific histopathology. Acta Neurochir. 2017; https://doi.org/10.1007/s00701-017-3127-y.
95. Willmann O, Wennberg R, May T, et al. The contribution of 18 FDG PET in preoperative epilepsy surgery evaluation for patients with temporal lobe epilepsy: a meta-analysis. Seizure. 2007;16:509–20.
96. LoPinto-Khoury C, Sperling MR, Skidmore C, et al. Surgical outcome in PET-positive, MRI-negative patients with temporal lobe epilepsy. Epilepsia. 2012;53:342–8.
97. Yang P-F, Pei J-S, Zhang H-J, et al. Long-term epilepsy surgery outcomes in patients with PET-positive. MRI-negative temporal lobe epilepsy. Epilepsy Behav. 2014;41:91–7.
98. Capraz IY, Kurt G, Akdemir O, et al. Surgical outcome in patients with MRI-negative. PET-positive temporal lobe epilepsy. Seizure. 2015;29:63–8.
99. Foldvary N, Lee N, Hanson MW, et al. Correlation of hippocampal neuronal density and FDG-PET in mesial temporal lobe epilepsy. Epilepsia. 1999;40:26–9.
100. Tonini C, Beghi E, Berg AT, et al. Predictors of epilepsy surgery outcome: a meta-analysis. Epilepsy Res. 2004;62:75–87.
101. Wang X, Zhang C, Wang Y, et al. Prognostic factors for seizure outcome in patients with MRI-negative temporal lobe epilepsy: a meta-analysis and systematic review. Seizure. 2016;38:54–62.
102. Englot DJ, Breshears JD, Sun PP, Chang EF, Auguste KI. Seizure outcomes after resective surgery for extra-temporal lobe epilepsy in pediatric patients. J Neurosurg Pediatr. 2013;12(2):126–33.

103. Barba C, Rheims S, Minotti L, et al. Temporal plus epilepsy is a major determinant of temporal lobe surgery failures. Brain 2016;139(Pt 2):444–51.
104. Schmeiser B, Hammen T, Steinhoff BJ, et al. Long-term outcome characteristics in mesial temporal lobe epilepsy with and without associated cortical dysplasia. Epilepsy Res. 2016:147–56.
105. Trenerry MR, Jack CR Jr, Ivnik RJ, Sharbrough FW, Cascino GD, Hirschorn KA, Marsh WR, Meyer WR, Meyer FB. MRI hippocampal volumes and memory function before and after temporal lobectomy. Neurology. 1993;43:1800–5.
106. Rausch R, Kraemer S, Pietras CJ, Le M, Vickrey BG, Passaro EA. Early and late cognitive changes following temporal lobe surgery for epilepsy. Neurology. 2003;60:951–9.
107. Stroup E, Langfitt J, Berg M, McDermott M, Pilcher W, Como P. Predicting verbal memory decline following anterior temporal lobectomy. Neurology. 2003;60:1266–73.
108. Shaheryar FA, Tubbs RS, Tery CL, Cohen-Gadol AA. Surgery for extratemporal nonlesional epilepsy in adults: an outcome meta-analysis. Acta Neurochir. 2010;152:1299–305.
109. Shaheryar FA, Maher CO, Tubbs RS, Terry CL, Cohen-Gadol AA. Surgery for extratemporal nonlesional epilepsy in children: a meta-analysis. Childs Nerv Syst. 2010;26:945–51.
110. Ansari SF, Tubbs RS, Terry CL, et al. Surgery for extratemporal nonlesional epilepsy in adults: an outcome meta-analysis. Acta Neurochir. 2010;152:1299–305.
111. Arya R, Leach JL, Horn PS, et al. Clinical factors predict surgical outcomes in pediatric MRI-negative drug-resistant epilepsy. Seizure. 2016;41:56–61.
112. Wetjen NM, Marsh WR, Meyer FB, Cascino GD, So E, Britton JW, Stead SM, Worrell GA. Intracranial electroencephalography seizure onset patterns and surgical outcomes in nonlesional extratemporal epilepsy. J Neurosurg. 2009;110:1147–52.
113. Bauman JA, Feoli E, Romanelli P, Doyle WK, Devinsky O, Weiner HL. Multistage epilepsy surgery: safety, efficacy, and utility of a novel approach in pediatric extratemporal epilepsy. Neurosurgery. 2005;56:318–34.
114. Centeno RS, Yacubian EM, Sakamoto AC, Ferraz AF, Junior HC, Cavalheiro S. Presurgical evaluation and surgical treatment in children with extratemporal epilepsy. Childs Nerv Syst. 2006;22:945–59.
115. Jeha LE, Najm I, Bingaman W, Dinner D, Widdess-Walsh P, Lüders H. Surgical outcome and prognostic factors of frontal lobe epilepsy surgery. Brain. 2007;130:574–84.
116. Siegel AM, Cascino GD, Meyer FB, Marsh WR, Scheithauer BW, Sharbrough FW. Surgical outcome and predictive factors in adult patients with intractable epilepsy and focal cortical dysplasia. Acta Neurol Scand. 2006;113:65–71.
117. Terra-Bustamante VC, Fernandes RM, Inuzuka LM, Velasco TR, Alexandre V Jr, Wichert-Ana L, Funayama S, Garzon E, Santos AC, Araujo D, Walz R, Assirati JA, Machado HR, Sakamoto AC. Surgically amenable epilepsies in children and adolescents: clinical, imaging, electrophysiological, and post-surgical outcome data. Childs Nerv Syst. 2005;21:546–51.
118. Elsharkawy AE, Pannek H, Schulz R, Hoppe M, Pahs G, Gyimesi C, et al. Outcome of extratemporal epilepsy surgery experience of a single center. Neurosurgery. 2008;63:516–25.
119. Kral T, Clusmann H, Blümcke I, Fimmers R, Ostertun B, Kurthen M, et al. Outcome of epilepsy surgery in focal cortical dysplasia. J Neurol Neurosurg Psychiatry. 2003;74:183–8.
120. Kutsy RL. Focal extratemporal epilepsy: clinical features, EEG patterns, and surgical approach. J Neurol Sci. 1999;166:1–15.
121. See S-J, Jehi LE, Vadera S, et al. Surgical outcomes in patients with extratemporal epilepsy and subtle or normal magnetic resonance imaging findings. Neurosurgery. 2013;73:68–77.
122. Noe K, Sulc V, Wong-Kisiel L, et al. Long-term outcomes after nonlesional extratemporal lobe epilepsy surgery. JAMA Neurol. 2013;70:1003–8.
123. Chiosa V, Granziera C, Spinelli L, et al. Successful surgical resection in non-lesional operculo-insular epilepsy without intracranial monitoring. Epileptic Disord. 2013;15:148–57.
124. Malak R, Bouthillier A, Carmant L, et al. Microsurgery of epileptic foci in the insular region: clinical article. J Neurosurg. 2009;110:1153–63.
125. Nguyen DK, Nguyen DB, Malak R, et al. Revisiting the role of the insula in refractory partial epilepsy. Epilepsia. 2009;50:510–20.
126. Shi J, Lacuey N, Lhatoo S. Surgical outcome of MRI-negative refractory extratemporal lobe epilepsy. Epilepsy Res. 2017;133:103–8. https://doi.org/10.1016/j.eplepsyres.2017.04.010.
127. Mosewich RK, So EL, O'Brien TJ, et al. Factors predictive of the outcome of frontal lobe epilepsy surgery. Epilepsia. 2000;41:843–9.
128. Kudr M, Krsek P, Marusic P, et al. SISCOM and FDG-PET in patients with non-lesional extratemporal epilepsy: correlation with intracranial EEG, histology, and seizure outcome. Epileptic Disord. 2013;15(1):3–13.
129. Park SA, Lim SR, Kim GS, et al. Ictal electrocorticographic findings related with surgical outcomes in nonlesional neocortical epilepsy. Epilepsy Res. 2002;48:199–206.
130. Cho EB, Joo EY, Seo D-W, Hong S-C, Hong SB. Prognostic role of functional neuroimaging after multilobar resection in patients with localization related epilepsy. PLoS One. 2015;10:e0136565.
131. Nilsson DT, Malmgren K, Flink R, Rydenhag B. Outcomes of multilobar resections for epilepsy in Sweden 1990-2013: a national population-based study. Acta Neurochir (Wien). 2016;158:1151–7.
132. Sarkis RA, Jehi L, Najm IM, Kotagal P, Bingaman WE. Seizure outcomes following multilobar epilepsy surgery. Epilepsia. 2012;53:44–50.

# 11 Pediatric Epilepsy Surgery

*The true measure of any society can be found in how it treats its most vulnerable members.*

*Mahatma Gandhi*

## Contents





J. Zentner, *Surgical Treatment of Epilepsies*, https://doi.org/10.1007/978-3-030-48748-5_11

Epilepsy is one of the most frequent neurologic diseases in the pediatric age group, particularly in the first years of life [1]. Cohort studies have shown that 50–70% of children achieve long-term seizure freedom under anticonvulsive drug treatment, while 20–25% present persistent seizures, and 10–15% fulfill the criteria of pharmacoresistance [2]. Pharmacoresistance presents early in the course of epilepsy, and its most reliable predictor is the presence of a structural brain lesion [3]. This emphasizes the importance of MR imaging, whereby interpretation of images is challenging in the very young age (see also below). In addition to the seizure burden, there is a noticeable disparity in cognitive development between children with epilepsy and their healthy peers. Epilepsy onset in the first years of life, with poor response to anti-seizure drugs and frequent epileptic seizures, will eventually result in developmental stagnation or even regression. This may be related to the underlying brain pathology causing the epilepsy. However, the most important negative impact certainly arises from the epileptic seizures themselves, the influence of epileptic activity on cognitive networks, and the effect of anti-seizure drugs on the developing brain since this disparity in cognitive development continuously increases with the duration of epilepsy [4–6].

Over 20 years ago, Asarnow et al. [7] were the first to demonstrate the superior seizure outcome of surgical treatment for infantile spasms compared to pharmacotherapy, thus advocating for epilepsy surgery in young children with severe epilepsy. In a multicenter, observational cohort study in Far-East Asia (the FACE study) comparing infants and young children with epileptic encephalopathy who underwent surgical or anti-seizure drug treatment, more favorable seizure outcomes were noted in those that had resective surgery [8]. These results have been confirmed in a randomized controlled trial providing unequivocal evidence of the superiority of epilepsy surgery in selected children and adolescents over further anti-seizure drug trials [9]. In addition to the relief of seizures, those studies clearly demonstrated beneficial effects of surgery on cognitive functions. Therefore, beyond seizure freedom, the postsurgical stabilization or even improvement of cognitive development constitutes a fundamental objective of epilepsy surgery in the pediatric age [4].

## 11.1 Special Features of Pediatric Epilepsy Surgery

Epilepsy surgery in the pediatric age features several special characteristics, such as the broad spectrum of age-specific epileptic syndromes, the typical range of predominant etiologies, and the age-dependent variability of clinical and electroencephalographic seizure patterns associated with focal lesions [10–14]. In addition, epilepsies in the first years of life pose special challenges (see also below). Currently, a shift towards epilepsy surgery in the pediatric age in general, and towards more complex cases in particular is faced [15–17]. This trend especially reflects advancements in MR imaging facilitating detection of cortical malformations in extratemporal location as the most frequent etiologies in the pediatric age. Moreover, the growing body of evidence that early epilepsy surgery in selected candidates has excellent results regarding both seizure control and cognitive development has led to a more open attitude and a lower threshold of pediatric neurologists and epileptologists towards epilepsy surgery and to refer children and adolescents to epilepsy centers in order to evaluate surgical options [11, 18–20].

### 11.1.1 Trend to Early Surgery

Several nationwide surveys document a noticeable increase in the volume of pediatric epilepsy surgery in recent years [15, 17, 21]. Barba et al. [22] reported data of 20 epilepsy centers in 10 European countries including 1859 pediatric operations between 2008 and 2015. The proportion of surgeries significantly increased over time with an enormous increase in extratemporal and a decrease in temporal surgeries [22]. In a high-volume tertiary epilepsy center with 580 pediatric epilepsy surgery cases over almost 20 years, pediatric surgical cases doubled in the later years (1998–2008) compared to the earlier years (1986–1997) [16]. The shift to younger ages within the spectrum of epilepsy surgery candidates is supported by the current trend to offer surgery as soon as intractability is ascertained, including the first years of life [8, 11, 13, 18–20, 23, 24]. In contrast to the growing numbers of pediatric epilepsy surgery, frequency of epilepsy surgery in the adult age is relatively stagnant or even decreasing as shown in a recent large monocentric study [25].

### 11.1.2 Etiology

The most frequent etiologies of pediatric focal epilepsy amenable to surgery are developmental lesions, including focal cortical dysplasias (FCD) and glioneuronal tumors, such as dysembryoblastic neuroepithelial tumors (DNET) and gangliogliomas (GG). The ILAE survey of 2004, comprising 401 children and adolescents from 20 epilepsy centers worldwide, noted the following etiologies in descending order: FCD (42%), glioneuronal tumors (19%), perinatal ischemic lesions (10%), phacomatosis (tuberous sclerosis, Sturge–Weber syndrome), hemispheric syndromes (Rasmussen's encephalitis, hemimegalencephaly), and hypothalamic hamartomas [26]. Similar pathological results have been reported by the European Epilepsy Brain Bank (EEBB) comprising 2623 children and adolescents [27]: Cortical malformations (39%), glioneuronal tumors (27%), hippocampal sclerosis (15%), glial scar (6%), encephalitis (3%), vascular malformations (3%), and no specific lesion (6%). In line with these studies, the etiological spectrum of children and adolescents who underwent epilepsy surgery in the Freiburg series included mainly FCD (55%), glioneuronal and rarely other low-grade tumors (20%), and perinatal ischemic lesions (11%), while other etiologies, such as Rasmussen's encephalitis, tuberous sclerosis, post-traumatic or post-infectious scars, and hypothalamic hamartomas amounted to around 3% [11, 12, 28, 29]. It should be noted that less than 3% of children undergoing epilepsy surgery had hippocampal sclerosis as their sole etiology [11, 29]. Similar data have been reported in previous studies of tertiary pediatric epilepsy surgery centers worldwide [16, 30]. Barba et al. [15] noted in an Italian nationwide survey including 527 children and adolescents FCD type II in 20.3% and glioneuronal tumors in 19.9% of cases. Figures 11.1 and 11.2 demonstrate typical etiologies of drug-resistant epilepsies in infancy and childhood.

### 11.1.3 Presurgical Assessment

Improved imaging techniques with high-field MRI [31], advanced epilepsy protocols, imaging post-processing, and repeated MRI [32], as well as refined surgical approaches enable a better appreciation of multiple facets of focal epilepsies in the pediatric age, facilitating the identification of children and adolescents that would otherwise not be considered as candidates for epilepsy surgery. In addition, the increased accessibility of radionuclide imaging, such as PET and SPECT [33], the advances in source localization techniques [34–36], and the availability of different approaches to intracranial EEG explorations (subdural electrodes, stereo-electroencephalography, SEEG) according to the individual features of each case [36–39] have proven to be useful tools in epilepsy surgery programs to address complexity of pediatric cases (Fig. 11.3).

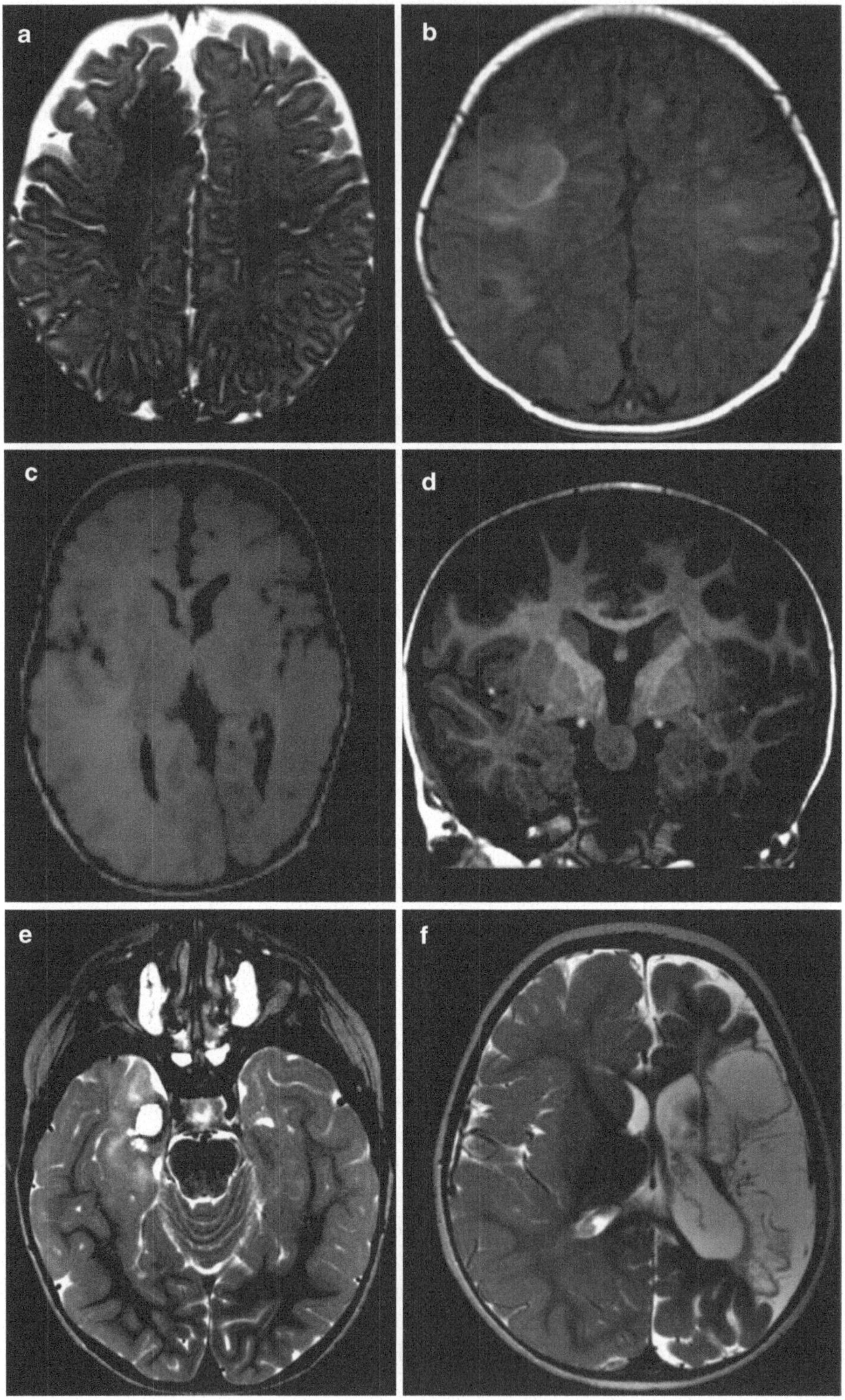


**Fig. 11.1** Most frequent etiologies of drug-resistant structural epilepsies during infancy. (**a**) Focal cortical dysplasia (FCD) right frontal; (**b**) Multiple cortical tubera in tuberous sclerosis; (**c**) Hemimegalencephaly right hemisphere; (**d**) Hypothalamic hamartoma; (**e**) Glioneuronal tumor right temporal; (**f**) Perinatal middle cerebral artery infarct left side (with courtesy of G. Ramantani, Zürich)

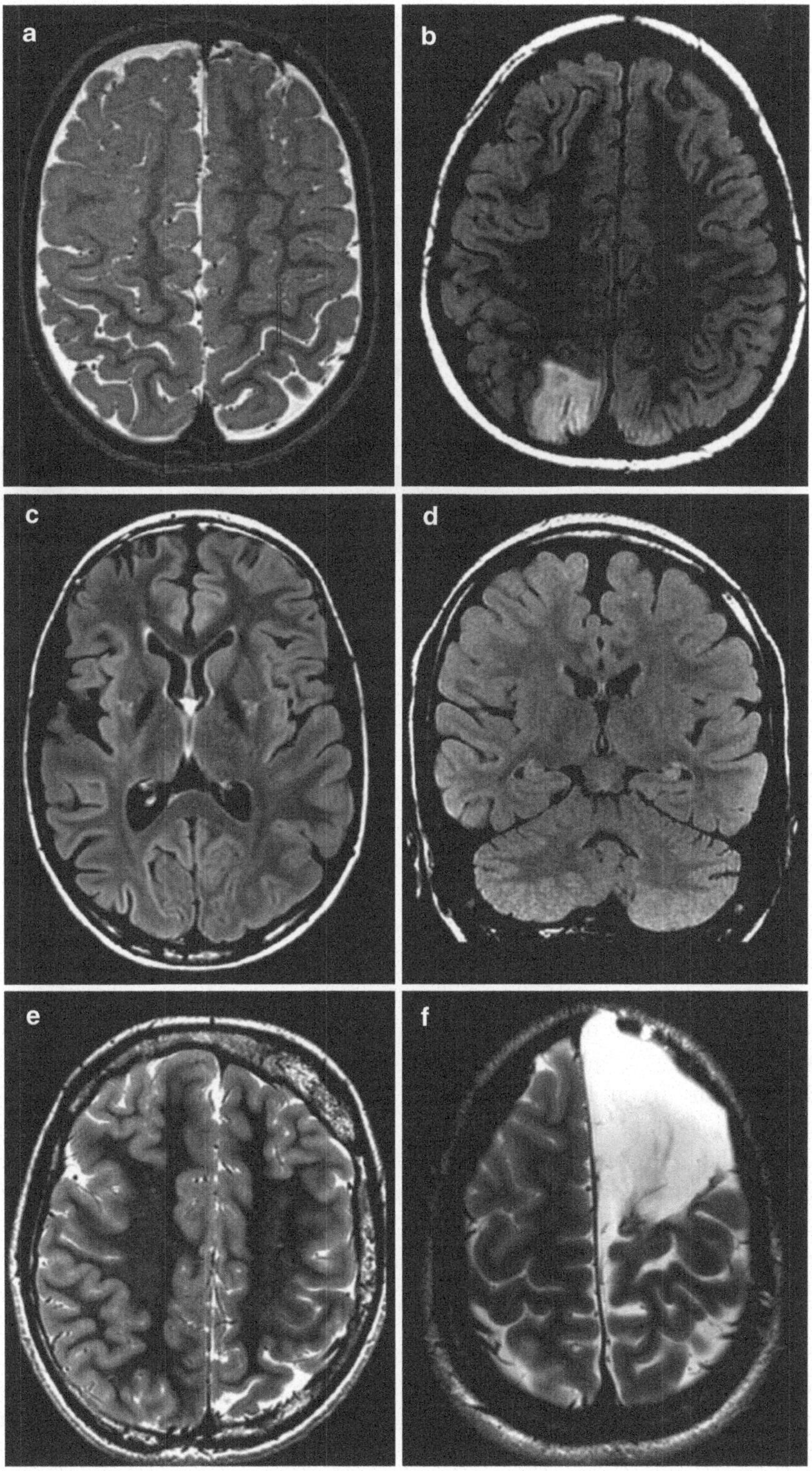


**Fig. 11.2** Most frequent etiologies of drug-resistant structural epilepsies in childhood. (**a**) Focal cortical dysplasia (FCD) right frontal; (**b**) Dysembryoplastic neuroepithelial tumor (DNET) right parietal; (**c**) Rasmussen's encephalitis right hemisphere; (**d**) Hippocampal sclerosis left temporal after meningoencephalitis during infancy; (**e**) Sturge–Weber syndrome left parieto-occipital; (**f**) Left frontal defect after perinatal hemorrhage (with courtesy of G. Ramantani, Zürich)

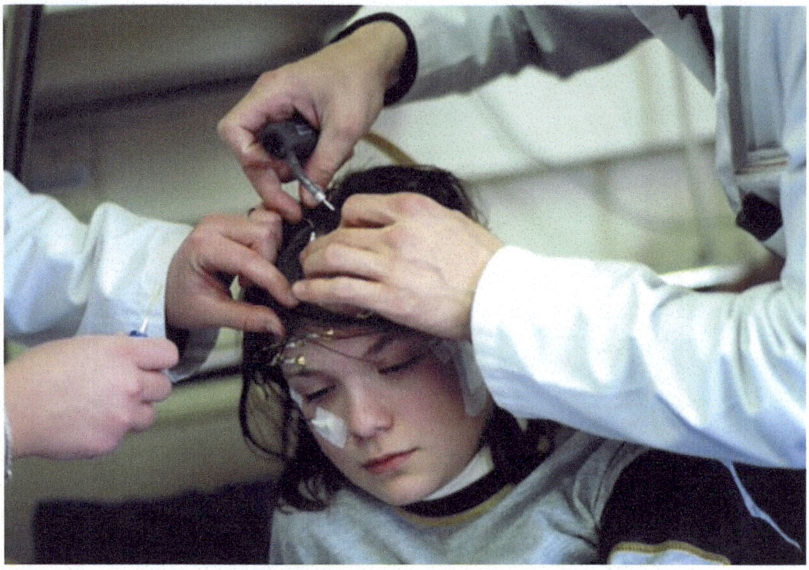

**Fig. 11.3** Placement and fixation of superficial electrodes in a 11-year-old girl (with courtesy of A. Schulze-Bonhage, Dpt. of Epileptology, Freiburg, and with permission of the patient)

## 11.2 Surgical Procedures

Since cortical malformations, often extensive or diffuse, are the predominant substrate of focal epilepsy in children and adolescents amenable to surgery, considerably more extensive resections are required, compared to those performed in the adult age [12, 28]. According to the international ILAE survey of pediatric epilepsy surgery in 2004 comprising 401 children and adolescents from 20 epilepsy centers [26], 21% of resective procedures were hemispheric and 18% multilobar, whereas the remaining 61% intralobar procedures encompassed mainly temporal (51%) and frontal (39%) resections. In line with these data, the Freiburg series including 378 children and adolescents shows the following percentage distribution: hemispheric procedures (19%), multilobar resections (19%), unilobar resections (60%), and other procedures such as for hypothalamic hamartomas (2%) [12, 28]. Among unilobar procedures, 50% were temporal, 36% frontal, and 13% were parietal or occipital [29, 40]. Comparable rates of hemispheric, multilobar and unilobar procedures have been reported for different pediatric epilepsy surgery cohorts, and some discrepancies can be readily attributed to differences in age distribution between cohorts as well as to dissimilar strategies employed in each epilepsy center [15, 17, 30, 41].

## 11.3 Outcome

Besides seizure outcome, cognitive as well as intellectual development [42, 43] and quality of life (QOL) [44–46] constitute important outcome measures in the pediatric age.

### 11.3.1 Seizure Outcome

#### 11.3.1.1 Overall outcome

Dwivedi et al. [9] randomized in a single-center trial including 116 children and adolescents 57 cases to surgery and 59 to a waiting list for surgery while receiving medical therapy alone. At 12 months follow-up, seizure freedom was noted in 44 patients (77%) in the surgical therapy group, but only in 4 (7%) in the medical therapy group ($p < 0.001$).

An Italian nationwide survey including 527 children and adolescents who underwent temporal and extratemporal resections between 2008 and 2014 reported seizure freedom (Engel I) in 74% with no significant changes over the years [15]. Similarly, in the nationwide Dutch series comprising 234 children and adolescents operated between 1990 and 2011, complete seizure freedom (Engel Ia) was achieved in 74% at 2-years follow-up without significant differences over time [17]. These findings are in line with the long-term seizure outcomes reported in a large monocentric study from North America published almost 10 years ago [16]. Seizure freedom rates have been found to be similar for infancy, childhood, and adolescence [16]. Different factors have been identified influencing seizure outcome.

#### 11.3.1.2 Type of surgery

The extent of the epileptogenic zone and, thus, of the necessary resection or disconnection, may influence seizure outcome. Seizure freedom ranges from 58% to 78% in intralobar [29, 30, 40, 47], from 22% to 65% in multilobar [11, 16, 30, 48], and from 43% to 83% in hemispheric [35, 49, 50] procedures. Analyzing 1859 pediatric surgeries, Barba et al. [22] noted a seizure-free outcome (Engel I) of 69.1% with no statistically significant correlation to any type of surgery.

#### 11.3.1.3 Etiology

Most importantly, seizure outcome depends on the underlying etiology. Mean seizure freedom rates following surgery in patients with glioneuronal tumors are given with 71% (range 36–100%) [51, 52], compared to 60% (range 46–70%) in patients with FCD [53, 54]. In the Freiburg cohort, 86% of children with glioneuronal tumor-associated epilepsy were seizure-free (Engel I) at the 12-months follow-up, and 14% had marked seizure reduction (Engel II). In the long-term follow-up of 1.3–12.3 years, 76% of children remained seizure-free (Engel I); of these children, two-thirds were of AED [52, 55]. With FCD-associated epilepsy, complete seizure control (Engel Ia) was achieved in 56% of children at the 24-months follow-up, 52% at the 5-years follow-up, and 50% at the last follow-up of 1.5–17 years in the Freiburg series [56].

#### 11.3.1.4 Extent of Lesion Resection

In the case of tumors or FCD, the completeness of resection of the epileptogenic lesion is the single most important predictor of long-lasting postsurgical seizure freedom [29, 40, 52, 57–59]. This rule does not hold true in case of other cortical malformations, such as polymicrogyria, that show a variable degree of involvement in the epileptogenic zone. In fact, the partial or lack of involvement of the polymicrogyria in the epileptogenic zone [38, 60, 61] is in contrast to the more concordance of the cortical malformation with the epileptogenic zone as encountered in FCD type II, the most common surgically treatable malformation [62]. FCD type II is highly epileptogenic, with several studies demonstrating that the epileptogenic zone mostly co-localizes with the dysplastic tissue [47, 63, 64]. In tumor-associated epilepsy, a recent large pediatric study suggested that the use of intraoperative ECoG to tailor resection does not provide improved seizure freedom compared to lesionectomy and extended lesionectomy alone [65].

#### 11.3.1.5 EEG and MRI findings

The concordance of presurgical EEG and MRI findings has been acknowledged as an independent predictor of postsurgical seizure freedom in the Cochrane review of epilepsy surgery that considered both pediatric and adult cohorts [66]. On the contrary, normal presurgical MRI, the need for long-term invasive EEG, and the presence of FCD have been identified as independent predictors of seizure recurrence in this review [66]. However, several pediatric studies have shown that this rule does not hold true for children undergoing epilepsy surgery, particularly those with early-onset catastrophic epilepsies. In this age group, in strong contrast to adult cohorts, there is no evidence of superior seizure outcome for patients with focal interictal epileptic discharges and initial discharges compared to patients with more widespread EEG abnormalities [11–13]. Diffuse EEG abnormalities, particularly in early-onset catastrophic epilepsy, are long known to be compatible with focal lesions that can be cured by surgery [14]. This highlights the paramount importance of MRI in pediatric epilepsies, while significance of EEG is limited, particularly in the very young age.

In pediatric epilepsy surgery, postsurgical outcomes may not be compromised by bilateral epileptic discharges in very extensive lesions and/or in very young children [11, 13, 14]. Novel concepts in epilepsy surgery support that postsurgical seizure freedom can be attained at the presence of EEG or

MRI abnormalities that are more widespread than the region that can be safely resected [67]. This is evident in the following scenarios [67]: (1) In early life, a localized or lateralized brain lesion may manifest with generalized semiology [10] and diffuse EEG abnormalities [11], (2) in tuberous sclerosis, seizure control may be achieved by the resection of the most epileptogenic of multiple lesions [68], and (3) in polymicrogyria, a partial lesionectomy based on an invasive exploration, may lead to seizure freedom [38].

#### 11.3.1.6 Left-sided Resection

Left-sided resections have been identified as a predictor of seizure recurrence in the Cochrane review of epilepsy surgery of West et al. [66]. This is not surprising since the proximity to eloquent cortex inevitably poses considerable restraints for resections performed in the dominant hemisphere. This limitation to surgical success in left-sided foci has been demonstrated in the case of both frontal [69] and posterior cortex [40] epilepsy surgery in children and adolescents. The distance between the epileptogenic lesion and the eloquent cortex is indeed crucial for postsurgical seizure freedom, whereas the overlapping of the epileptogenic zone and/or lesion with eloquent cortex is a major obstacle for seizure control [29].

The risk of surgical failure due to functional considerations is highly pertinent in extensive FCD, where complete resections may involve partially functional cortex [11, 13, 28]. Younger age at surgery may permit more radical surgical approaches aiming at the complete resection of the epileptogenic lesion since expected functional deficits can be overcome by more potent plasticity mechanisms [11, 29, 70].

#### 11.3.1.7 Duration of Epilepsy

Longer duration of epilepsy to surgery has been acknowledged as a negative predictor of seizure outcome in several studies [17, 25, 29, 40, 51, 58, 69, 71–73]. The negative effect of epilepsy duration may be associated with a progressive establishment of epileptogenic networks in the immature brain over time, culminating in secondary epileptogenesis [40]. In addition to the negative effect of longer epilepsy duration to seizure outcomes, it has been previously demonstrated that longer epilepsy duration has also a negative effect to cognitive outcomes [11, 18, 20, 29].

#### 11.3.1.8 Postoperative Seizures

Acute postsurgical seizures, conventionally defined as occurring during the first week after resective epilepsy surgery [74], have been acknowledged as predictors of seizure recurrence in various pediatric epilepsy surgery cohorts [12, 29, 75–77]. Similar seizure semiology pre- and post-surgery may be a more specific predictor of poor seizure outcome than acute postsurgical seizures alone, but this has not been demonstrated in pediatric cohorts so far, possibly due to the limitations in defining seizure semiology (i.e., auras) in very young children [75]. Acute postsurgical seizures have been associated with epileptic discharges in postsurgical EEG that, in turn, have been previously identified as predictors of poor seizure control in pediatric frontal [29] and posterior cortex [58] epilepsy surgery cohorts although epileptic discharges in postsurgical EEG have not reached statistical significance in the respective Cochrane review [66]. These features apparently correspond to residual epileptogenicity following an incomplete resection and are crucial for the appreciation of a surgical failure, and, eventually, for the initiation of reevaluation and, potentially, of reoperation [12, 28, 29]. On the other hand, seizures occurring within few days after resective surgery may to be linked to the immediate effects of the resection, to surgical or medical complications, metabolic derangements, infections, or abrupt shifts in antiepileptic drug levels and hence may not indicate long-term surgical failure [75].

### 11.3.2 Cognitive Outcome

In the prospective randomized controlled trial of Dwivedi et al. [9], children and adolescents who had undergone surgery had better postoperative scores with respect to behavior and quality of life than those who continued medical therapy.

Helmstaedter et al. [78] assessed neuropsychological performance of 306 children and adolescents before and 1 year after surgery for temporal, extratemporal, and hemispheric epilepsies. Preoperatively, 85% of the patients had cognitive impairments and 71% behavioral problems which is in line with others [79]. Longer epilepsy duration, higher drug load, and larger cerebral damage predicted worse presurgical performance. At 1 year after surgery, 21–50% of the children experienced functional recovery, and twice as much patients experienced gains than losses in the domains of motor functions, attention, language, visuospatial functions as well as in behavior. Improvement in IQ, figural and verbal memory was noted in 34–37%, while 29–39% of cases declined. A better baseline performance reflecting higher mental reserve capacity, shorter epilepsy duration, seizure control, and reduced postoperative drug load were predictive for favorable outcomes. Regarding surgery sides as well as sites, both presurgical impairments and postoperative changes were rather nonspecific than specific [78]. In addition, it has been shown that mental reserve capacity and functional plasticity [80], preservation of functional tissue [81–83], as well as seizure control and reduction of the antiepileptic drug load [43, 84, 85] are decisive for functional recovery [78]. In line with the results of standardized testings, Hoppe et al. [86] reported that parents acknowledged the overall positive neurocognitive development after pediatric epilepsy surgery.

### 11.3.3 Quality of Life (QOL)

Maragkos et al. [46] provided a systematic review and meta-analysis comprising 890 pediatric patients to assess QOL long-term outcomes. Following surgery, children showed improvement of QOL compared to their preoperative state and a better QOL than matched controls treated medically. IQ had increased after surgery by about 10 points on the average. Improvement of QOL was statistically significant in seizure-free cases, but not in individuals with persisting seizures [46]. It may be argued that the extent of seizure control and reduction of antiepileptic medication constitute the key factors for improvement of both psychosocial development and QOL after surgery [46]. These results are in line with previous studies demonstrating better IQ and improvement of QOL after successful epilepsy surgery [87]. Thus, seizure freedom remains the central desirable goal since it is the most important factor predicting improvement in QOL [46].

### 11.3.4 Temporal Resections

Temporal lobe epilepsy (TLE), particularly when related to the mesial temporal structures, commonly has its onset in the first years of life [88], with a substantial percentage of children presenting with pharmacoresistance at an early stage [89]. Temporal resections comprised 30% of all resections in an international survey of pediatric epilepsy surgery conducted 15 years ago and were thus marginally more frequent than frontal lobe resections that comprised 23% [26]. The last decade has witnessed a slow but steady decrease in the proportion of temporal resections in pediatric epilepsy surgery programs [15, 17]. Improved management of complex febrile seizures and febrile status epilepticus as well as the lower incidence and improved treatment of brain infections have resulted in overall declining referrals for mesial temporal lobe epilepsy [15]. Thus, the era of epilepsy surgery for hippocampal sclerosis (HS) related to febrile seizures and brain infections in early life seems slowly to come to an end, at least in developed countries [90].

#### 11.3.4.1 Etiology

In the survey of Harvey et al. [26], the most frequently identified pathological substrates in pediatric temporal resections were glioneuronal tumors (40%) followed by cortical dysplasia (30%). It should be noted that hippocampal sclerosis, still identified as the underlying etiology in one-third of cases in contemporary adult epilepsy surgery cohorts [25], is found in less than 15% of cases in actual pediatric surgical series [16, 17, 91]. Dual pathology, referring to the coexistence of HS with an extrahippocampal potentially epileptogenic lesion, is a more frequent finding in children than in adults, commonly including cortical dysplasia [30, 92]. With cortical dysplasia constituting the predominant epilepsy substrate in pediatric epilepsy surgery cohorts [11, 13, 29, 40, 53], it has been noted that in temporal location more often mild, type I dysplasia, is observed in contrast to extratemporal location where more often severe, type II dysplasia, is found [93].

#### 11.3.4.2 Overall Seizure Outcome

In a meta-analysis of pediatric TLE surgery [94], 76% of patients achieved seizure freedom, with significantly higher rates of seizure control in patients with an MRI-detectable lesion. In line with this meta-analysis, the Freiburg cohort of 106 children and adolescents undergoing TLE surgery, showed 75% seizure-free patients in the long-term follow-up. It should be noted that, in order to achieve seizure freedom, a higher proportion of children compared to adults undergo repeat temporal lobe resections. In these cases, initial surgical failure may be linked to an incomplete resection of the mesial temporal structures, as shown in a recent study of reoperations in a pediatric epilepsy surgery cohort [28]. In the Bonn series including 183 patients [95], seizure-free outcome (Engel I) was noted in 78.8%, and a favorable outcome (Engel I–II) in 84.8%. Reviewing the literature including 2089 temporal resections, Engel I–II outcome occurred in 79% of children and adolescents [95]. Overall, postsurgical seizure-free outcome has been found to range between 65% and 85%, and results are similar from early childhood through to adolescence, with some variation according to etiologic substrate [96–98].

#### 11.3.4.3 Seizure Outcome in Children Versus Adults

A meta-analysis [99] reported a median rate of long-term seizure freedom of 66% with temporal lobe resections with a trend for superior seizure outcomes in children compared to adults. This observation was confirmed by a study that compared the postsurgical seizure outcome of children and adults with TLE matched for pathology, epilepsy onset, side and type of surgery [80]. In this study, 80% children but only 63% adults were seizure-free at 1 year after surgery [80]. The superior outcomes of temporal lobe resections in pediatric cohorts were further illustrated by a recent monocentric epilepsy surgery study in a pediatric and adult population that showed significantly higher seizure freedom rates in children compared to adults, particularly in the subgroup of patients with mesial temporal sclerosis [25].

#### 11.3.4.4 Developmental and Cognitive Outcome

Several studies have focused on the developmental and cognitive outcomes of temporal lobe resections in childhood and adolescence. In a study comparing pre- and postsurgical verbal memory in children and adolescents with TLE [100], a significant decline linked to left-sided resections and higher presurgical functioning was observed at 3 months after surgery, followed by a full recovery 1 year after surgery. In a further study comparing children with adults matched for etiology, age at epilepsy onset, as well as side and type of surgery, adults had lower presurgical scores for verbal memory, probably due to the longer epilepsy duration, and failed to recover after surgery [80]. Additionally, children had superior outcomes regarding attentional functions compared to adults, with their vast majority improving 1 year after surgery. Recoveries following surgery that occurred exclusively in children and adolescents were attributed to the higher plasticity of the developing brain, defined as the brain capacity to be formed by experience, to learn and remember and, most importantly, to reorganize after injury [80].

In an observational study of pediatric TLE surgery, improved cognitive functioning in the long-term follow-up was found in the surgical group, in contrast to a well-matched non-surgical control group [43]. Long-term cognitive improvements were established after more than 6 years following surgery, which is in line with studies indicating that cognitive recovery and subsequent developmental progress require a long time [4, 5, 101]. In this study [43], cognitive improvements were linked to the tapering of AED, underling the importance of timely AED withdrawal in selected patients to enable an optimal cognitive development as confirmed by others [84]. Children with low presurgical cognitive functioning improved more after surgery compared to those with average or high presurgical functioning [43], in line with other studies addressing the developmental and cognitive outcomes of pediatric epilepsy surgery [101, 102]. The follow-up study from the same group [103] replicated the superior outcomes of the surgical versus the non-surgical group and reported improvements in 39% of surgically treated children and declines in 10%. However, complete seizure control and AED cessation were not predictive of improvements in IQ [103].

### 11.3.5 Extratemporal Resections

While TLE is predominant in adult cohorts, extratemporal epilepsy (ETE) is equally or even more frequent as TLE in pediatric cohorts [26]. Frontal lobe resections account for 36% of intralobar resections in pediatric epilepsy surgery, whereas posterior cortex resections, involving the parietal and/or occipital lobe and sometimes extending to the posterior border of the temporal lobe, account for 10% [26]. Similar to the adult age, results of extratemporal resections in children and adolescents have significantly improved over time leading to variable seizure control rates when actual series are compared with previous studies. This progress in pediatric epilepsy surgery mainly reflects advances in quality of MR imaging.

**Etiology**

FCD is the most predominant etiology, and extensive presurgical investigations, including invasive EEG recordings, are often required to guide surgical decision [29, 40, 58, 104]. In addition, epilepsies arising from FCD within the frontal, parietal, and occipital neocortex have a propensity for reorganization and thus for seizure recurrence over time [105]. In the study of Liava et al. [106] including 62 children and adolescents who underwent posterior cortex resections, FCD was the most frequent histopathological diagnosis (50%), followed by tumors (24%). Similarly, Ramantani et al. [40] comprising 50 pediatric posterior cortex epilepsies, noted FCD in 42% and tumors in 32% of cases.

**Overall Seizure Outcome**

In a meta-analysis of pediatric ETE surgery comprising 1259 cases [107], 56% of children and adolescents were seizure-free (Engel I) following surgery, regardless of the lobar localization of the epileptogenic zone. The presence of an MRI-detectable lesion and its complete resection have proven to be significant prognostic factors indicating a favorable seizure outcome. In addition, epilepsy duration of less than 7 years correlated with higher chances of postsurgical seizure freedom, thus underlining the importance of early referral and, consequently, of early surgical intervention [107].

#### 11.3.5.1 Frontal Resections

**Seizure Outcome**

In frontal lobe epilepsy (FLE) surgery, seizure freedom is achieved in up to 66% of selected children and adolescents [108–110]. In the study of Ramantani et al. [29], two-thirds of children remained seizure-free at a mean follow-up of 8.1 years, and one-third of them had discontinued AED.

**Predictors**

In line with mixed pediatric/adult cohorts, the following predictors for seizure freedom in pediatric frontal resections have been identified: a well-defined structural lesion distant from eloquent cortex that can be completely resected [29, 111–114], strictly regional epileptic discharges in scalp EEG [29, 69, 112–114], and shorter epilepsy duration [29]. Conversely, early postsurgical seizures and epileptic discharges in postsurgical scalp EEG predicted seizure recurrence [29, 69, 112–114]. The meta-analysis of Englot et al. [111] including both children and adults with FLE surgery, however, did not show any predictive value of time variables [111], whereas two later monocentric studies supported the significance of shorter epilepsy duration [69, 114] and younger age at surgery [69] for seizure freedom.

#### 11.3.5.2 Posterior Cortex Resections

**Seizure Outcome**

In posterior cortex epilepsy (PCE) surgery, the rates of seizure freedom have risen from 43–47% in the 1990s [115, 116] to 61–75% in the last decade [117, 118]. In the same time period, the percentage of MRI-negative patients dropped from 13% to 5% indicating the influence of MR imaging on outcome. In line with the lower rate of PCE surgery compared to other lobar localizations, the current literature relevant to the pediatric population is sparse and, to some extent, contradictory. However, two large pediatric studies have been published [40, 106], addressing this field. In the Italian study that included 62 children and adolescents [106], 86% of patients remained seizure-free (Engel I) following surgery at a mean follow-up of 6.9 years, and two-thirds discontinued AED. The study of Ramantani et al. [40] including 50 children and adolescents reported 60% seizure-free (Engel I) patients at a mean follow-up of 8 years, and one-third discontinued AED.

#### Predictors

In the study of Liava et al. [106], older age at epilepsy onset, the presence of a restricted MRI visible lesion, and complete resection of the lesion were predictive of seizure freedom, and none of the MRI-negative patients achieved postsurgical seizure-free outcome. Furthermore, the authors underlined the value of invasive explorations in achieving optimal postsurgical seizure outcomes [106]. Left-sided, parietal epileptogenic zones and resections, as well as longer epilepsy duration have been identified as independent predictors of seizure recurrence, thus supporting the early consideration of surgical intervention in children and adolescents with refractory PCE [40].

## 11.3.6 Multilobar Resections

Multilobar resections are performed more often in childhood and adolescence [16, 59, 119] than later in life [72] and amount to 18% of pediatric epilepsy surgery according to the 2004 international survey [26]. The higher rate of multilobar resections in the pediatric age as compared to adults is linked to the higher prevalence of (often widespread) FCD, the most common etiology leading to surgery in this age group [26, 27]. In fact, in the study on FCD-related pediatric epilepsy surgery [56], hemispheric or multilobar FCD was identified in 26 of 57 patients (46%) with epilepsy onset in the first 2 years of life compared to 10 of 56 patients (18%) with later epilepsy onset. This observation is in line with studies that identified FCD as the predominant etiology in very young children, with an incidence of 80% in the first 3 years of life [120]. Younger children are more likely to have multilobar and severe forms of FCD compared with older patients that feature mostly focal and mild FCD [93, 120, 121]. Of the 133 children in the study on FCD-related pediatric epilepsy surgery of Martinez-Lizana et al. [56], 16% underwent multilobar resections and 7% hemispherotomy (Fig. 11.4). Kalbhenn et al. [122] suggested that multilobar lesions affecting the temporal, occipital, and parietal lobes may be treated by a procedure that they termed "posterior disconnection."

In the presence of a hemispheric lesion, not uncommonly the dilemma is faced between the necessity to proceed with hemispherectomy/hemispherotomy in order to achieve seizure control and to prevent progressive cognitive deterioration on the one hand and to perform a limited resection in order to preserve intact functions on the other hand (see also Chaps. 8 and 12). A typical case demonstrating this dilemma is shown in Fig. 11.5. In principle, an early hemispherical procedure can be recommended in such cases accepting additional neurological deficits but preventing progressive cognitive deterioration and seizing the chance of a functional recovery due to brain plasticity. However, decision-making has to be based on a case-by-case assessment of risks and benefits, and, in the end, the decision remains with the parents.

### 11.3.6.1 Seizure Outcome

Despite their high relevance for the pediatric population, multilobar resections are less well studied than intralobar or hemispheric procedures. The available data mainly stem from subsets of large pediatric [16, 30, 59, 119, 123] or mixed pediatric and adult [48, 72] surgical series that report widely variable seizure freedom rates of 18–60%, all emphasizing worse long-term outcomes following multilobar as

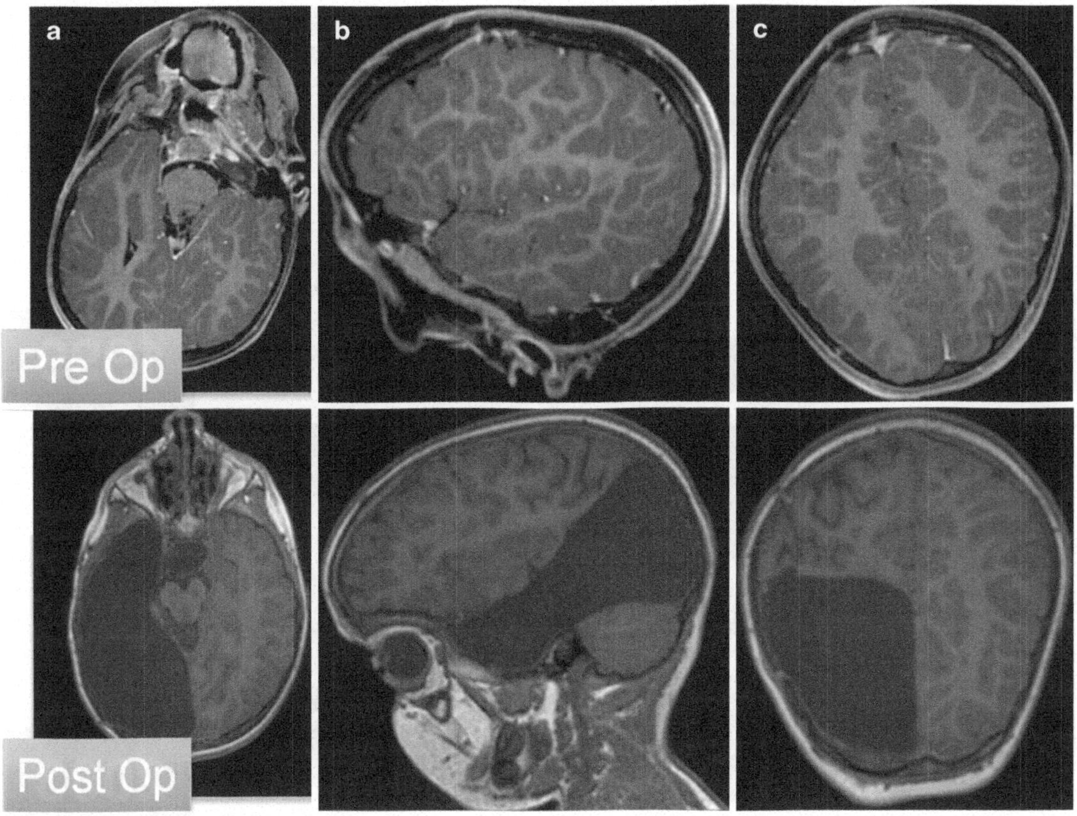


**Fig. 11.4** Pre- and postsurgical MRI in axial (**a**), sagittal (**b**), and coronal (**c**) view of a 2-year-old girl with epilepsy onset in the second month of life and severe developmental delay. At the time of surgery, the child had already been treated with corticosteroids and ketogenic diet for infantile spasms and had received a total of 8 anti-seizure drugs, but continued to seize several times per hour. Preoperative MRI (upper sequence) show a multilobar cortical dysplasia stretching over the posterior right quadrant. At the age of 2 years, a multilobectomy was performed. Postoperative MRI (lower sequence) demonstrate complete resection of the right temporal and occipital lobes as well as subtotal resection of the parietal lobe. Histology revealed FCD type IIa. Postoperatively, the patient was not completely seizure-free (Engel II)

opposed to intralobar resections [59]. Sarkis et al. [48] noted in a mixed pediatric/adult series of 63 patients seizure-free rates of 71% at 6 months, 64% at 1 year, 52% at 5 years, and 41% at 10 years after surgery. Nine patients (14%) required reoperation. In the Freiburg cohort including 69 children and adolescents that underwent multilobar resections, 48% patients were seizure-free at last follow-up of median 9 years, and 33% were off AED. Ten percent of patients, all with dysplastic etiology, required reoperations, and the majority achieved seizure freedom [124].

#### 11.3.6.2 Predictors

Left-sided as well as fronto-temporal and temporo-parietal resections, residual lesions in postsurgical MRI, and spikes in postsurgical EEG have been identified as predictors of seizure recurrence [48, 125]. On the other hand, seizure freedom has been found to be strongly associated with the complete resection of the MRI visible lesion [124]. Therefore, in younger children, early intervention and more radical and thus complete lesion resection, given the obvious benefits of functional plasticity in

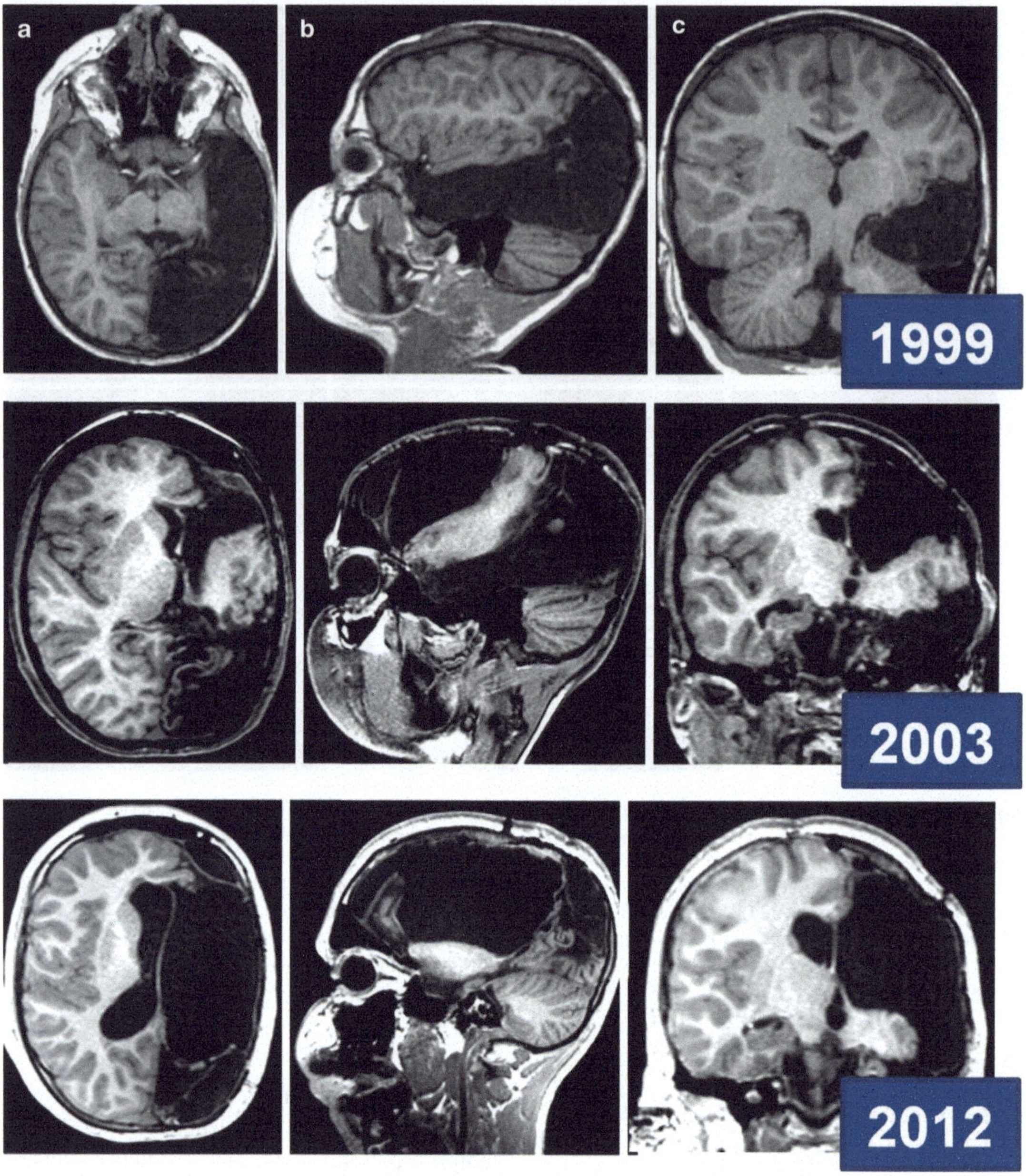


**Fig. 11.5** Left hemispheric FCD type Ia. The patient presented with tonic seizures starting from the first months of life. He underwent a first temporo-parieto-occipital resection at the age of 1.5 years, guided by an invasive evaluation with subdural grid electrodes (upper sequence; 1999). Seizures recurred with unchanged semiology few weeks after surgery and were refractory to several drugs. At the age of 5 years, the boy showed a severe developmental delay, particularly regarding language functions. At that time, parents feared additional neurological deficits, particularly motor impairment, and were not ready to agree with hemispheric surgery. The child underwent a repeat invasive evaluation and surgery, including removal of the frontal lobe and multiple subpial transections of the motor cortex (middle sequence; 2003). Postoperative motor function remained intact. However, daily tonic seizures continued to occur in the next 9 years. The boy was able to walk but could not speak. Finally, the parents agreed to complete anatomical hemispherectomy (lower sequence; 2012). The child was seizure-free after the last surgery, even after drug withdrawal. He could walk, but had a paralysis of his right hand and retained cognitive impairment. Language functions did not recover. MRI in axial (**a**), coronal (**b**), and sagittal (**c**) view after the first (1999), the second (2003), and the third (2012) resection are shown

overcoming anticipated functional deficit is strongly advocated [124].

## 11.4 Epilepsy Surgery in the First Years of Life

Characteristic features of epilepsy surgery in the first years of life include poor specificity of electroclinical correlations [10, 14], challenging interpretation of MR images [126], and lesional epilepsy with a predominance of malformations of cortical development requiring extensive resections [11, 13].

Under the age of 2 years, seizure semiology is frequently generalized and unspecific [10, 127]. EEG shows mainly diffuse or bilateral interictal and ictal patterns [14]. In addition, interpretation of MR images is rendered difficult due to the ongoing brain development, in particular of myelination [128]. Less conspicuous lesions can often only be detected at the age of 2 years, finer ones even later [126]. Thus, what is called MRI-negative is highly age dependent, and MRI studies have to be repeated several times.

On the other hand, cortical malformations, in particular FCD as most frequently seen in the young age group, often require extensive, multilobar, or hemispheric procedures [11, 13]. In other words: The younger the child, the more difficult diagnostics, and the larger the resection. In the study of Kadish et al. [11] considering 48 children in the first 3 years of life, hemispherectomy/hemispherotomy has been performed in 52%, multilobar resection in 13%, and intralobar resection in 35%. Etiology included cortical malformations in 71%, and peri- or postnatal ischemic lesions in 13% of the patients.

### 11.4.1 Seizure Outcome

Seizure freedom following epilepsy surgery in early life is achieved in up to two-thirds of children [11, 13, 18, 20, 23, 24, 129–133]. Analyzing 48 children, Kadish et al. [11] noted seizure freedom in 60% at the mean follow-up of 4.3 years, and one-third of children had discontinued AED. Intralobar (or lobar) resections resulted more often in seizure control than multilobar or hemispheric surgery: 76% of children after intralobar resections, but only 56% after multilobar or hemispheric procedures were seizure-free. Postsurgical seizure freedom was determined by the completeness of lesion resection [11], as previously demonstrated for older children and adolescents [29, 40, 52, 57].

### 11.4.2 Development and Cognitive Outcome

Additional to seizure alleviation, epilepsy surgery in early life has the potential to successfully address the developmental delay associated with early epilepsy onset [134], longer epilepsy duration [19], high seizure frequency [135], continuous epileptic discharges [136], and AED [137]. In the study of Kadish et al. [11], presurgical cognitive development was impaired in 89% of children, and this correlated strongly with the postsurgical cognitive development. Longer epilepsy duration and larger lesion extent were detrimental to presurgical development, which, in turn, determined the postsurgical developmental outcome. With epilepsy duration constituting the only modifiable developmental predictor, these findings underscore the importance of early surgical intervention, in line with previous studies [18–20, 138, 139].

**Concluding Remarks**

- ***Shift towards pediatric epilepsy surgery.*** *Advances in MR imaging facilitating detection of cortical malformations as the most important structural abnormalities in the young age and a more open attitude of pediatric neurologists and epileptologists towards epilepsy surgery with respect to favorable results in terms of seizure and developmental outcome have promoted pediatric epilepsy surgery with increasing numbers of surgical, and particularly, extratemporal, multilobar, and hemispheric procedures.*

- ***Diagnostic challenges in early life.*** *Due to the ongoing brain development and myelinization, interpretation of MR images is rendered difficult in the first years of life, and repeat MRI studies in negative cases are required. In addition, clinical and electrophysiological presurgical assessment is impeded in early life by unspecific seizure semiology and diffuse or bilateral EEG patterns.*
- ***Seizure outcome.*** *Seizure-free (Engel I) outcome is achieved in 60–80% of children with intralobar resections, while results of multilobar procedures are less favorable with long-term seizure control rates of 40–60% and a significant percentage of patients requiring reoperation.*
- ***Timing of surgery.*** *There is a general consensus to offer surgery as soon as intractability of epilepsy is ascertained, including in the first years of life, in order to achieve seizure freedom and facilitate undisturbed development at sensitive windows of brain maturation. Given the obvious benefits of plasticity in overcoming anticipated functional deficits, early intervention and more radical and thus complete lesion resection is justified.*

## References

1. Aaberg KM, Gunnes N, Bakken IJ, Lund Søraas C, Berntsen A, Magnus P, et al. Incidence and prevalence of childhood epilepsy: a nationwide cohort study. Pediatrics. 2017;139(5):e20163908.
2. Arts WF, Geerts AT. When to start drug treatment for childhood epilepsy: the clinical-epidemiological evidence. Eur J Paediatr Neurol. 2009;13(2):93–101.
3. Berg AT, Mathern GW, Bronen RA, Fulbright RK, DiMario F, Testa FM, et al. Frequency, prognosis and surgical treatment of structural abnormalities seen with magnetic resonance imaging in childhood epilepsy. Brain J Neurol. 2009;132(Pt 10):2785–97.
4. Ramantani G, Reuner G. Cognitive development in pediatric epilepsy surgery. Neuropediatrics. 2018;49(2):93–103.
5. Roulet-Perez E, Davidoff V, Mayor-Dubois C, Maeder-Ingvar M, Seeck M, Ruffieux C, et al. Impact of severe epilepsy on development: recovery potential after successful early epilepsy surgery. Epilepsia. 2010;51(7):1266–76.
6. Van Schooneveld MMJ, Braun KPJ. Cognitive outcome after epilepsy surgery in children. Brain Dev. 2013;35(8):721–9.
7. Asarnow RF, LoPresti C, Guthrie D, Elliott T, Cynn V, Shields WD, et al. Developmental outcomes in children receiving resection surgery for medically intractable infantile spasms. Dev Med Child Neurol. 1997;39(7):430–40.
8. Otsuki T, Kim H-D, Luan G, Inoue Y, Baba H, Oguni H, et al. Surgical versus medical treatment for children with epileptic encephalopathy in infancy and early childhood: Results of an international multicenter cohort study in Far-East Asia (the FACE study). Brain Dev. 2016;38:449–60.
9. Dwivedi R, Ramanujam B, Chandra PS, Sapra S, Gulati S, Kalaivani M, et al. Surgery for drug-resistant epilepsy in children. N Engl J Med. 2017;377(17):1639–47.
10. Hamer HM, Wyllie E, Lüders HO, Kotagal P, Acharya J. Symptomatology of epileptic seizures in the first three years of life. Epilepsia. 1999;40(7):837–44.
11. Kadish NE, Bast T, Reuner G, Wagner K, Mayer H, Schubert-Bast S, et al. Epilepsy surgery in the first 3 years of life: predictors of seizure freedom and cognitive development. Neurosurgery. 2019;84(6):E368–77. https://doi.org/10.1093/neuros/nyy376.
12. Ramantani G, Kadish NE, Brandt A, Strobl K, Stathi A, Wiegand G, et al. Seizure control and developmental trajectories after hemispherotomy for refractory epilepsy in childhood and adolescence. Epilepsia. 2013;54(6):1046–55.
13. Ramantani G, Kadish NE, Strobl K, Brandt A, Stathi A, Mayer H, et al. Seizure and cognitive outcomes of epilepsy surgery in infancy and early childhood. Eur J Paediatr Neurol. 2013;17(5):498–506.
14. Wyllie E, Lachhwani DK, Gupta A, Chirla A, Cosmo G, Worley S, et al. Successful surgery for epilepsy due to early brain lesions despite generalized EEG findings. Neurology. 2007;69(4):389–97.
15. Barba C, Specchio N, Guerrini R, Tassi L, De Masi S, Cardinale F, et al. Increasing volume and complexity of pediatric epilepsy surgery with stable seizure outcome between 2008 and 2014: a nationwide multicenter study. Epilepsy Behav. 2017;75:151–7.
16. Hemb M, Velasco TR, Parnes MS, Wu JY, Lerner JT, Matsumoto JH, et al. Improved outcomes in pediatric epilepsy surgery: the UCLA experience, 1986-2008. Neurology. 2010;74(22):1768–75.
17. Lamberink HJ, Boshuisen K, van Rijen PC, Gosselaar PH, Braun KPJ, Dutch Collaborative Epilepsy Surgery Program (DCESP). Changing profiles of pediatric epilepsy surgery candidates over time: a nationwide single-center experience from 1990 to 2011. Epilepsia. 2015;56(5):717–25.
18. Honda R, Kaido T, Sugai K, Takahashi A, Kaneko Y, Nakagwa E, et al. Long-term developmental outcome after early hemispherotomy for hemimegalen-

cephaly in infants with epileptic encephalopathy. Epilepsy Behav. 2013;29(1):30–5.
19. Jonas R, Asarnow RF, LoPresti C, Yudovin S, Koh S, Wu JY, et al. Surgery for symptomatic infant-onset epileptic encephalopathy with and without infantile spasms. Neurology. 2005;64(4):746–50.
20. Loddenkemper T, Holland KD, Stanford LD, Kotagal P, Bingaman W, Wyllie E. Developmental outcome after epilepsy surgery in infancy. Pediatrics. 2007;119(5):930–5.
21. Pestana Knight EM, Schiltz NK, Bakaki PM, Koroukian SM, Lhatoo SD, Kaiboriboon K. Increasing utilization of pediatric epilepsy surgery in the United States between 1997 and 2009. Epilepsia. 2015;56(3):375–81.
22. Barba C, Cross JH, Brain K, et al. Trends in pediatric epilepsy surgery in Europe between 2008 and 2015: Country-, center-, and age-specific variation. Epilepsia. 2020;61(2):216–27.
23. Dunkley C, Kung J, Scott RC, Nicolaides P, Neville B, Aylett SE, et al. Epilepsy surgery in children under 3 years. Epilepsy Res. 2011;93(2–3):96–106.
24. Steinbok P, Gan PYC, Connolly MB, Carmant L, Barry Sinclair D, Rutka J, et al. Epilepsy surgery in the first 3 years of life: a Canadian survey. Epilepsia. 2009;50(6):1442–9.
25. Cloppenborg T, May TW, Blümcke I, Fauser S, Grewe P, Hopf JL, et al. Differences in pediatric and adult epilepsy surgery: a comparison at one center from 1990 to 2014. Epilepsia. 2019;60(2):233–45.
26. Harvey AS, Cross JH, Shinnar S, Mathern GW, Mathern BW, ILAE Pediatric Epilepsy Surgery Survey Taskforce. Defining the spectrum of international practice in pediatric epilepsy surgery patients. Epilepsia. 2008;49(1):146–55.
27. Blümcke I, Spreafico R, Haaker G, Coras R, Kobow K, Bien CG, et al. Histopathological findings in brain tissue obtained during epilepsy surgery. N Engl J Med. 2017;377(17):1648–56.
28. Ramantani G, Strobl K, Stathi A, Brandt A, Schubert-Bast S, Wiegand G, et al. Reoperation for refractory epilepsy in childhood: a second chance for selected patients. Neurosurgery. 2013;73(4):695–704.
29. Ramantani G, Kadish NE, Mayer H, Anastasopoulos C, Wagner K, Reuner G, et al. Frontal lobe epilepsy surgery in childhood and adolescence: predictors of long-term seizure freedom, overall cognitive and adaptive functioning. Neurosurgery. 2018;83(1):93–103.
30. Cossu M, Lo Russo G, Francione S, Mai R, Nobili L, Sartori I, et al. Epilepsy surgery in children: results and predictors of outcome on seizures. Epilepsia. 2008;49(1):65–72.
31. Veersema TJ, van Eijsden P, Gosselaar PH, Hendrikse J, Zwanenburg JJM, Spliet WGM, et al. 7 tesla T2*-weighted MRI as a tool to improve detection of focal cortical dysplasia. Epileptic Disord. 2016;18(3):315–23.
32. Adler S, Wagstyl K, Gunny R, Ronan L, Carmichael D, Cross JH, et al. Novel surface features for automated detection of focal cortical dysplasias in paediatric epilepsy. Neuroimage Clin. 2017;14:18–27.
33. Jayakar P, Gaillard WD, Tripathi M, Libenson MH, Mathern GW, Cross JH, et al. Diagnostic test utilization in evaluation for resective epilepsy surgery in children. Epilepsia. 2014;55(4):507–18.
34. Cosandier-Rimélé D, Ramantani G, Zentner J, Schulze-Bonhage A, Duempelmann M. A realistic multimodal modeling approach for the evaluation of distributed source analysis: application to sLORETA. J Neural Eng. 2017; https://doi.org/10.1088/1741-2552/aa7db1.
35. Ramantani G, Cosandier-Rimélé D, Schulze-Bonhage A, Maillard L, Zentner J, Dümpelmann M. Source reconstruction based on subdural EEG recordings adds to the presurgical evaluation in refractory frontal lobe epilepsy. Clin Neurophysiol. 2013;124(3):481–91.
36. Ramantani G, Dümpelmann M, Koessler L, Brandt A, Cosandier-Rimélé D, Zentner J, et al. Simultaneous subdural and scalp EEG correlates of frontal lobe epileptic sources. Epilepsia. 2014;55(2):278–88.
37. Koessler L, Cecchin T, Colnat-Coulbois S, Vignal J-P, Jonas J, Vespignani H, et al. Catching the invisible: mesial temporal source contribution to simultaneous EEG and SEEG recordings. Brain Topogr. 2015;28(1):5–20.
38. Maillard LG, Tassi L, Bartolomei F, Catenoix H, Dubeau F, Szurhaj W, et al. Stereoelectroencephalography and surgical outcome in polymicrogyria-related epilepsy: a multicentric study. Ann Neurol. 2017;82(5):781–94.
39. Rikir E, Koessler L, Gavaret M, Bartolomei F, Colnat-Coulbois S, Vignal J-P, et al. Electrical source imaging in cortical malformation-related epilepsy: a prospective EEG-SEEG concordance study. Epilepsia. 2014;55(6):918–32.
40. Ramantani G, Stathi A, Brandt A, Strobl K, Schubert-Bast S, Wiegand G, et al. Posterior cortex epilepsy surgery in childhood and adolescence: predictors of long-term seizure outcome. Epilepsia. 2017;58(3):412–9.
41. Wyllie E, Comair YG, Kotagal P, Bulacio J, Bingaman W, Ruggieri P. Seizure outcome after epilepsy surgery in children and adolescents. Ann Neurol. 1998;44(5):740–8.
42. Chen HH, Chen C, Hung SC, et al. Cognitive and epilepsy outcomes after epilepsy surgery caused by focal cortical dysplasia in children: early intervention maybe better. Child Nerv Syst. 2014;30(11):1885–95.
43. Skirrow C, Cross JH, Cormack F, Harkness W, Vargha-Khadem F, Baldeweg T. Long-term intellectual outcome after temporal lobe surgery in childhood. Neurology. 2011;76(15):1330–7.
44. Dagar A, Chandra PS, Chaudhary K, et al. Epilepsy surgery in a pediatric population: a retrospective study of 129 children from a tertiary care hospital in a developing country along with assessment of quality of life. Pediatr Neurosurg. 2011;47(3):186–93.

45. Griffiths SY, Sherman EM, Slick DJ, et al. Postsurgical health-related quality of life (HRQOL) in children following hemispherectomy for intractable epilepsy. Epilepsia. 2007;48(3):564–70.
46. Maragkos GA, Geropoulos G, Kechagias K, et al. Quality of life after epilepsy surgery in children: a systematic review and meta-analysis. Neurosurgery. 2019;85:741–9.
47. Krsek P, Maton B, Korman B, Pacheco-Jacome E, Jayakar P, Dunoyer C, et al. Different features of histopathological subtypes of pediatric focal cortical dysplasia. Ann Neurol. 2008;63(6):758–69.
48. Sarkis RA, Jehi L, Najm IM, Kotagal P, Bingaman WE. Seizure outcomes following multilobar epilepsy surgery. Epilepsia. 2012;53(1):44–50.
49. Boshuisen K, van Schooneveld MMJ, Leijten FSS, de Kort GAP, van Rijen PC, Gosselaar PH, et al. Contralateral MRI abnormalities affect seizure and cognitive outcome after hemispherectomy. Neurology. 2010;75(18):1623–30.
50. Moosa ANV, Gupta A, Jehi L, Marashly A, Cosmo G, Lachhwani D, et al. Longitudinal seizure outcome and prognostic predictors after hemispherectomy in 170 children. Neurology. 2013;80(3):253–60.
51. Englot DJ, Berger MS, Barbaro NM, Chang EF. Predictors of seizure freedom after resection of supratentorial low-grade gliomas. A review. J Neurosurg. 2011;115(2):240–4.
52. Ramantani G, Kadish NE, Anastasopoulos C, Brandt A, Wagner K, Strobl K, et al. Epilepsy surgery for glioneuronal tumors in childhood: avoid loss of time. Neurosurgery. 2014;74(6):648–57; discussion 657.
53. Bast T, Ramantani G, Seitz A, Rating D. Focal cortical dysplasia: prevalence, clinical presentation and epilepsy in children and adults. Acta Neurol Scand. 2006;113(2):72–81.
54. Chern JJ, Patel AJ, Jea A, Curry DJ, Comair YG. Surgical outcome for focal cortical dysplasia: an analysis of recent surgical series. J Neurosurg Pediatr. 2010;6(5):452–8.
55. Ramantani G, Zentner J. In reply: avoid loss of time. Neurosurgery. 2014;75(2):E197–8.
56. Martinez-Lizana E, Fauser S, Brandt A, Schuler E, Wiegand G, Doostkam S, et al. Long-term seizure outcome in pediatric patients with focal cortical dysplasia undergoing tailored and standard surgical resections. Seizure. 2018;62:66–73.
57. Krsek P, Maton B, Jayakar P, Dean P, Korman B, Rey G, et al. Incomplete resection of focal cortical dysplasia is the main predictor of poor postsurgical outcome. Neurology. 2009;72(3):217–23.
58. Liava A, Francione S, Tassi L, Lo Russo G, Cossu M, Mai R, et al. Individually tailored extratemporal epilepsy surgery in children: anatomo-electro-clinical features and outcome predictors in a population of 53 cases. Epilepsy Behav. 2012;25(1):68–80.
59. Paolicchi JM, Jayakar P, Dean P, Yaylali I, Morrison G, Prats A, et al. Predictors of outcome in pediatric epilepsy surgery. Neurology. 2000;54(3):642–7.
60. Maillard L, Ramantani G. Epilepsy surgery for polymicrogyria: a challenge to be undertaken. Epileptic Disord. 2018;20(5):319–38.
61. Ramantani G, Koessler L, Colnat-Coulbois S, Vignal J-P, Isnard J, Catenoix H, et al. Intracranial evaluation of the epileptogenic zone in regional infrasylvian polymicrogyria. Epilepsia. 2013;54(2):296–304.
62. Guerrini R, Duchowny M, Jayakar P, Krsek P, Kahane P, Tassi L, et al. Diagnostic methods and treatment options for focal cortical dysplasia. Epilepsia. 2015;56(11):1669–86.
63. Chassoux F, Landré E, Mellerio C, Turak B, Mann MW, Daumas-Duport C, et al. Type II focal cortical dysplasia: electroclinical phenotype and surgical outcome related to imaging. Epilepsia. 2012;53(2):349–58.
64. Tassi L, Pasquier B, Minotti L, Garbelli R, Kahane P, Benabid AL, et al. Cortical dysplasia: electroclinical, imaging, and neuropathologic study of 13 patients. Epilepsia. 2001;42(9):1112–23.
65. Robertson FC, Ullrich NJ, Manley PE, Al-Sayegh H, Ma C, Goumnerova LC. The impact of intraoperative electrocorticography on seizure outcome after resection of pediatric brain tumors: a cohort study. Neurosurgery. 2019;85(3):375–83.
66. West S, Nolan SJ, Newton R. Surgery for epilepsy: a systematic review of current evidence. Epileptic Disord. 2016;18(2):113–21.
67. Ryvlin P, Cross JH, Rheims S. Epilepsy surgery in children and adults. Lancet Neurol. 2014;13(11):1114–26.
68. Arya R, Tenney JR, Horn PS, Greiner HM, Holland KD, Leach JL, et al. Long-term outcomes of resective epilepsy surgery after invasive presurgical evaluation in children with tuberous sclerosis complex and bilateral multiple lesions. J Neurosurg Pediatr. 2015;15(1):26–33.
69. Simasathien T, Vadera S, Najm I, Gupta A, Bingaman W, Jehi L. Improved outcomes with earlier surgery for intractable frontal lobe epilepsy. Ann Neurol. 2013;73(5):646–54.
70. Cross JH, Jayakar P, Nordli D, Delalande O, Duchowny M, Wieser HG, et al. Proposed criteria for referral and evaluation of children for epilepsy surgery: recommendations of the Subcommission for Pediatric Epilepsy Surgery. Epilepsia. 2006;47(6):952–9.
71. Dalmagro CL, Bianchin MM, Velasco TR, Alexandre V, Walz R, Terra-Bustamante VC, et al. Clinical features of patients with posterior cortex epilepsies and predictors of surgical outcome. Epilepsia. 2005;46(9):1442–9.
72. Edelvik A, Rydenhag B, Olsson I, Flink R, Kumlien E, Källén K, et al. Long-term outcomes of epilepsy

surgery in Sweden: a national prospective and longitudinal study. Neurology. 2013;81(14):1244–51.
73. Englot DJ, Chang EF. Rates and predictors of seizure freedom in resective epilepsy surgery: an update. Neurosurg Rev. 2014;37(3):389–404; discussion 404–5.
74. Engel J Jr, Van Ness PC, Rasmussen TB, Ojemann LM. Outcome with respect to epileptic seizures. In: Engel Jr J, editor. Surgical treatment of the epilepsies. New York: Raven Press; 1993. p. 609–21.
75. Greiner HM, Horn PS, Arya R, Holland K, Turner M, Alsaidi MH, et al. Acute postoperative seizures and long-term outcome following pediatric epilepsy surgery. Seizure. 2014;23(6):483–6.
76. Mani J, Gupta A, Mascha E, Lachhwani D, Prakash K, Bingaman W, et al. Postoperative seizures after extratemporal resections and hemispherectomy in pediatric epilepsy. Neurology. 2006;66(7):1038–43.
77. Park K, Buchhalter J, McClelland R, Raffel C. Frequency and significance of acute postoperative seizures following epilepsy surgery in children and adolescents. Epilepsia. 2002;43(8):874–81.
78. Helmstaedter C, Beeres K, Elger CE, et al. Cognitive outcome of pediatric epilepsy surgery across ages and different types of surgeries: a monocentric 1-year follow-up study in 306 patients of school age. Eur J Epilepsy. 2019; https://doi.org/10.1016/j.seizure.2019.07.021.
79. Hermann BP, Seidenberg M, Bell B. The neurodevelopmental impact of childhood onset temporal lobe epilepsy on brain structure and function and the risk of progressive cognitive effects. Brain Res. 2002;135:429–38.
80. Gleissner U, Sassen R, Schramm J, Elger CE, Helmstaedter C. Greater functional recovery after temporal lobe epilepsy surgery in children. Brain J Neurol. 2005;128(Pt 12):2822–9.
81. Helmstaedter C, Roeske S, Kaaden S, Elger CE, Schramm J. Hippocampal resection length and memory outcome in selective epilepsy surgery. J Neurol Neurosurg Psychiatry. 2011;82(12):1375–81.
82. Helmstaedter C, Roeske S, Kaaden S, et al. Hippocampal resection length and memory outcome in selective epilepsy surgery. J Neurol Neurosurg Psychiatry. 2011; https://doi.org/10.1136/jnnp.2010.240176.
83. Helmstaedter C, Petzold I, Bien CG. The cognitive consequence of resecting nonlesional tissues in epilepsy surgery–results from MRI- and histopathology-negative patients with temporal lobe epilepsy. Epilepsia. 2011;52(8):1402–8.
84. Boshuisen K, van Schooneveld MMJ, Uiterwaal CSPM, Cross JH, Harrison S, Polster T, et al. Intelligence quotient improves after antiepileptic drug withdrawal following pediatric epilepsy surgery. Ann Neurol. 2015;78(1):104–14.
85. Helmstaedter C, Elger CE, Witt JA.The effect of quantitative and qualitative antiepileptic drug changes on cognitive recovery after epilepsy surgery. Seizure. 2016;36:63–9.
86. Hoppe C, Porebska I, Beeres K, et al. Parents' view of the cognitive outcome one year after pediatric epilepsy surgery. Epilepsy Behav. 2019; https://doi.org/10.1016/j.yebeh.2019.106552.
87. Clary LE, Vander Wal JS, Titus JB. Examining health-related quality of life, adaptive skills, and psychological functioning in children and adolescents with epilepsy presenting for a neuropsychological evaluation. Epilepsy Behav. 2010;19(3):487–93.
88. Spooner CG, Berkovic SF, Mitchell LA, Wrennall JA, Harvey AS. New-onset temporal lobe epilepsy in children: lesion on MRI predicts poor seizure outcome. Neurology. 2006;67(12):2147–53.
89. Wirrell EC. Predicting pharmacoresistance in pediatric epilepsy. Epilepsia. 2013;54(Suppl 2):19–22.
90. Ramantani G, Holthausen H. Epilepsy after cerebral infection: review of the literature and the potential for surgery. Epileptic Disord. 2017;19(2):117–36.
91. Neligan A, Haliasos N, Pettorini B, Harkness WFJ, Solomon JK. A survey of adult and pediatric epilepsy surgery in the United Kingdom. Epilepsia. 2013;54(5):e62–5.
92. Mohamed A, Wyllie E, Ruggieri P, Kotagal P, Babb T, Hilbig A, et al. Temporal lobe epilepsy due to hippocampal sclerosis in pediatric candidates for epilepsy surgery. Neurology. 2001;56(12):1643–9.
93. Hauptman JS, Mathern GW. Surgical treatment of epilepsy associated with cortical dysplasia: 2012 update. Epilepsia. 2012;53(Suppl 4):98–104.
94. Englot DJ, Rolston JD, Wang DD, Sun PP, Chang EF, Auguste KI. Seizure outcomes after temporal lobectomy in pediatric patients. J Neurosurg Pediatr. 2013;12(2):134–41.
95. Ormond DR, Clusmann H, Sassen R, et al. Pediatric Temporal Lobe Epilepsy Surgery in Bonn and Review of the Literature. Neurosurgery. 2018; https://doi.org/10.1093/neuros/nyy125.
96. Benifla M, Otsubo H, Ochi A, Weiss SK, Donner EJ, Shroff M, et al. Temporal lobe surgery for intractable epilepsy in children: an analysis of outcomes in 126 children. Neurosurgery. 2006;59(6):1203–13; discussion 1213–14.
97. Miserocchi A, Cascardo B, Piroddi C, Fuschillo D, Cardinale F, Nobili L, et al. Surgery for temporal lobe epilepsy in children: relevance of presurgical evaluation and analysis of outcome. J Neurosurg Pediatr. 2013;11(3):256–67.
98. Smyth MD, Limbrick DD, Ojemann JG, Zempel J, Robinson S, O'Brien DF, et al. Outcome following surgery for temporal lobe epilepsy with hippocampal involvement in preadolescent children: emphasis on mesial temporal sclerosis. J Neurosurg. 2007;106(3 Suppl):205–10.
99. Téllez-Zenteno JF, Dhar R, Wiebe S. Long-term seizure outcomes following epilepsy surgery: a sys-

tematic review and meta-analysis. Brain J Neurol. 2005;128(Pt 5):1188–98.
100. Gleissner U, Sassen R, Lendt M, Clusmann H, Elger CE, Helmstaedter C. Pre- and postoperative verbal memory in pediatric patients with temporal lobe epilepsy. Epilepsy Res. 2002;51(3):287–96.
101. Freitag H, Tuxhorn I. Cognitive function in preschool children after epilepsy surgery: rationale for early intervention. Epilepsia. 2005;46(4):561–7.
102. Gleissner U, Clusmann H, Sassen R, Elger CE, Helmstaedter C. Postsurgical outcome in pediatric patients with epilepsy: a comparison of patients with intellectual disabilities, subaverage intelligence, and average-range intelligence. Epilepsia. 2006;47(2):406–14.
103. Skirrow C, Cross JH, Owens R, Weiss-Croft L, Martin-Sanfilippo P, Banks T, et al. Determinants of IQ outcome after focal epilepsy surgery in childhood: a longitudinal case-control neuroimaging study. Epilepsia. 2019;60(5):872–84.
104. D'Argenzio L, Colonnelli MC, Harrison S, Jacques TS, Harkness W, Scott RC, et al. Seizure outcome after extratemporal epilepsy surgery in childhood. Dev Med Child Neurol. 2012;54(11):995–1000.
105. Blount JP. Extratemporal resections in pediatric epilepsy surgery-an overview. Epilepsia. 2017;58(Suppl 1):19–27.
106. Liava A, Mai R, Tassi L, Cossu M, Sartori I, Nobili L, et al. Paediatric epilepsy surgery in the posterior cortex: a study of 62 cases. Epileptic Disord. 2014;16(2):141–64.
107. Englot DJ, Breshears JD, Sun PP, Chang EF, Auguste KI. Seizure outcomes after resective surgery for extra-temporal lobe epilepsy in pediatric patients. J Neurosurg Pediatr. 2013;12(2):126–33.
108. Kasasbeh AS, Yarbrough CK, Limbrick DD, Steger-May K, Leach JL, Mangano FT, et al. Characterization of the supplementary motor area syndrome and seizure outcome after medial frontal lobe resections in pediatric epilepsy surgery. Neurosurgery. 2012;70(5):1152–68.
109. Kral T, Kuczaty S, Blümcke I, Urbach H, Clusmann H, Wiestler OD, et al. Postsurgical outcome of children and adolescents with medically refractory frontal lobe epilepsies. Childs Nerv Syst. 2001;17(10):595–601.
110. Vachhrajani S, de Ribaupierre S, Otsubo H, Ochi A, Weiss SK, Donner EJ, et al. Neurosurgical management of frontal lobe epilepsy in children. J Neurosurg Pediatr. 2012;10(3):206–16.
111. Englot DJ, Wang DD, Rolston JD, Shih TT, Chang EF. Rates and predictors of long-term seizure freedom after frontal lobe epilepsy surgery: a systematic review and meta-analysis. J Neurosurg. 2012;116(5):1042–8.
112. Janszky J, Jokeit H, Schulz R, Hoppe M, Ebner A. EEG predicts surgical outcome in lesional frontal lobe epilepsy. Neurology. 2000;54(7):1470–6.
113. Jeha LE, Najm I, Bingaman W, Dinner D, Widdess-Walsh P, Lüders H. Surgical outcome and prognostic factors of frontal lobe epilepsy surgery. Brain. 2007;130(Pt 2):574–84.
114. Pinheiro-Martins AP, Bianchin MM, Velasco TR, Terra VC, Araújo D, Wichert-Ana L, et al. Independent predictors and a prognostic model for surgical outcome in refractory frontal lobe epilepsy. Epilepsy Res. 2012;99(1–2):55–63.
115. D'Agostino MD, Bastos A, Piras C, Bernasconi A, Grisar T, Tsur VG, et al. Posterior quadrantic dysplasia or hemi-hemimegalencephaly: a characteristic brain malformation. Neurology. 2004;62(12):2214–20.
116. Sinclair DB, Wheatley M, Snyder T, Gross D, Ahmed N. Posterior resection for childhood epilepsy. Pediatr Neurol. 2005;32(4):257–63.
117. Ibrahim GM, Fallah A, Albert GW, Withers T, Otsubo H, Ochi A, et al. Occipital lobe epilepsy in children: characterization, evaluation and surgical outcomes. Epilepsy Res. 2012;99(3):335–45.
118. Yang P-F, Mei Z, Lin Q, Pei J-S, Zhang H-J, Zhong Z-H, et al. Disconnective surgery in posterior quadrantic epilepsy: a series of 12 paediatric patients. Epileptic Disord. 2014;16(3):296–304.
119. Teutonico F, Mai R, Veggiotti P, Francione S, Tassi L, Borrelli P, et al. Epilepsy surgery in children: evaluation of seizure outcome and predictive elements. Epilepsia. 2013;54(Suppl 7):70–6.
120. Cepeda C, André VM, Levine MS, Salamon N, Miyata H, Vinters HV, et al. Epileptogenesis in pediatric cortical dysplasia: the dysmature cerebral developmental hypothesis. Epilepsy Behav. 2006;9(2):219–35.
121. Lerner JT, Salamon N, Hauptman JS, Velasco TR, Hemb M, Wu JY, et al. Assessment and surgical outcomes for mild type I and severe type II cortical dysplasia: a critical review and the UCLA experience. Epilepsia. 2009;50(6):1310–35.
122. Kalbhenn T, Cloppenborg T, Wörmann FG, et al. Operative posterior disconnection in epilepsy surgery: Experience with 29 patients. Epilepsia. 2019;60:1973–83.
123. Jayakar P, Dunoyer C, Dean P, Ragheb J, Resnick T, Morrison G, et al. Epilepsy surgery in patients with normal or nonfocal MRI scans: integrative strategies offer long-term seizure relief. Epilepsia. 2008;49(5):758–64.
124. Kogias E, Schmeiser B, Doostkam S, Brandt A, Hammen T, Zentner J, et al. Multilobar resections for 3T MRI-negative epilepsy: worth the trouble? World Neurosurg. 2019; https://doi.org/10.1016/j.wneu.2018.11.170.
125. Cho EB, Joo EY, Seo D-W, Hong S-C, Hong SB. Prognostic role of functional neuroimaging after multilobar resection in patients with localization-related epilepsy. PLoS One. 2015;10(8):e0136565.

126. Gaillard WD, Chiron C, Cross JH, Harvey AS, Kuzniecky R, Hertz-Pannier L, et al. Guidelines for imaging infants and children with recent-onset epilepsy. Epilepsia. 2009;50(9):2147–53.
127. Brockhaus A, Elger CE. Complex partial seizures of temporal lobe origin in chil- dren of different age groups. Epilepsia. 1995;36:1173–81.
128. Vasung L, Fischi-Gomez E, Hüppi PS. Multimodality evaluation of the pediatric brain: DTI and its competitors. Pediatr Radiol. 2013;43(1):60–8.
129. Bittar RG, Rosenfeld JV, Klug GL, Hopkins IJ, Harvey AS. Resective surgery in infants and young children with intractable epilepsy. J Clin Neurosci. 2002;9(2):142–6.
130. Cossu M, Schiariti M, Francione S, Fuschillo D, Gozzo F, Nobili L, et al. Stereoelectroencephalography in the presurgical evaluation of focal epilepsy in infancy and early childhood. J Neurosurg Pediatr. 2012;9(3):290–300.
131. Gowda S, Salazar F, Bingaman WE, Kotagal P, Lachhwani DL, Gupta A, et al. Surgery for catastrophic epilepsy in infants 6 months of age and younger. J Neurosurg Pediatr. 2010;5(6):603–7.
132. Taussig D, Dorfmüller G, Fohlen M, Jalin C, Bulteau C, Ferrand-Sorbets S, et al. Invasive explorations in children younger than 3 years. Seizure. 2012;21(8):631–8.
133. Weiss HK, Bandt SK. Epilepsy Surgery in Children Under Three Years of Age. Pediatr Neurol Briefs. 2019;33:3.
134. Vasconcellos E, Wyllie E, Sullivan S, Stanford L, Bulacio J, Kotagal P, et al. Mental retardation in pediatric candidates for epilepsy surgery: the role of early seizure onset. Epilepsia. 2001;42(2):268–74.
135. Nabbout R, Dulac O. Epileptic encephalopathies: a brief overview. J Clin Neurophysiol. 2003;20(6):393–7.
136. Ebus S, Arends J, Hendriksen J, van der Horst E, de la Parra N, Hendriksen R, et al. Cognitive effects of interictal epileptiform discharges in children. Eur J Paediatr Neurol. 2012;16(6):697–706.
137. Nolan MA, Redoblado MA, Lah S, Sabaz M, Lawson JA, Cunningham AM, et al. Intelligence in childhood epilepsy syndromes. Epilepsy Res. 2003;53(1–2):139–50.
138. Vendrame M, Alexopoulos AV, Boyer K, Gregas M, Haut J, Lineweaver T, et al. Longer duration of epilepsy and earlier age at epilepsy onset correlate with impaired cognitive development in infancy. Epilepsy Behav. 2009;16(3):431–5.
139. Cossu M, Cardinale F, Castana L, Nobili L, Sartori I, Lo Russo G. Stereo-EEG in chil- dren. Childs Nerv Syst. 2006;22:766–78.

# 12 Reoperations After Failed Resective Surgery

*True wisdom comes to each of us when we realize how little we understand about life, ourselves, and the world around us.*

*Socrates*

## Contents



Resective epilepsy surgery leads to a favorable seizure outcome (Engel I–II, ILAE 1–2) in 70–90% of patients indicating that 10–30% continue to have disabling seizures after surgery. Patients with persisting seizures may show a different course: Some achieve spontaneously seizure control by the "running down phenomenon" [1], others may benefit from modified anticonvulsive medication or alternative treatment options, while in a significant percentage epilepsy will persist despite various efforts. In these patients who continue to have more than rarely seizures after a resective procedure corresponding to the outcome classes Engel III–IV [2] and ILAE 3–6 [3], epilepsy surgery is considered as a failure.

In addition to persisting seizures and missed expectations such as psychosocial and psychological improvement and a better quality of life, some of those patients may significantly decline in memory, e.g., after left temporal resections, and fail to recover from this impairment in the long run [4]. These "double loosers," 8% in the study of Langfitt et al. [5], reveal the most severe deteriorations in health-related quality of life (HRQOL). Failed surgery emphasizes the need for careful




J. Zentner, *Surgical Treatment of Epilepsies*, https://doi.org/10.1007/978-3-030-48748-5_12

patient selection, comprehensive presurgical diagnostics, and advising patients about the chances and risks of surgery [6]. Given this unsuccessful course of the disease, questions arise as to the causes of failed surgery and appropriate strategies to consider re-evaluation with the option of a second resective surgery [7].

## 12.1 Causes of Failed Resective Surgery

As mentioned by Surges and Elger [7], there are several possible causes for failed resective epilepsy surgery: (1) Surgery is based on an incorrect hypothesis and localization of the seizure focus [8], (2) too limited resection has been planned due to close relationships of the epileptogenic zone with eloquent areas [9–11], (3) the resection performed does not correspond to the planning with respect to localization and/or extent, e.g., persistent seizures may be caused by residual entorhinal cortex, hippocampus, or dysplastic tissue, resection of which has been planned but not carried out [10–14], and (4) there is a more widespread ictogenic network such as in the presence of a dual pathology [9, 15, 16], rapid seizure spread [17], or in case of a "temporal plus epilepsy" [18–23]. In fact, in all these circumstances, definition and/or removal of the epileptogenic area or disruption of the epileptogenic network was not successful. In addition, the nature of the underlying disease can cause failed resective surgery leading to a recurrent seizure focus (e.g., tumor recurrence) [9, 24], a new seizure focus (e.g., involvement of the contralateral hippocampus) [25], or by unrecognized coexistence of two syndromes (e.g., TLE and idiopathic generalized epilepsy) [7, 26, 27]. Overall, insufficient resection has been suggested to be the most common reason for recurrent seizures [7, 9–11, 28]. Figures 12.1 and 12.2 show typical examples.

## 12.2 Re-evaluation and Reoperation

In most cases, seizures recur within the first year after the primary procedure [7, 28]. According to the review of 15 adult case series by Surges and Elger [7], criteria to select candidates for re-evaluation vary from center to center and include mainly type of epilepsy, underlying pathology,

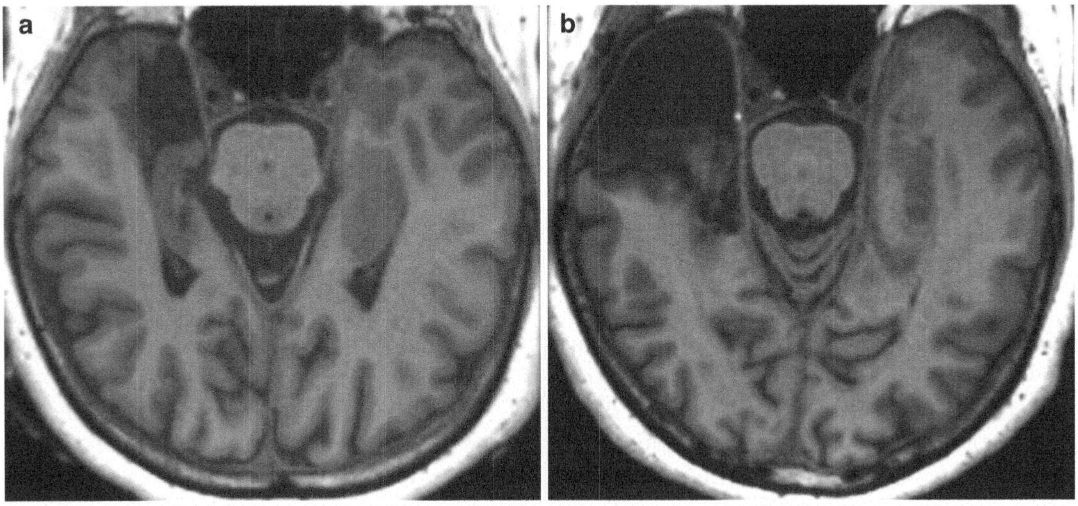


**Fig. 12.1** Thirty-seven-year-old female patient with a right temporomesial epilepsy. Amygdalohippocampectomy has been planned in a hospital without an epilepsy surgical program. (**a**) Postoperative axial T1-weighted MRI show the limited resection. Only marginal parts of the hippocampus have been removed. Due to recurrent seizures, the patient has been reoperated 21 years later. (**b**) Axial T1-weighted MRI after reoperation shows ATL with amygdalohippocampectomy

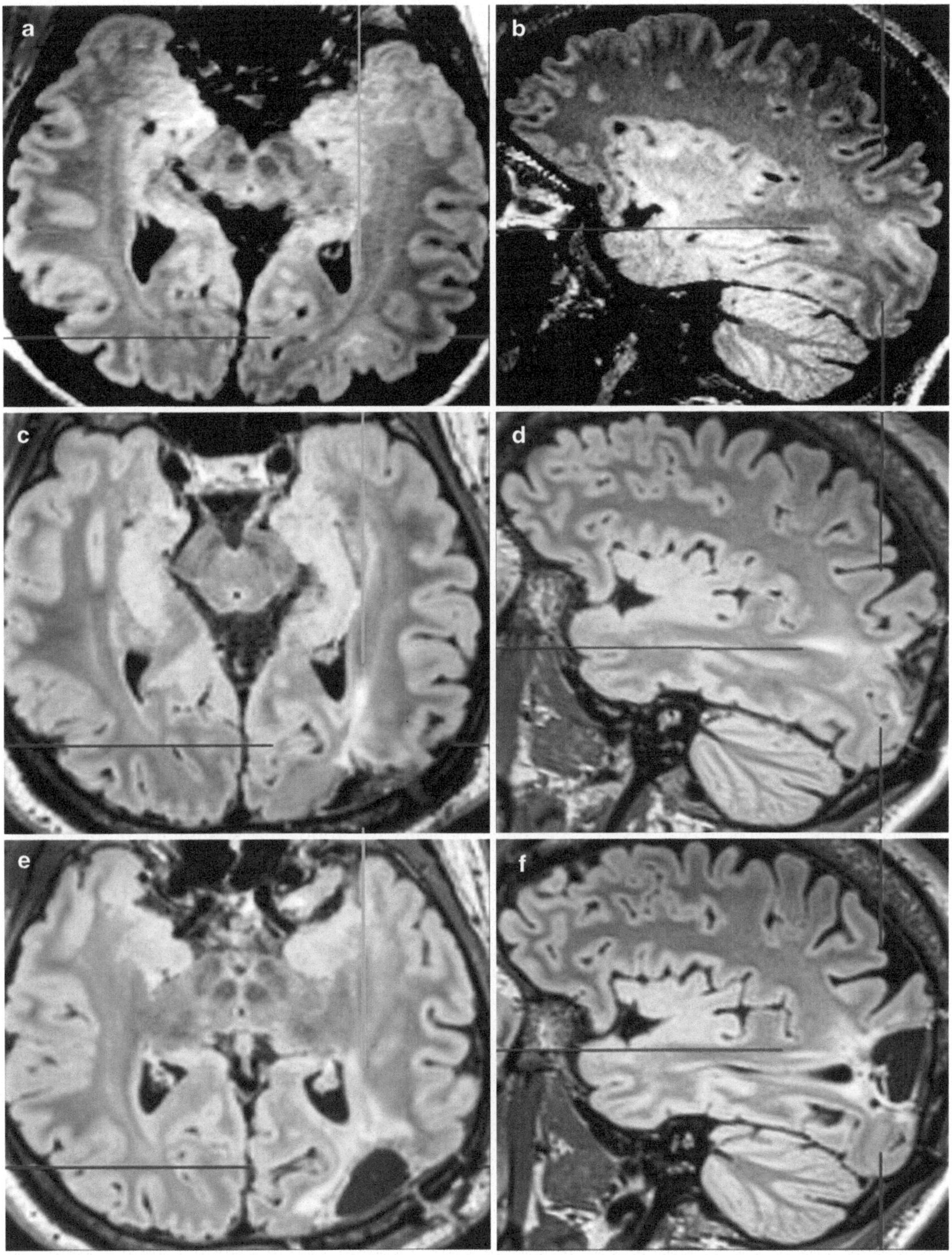


**Fig. 12.2** Thirty-four-year-old male patient with a left occipital FCD. Axial (left) and sagittal (right) MRI (FLAIR) are shown. (**a**, **b**) Preoperative MRI demonstrate the lesion in the left occipital lobe (the lesion is marked with a crosshair). (**c**, **d**) After the first procedure, parts of the lesion (crosshair) can still be seen in front of the resection site. Histological analysis revealed FCD type IIa. Postoperatively, visual fields were intact. (**e**, **f**) Due to recurrent seizures, reoperation with complete removal of the lesion was performed 39 months after the first procedure. Histopathological analysis demonstrated FCD type IIb. Postoperatively, there was a lower quadrant hemianopia. The patient was seizure-free

and postsurgical MRI findings. The rate of re-evaluated failed cases ranged from 32% to 100% among different centers, and 22.1–73.3% of re-evaluated cases proceeded to a second operation. Thus, reoperation rates ranged between 35.9% and 65.2% of patients with unfavorable outcome after primary surgery [7]. Others noted that 3.8–14% of all patients who had resective epilepsy surgery underwent a second operation [12, 25, 28–34]. Reoperation was performed on the average between 2 and 5.5 years after the first surgery in the review of Surges and Elger [7]. Grote et al. [28] noted a mean time interval between the primary and the second surgery of 5.6 years. In accordance to the frequency distribution of the primary epileptic foci and the causes of failed surgery, the majority of reoperations referred to the temporal and frontal lobe and consisted in the extension of the first operation [7, 9–11, 28].

## 12.3 Outcome After Reoperation

### 12.3.1 Systematic Reviews and Meta-analyses

Krucoff et al. [35] published a meta-analysis comprising 36 studies and 782 pediatric and adult patients who underwent repeat surgery. Overall, Engel I outcome was observed in 47% of patients. Surges and Elger [7] reviewed 15 case series including a total of 402 reoperated adults. At a follow-up of 6 months to 4 years after the second procedure, Engel I outcome was noted in 36.6% of patients (range: 9.5–57.1%). In larger of those cohorts including 31–64 reoperated cases, Engel I outcome was 34% [34], 48% [36], 53% [37], and 39% [38].

### 12.3.2 Observational Studies

Analyzing the Bonn series of 66 reoperations with a median follow-up of 10.3 years, Grote et al. [28] noted complete seizure freedom (ILAE 1) in 46 patients (70%). Similarly, seizure-free outcome was achieved in 10 of 16 reoperated cases (63%) reported by Englot et al. [10, 11], in 6 of 10 patients (60%) observed by Schmeiser et al. [39], and in 10 of 17 cases (59%) documented by Reed et al. [9]. After additional resection of remaining temporomesial structures, Salanova et al. [32] noted seizure freedom in 64% of their cases. It seems to be noteworthy that 4.7–14.1% of the patients who were reoperated without success were operated a third time, and seizure freedom was achieved in 44–100% of the cases [29, 34, 37–40]. Analyzing 110 reoperations, Yardi et al. [41] reported seizure-free outcome in 42% of patients who had one previous surgery and in 33% with two or more prior resections.

### 12.3.3 Predictors for Successful Repeat Surgery

The following predictors of a favorable seizure outcome after reoperation have been identified: MRI visible tumor [28, 38, 41, 42], shorter duration of epilepsy before the first operation as well as the presence of focal interictal discharges (IED) prior to first surgery [9, 34], younger age [9, 28], absence of preoperative invasive diagnostics [28], and reoperations extending previous resections [29, 36, 43]. Krucoff et al. [35] noted in their meta-analysis of 36 studies and 782 patients the following significant predictors of seizure freedom: congruent electrophysiological data, lesional epilepsy, and insufficient resection at the first procedure. Seizure-free outcome increased from 47% to 58% in patients who had at least one of these positive predictors. In addition, temporal location and abnormal preoperative MRI, although not significant, showed trends towards seizure freedom. Gender, epilepsy duration, age at either surgery, time interval between resections, laterality of resections, and seizure generalization did not significantly correlate with outcome [35].

### 12.3.4 Predictors for Failed Repeat Surgery

Predictors indicating poor outcome after repeat surgery include: normal MRI findings [10, 11,

27, 34, 44], recurrent or new epileptiform areas despite adequate achievement of primary surgical targets [45], distant or multifocal epileptiform discharges as well as secondary propagation of ictal activity to the contralateral hemisphere [33, 37, 45, 46], early recurrence of seizures after initial surgery [46], history of encephalitis [29], history of traumatic brain injury [47], and FCD as pathology [38]. In addition, invasive preoperative monitoring correlated significantly with a worse seizure outcome in the review of Krucoff et al. [35], and the presence of generalized seizures showed a trend towards a worse outcome, but this association did not reach statistical significance. Yardi et al. [41] noted that the chances of success diminish with every subsequent resection.

## 12.4 Special Considerations in Children and Adolescents

A particular feature of epilepsy surgery in the pediatric age is the high rate of reoperations. This relates to FCD as the most frequent etiology and to the inherent difficulties in its accurate delineation, especially in catastrophic epilepsies in early life (see also Chap. 11). Englot et al. [10, 11] found that limited resection is the most important cause of failed surgery as observed in 72% (26 of 36 cases) in his report, while an additional epileptogenic zone distant from the resection caused recurrent seizures in 10 of 36 patients (28%). In line, incomplete resection has been recognized as the single most important risk factor for seizure recurrence in several other pediatric studies [48–51]. This holds particularly true in extensive or even hemispheric dysplasia, where complete resections would involve functional cortex.

### 12.4.1 Frequency of Repeat Surgery

As a result of limited primary resection of hardly definable extensive seizure foci, a higher proportion of children compared to adults undergo repeat surgery [52–54]. Repeat surgery is required in 17–23% of very young children [48, 53, 55, 56], in 9–10% of children and adolescents [57, 58], and in 13% of pediatric and adult cohorts with FCD [49]. On the other hand, it should be noted that, of the 10–30% of children who do not reach a favorable outcome (Engel I–II, ILAE 1–2) after the first surgery, only 5–20% undergo repeat resection [48–51, 53, 55, 57–59].

### 12.4.2 Seizure Outcome

In the study of Ramantani et al. [46] comprising 23 children and adolescents (83% of them with FCD as the underlying etiology), 61% were seizure-free after reoperation, 26% showed significant or worthwhile improvement, and only 13% failed to respond to repeat surgery. Similar favorable results after reoperation have been reported by others [60, 61]. In children and adolescents undergoing repeat temporal resections, long-term seizure freedom has been reported in 4 of 4 [62], and in 14 of 23 (61%) [63] cases. Patients with ipsilateral mesial or basal temporal recurrences have been thought to represent ideal candidates for reoperation [43]. Overall, results demonstrate that the majority of children and adolescents with recurrent seizures following an initial resection can benefit from a repeat procedure.

### 12.4.3 Predictors

In the study of Englot et al. [10, 11], the most important positive predictor for favorable long-term seizure and neuropsychological outcome was early reoperation with complete lesion resection. In addition, children presenting fewer than 14 seizures per week preoperatively were more likely to become seizure-free after a new surgery [10, 11]. Reoperation is especially beneficial for patients with an extensive epileptogenic zone who have not responded to the initial limited resection but may achieve seizure freedom after a multilobar of even hemispheric procedure. The decision to proceed to repeat surgery should be considered shortly after seizure recurrence since early postsurgical seizures predict poor long-term seizure control [10, 11, 64]. Infancy and early childhood carry a unique potential of significant functional reorganization, and congenital or early acquired etiologies enable the inter- or intrahemispheric transfer of eloquent functions. In contrast, surgical approaches aiming to spare eloquent cortex bear the risk of unfavorable seizure outcomes [46, 53, 64, 65].

**Concluding Remarks**

- ***Failed surgery.*** *Failed epilepsy surgery refers to patients with persistent disabling seizures (Engel III–IV and ILAE 3–6, respectively) after a resective procedure. In addition to persistent seizures, some of those patients may significantly decline in memory and fail to recover ("double loosers").*
- ***Reoperations.*** *The main cause of failed surgery is insufficient resection, frequently not corresponding to the planning. Repeat surgery with extended resection has proven to provide seizure control in 50–70% of those patients.*
- ***Pediatric age.*** *Due to cortical dysplasia as the most frequent pathology, reoperation is required in around 20% of very young and in 10% of older children, and seizure control is achieved in the majority (around 60%) of cases.*

## References


1. Salanova V, Andermann F, Rasmussen T, Olivier A, Quesney L. The running down phenomenon in temporal lobe epilepsy. Brain. 1996;119:989–96.
2. Engel J, van Ness PC, Rasmussen T, Ojemann LM. Outcome with respect to epileptic seizures. In: Engel J, editor. Surgical treatment of the epilepsies. New York: Raven Press; 1993. p. 609–21.
3. Wieser HG, Blume WT, Fish D, et al. ILAE Commission Report. Proposal for a new classification of outcome with respect to epileptic seizures following epilepsy surgery. Epilepsia. 2001;42(2):282–6.
4. Helmstaedter C, Elger CE, Vogt VL. Cognitive outcomes more than 5 years after temporal lobe epilepsy surgery: Remarkable functional recovery when seizures are controlled. Seizure. 2018;62:116–23.
5. Langfitt JT, Westerveld M, Hamberger MJ, et al. Worsening of quality of life after epilepsy surgery: effect of seizures and memory decline. Neurology. 2007;68(23):1988–94.
6. Vakharia VN, Duncan JS, Witt J-A, et al. Getting the best outcomes from epilepsy surgery. Annals of Neurology. 2018;83(4):676–90.
7. Surges R, Elger CE. Reoperation after failed resective epilepsy surgery. Seizure. 2013;22:493–501.
8. Sperling MR. Clinical challenges in invasive monitoring in epilepsy surgery. Epilepsia. 1997;38(Suppl 4):S6–S12.
9. Reed C, Dewar S, Fried I, et al. Failed epilepsy surgery deserves a second chance. Clin Neurol Neurosurg. 2017; https://doi.org/10.1016/j.clineuro.2017.10.023.
10. Englot DJ, Raygor KP, Molinaro AM, Garcia PA, Knowlton RC, Auguste KI, Chang EF. Factors associated with failed focal neocortical epilepsy surgery. Neurosurgery. 2014;75:648–55.
11. Englot DJ, Han SJ, Rolston JD, Ivan ME, Kuperman RA, Chang EF, Gupta N, Sullivan JE, Auguste KI. Epilepsy surgery failure in children: a quantitative and qualitative analysis. J Neurosurg Pediatr. 2014;14:386–95.
12. Awad IA, Nayel MH, Lüders H. Second operation after the failure of previous resection for epilepsy. Neurosurgery. 1991;28:510–8.
13. Hennessy MJ, Elwes RD, Binnie CD, Polkey CE. Failed surgery for epilepsy. A study of persistence and recurrence of seizures following temporal resection. Brain. 2000;123:2445–66.
14. Zachenhofer I, Novak K, Baumgartner C, Prayer D, Czech T. Reoperation after selective amygdalohippocampectomy: an MRI analysis of the extent of temporomesial resection in ten cases. Acta Neurochir (Wien). 2011;153:239–48.
15. Fauser S, Schulze-Bonhage A. Epileptogenicity of cortical dysplasia in temporal lobe dual pathology: an electrophysiological study with invasive recordings. Brain. 2006;129:82–95.
16. Schmeiser B, Zentner J, Steinhoff BJ, et al. The role fo presurgical EEG parameters and of reoperation for seizure outcome in temporal lobe epilepsy. Seizure. 2017;51:174–9.
17. Andrews JP, Gummadavelli A, Farooque P, et al. Association of seizure spread with surgical failure in epilepsy. JAMA Neurol. 2019;76(4):462–9.
18. Devinsky O, Morrell MJ, Vogt BA. Contributions of anterior cingulate cortex to behaviour. Brain. 1995;118(Pt 1):279–306.
19. Isnard J, Guenot M, Ostrowsky K, Sindou M, Mauguiere F. The role of the insular cortex in temporal lobe epilepsy. Ann Neurol. 2000;48:614–23.
20. Lee KH, Park YD, King DW, Meador KJ, Loring DW, Murro AM, Smith JW. Prognostic implication of contralateral secondary electrographic seizures in temporal lobe epilepsy. Epilepsia. 2000;41:1444–9.
21. Ryvlin P, Kahane P. The hidden causes of surgery-resistant temporal lobe epilepsy: extratemporal or temporal plus? Curr Opin Neurol. 2005;18:125–7.
22. Shihabuddin B, Abou-Khalil B, Delbeke D, Fakhoury T. Orbito-frontal epilepsy masquerading as temporal lobe epilepsy-a case report. Seizure. 2001;10:134–8.

23. Barba C, Rheims S, Minotti L, et al. Temporal plus epilepsy is a major determinant of temporal lobe surgery failures. Brain. 2016;139(Pt 2):444–51.
24. Maschio M. Brain tumor-related epilepsy. Curr Neuropharmacol. 2012;10:124–33.
25. Ramos E, Benbadis S, Vale FL. Failure of temporal lobe resection for epilepsy in patients with mesial temporal sclerosis: results and treatment options. J Neurosurg. 2009;110:1127–34.
26. Sadler RM, Blume WT. Significance of bisynchronous spike-waves in patients with temporal lobe spikes. Epilepsia. 1989;30:143–6.
27. Tahry RE, Wang IZ. Failed epilepsy surgery: is this the end? Acta Neurol Belg. 2017; https://doi.org/10.1007/s13760-017-0769-8.
28. Grote A, Witt JA, Surges R, von Lehe M, Pieper M, Elger CE, Helmstaedter C, Ormond DR, Schramm J, Delev D. A second chance—reoperation in patients with failed surgery for intractable epilepsy: long-term outcome, neuropsychology and complications. J Neurol Neurosurg Psychiatry. 2016;87:379–85.
29. Holmes MD, Wilensky AJ, Ojemann LM, Ojemann GA. Predicting outcome following reoperation for medically intractable epilepsy. Seizure. 1999;8:103–6.
30. Pati S, Abla AA, Rekate HL, Ng YT. Repeat surgery for hypothalamic hamartoma in refractory epilepsy. Neurosurg Focus. 2011;30:E3.
31. Salanova V, Quesney LF, Rasmussen T, Andermann F, Olivier A. Reevaluation of surgical failures and the role of reoperation in 39 patients with frontal lobe epilepsy. Epilepsia. 1994;35:70–80.
32. Salanova V, Markand O, Worth R. Temporal lobe epilepsy: analysis of failures and the role of reoperation. Acta Neurol Scand. 2005;111:126–33.
33. Schulz R, Hoppe M, Boesebeck F, Gyimesi C, Pannek HW, Woermann FG, et al. Analysis of reoperation in mesial temporal lobe epilepsy with hippocampal sclerosis. Neurosurgery. 2011;68:89–97.
34. Siegel AM, Cascino GD, Meyer FB, McClelland RL, So EL, Marsh WR, et al. Resective reoperation for failed epilepsy surgery: seizure outcome in 64 patients. Neurology. 2004;63:2298–302.
35. Krucoff MO, Chan AY, Harward SC, et al. Rates and predictors of success and failure in repeat epilepsy surgery: a meta-analysis and systematic review. Epilepsia. 2017;58(12):2133–42.
36. Wyler AR, Hermann BP, Richey ET. Results of reoperation for failed epilepsy surgery. J Neurosurg. 1989;71:815–9.
37. Germano IM, Poulin N, Olivier A. Reoperation for recurrent temporal lobe epilepsy. J Neurosurg. 1994;81:31–6.
38. González-Martínez JA, Srikijvilaikul T, Nair D, Bingaman WE. Long-term seizure outcome in reoperation after failure of epilepsy surgery. Neurosurgery. 2007;60:873–80.
39. Schmeiser B, Zentner J, Steinhoff BJ, et al. The role fo presurgical EEG parameters and of reoperation for seizure outcome in temporal lobe epilepsy. Seizure. 2017;51:174–9.
40. Erdem A, Kahilogullari G, Erbas YC, Karatas A, Bilir E. Reoperation of a recurrent temporal lobe epilepsy: a technical case report. Surg Neurol. 2005;64(Suppl. 2):S102–5.
41. Yardi R, Morita-Sherman ME, Fithgerald Z, et al. Long-term outcomes of reoperations in epilepsy surgery. Epilepsy. 2020; https://doi.org/10.1111/epi.16452.
42. Schwartz TH, Spencer DD. Strategies for reoperation after comprehensive epilepsy surgery. J Neurosurg. 2001;95:615–23.
43. Jehi LE, Silveira DC, Bingman W, et al. Temporal lobe epilepsy surgery failures: predictors of seizure recurrence, yield of reevaluation, and outcome following reoperation. J Neurosurg. 2010;113:1186–94.
44. Janszky J, Pannek HW, Janszky I, Schulz R, Behne F, Hoppe M, Ebner A. Failed surgery for temporal lobe epilepsy: predictors of long-term seizure-free course. Epilepsy Res. 2005;64:35–44.
45. Schwartz TH, Spencer DD. Strategies for reoperation after comprehensive epilepsy surgery. J Neurosurg. 2001;95:615–23.
46. Ramantani G, Strobl K, Stathi A, Brandt A, Schubert-Bast S, Wiegand G, et al. Reoperation for refractory epilepsy in childhood: a second chance for selected patients. Neurosurgery. 2013;73(4):695–704.
47. Jung R, Aull-Watschinger S, Moser D, et al. Is reoperation an option for patients with temporal lobe epilepsy after failure of surgery? Seizure. 2013;22:502–6.
48. Kadish NE, Bast T, Reuner G, Wagner K, Mayer H, Schubert-Bast S, et al. Epilepsy surgery in the first 3 years of life: predictors of seizure freedom and cognitive development. Neurosurgery. 2019;84(6):E368–77.
49. Krsek P, Maton B, Jayakar P, Dean P, Korman B, Rey G, et al. Incomplete resection of focal cortical dysplasia is the main predictor of poor postsurgical outcome. Neurology. 2009;72(3):217–23.
50. Ramantani G, Stathi A, Brandt A, Strobl K, Schubert-Bast S, Wiegand G, et al. Posterior cortex epilepsy surgery in childhood and adolescence: Predictors of long-term seizure outcome. Epilepsia. 2017;58(3):412–9.
51. Ramantani G, Kadish NE, Mayer H, Anastasopoulos C, Wagner K, Reuner G, et al. Frontal lobe epilepsy surgery in childhood and adolescence: predictors of long-term seizure freedom, overall cognitive and adaptive functioning. Neurosurgery. 2018;83(1):93–103.
52. Ramantani G, Cosandier-Rimélé D, Schulze-Bonhage A, Maillard L, Zentner J, Dümpelmann M. Source reconstruction based on subdural EEG recordings adds to the presurgical evaluation in refractory frontal lobe epilepsy. Clin Neurophysiol. 2013;124(3):481–91.

53. Ramantani G, Kadish NE, Strobl K, Brandt A, Stathi A, Mayer H, et al. Seizure and cognitive outcomes of epilepsy surgery in infancy and early childhood. Eur J Paediatr Neurol. 2013;17(5):498–506.
54. Ramantani G, Dümpelmann M, Koessler L, Brandt A, Cosandier-Rimélé D, Zentner J, et al. Simultaneous subdural and scalp EEG correlates of frontal lobe epileptic sources. Epilepsia. 2014;55(2):278–88.
55. Dunkley C, Kung J, Scott RC, Nicolaides P, Neville B, Aylett SE, et al. Epilepsy surgery in children under 3 years. Epilepsy Res. 2011;93(2–3):96–106.
56. Steinbok P, Gan PYC, Connolly MB, Carmant L, Barry Sinclair D, Rutka J, et al. Epilepsy surgery in the first 3 years of life: a Canadian survey. Epilepsia. 2009;50(6):1442–9.
57. Cossu M, Lo Russo G, Francione S, Mai R, Nobili L, Sartori I, et al. Epilepsy surgery in children: results and predictors of outcome on seizures. Epilepsia. 2008;49(1):65–72.
58. Hemb M, Velasco TR, Parnes MS, Wu JY, Lerner JT, Matsumoto JH, et al. Improved outcomes in pediatric epilepsy surgery: the UCLA experience, 1986-2008. Neurology. 2010;74(22):1768–75.
59. Ramantani G, Kadish NE, Anastasopoulos C, Brandt A, Wagner K, Strobl K, et al. Epilepsy surgery for glioneuronal tumors in childhood: avoid loss of time. Neurosurgery. 2014;74(6):648–57; discussion 657.
60. Bower RS, Wirrell EC, Eckel LJ, Wong-Kisiel LC, Nickels KC, Wetjen NM. Repeat resective surgery in complex pediatric refractory epilepsy: lessons learned. J Neurosurg Pediatr. 2015;16(1):94–100.
61. Muthaffar O, Puka K, Rubinger L, Go C, Snead OC, Rutka JT, et al. Reoperation after failed resective epilepsy surgery in children. J Neurosurg Pediatr. 2017;20(2):134–40.
62. Mittal S, Montes JL, Farmer JP, et al.: Long-term outcome after surgical treatment of temporal lobe epilepsy in children. J Neurosurg. 2005;103;401–12.
63. Benifla M, Otsubo H, Ochi A, Weiss SK, Donner EJ, Shroff M, et al. Temporal lobe surgery for intractable epilepsy in children: an analysis of outcomes in 126children. Neurosurgery. 2006;59(6):1203–13; discussion 1213-14.
64. Kadish NE, Bast T, Reuner G, Wagner K, Mayer H, Schubert-Bast S, et al. Epilepsy Surgery in the First 3 Years of Life: Predictors of Seizure Freedom and Cognitive Development. Neurosurgery. 2019;84(6):E368-E377.
65. Ramantani G, Kadish NE, Brandt A, Strobl K, Stathi A, Wiegand G, et al. Seizure control and developmental trajectories after hemispherotomy for refractory epilepsy in childhood and adolescence. Epilepsia. 2013;54(6):1046–55.

# Pathology in Epilepsy Surgery 13

*My therapist read my pathology report and said: There's only one way you can beat your tumor. What's that? You have to find out what caused it.*

*Kathy Acker*

## Contents



In may be postulated that every focal epilepsy is based on structural abnormalities of the brain. In fact, since the description of Ammon's horn sclerosis in 1880 by Sommer [1], histopathological analysis of specimens obtained from epilepsy surgery revealed a large amount of lesions including hippocampal sclerosis, malformative, neoplastic, ischemic, and traumatic lesions, as well as cerebrovascular and infectious diseases [2–11]. Advances have been made in understanding the functional implications of different structural abnormalities as a cause of seizures which may arise within the lesion, in the surrounding tissue, or remote of the lesion [12–16]. Moreover, clinicopathological correlations have demonstrated prognostic relevance of pathological findings in terms of seizure outcome [17]. Thus, pathological analysis of surgical specimens is important both for understanding mechanisms of epileptogenesis and postoperative care of patients.



J. Zentner, *Surgical Treatment of Epilepsies*, https://doi.org/10.1007/978-3-030-48748-5_13

## 13.1 Classification of Structural Abnormalities: The European Epilepsy Brain Bank (EEBB)

In order to emphasize the role of pathology in epilepsy surgery and to contribute to standardized analysis and classification of structural abnormalities facilitating multicenter collaborating studies for both clinical care and research, the European Epilepsy Brain Bank (EEBB) has been established in 2006 under the direction of the Framework Program of the European Union. The data of the EEBB comprising specimens of 9523 patients (4944 men, 4579 women; 6900 adults, 2623 children) who underwent resective surgery for drug-resistant seizures in 36 centers of 12 European countries over 25 years have been published by Blümcke et al. in 2017 [17]. Overall, the most common categories were hippocampal sclerosis (HS) as found in 36.4% of the patients (88.7% of cases were adults), tumors (mainly gangliogliomas) detected in 23.6%, and malformations of cortical development (MCD) as observed in 19.8% of patients (FCD was the most common type, 52.7% of cases were children). No histopathological diagnosis could be established for 7.7% of the patients. The ten most frequent histopathological diagnoses accounted for 86.7% of cases [17].

### 13.1.1 Hippocampal Sclerosis (HS)

Hippocampal sclerosis, also referred to as mesial temporal sclerosis (MTS) or Ammon's horn sclerosis (AHS) is characterized by atrophy of the hippocampus with loss of pyramidal neurons, granule cell dispersion and gliosis [2, 18–21]. The 2013 International League Against Epilepsy (ILAE) classification distinguishes between typical (HS type 1) and atypical (HS types 2 and 3) forms, based on the histopathological patterns of subfield neuronal loss and gliosis. ILAE type 1 (classical HS) includes neuronal cell loss and gliosis in all subfields (extensive HS) or in CA1 > CA4, CA3, sparing CA2, while neuronal cell loss and gliosis are predominant in CA1 with ILAE type 2, and in CA4 with ILAE type 3 [22] (Fig. 13.1). In addition to cell loss and gliosis, granule cell reorganization and alterations of interneuronal populations, neuropeptide fiber networks, and mossy fiber sprouting are distinctive features of HS associated with epilepsies [23]. HS is thought to constitute an acquired structural abnormality on a multifactorial basis and may be caused by prolonged febrile seizures or other precipitating injuries (see also Chap. 6). Moreover, genetic susceptibility, inflammatory, and neurodevelopmental factors are discussed [23]. The study of Na et al. [24] demonstrated a significant correlation between ILAE types of HS and long-term postoperative seizure outcome in patients with MTLE due to HS. The most favorable outcome was noted with HS type 1. There were no significant differences in seizure outcome between HS types 2 and 3 patients [24].

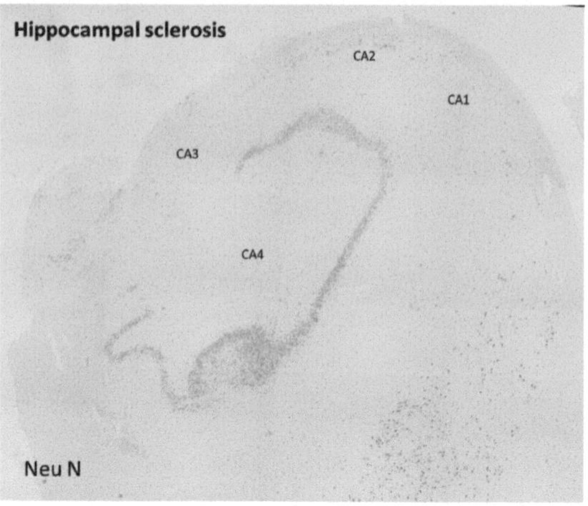


**Fig. 13.1** Hippocampal sclerosis (HS), ILAE type 1, with segmental pyramidal cell loss in CA1 and CA4 sectors representing the most common type of HS in MTLE. In this type, CA3 is less affected, while CA2 is largely unaffected. (With courtesy of S. Doostkam, Dpt. of Neuropathology, Freiburg)

### 13.1.2 Epilepsy-Associated Tumors

A variety of tumors, particularly with cortical extension, cause focal seizures in a high percentage. Glioneuronal tumors include gangliogliomas

(GG) and dysembryoplastic neuroepithelial tumors (DNET). Other WHO-grade I glial tumors frequently associated with epilepsy may also have a minor neuronal component, including pleomorphic xanthoastrocytomas (PXA), pilocytic astrocytomas, isomorphic astrocytomas, the angiocentric neuroepithelial tumor, papillary glioneuronal tumors, and extraventricular neurocytomas [25, 26] (Figs. 13.2, 13.3, 13.4, 13.5, and 13.6). WHO-grade II tumors causing drug-resistant epilepsy in a lower percentage include diffuse astrocytomas and oligodendrogliomas [26–30] (Figs. 13.7, 13.8, 13.9, and 13.10). For those epilepsy-associated tumors which typically occur in young age and show a stable course over years, the terms "long-term epilepsy-associated tumors, LEATs" [31] or "low-grade epilepsy-associated neuroepithelial tumors" [32] have been suggested (see also Chap. 9). Depending on tumors characteristics, 10-years survival rates of 90–100% can be achieved with surgical removal of LEATs [29, 31, 33–38]. Malignant transformation has been described in rare cases [26, 28, 31, 37, 39–41].

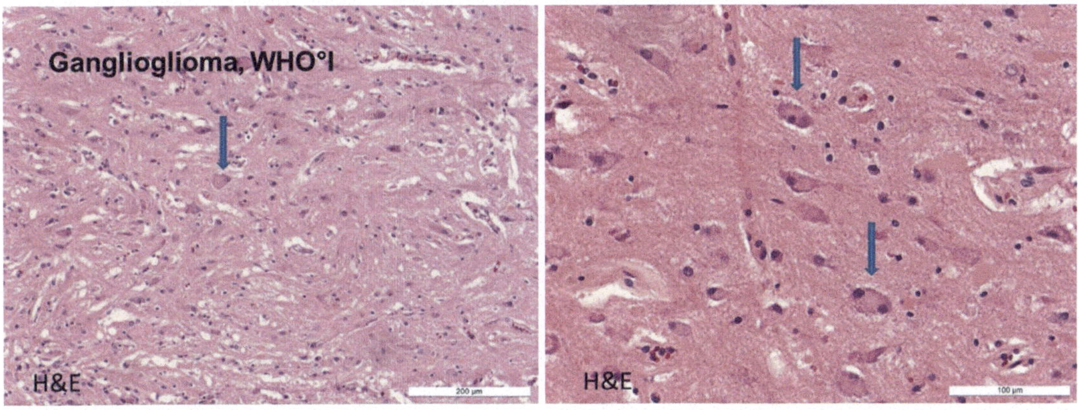


**Fig. 13.2** Ganglioglioma WHO-grade I (H&E). This low-grade neuroepithelial tumor shows both glial and neuronal components. Binucleated and dysplastic neurons (arrow) are interspersed in glial components resembling a pilocytic astrocytoma, fibrillar astrocytoma, or oligodendroglioma. There are no criteria of malignancy. (With courtesy of S. Doostkam, Dpt. of Neuropathology, Freiburg)

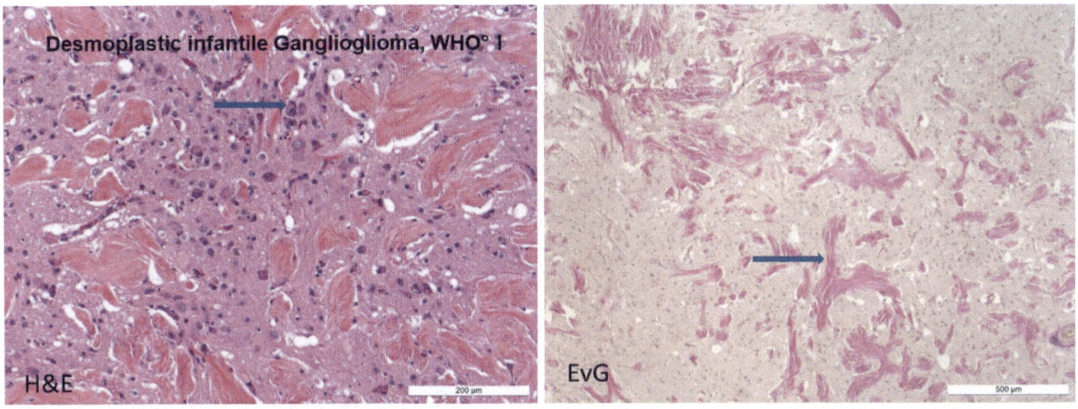


**Fig. 13.3** Desmoplastic infantile ganglioglioma WHO-grade I (H&E, left, and EvG, right). The tumor shows a desmoplastic leptomeningeal and a ganglioglioma component with abnormal dysplastic and binuclear neurons. (With courtesy of S. Doostkam, Dpt. of Neuropathology, Freiburg)

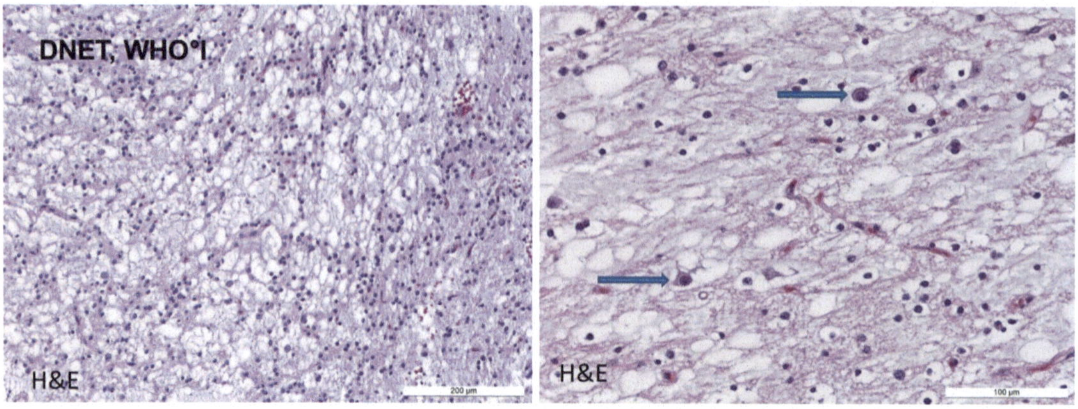


**Fig. 13.4** Dysembryoplastic neuroepithelial tumor (DNET) WHO-grade I (H&E). The widened cortex is enforced with the so-called specific glioneural element, a mucoid loosened matrix consisting of astrocytes, oligodendrocytes, and neurons (floating neurons). (With courtesy of S. Doostkam, Dpt. of Neuropathology, Freiburg)

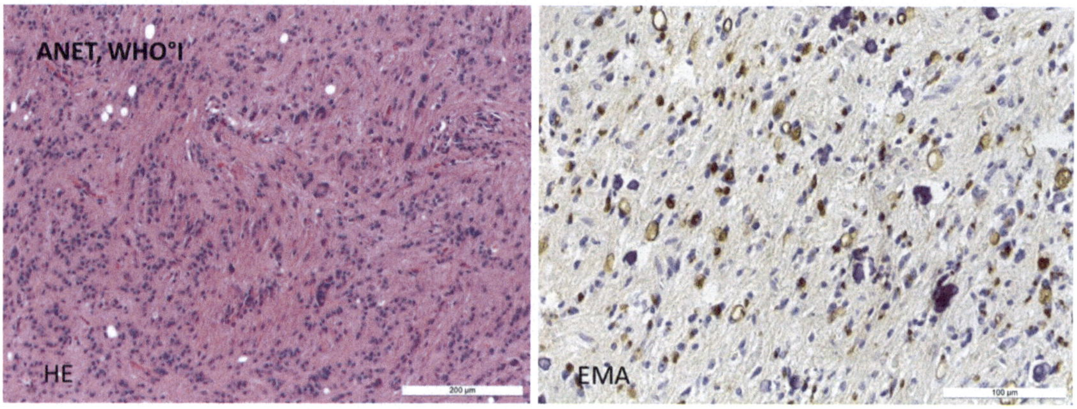


**Fig. 13.5** Angiocentric neuroepithelial tumor (ANET) WHO-grade I (H&E, left, and EMA, right). Monomorphous, slowly growing glial tumor with bipolar elongated glial cells oriented around cortical blood vessels. There is a typical punctual intracytoplasmic immunoreactivity for EMA. (With courtesy of S. Doostkam, Dpt. of Neuropathology, Freiburg)

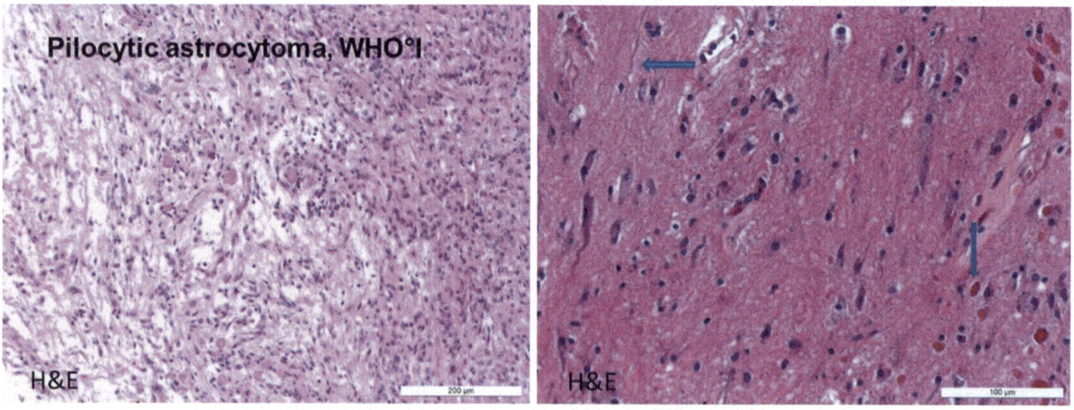


**Fig. 13.6** Pilocytic astrocytoma WHO-grade I (H&E). Uniform astrocytic differentiated tumor with bipolar elongated tumor cells, Rosenthal fibers, and protein droplets. (With courtesy of S. Doostkam, Dpt. of Neuropathology, Freiburg)

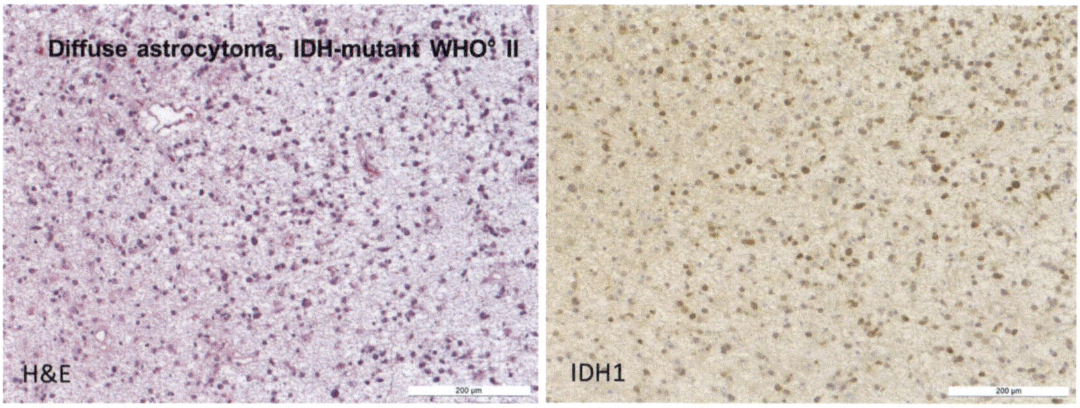


**Fig. 13.7** Diffuse astrocytoma WHO-grade II (H&E, left, and IDH1 immunohistochemistry, right). Diffuse infiltrating astrocytic tumor, mostly ATRX and IDH mutated. No significantly increased mitotic or proliferation rate. (With courtesy of S. Doostkam, Dpt. of Neuropathology, Freiburg)

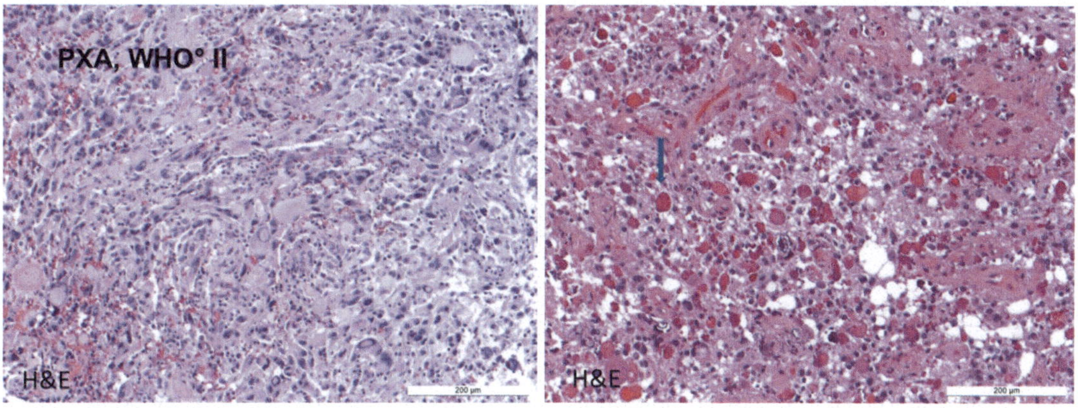


**Fig. 13.8** Pleomorphic xanthoastrocytoma (PXA) WHO-grade II (H&E). Astrocytic tumor with pleomorphic as well as double and multinucleated giant cells, frequently with evidence of granular bodies (arrow). No increased mitosis or proliferation rate. No further malignancy criteria. (With courtesy of S. Doostkam, Dpt. of Neuropathology, Freiburg)

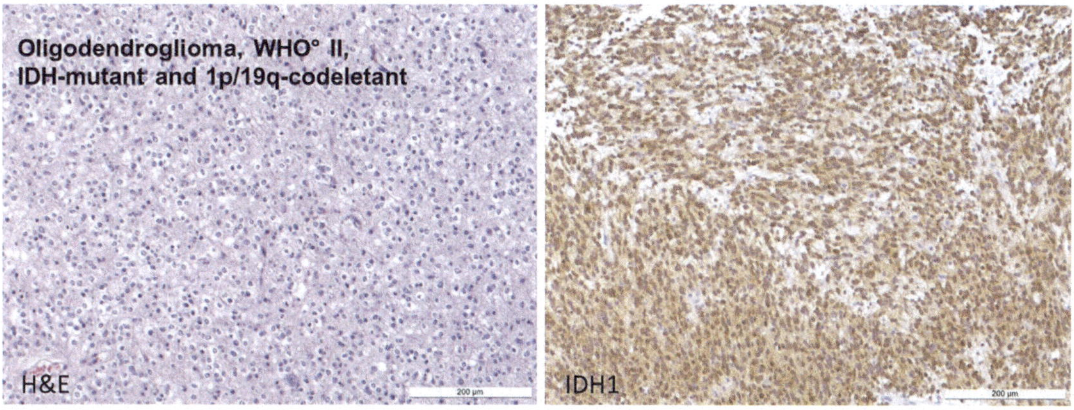


**Fig. 13.9** Oligodendroglioma WHO-grade II (H&E, left, and IDH1 immunohistochemistry, right). Uniform oligodendroglially differentiated tumor with IDH mutation and 1p/19q codeletion. Typical perinuclear optically empty spaces (honeycomb or fried-egg pattern). No increased rate of mitosis or proliferation tendency. (With courtesy of S. Doostkam, Dpt. of Neuropathology, Freiburg)

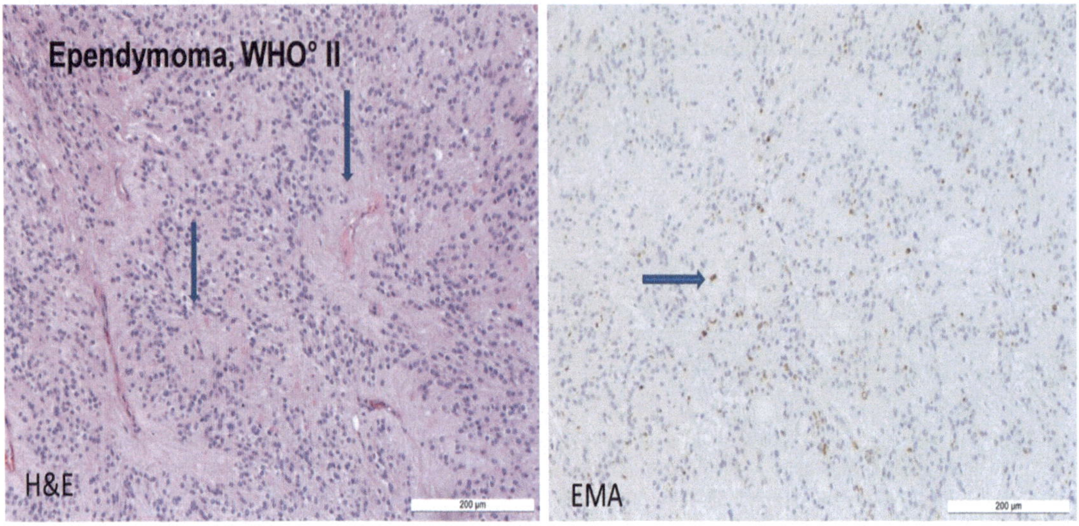


**Fig. 13.10** Ependymoma WHO-grade II (H&E, left, and EMA, right). Characteristic perivascular anucleate spaces (pseudorosettes). Punctual intracytoplasmic immunoreactivity for EMA (microrosettes). (With courtesy of S. Doostkam, Dpt. of Neuropathology, Freiburg)

### 13.1.3 Malformations of Cortical Development (MCD)

The histopathological spectrum of MCD includes hemimegalencephaly, polymicrogyria, hamartia/hamartoma, and in particular focal cortical dysplasia (FCD) [3]. FCD constitutes around 40% of lesions observed in pediatric epilepsy surgical series [42–46]. Different classification systems for FCD have been proposed relying either on histopathological examination [47], imaging and genetic findings [42], or a combination of clinical and histopathological patterns [48]. Palmini et al. [48] distinguished two types of FCD: type I (cytoarchitectural abnormalities without balloon cells or dysmorphic neurons), and type II (cytoarchitectural abnormalities with abnormal neurons or balloon cells) including subgroups depending on severity of dysplasia (Fig. 13.11). In 2011, the ILAE Consensus Commission published a revised classification of FCD introducing type III as a new category which means the association of FCD with a second pathology (including hippocampal sclerosis, tumors, scars, and vascular lesions), thus to separate isolated FCD (types I and II) from associated dysplasias which may represent acquired changes in the developed cortex rather than developmental lesions [12, 26].

Analyzing 9523 patients, Blümcke et al. [17] found mild malformations of cortical development (mMCD) in 2.9%, FCD type I in 2.8%, FCD type II in 9.0%, and unclassified FCD in 2.2%. Compared to FCD types I and II, patients with mMCD develop seizures later in life with a predilection for the temporal lobe and a lower seizure-free outcome rate. The inferior outcome after surgery in mMCD is likely due to difficulties in accurate identification and complete removal of those lesions [49]. Analyzing 88 patients with MCD, Veersema et al. [49] found complete seizure freedom (Engel Ia) in 32% of cases with mMCD as compared to 59% in patients with FCD. Similarly, Kim et al. [50] noted seizure-free outcome (Engel I) in 43% of mMCD patients and in 59% with FCD. Fauser et al. [51] found Engel Ia outcome in 67% with FCD type Ia, in 55% with FCD type Ib, but only in 43% with FCD type IIa, and in 50% with FCD type IIb (Taylor type) which represents the most frequently recognized FCD entity. Correspondingly, seizure reduction by less than 75% (Engel IV)

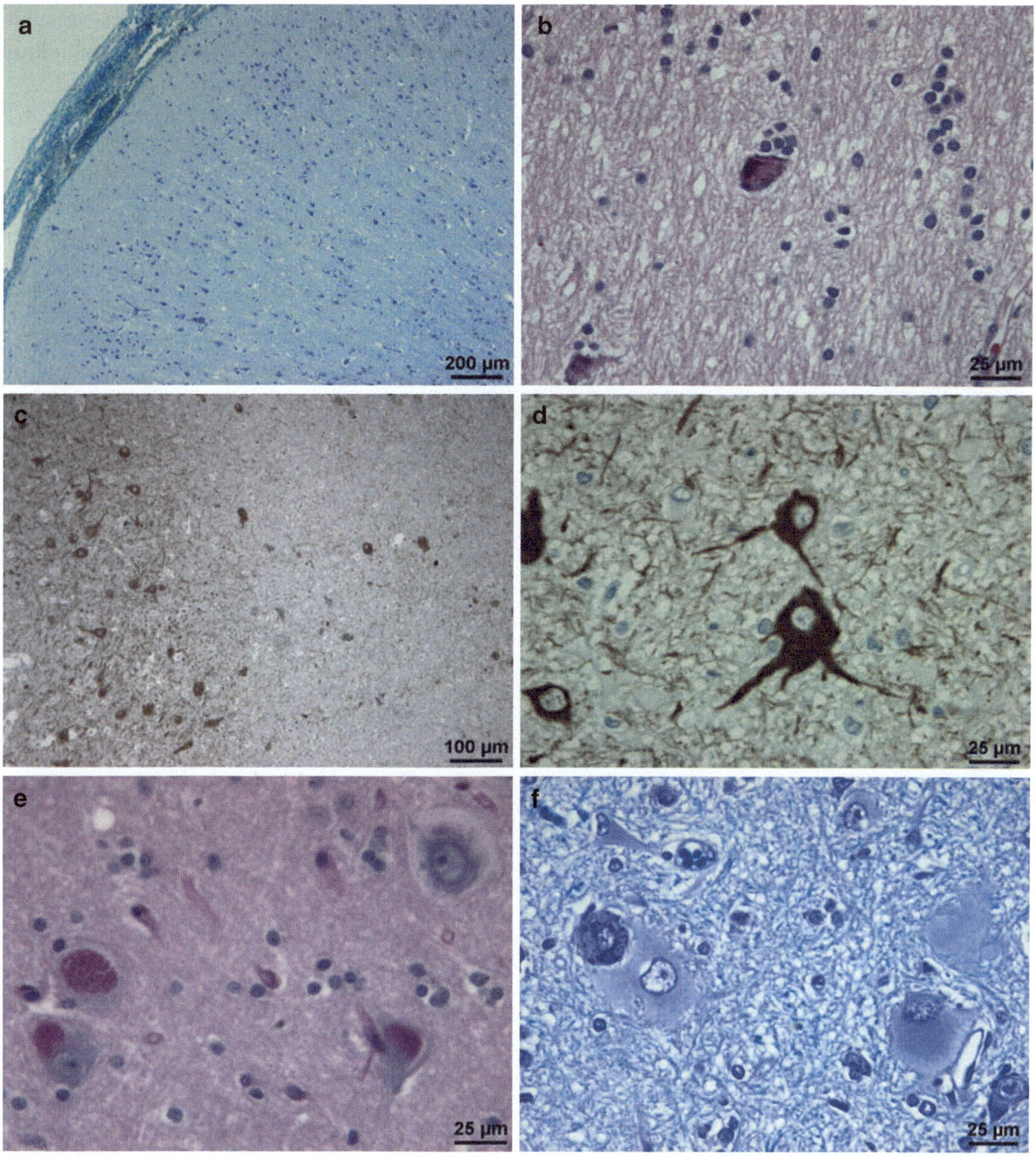


**Fig. 13.11** Focal cortical dysplasia (FCD). Cytoarchitectural abnormalities in different histopathological types of FCD are shown. (**a**) FCD Ia. Columnar arrangement of neurons (Klüver–Barrera). (**b**) FCD Ia. Clusters of oligodendrocytes (hematoxylin and eosin). (**c**) FCD Ib. Severe dyslamination with immature neurons in the deeper layers of the cortex and heterotopic neurons in the white matter (neurofilament). (**d**) FCD IIa. Dysmorphic neurons (neurofilament). (**e**) FCD IIa. Dysmorphic neurons with aggregates of Nissl substance and lipofuscin (periodic acid Schiff). (**f**) FCD IIb. Balloon cells and dysmorphic neurons (Klüver–Barrera). (From Fauser et al. [51], with permission)

was noted more frequently in patients with FCD type IIa than with other subgroups. Dual pathology did not imply a worse seizure outcome [51]. Others have demonstrated excellent results in patients with FCD IIb with seizure-free outcome rates of up to 90% [49, 52]. Overall, the quality of MRI to detect and delineate malformations of cortical development constitutes the decisive factor influencing seizure outcome and may explain different results in previous studies.

## 13.2 Temporal and Extratemporal Epilepsies

### 13.2.1 Temporal Lobe Epilepsies (TLE)

Analyzing 6358 TLE patients with specific structural abnormalities of the European Epilepsy Brain Bank (EEBB), Blümcke et al. [17] observed hippocampal sclerosis (HS) in 54.4% of temporal specimens (58.8% in adults, and 34.7% in children and adolescents), tumors in 22.3% (18.7% in adults, and 39.1% in children and adolescents), and MCD in 7.5% (5.6% in adults, and 16.0% in children and adolescents). A second histopathological diagnosis (dual pathology) was found in 1.5% of specimens with HS including ganglioglioma (25.2%), glial scars (23.7%), focal cortical dysplasia (8.6%), dysembryoplastic neuroepithelial tumors (8.6%), encephalitis (7.2%), and cavernous angioma (5.8%) [17].

In the literature, dual pathology has been reported in 5–30% of temporal lobe resections [53–56] and refers mainly to the coexistence of HS with malformations of cortical development, most commonly with FCD [51, 55, 57–59]. Salanova [60] found dual pathology in 15%, Fauser et al. [51] in 43%, and Eriksson et al. [57] in 48% of HS patients. However, dual pathology has been diagnosed in up to 100% of patients with HS evaluating minor microscopical extrahippocampal abnormalities [61–63]. Major differences regarding the incidence of dual pathology may result both from pathological evaluation and from inconsistent neurosurgical sampling [17].

### 13.2.2 Extratemporal Epilepsies (ETE)

FCD represents the most frequent etiology of ETE observed in 20–80% of patients, followed by tumors (15–35%), gliosis including post-traumatic and ischemic lesions (10–30%), and vascular malformations (5–15%) [64–68]. Similarly, Aykut-Bingol et al. [69] and Olivier et al. [70] found a predominance of MCD and tumors in posterior cortex epilepsies (PCE), while Binder et al. [71] noted that the spectrum of lesions in PCE may be different from other areas predominantly showing glial scars/gliosis (29%), followed by vascular malformations (25%), FCD (17%), gangliogliomas (17%), and other tumors (12%) [71].

Evaluating 1690 ETE patients with specific pathologies of the European Epilepsy Brain Bank (EEBB), Blümcke et al. [17] observed in extratemporal location MCD in 47.9% (40.6% in adults, and 56.4% in children and adolescents) and tumors in 23.0% (25.8% in adults, and 19.8% in children and adolescents). With multilobar resections (797 patients with specific histopathological diagnoses), MCD were noted in 35.6% (27.8% in adults, and 39.7% in children and adolescents) and tumors in 18.6% (27.1% in adults, and 14.1% in children and adolescents). FCD was the most common malformation of cortical development, accounting for 70.6% of cases. Most frequently, the combination of dysmorphic neurons and balloon cells, which is characteristic of FCD type II was found amounting to 45.3% of cases [17].

## 13.3 MRI-Negative Epilepsies

### 13.3.1 Temporal Lobe Epilepsies

Hippocampal sclerosis (HS) has been detected on histopathological evaluation in between 9% and 49% of MRI-negative TLE cases based on 1.5/3T MRI [72–74]. Bell et al. [75] found HS in 18%, and gliosis in up to 80% of MRI-negative cases. In another series of 399 epilepsy patients with predominantly MRI-negative TLE, gliosis was the underlying pathology in 59%, and HS in 28% of cases [72]. Overall, nonspecific gliosis constitutes the most common pathology in MRI-negative TLE [73, 75–80].

### 13.3.2 Temporal/Extratemporal Epilepsies

Wang et al. [74] evaluated histopathological findings in 95 MRI-negative patients with temporal and extratemporal epilepsies. Most common lesions included FCD (45%), gliosis (22%), hamartia and gliosis (13%), and HS (9%). The majority of FCD showed ILAE or Palmini type I. Only 7% of the patients had no identifiable pathological abnormalities [74]. Similarly, FCD has been found to represent the most frequent pathology in MRI-negative extratemporal cases by others [81–85]. Kogias et al. [86] reported histopathological findings in 20 specimens of 3T MRI-negative epilepsies. Results showed gliosis in 11 patients, mMCD in 5 cases, and FCD type I in 4 individuals. In pediatric series, FCD has been mainly found [87, 88]. Overall, the most common epilepsy substrate in MRI-negative ETE is FCD [81–85].

## 13.4 Unspecific Pathological Findings

According to the data of the EEBB comprising 9523 patients [17], no specific lesion (or only nonspecific reactive gliosis) could be identified by microscopic inspection in 7.7% of patients (8.4% of adults and 6.1% of children). Relating seizure-free outcome at 1-year after surgery to pathological findings shows the following results: With hippocampal sclerosis, the rate of seizure-free outcome was 61.4%, with tumors 68.4% (79.9% of children and 63.5% of adults), with malformations of cortical development 57.6% (59.9% of children and 54.6% of adults), and without any specific lesion 50.2% (55.2% of children and 48.7% of adults) (EEBB [17]). Thus, differences in seizure-free outcome between patients with and without specific pathological findings are not as high as one might have expected. In fact, seizure freedom as observed in around half of nonlesional patients indicates that the tissue removed was involved in epileptogenesis in these cases.

Nonspecific histopathological findings may in part result from inconsistent neurosurgical sampling [17], or from histopathological entities that have still to be characterized such as oligodendroglial hyperplasia in white matter and hyaline protoplasmic astrocytopathy [89, 90]. However, in non-lesional cases also successful interruption of a functional epileptogenic network has to be discussed. Gil et al. [91] demonstrated in a study on 21 extratemporal and mainly MRI-negative patients epileptic networks that were composed of a large number of elements interacting dynamically to generate interictal epileptic activity and epileptic seizures. Some elements of these functional networks were thought to exhibit intrinsic epileptogenicity, while others might propagate epileptic activity. Those networks could also contribute to the understanding of the impact of focal epilepsy on epilepsy-related cognitive disturbances [91]. In all, the relative high number of successfully treated patients without evidence of a specific structural abnormality rises questions to the classical concept of epileptogenesis (see also Chap. 3) and supports the existence of functional epileptogenic networks.

**Concluding Remarks**

- ***Significance of neuropathological assessment.*** *Advances in neuropathological diagnosis and classification of epileptogenic brain lesions contribute to the understanding of epileptogenesis and are helpful for clinical correlation, outcome stratification, and patient care. The efforts of the Task Force of Neuropathology of the ILAE Commission on Diagnostic Methods in developing a consensus standard operational procedure (SOP) for tissue inspection, distribution, and processing can be expected to provide a systematic framework for histopathological assessment of operative specimens, facilitating collaborating studies for both clinical care and research.*
- ***Demands on surgical dissection and handling.*** *In order to support those efforts in neuropathology, anatomically intact surgical specimens representing all aspects of the pathology and facilitating systematic analysis should be provided by the surgeon whenever possible, e.g., the hippocampal formation should be dissected en bloc allowing correct orientation in relation to preoperative imaging and neurophysiological studies. A good communication between pathology and the neurosurgical team is required. The surgical tissue should be sent immediately and fresh to the laboratory, thus allowing appropriate freezing, fixing, and banking of tissue samples for both diagnostic and research purposes.*
- ***Concept of epileptogenesis.*** *The relatively high rate of seizure-free outcome in patients without specific histopathological findings (around 50%) rises questions as to the classical concept of epileptogenesis based on specific structural abnormalities indicating successful surgical interruption of functional epileptogenic networks.*

## References


1. Sommer W. Erkrankung des Ammonshorns als aetiologisches Moment der Epilepsie. Arch Psychiatr Nervenkr. 1880;10:631–75.
2. Babb TL, Brown WJ, Pretorius J, et al. Temporal lobe volumetric cell densities in temporal lobe epilepsy. Epilepsia. 1984;25(6):729–40.
3. Blümcke I, Vinters HV, Armstrong D, et al. Malformations of cortical development and epilepsies: neuropathological findings with emphasis on focal cortical dysplasia. Epileptic Disord. 2009;11(3):181–93.
4. De Lanerolle NC, Lee T-S, Spencer DD. Histopathology of human epilepsy. In: Noebels J, Avoli M, Rogawski M, Olsen R, Delgado-Escueta A, editors. Jasper's basic mechanisms of the epilepsies. New York: Oxford University Press; 2012. Print ISBN-13: 9780199746545.
5. Dlugos DJ, Jaggi J, O'Connor WM, Ding XS, Reivich M, O'Connor MJ, Sperling MR. Hippocampal cell density and subcortical metabolism in temporal lobe epilepsy. Epilepsia. 1999;40:408–13.
6. Engel J, Brown WJ, Kuhl DE, Phelps ME, Mazziota JC, Crandall PH. Pathological findings underlying focal temporal lobe hypometabolism in partial epilepsy. Ann Neurol. 1982;12:518–28.
7. Falconer MA. The significance of mesial temporal sclerosis (Ammon's horn sclerosis) in epilepsy. Guys Hosp Rep. 1968;117:1–12.
8. Kim JH. Pathology of seizure disorders. Neuroimaging Clin N Am. 1995;5:527–45.
9. Kim JH. Pathology of epilepsy. Exp Mol Pathol. 2001;70:345–67.
10. Vinters HV, Armstrong DL, Babb TL, et al. The neuropathology of human symptomatic epilepsy. In: Engel J, editor. Surgical treatment of the epilepsies. New York: Raven Press; 1993. p. 593–608.
11. Al Sufiani FA, Ang LC. Neuropathology of temporal lobe epilepsy. Epilepsy Res Treat. 2012; https://doi.org/10.1155/2012/624519.
12. Blümcke I, Thom M, Aronica E, et al. The clinicopathologic spectrum of focal cortical dysplasias: a consensus classification proposed by an ad hoc Task Force of the ILAE Diagnostic Methods Commission. Epilepsia. 2011;52:158–74.
13. Dudek FE, Sutula TP. Epileptogenesis in the dentate gyrus: a critical perspective. Prog Brain Res. 2007;163:755–73.
14. Haas CA, Dudeck O, Kirsch M, Huszka C, Kann G, Pollak S, Zentner J, Frotscher M. Role for reelin in the development of granule cells dispersion in temporal lobe epilepsy. J Neurosci. 2002;22:5797–802.
15. Sloviter RS, Sollas AL, Barbaro NM, Laxer KD. Calcium-binding protein (Calbindin-D28K) and parvalbumin immunocytochemistry in the normal and epileptic human hippocampus. J Comp Neurol. 1991;308:381–96.
16. Soriano E, Frotscher M. Mossy cells of the rat fascia dentata are glutamate-immunoreactive. Hippocampus. 1994;4:65–9.
17. Blümcke I, Spreafico R, Haaker G, et al. Histopathological findings in brain tissue obtained during epilepsy surgery. N Engl J Med. 2017;377:1648–56.
18. Babb TL, Wilson CL, Isokawa-Akesson M. Firing patterns of human limbic neurons during stereoencephalography (SEEG) and clinical temporal lobe seizures. Electroencephalogr Clin Neurophysiol. 1987;66(6):467–82.
19. Rausch R, Babb TL. Hippocampal neuron loss and memory scores before and after temporal lobe surgery for epilepsy. Arch Neurol. 1993;50(8):812–7.
20. Vivash L, Tostevin A, Liu DS, Dalic L, Dedeurwaerdere S, Hicks RJ, Williams DA, Myers DE, O'Brien TJ. Changes in hippocampal GABAA/cBZR density during limbic epileptogenesis: relationship to cell loss and mossy fibre sprouting. Neurobiol Dis. 2011;41(2):227–36. https://doi.org/10.1016/j.nbd.2010.08.021.
21. Borges K, Gearing M, McDermott DL, Smith AB, Almonte AG, Wainer BH, Dingledine R. Neuronal and glial pathological changes during epileptogenesis in the mouse pilocarpine model. Exp Neurol. 2003;182(1):21–34.
22. Blümcke I, Thom M, Aronica E, et al. International consensus classification of hippocampal sclerosis in temporal lobe epilepsy: a Task Force report from the ILAE Commission on Diagnostic Methods. Epilepsia. 2013;54:1315–29.
23. Thom M. Review: Hippocampal sclerosis in epilepsy: a neuropathology review. Neuropathol Appl Neurobiol. 2014;40(5):520–43.
24. Na M, Ge H, Shi C. Long-term seizure outcome for international consensus classification of hippocampal sclerosis: a survival analysis. Seizure. 2015;25:141–6.
25. Blümcke I, Aronica E, Urbach H, et al. A neuropathology-based approach to epilepsy surgery in brain tumors and proposal for a new terminology use for long-term epilepsy-associated brain tumors. Acta Neuropathol. 2014;128(1):39–54.
26. Thom M, Blümcke I, Aronica E. Long-term epilepsy-associated tumors. Brain Pathol. 2012;22:350–79.
27. Giulioni M, Marucci G, Pelliccia V, Gozzo F, Barba C, et al. Epilepsy surgery of "low grade epilepsy associated neuroepithelial tumors": a retrospective nationwide Italian study. Epilepsia. 2017; https://doi.org/10.1111/epi.13866.
28. Louis DN, Ohgaki H, Wiestler OD, et al. WHO classification of tumours of the central nervous system. Lyon: IARC; 2016.
29. Pelliccia V, Deleo F, Gozzo F, et al. Early and late epilepsy surgery in focal epilepsies associated with long-term epilepsy-associated tumors. J Neurosurg. 2017;127(5):1147–52.
30. Prayson R, Fong J, Najm I. Coexistent pathology in chronic epilepsy patients with neoplasms. Mod Pathol. 2010;23:1097–103.
31. Luyken C, Blümcke I, Fimmers R, Urbach H, Elger CE, Wiestler OD, Schramm J. The spectrum of long-term epilepsy-associated tumors: long-term seizure and tumor outcome and neurosurgical aspects. Epilepsia. 2003;44:822–30.

32. Blümcke I, Aronica E, Miyata H, et al. International recommendation for a comprehensive neuropathologic workup of epilepsy surgery brain tissue: a consensus Task Force report from the ILAE Commission on Diagnostic Methods. Epilepsia. 2016;47(3):348–58.
33. Englot DJ, Berger MS, Barbaro NM, Chang EF. Factors associated with seizure freedom in the surgical resection of glioneuronal tumors. Epilepsia. 2012;53:51–7.
34. Chassoux F, Landré E, Mellerio C, Turak B, Mann MW, Daumas-Duport C, et al. Type II focal cortical dysplasia: electroclinical phenotype and surgical outcome related to imaging. Epilepsia. 2012;53(2):349–58.
35. Giulioni M, Marucci G, Martinoni M, et al. Seizure outcome in surgically treated drug-resistant mesial temporal lobe epilepsy based on the recent histopathological classifications. J Neurosurg. 2013;119: 37–47.
36. Giulioni M, Marucci G, Martinoni M, et al. Epilepsy associated tumors: review article. World J Clin Cases. 2014;2:623–41.
37. Tomita T, Volk JM, Shen W, et al. Glioneuronal tumors of cerebral hemisphere in children: correlation of surgical resection with seizure outcomes and tumor recurrences. Child's Nerv Syst. 2016;32:1839–48.
38. Clusmann H, Schramm J, Kral T, et al. Prognostic factors and outcome after different types of resection for temporal lobe epilepsy. J Neurosurg. 2002;97(5):1131–41.
39. Majores M, von Lehe M, Fassunke J, et al. Tumor recurrence and malignant progression of gangliogliomas. Cancer. 2008;113:3355–63.
40. Bonney PA, Glenn CA, Ebeling PA, et al. Literature review seizure freedom rates and prognostic indicators after resection of gangliogliomas: a review. World Neurosurg. 2015;84:1988–96.
41. Hirsch M, Coenen VA, Heiland DH, Lützen N, Straszewski O, Schulze-Bonhage A. Epilepsieassoziierte Tumoren des Zentralnervensystems. Nervenarzt. 2015; https://doi.org/10.1007/s00115-015-0031-7.
42. Barkovitch AJ, Kuzniecky RI, et al. A developmental and genetic classification for malformations of cortical development. Neurology. 2005;65:1873–87.
43. Cloppenborg T, May TW, Blümcke I, et al. Trends in epilepsy surgery: stable surgical numbers despite increasing presurgical volumes. J Neurol Neurosurg Psychiatry. 2016;87:1322–9.
44. Hemb M, Velasco TR, Parnes MS, et al. Improved outcomes in pediatric epilepsy surgery: the UCLA experience, 1986-2008. Neurology. 2010;74:1768–75.
45. Lamberink HJ, Boshuisen K, van Rijen PC, Gosselaar PH, Braun KP. Changing profiles of pediatric epilepsy surgery candidates over time: a nationwide single-center experience from 1990 to 2011. Epilepsia. 2015;56:717–25.
46. Harvey AS, Cross JH, Shinnar S, Mathern GW, Mathern BW. ILAE Pediatric Epilepsy Surgery Survey Taskforce. Defining the spectrum of international practice in pediatric epilepsy surgery patients. Epilepsia. 2008;49(1):146–55.
47. Mischel PS, Nguyen LP, Vinters HV. Cerebral cortical dysplasia associated with pediatric epilepsy. Review of neuropathologic features and proposal for a grading system. J Neuropathol Exp Neurol. 1995;54:137–53.
48. Palmini A, Najm I, Avanzini G, et al. Terminology and classification of the cortical dysplasias. Neurology. 2004;62:S2–8.
49. Veersema TJ, Swampillai B, Ferrier CH, et al. Long-term seizure outcome after epilepsy surgery in patients with mild malformation of cortical development and focal cortical dysplasia. Epilepsia. 2019; https://doi.org/10.1002/epi4.12289.
50. Kim DW, Lee SK, Chu K, et al. Predictors of surgical outcome and pathologic considerations in focal cortical dysplasia. Neurology. 2009;72:211–6.
51. Fauser S, Schulze-Bonhage A, Honegger J, et al. Focal cortical dysplasias: surgical outcome in 67 patients in relation to histological subtypes and dual pathology. Brain. 2004;127:2406–18.
52. Wagner J, Urbach H, Niehusmann P, von Lehe M, Elger CE, Wellmer J. Focal cortical dysplasia type IIb: completeness of cortical, not subcortical, resection is necessary for seizure freedom. Epilepsia. 2011;52:1418–24.
53. Cendes F, Cook MJ, Watson C, et al. Frequency and characteristics of dual pathology in patients with lesional epilepsy. Neurology. 1995;45:2058–64.
54. Lévesque MF, Nakasato N, Vinters HV, Babb TL. Surgical treatment of limbic epilepsy associated with extrahippocampal lesions: the problem of dual pathology. J Neurosurg. 1991;75:364–70.
55. Li LM, Cendes F, Andermann F, et al. Surgical outcome in patients with epilepsy and dual pathology. Brain. 1999;122:799–805.
56. Raymond AA, Fish DR, Stevens JM, Cook MJ, Sisodiya SM, Shorvon SD. Association of hippocampal sclerosis with cortical dysgenesis in patients with epilepsy. Neurology. 1994;44:1841–5.
57. Eriksson SH, Nordborg D, Rydenhag B, et al. Parenchymal lesions in pharmacoresistant temporal lobe epilepsy: dual and multiple pathology. Acta Neurol Scand. 2005;112:151–6.
58. Kral T, Clusmann H, Blumcke I, Fimmers R, Ostertun B, Kurthen M, Schramm J. Outcome of epilepsy surgery in focal cortical dysplasia. J Neurol Neurosurg Psychiatry. 2003;74:183–8.
59. Srikijvilaikul T, Najm IM, Hovinga CA, Prayson RA, Gonzalez-Martinez J, Bingaman WE. Seizure outcome after temporal lobectomy in temporal lobe cortical dysplasia. Epilepsia. 2003;44:1420–4.
60. Salanova V. Temporal lobe epilepsy: analysis of patients with dual pathology. Acta Neurol Scand. 2004;109(2):126–31.
61. Jay V, Becker LE, Otsubo H, Hwang PA, Homan HJ, Harwood-Nash D. Pathology of temporal lobectomy for refractory seizures in children. Review of 20 cases including some unique malformative lesions. J Neurosurg. 1993;79:53–61.
62. Nishio S, Morioka T, Hisada K, Fukui M. Temporal lobe epilepsy: a clinicopathological study with special reference to temporal neocortical changes. Neurosurg Rev. 2000;23:84–9.

63. Watson C, Chen W, Kupsky W, et al. The characteristics of microscopic dual pathology: a volumetric MRI and histopathological study. Epilepsia. 1999;40:200.
64. Ferrier CH, Engelsman J, Alarcon G, et al. Prognostic factors in presurgical assessment of frontal lobe epilepsy. J Neurol Neurosurg Psychiatry. 1999;66:350–6.
65. Frater JL, Prayson RA, Morris HH 3rd., et al. Surgical pathologic findings of extratemporal-based intractable epilepsy: a study of 133 consecutive resections. Arch Pathol Lab Med. 2000;124:545–9.
66. Jobst BC, Siegel AM, Thadani VM, et al. Intractable seizures of frontal lobe origin: clinical characteristics, localizing signs, and results of surgery. Epilepsia. 2000;41:1139–52.
67. Schramm J, Kral T, Kurthen M, et al. Surgery to treat focal frontal lobe epilepsy in adults. Neurosurgery. 2002;51:644–54.
68. Jeha LE, Najm I, Bingaman W, Dinner D, Widdess-Walsh P, Lüders H. Surgical outcome and prognostic factors of frontal lobe epilepsy surgery. Brain. 2007;130:574–84.
69. Aykut-Bingol C, Bronen RA, Kim JH, Spencer DD, Spencer SS. Surgical outcome in occipital lobe epilepsy: implications for pathophysiology. Ann Neurol. 1998;44:60–9.
70. Olivier A, Boling W Jr. Surgery of parietal and occipital lobe epilepsy. Adv Neurol. 2000;84:533–75.
71. Binder DK, Lehe v M, Kral T, et al. Surgical treatment of occipital lobe epilepsy. J Neurosurg. 2008;109(1):57–69.
72. Cohen-Gadol AA, Bradley CC, Williamson A, Kim JH, Westerveld M, Duckrow RB, Spencer DD. Normal magnetic resonance imaging and medial temporal lobe epilepsy: the clinical syndrome of paradoxical temporal lobe epilepsy. J Neurosurg. 2005;102:902–9.
73. Vale FL, Effio E, Arredondo N, et al. Efficacy of temporal lobe surgery for epilepsy in patients with negative MRI for mesial temporal lobe sclerosis. J Clin Neurosci. 2012;19:101–6.
74. Wang ZI, Alexopouzlos AV, Jones SE, et al. The pathology of magnetic-resonance imaging-negative epilepsy. Mod Pathol. 2013;26:1051–8.
75. Bell ML, Rao S, So EL, et al. Epilepsy surgery outcomes in temporal lobe epilepsy with a normal MRI. Epilepsia. 2009;50:2053–60.
76. Burkholder DB, Sulc V, Hoffman EM, et al. Interictal scalp electroencephalography and intraoperative electrocorticography in magnetic resonance imaging-negative temporal lobe epilepsy surgery. JAMA Neurol. 2014;71:702–9.
77. Cukiert A, Burattini JA, Mariani PP, et al. Outcome after corticoamygdalohippocampectomy in patients with temporal lobe epilepsy and normal MRI. Seizure. 2010;19:319–23.
78. Fong JS, Lehi L, Najm I, et al. Seizure outcome and its predictors after temporal lobe epilepsy surgery in patients with normal MRI. Epilepsia. 2011;52:1393–401. https://doi.org/10.1111/j.1528-1167.2011.03091.x.
79. Smith AP, Sani S, Kanner AM, et al. Medically intractable temporal lobe epilepsy in patients with normal MRI: surgical outcome in twenty-one consecutive patients. Seizure. 2011;20:475–9.
80. Sylaja PN, Radhakrishnan K, Kesavadas C, Sarma PS. Seizure outcome after anterior temporal lobectomy and its predictors in patients with apparent temporal lobe epilepsy and normal MRI. Epilepsia. 2004;45(7):803–8.
81. Carne RP, O'Brien TJ, Kilpatrick CJ, MacGregor LR, Hicks RJ, Murphy MA, Bowden SC, Kaye AH, Cook MJ. MRI-negative PET-positive temporal lobe epilepsy: a distinct surgically remediable syndrome. Brain. 2004;127:2276–85.
82. Cascino GD, Jack CRJ, Parisi JE, et al. Magnetic resonance imaging-based volume studies in temporal lobe epilepsy: pathological correlations. Ann Neurol. 1991;30:31–6.
83. Hong KS, Lee SK, Kim JY, Lee DS, Chung CK. 2002. Presurgical evaluation and surgical outcome of 41 patients with nonlesional neocortical epilepsy. Seizure. 2002;11:184–92.
84. Kutsy RL. Focal extratemporal epilepsy: clinical features, EEG patterns, and surgical approach. J Neurol Sci. 1999;166:1–15.
85. Semah F, Picot MC, Adam C, et al. Is the underlying cause of epilepsy a major prognostic factor for recurrence? Neurology. 1998;51:1256–62.
86. Kogias E, Altenmüler D-M, Klingler J-H, et al. Histopathology of 3 Tesla MRI-negative extratemporal focal epilepsies. J Clin Neurosci. 2018;50:232–6.
87. Guerrini R, Duchowny M, Jayakar P, Krsek P, Kahane P, Tassi L, et al. Diagnostic methods and treatment options for focal cortical dysplasia. Epilepsia. 2015;56(11):1669–86.
88. Adler S, Wagstyl K, Gunny R, Ronan L, Carmichael D, Cross JH, et al. Novel surface features for automated detection of focal cortical dysplasias in paediatric epilepsy. NeuroImage Clin. 2017;14:18–27.
89. Hedley-Whyte ET, Goldman JE, Nedergaard M, et al. Hyaline protoplasmic astrocytopathy of neocortex. J Neuropathol Exp Neurol. 2009;68:136–47.
90. Schurr J, Coras R, Rössler K, et al. Mild malformation of cortical development with oligodendroglial hyperplasia in frontal lobe epilepsy: a new clinico-pathological entity. Brain Pathol. 2017;27:26–35.
91. Gil F, Padilla N, Soria-Pastor S, et al. Beyond the epileptic focus: functional epileptic networks in focal epilepsy. Cereb Cortex. 2019; https://doi.org/10.1093/cercor/bhz243.

# Non-resective Epilepsy Surgery 14

*If you want new ideas, read old books*

*I. Pavlov*

## Contents



Today, surgical resection constitutes the gold standard for the treatment of medically intractable epilepsy. However, patients with poorly localized seizure foci, multiple epileptogenic zones, or foci co-localizing with eloquent areas may not be amenable to resective surgery [1, 2]. Furthermore, some patients harbor significant risk factors for a resective procedure or are averse to it. For these patients, several non-resective surgical options are available pursuing palliative or curative goals [3–5].

- *Palliative procedures*. Palliative procedures aim at reducing frequency and severity of seizures, in particular of most disabling seizures. Options include corpus callosotomy (CC) and multiple subpial transections (MST) which are called disconnective procedures, as well as vagal nerve stimulation (VNS), deep brain stimulation (DBS), responsive neurostimulation (RNS), and chronic subthreshold cortical stimulation (CSCS) which can be summarized under the term neurostimulation.
- *Curative procedures.* The goal of curative non-resective surgery is to achieve complete seizure freedom as with resection. Curative non-resective approaches include ablative procedures (radiofrequency thermocoagulation, RFTC; laser-induced thermotherapy, LITT; focused ultrasound ablation, FUS) and stereotactic radiosurgery (SRS).
- *Outcome measures.* As with resective surgery, seizure freedom rates are the primary outcome



J. Zentner, *Surgical Treatment of Epilepsies*, https://doi.org/10.1007/978-3-030-48748-5_14

measures reported for non-resective surgical options with curative goals. For palliative procedures, however, percent decrease in seizure frequency and rate of response to therapy (defined as ≥50% decrease in seizure frequency) are typically primary outcome measures. In addition, callosotomy studies often report reduced frequency of drop attacks [3–5].

## 14.1 Palliative Procedures

### 14.1.1 Disconnective Procedures

#### 14.1.1.1 Corpus Callosotomy (CC)

Sectioning of the posterior third of the corpus callosum was first used by Dandy [6] to approach tumors of the pineal region. Corpus callosotomy (CC) for the treatment of epilepsy was introduced by Van Wagenen and Herren in 1940 [7]. The idea underlying this procedure was that consciousness should not be lost if the seizure could be confined to one cerebral hemisphere. This hypothesis was based on their observation that generalized convulsions became less common when the corpus callosum had been destroyed by tumor or hemorrhage. Although psychiatric and psychological testing did not result in any gross disturbances, they observed a patient who stated, “I find myself trying to open a door with the right hand and at the same time trying to push it shut with the left.” Since this disorder was temporary and disappeared completely, they concluded their paper by stating, “section of the commissural pathways contained in the corpus callosum may be carried out without any untoward effect on the patient” [7]. Akelaitis [8] studying the callosotomy patients of Van Wagenen noted a difficulty with bimanual cooperation between the right and left hands as confirmed later on [9] with the availability of more sophisticated testing methods to assess interhemispheric transfer [10].

**Physiological Basis of Callosotomy and Early Clinical Experience**

Rationale

The rationale for callosotomy is based on the principles that (1) generalized motor seizures arise from the cortex, while subcortical structures are secondarily involved, (2) the corpus callosum mediates propagation of epileptiform discharges, and generalized seizures are preceded by bilateral synchrony leading to bilateral motor manifestations, and (3) sectioning of the corpus callosum diminishes or abolishes the synchrony of epileptiform discharges [11, 12].

Excitatory Activity

Using recordings from depth electrodes in humans, Bancaud et al. [13] and Goldring [14] showed that generalized motor seizures originate particularly from the frontal cortex, and that subcortical structures become involved secondarily, including the thalamus, the substantia nigra, and the reticular formation [15–19]. Moreover, a close association between generalized seizures and bilaterally synchronous interictal and ictal epileptiform paroxysms has been observed [18, 20–24]. Transmission of impulses from one hemisphere to the other via the corpus callosum and inhibition of propagation by callosal section has been demonstrated in animal experiments [25–29]. Thus, the clinical and experimental literature suggested a role of the corpus callosum for spread and synchronization of epileptic activity.

Inhibitory Activity

Further studies have suggested that the corpus callosum transmits not only excitatory activity between hemispheres but also inhibitory signals [30, 31]. Therefore, it has been argued that although corpus callosotomy may inhibit propagation of epileptic discharges and disrupt synchrony, such procedure may also increase focal epileptogenicity [12, 32–35].

Early Clinical Experience

Stimulated by animal experimental evidence that the corpus callosum plays an important role in secondary epileptogenesis [26–29, 33, 36–39] and the promising clinical results presented by Bogen [40–42], callosotomy has received increased awareness. Wilson et al. [43] reporting several patient series developed microsurgical techniques for partial and complete callosotomy [43–46]. Luessenhop et al. [47] described for the first time surgical disconnection of the cerebral hemispheres in children. Milestones in promotion of callosotomy were the Dartmouth Conference in 1982 [48] and the Dartmouth International Workshop in 1991 [49]. Although the physiological basis and neurobehavioral consequences of corpus callosum section were not completely understood, this procedure became a widely accepted option for the treatment of certain types of severe and uncontrolled seizures in patients who were not considered to be candidates for resective approaches [34, 35, 50, 51]. A multicenter survey in 1987 noted 197 patients who had undergone corpus callosum section [52]. In parallel, favorable experience with epilepsy has encouraged the use of callosotomy as an approach to the third ventricle and other midline structures [53–55].

### Selection of Surgical Candidates

The indications for corpus callosotomy (CC) are less generally accepted and vary considerably from center to center [56, 57]. Callosotomy may be considered for patients with intractable generalized seizures in the absence of a resectable epileptic focus, frontal epileptic foci demonstrating rapid secondary bilateral synchrony, recurrent episodes of status epilepticus, and for patients with multifocal or widespread lesions [46, 48, 58–69]. Among the different types of generalized seizures, tonic and atonic drop attacks are the most common indication for CC [46, 48, 58, 59, 62, 65, 66, 70–79]. Others have advocated CC also for patients with generalized tonic-clonic and absence seizures [71, 80], and for selected children with Lennox–Gastaut syndrome demonstrating tonic, atonic, or tonic-clonic seizures [69, 70, 81–83], while its role in complex partial seizures and simple partial motor seizures has been discussed controversially [34, 35, 48, 58, 65, 66, 84]. In contrast to earlier series, mental retardation is not considered as a contraindication for surgery [12, 57, 66, 67, 85]. However, caution is called for patients in whom language function is localized in the nondominant hemisphere for handedness (mixed hemispheric dominance), since these patients are at risk for language impairment after callosotomy [57, 67, 86], and some feel that callosotomy is contraindicated in these cases [34, 35] (see also the section "Operative Sequelae"). Today, corpus callosotomy is mainly reserved for children and adolescents with frequent drop attacks, but can also be used in adult patients to treat rapidly generalizing seizures [87].

### Surgical Approaches and Structures Sectioned

#### Historical Aspects

Van Wagenen and Herren [7] performed partial and complete callosal section with and without division of the anterior commissure and the fornix. The corpus callosum was approached through a large, right fronto-parietal craniotomy, and frequently the sagittal sinus and anterior falx were divided in order to obtain adequate exposure. For complete callosotomy, Bogen [40] used two rectangular craniotomies leaving a 5 cm strip in between over the central area. The procedure allowing both anterior and posterior approach included division of the anterior and hippocampal commissures, and, in some instances, of the massa intermedia. Luessenhop et al. [47], using a fronto-parietal craniotomy, exposed the full length of the corpus callosum and divided it lateral to the midline including the anterior commissure and—in most cases—the right fornix. Wilson et al. [43] initially sectioned the anterior and hippocampal commissures as well as one fornix. They changed their technique in the mid-1970s after a 50% incidence of ventriculitis (chemical and/or bacterial), hydrocephalus, and death in one patient. The revised procedure involved division of only the corpus callosum and the hippocampal commissure leaving the ependymal lining intact and staying extraventricularly as much as possible [45]. In a further modification, Wilson began to perform the division in two stages, usually separated by 2 months, a procedure which was found to further reduce postoperative sequelae [46]. Thus, the callosum section has undergone continuous change. The number of structures divided has steadily decreased over time, since it has become obvious that division of the corpus callosum alone is sufficient, and that division of additional structures does not significantly improve epileptological outcome, but may contribute to complications.

### Current Approaches

At the present time, the anterior commissure, fornix, and massa intermedia are spared. Many centers advocate complete one-staged callosotomy, since results from partial section have not been thought to match those achieved by complete section, although complete section may neuropsychologically be more risky than partial section [88, 89]. Some centers prefer to cut the anterior two-thirds to three quarters of the corpus callosum [66, 90, 91], while others perform strictly anterior or posterior section first, followed by completion of the callosotomy in a second stage, when the desired effect on seizures is not realized [11, 34, 35, 58]. Posterior callosotomy alone is rarely indicated, since epileptiform discharges are usually predominant over the frontal lobes which are connected via the anterior half of the corpus callosum [91].

Definition of extent of callosal sectioning by anatomical landmarks is largely uncertain. The posterior aspect of the septum pellucidum, callosal length as well as its shape and thickness (Fig. 14.1), and the area where the fornix attaches the corpus callosum (Fig. 14.2) are highly variable. MRI-based neuronavigation provides a useful tool to define the extent of section. Alternatively, a simple ruler may be sufficient.

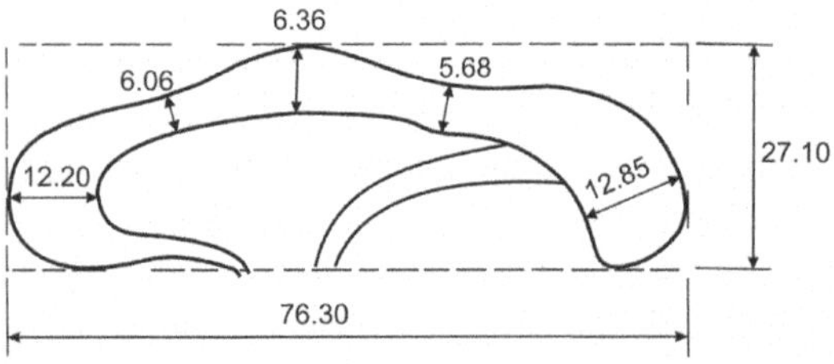


**Fig. 14.1** Schematic illustration and measures of corpus callosum based on the analysis of 150 MRI of normal individuals over 6 years of age and 25 anatomical sections (mean values in mm). (From Yasargil [92], with permission)

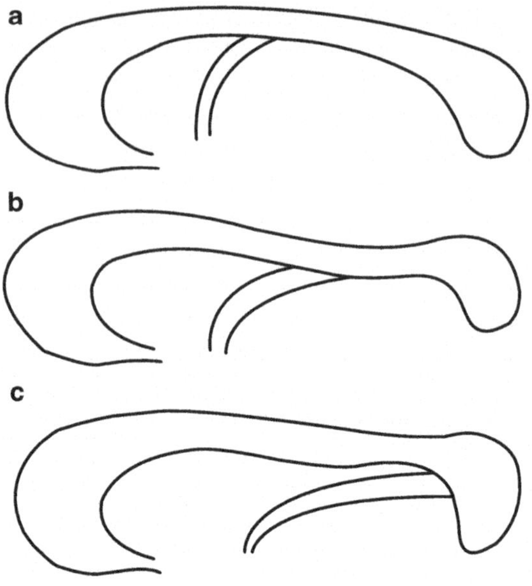


**Fig. 14.2** Schematic illustration of variants of relationship between the corpus callosum and the fornices. The most frequent situation as observed in 77% of patients is shown in (**b**), variant (**a**) is found in 4%, and variant (**c**) in 19%. (From Lang and Ederer [93] and Zentner [94], with permission)

## Surgical Steps

The most widespread technique of corpus callosotomy actually used includes the following main steps:

- The patient is placed in supine position with a 45° inclination of the head for anterior, and a 30° inclination for complete callosotomy, and in prone position with a 30° retroflexion of the head for posterior callosotomy. Skin incision may be rectangular for the anterior approach and linear for posterior one, or linear for both. At the time of scalp incision, mannitol (1 g/kg) is administered intravenously.
- For the anterior procedures, a right frontal bone flap measuring 6 by 5 cm that runs 1 cm dorsal and 5 cm anterior to the bregma and slightly crosses the midline is fashioned. The corresponding bone flap for the posterior approach, also measuring 6 by 5 cm, extends 1 cm posterior and 5 cm anterior to the lambda again slightly crossing the midline. It is advisable not to shorten the anterior-posterior extension of the craniotomy below 6 cm, since the individual venous architecture may require

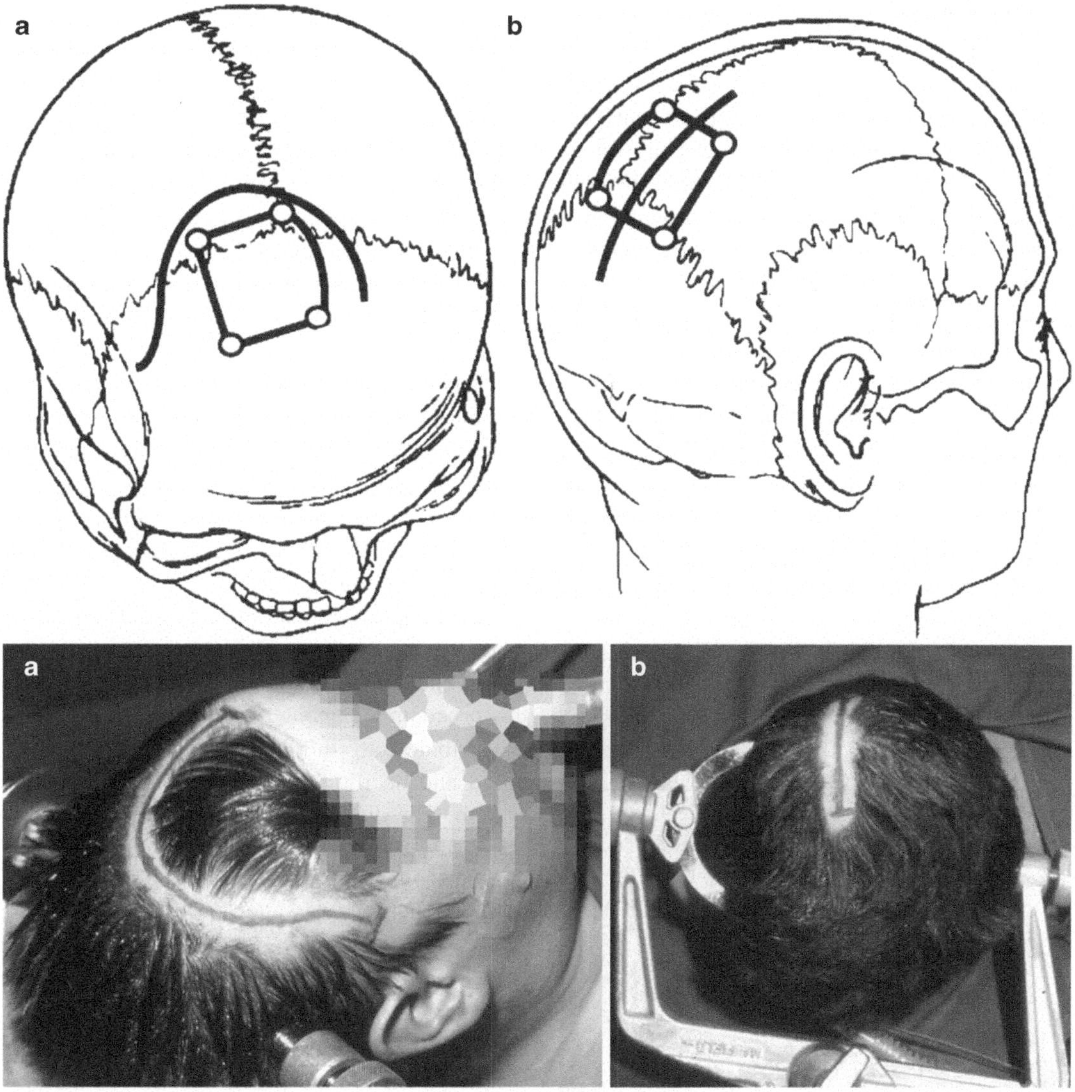

**Fig. 14.3** (**a**) Anterior/complete and (**b**) posterior callosotomy. Above: Schematic illustration of skin incision and trephination. Below: Positioning of the head fixed in the Mayfield clamp. (From Zentner [94], with permission)

modification of the actual approach for which 3–4 cm certainly are sufficient (Fig. 14.3).

- The dura is opened in a curvilinear fashion and reflected to the sagittal sinus. While dissecting the interhemispheric fissure, it may be necessary to divide small bridging veins. However, division of larger veins posterior to the bregma is always avoided. The dissection down to the interhemispheric fissure is continued, dividing arachnoidal adhesions that are often encountered particularly at the level of the cingulate gyrus until the corpus callosum is reached. Corpus callosum is readily distinguished from the overlying cingulate cortex by its glistening, bright white color.
- The self-retaining retractor is inserted, and the pericallosal arteries are identified. Gentle retraction of the deeper falx by an additional self-retaining retractor is often unnecessary, but may significantly widen the exposure and lessen retraction of the right hemisphere. Further exposure of the callosum is accom-

plished following the pericallosal arteries anteriorly as well as posteriorly. In order to provide sufficient working space between both pericallosal arteries, small arterial vessels supplying the exposed corpus callosum as well as veins are coagulated and divided. Thereafter, the pericallosal arteries are protected with cotton wool, and the retractor is adjusted over the protected artery.

- Division of the corpus callosum is accomplished using the ultrasonic aspirator (CUSA). The dissection is carried down to the blue-gray ependymal lining which provides a barrier to the ventricles and should be preserved in its integrity (Fig. 14.4). In anterior procedures, sectioning is first performed forward through the genu and rostrum until the anterior commissure is reached, which is spared (Fig. 14.5). Thereafter, section is extended posteriorly as desired. If complete callosotomy is intended, division is carried out through the splenium to the tectorial arachnoid, until the vein of Galen is visualized. It is essential to keep the midline, thus not jeopardizing the fornices. Extent of sectioning is usually defined by MRI-based neuronavigation. The interhemispheric fissure is examined throughout its length to assure hemostasis.

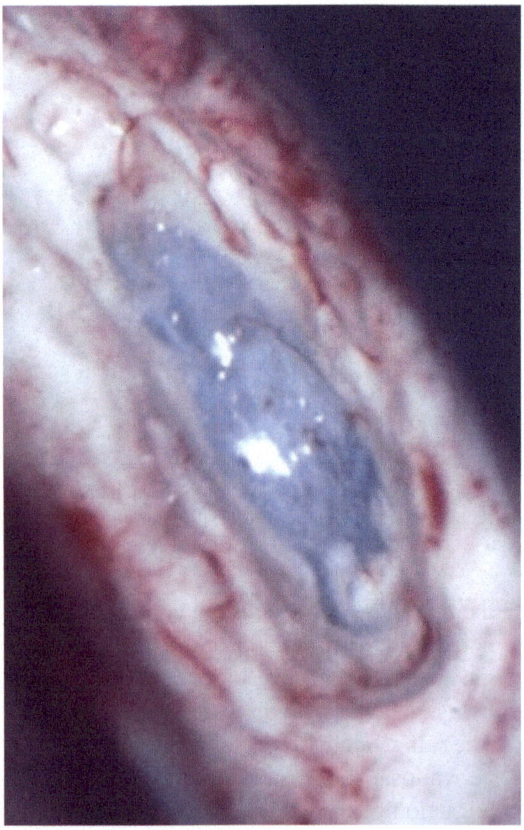

**Fig. 14.4** Operative view during sectioning of the corpus callosum. Note the intact bluish gleaming ependymal layer of the third ventricle which should remain intact as far as possible

Usually, the patient awakes promptly from anesthesia. However, he/she may continue to be unresponsive because of disconnection signs and symptoms, such as abulic speech and a paucity of responses on verbal commands. Postoperatively, T1-weighted MR images clearly demonstrate the extent of section (Fig. 14.6).

In principle, callosotomy represents an extraventricular procedure. However, opening of the tender ependymal layer frequently occurs during this procedure, causing *aseptic meningitis* which is attributed to intraoperative introduction of blood and necrotic material into the ventricular system. The differential diagnosis between *bacterial and abacterial meningitis* is most important and sometimes rendered difficult. Bacterial meningitis should be considered if there is a secondary increase in headaches and meningism, a rise in temperature along with progressive lethargy and confusion of the patient. High CSF cell counts (several thousands per $mm^3$) will support the diagnosis. In case of doubt, antibiotic therapy should be initiated despite negative CSF cultures.

## Modifications of Callosum Section

Main modifications of callosum section refer to positioning of the patient, surgical tools used, and techniques for guidance of sectioning.

### Patient Positioning

Some surgeons use the lateral decubitus position, which may allow gravity to assist in the interhemispheric dissection by pulling the dependent hemisphere away from the falx. In this case, the operating table is on an incline with the head slightly above the level of the feet, and a rectilin-

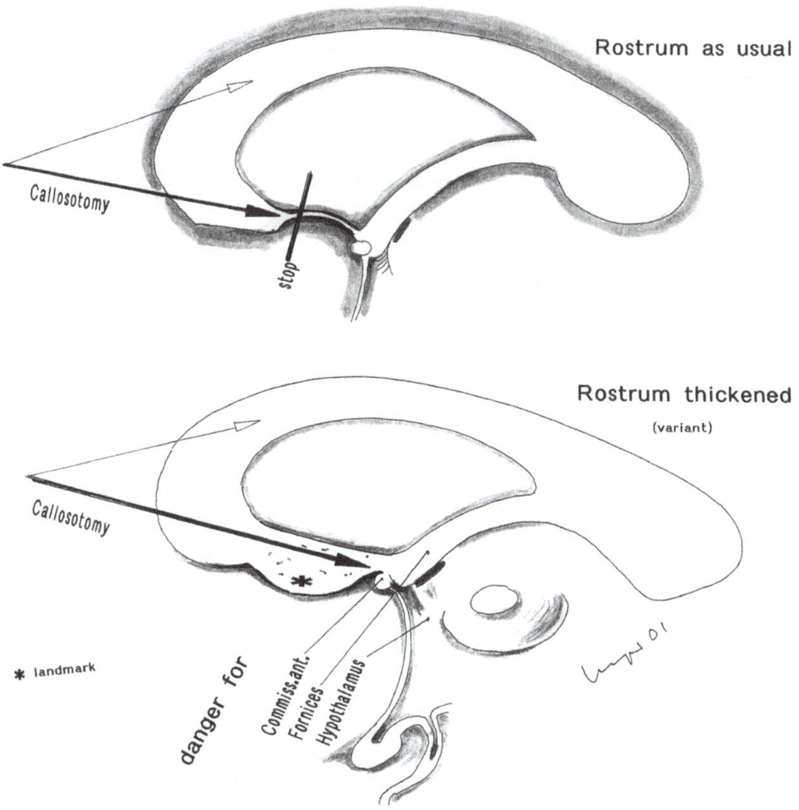


**Fig. 14.5** Basal limit of callosotomy. Section of the callosum is stopped as soon as the thin-walled rostrum corporis callosi, which as a variant may be thickened, is reached. In basal direction, commissura anterior, fornices, and hypothalamus are endangered. (From Seeger and Zentner [95], with permission)

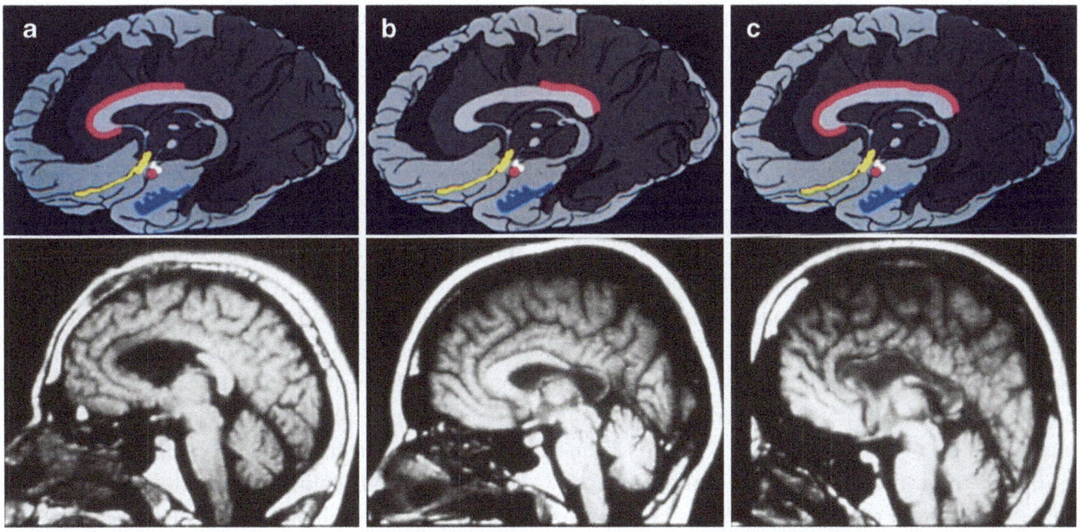


**Fig. 14.6** Variants of callosotomy. Schematic illustration (upper sequence) and postoperative T1-weighted MRI scans of three single patients (lower sequence). (**a**) Anterior two-thirds callosotomy, (**b**) posterior one-third callosotomy, (**c**) complete callosotomy. Red: Extent of callosal section. (From Zentner [94], with permission)

ear vertex scalp incision based approximately on the junction of the coronal and sagittal sutures is used [96].

#### Surgical Tools

The corpus callosum can be sectioned by bipolar cautery, microsuction, microdissection, or ultrasonic aspiration. Usually, ultrasonic aspiration is applied. Sood et al. [97] suggested an endoscopic approach for callosotomy. With this approach, interhemispheric dissection to the corpus callosum is done using the standard microsurgical technique through a 2–3 cm precoronal craniotomy. Subsequently, the bimanual technique with a suction device mounted on an endoscope is used to perform callosotomy. Sood et al. [97] found this approach to be as effective as conventional sectioning. Similar favorable experience using the endoscopic technique has been reported by Luat et al. [98] and Smyth et al. [99].

#### EEG and DTI Guidance of Sectioning

Location and extent of sectioning may be tailored and guided by EEG studies [100–103]. In addition, a new measure for the analysis of diffusion-weighted images called apparent fiber density (AFD) may facilitate to selectively cut callosal fibers in question, e.g., fibers connecting both motor cortices [104, 105].

### Minimal Invasive Techniques

#### Radiosurgery

Gamma Knife radiosurgery has been used in a total of 19 children and adults for anterior [106–109] and, less commonly, posterior [107, 110] callosotomy, frequently in Lennox–Gastaut syndrome. Radiation doses varied between 55 and 170 Gy. In all series significant improvement of most disabling seizures (generalized tonic-clonic seizures and/or drop attacks) has been reported. There were no serious adverse effects, and progress in mental and physical development was noted in many cases [111]. Improvement in seizure control occurred with a median delay of around 3 months [109]. Focal radionecrosis followed by atrophy of the corpus callosum has been shown on MRI, and DTI suggested that Gamma Knife radiosurgery produces axonal degeneration of callosal fibers [111, 112].

#### Radiofrequency Thermocoagulation (RFTC)

Marino and Gronich [113] and Marino et al. [114] reported on 12 patients undergoing stereotactic anterior callosotomy using radiofrequency thermocoagulation (RFTC). Lesions were generated during 60 s at 65–70 °C, spaced 0.5 cm from each other. The callosal section was carried out under continuous electrocorticographic monitoring by means of platinum electrodes placed over both medial hemispheres. Extension of section was defined by the disruption of secondary bilateral synchrony. No disconnection syndrome was observed, and neuropsychological abnormalities were less pronounced as compared to conventional microsurgical callosotomy [113, 114].

#### Laser-Induced Thermal Therapy (LITT)

A total of six cases in whom LITT was used for partial callosal sectioning have been reported [115–118]. It has been suggested that laser callosotomy may be a safe and effective alternative to microsurgical sectioning [115]. Analyzing 10 patients, Tao et al. [119] found stereotactic laser anterior corpus callosotomy for Lennox–Gastaut syndrome an effective technique with minimal postoperative discomfort and a short recovery period.

#### Stimulation

Marino and Gronich [113] evaluated the effect of corpus callosum stimulation. The rationale for this approach was to produce a functional but non-surgical interruption of the callosal fibers by depolarizing or inhibiting transmission of epileptic discharges from one hemisphere to the other. However, corpus callosum stimulation, produced by chronically implanted electrodes placed either by craniotomy or stereotactically, failed to control refractory generalized epilepsy in humans and also in experimentally produced penicillin epilepsy in cats [113]. Therefore, this technique has been abandoned.

**Table 14.1** Seizure outcome per seizure type after callosotomy

| Seizure type | Seizure outcome | Maehara and Shimizu [75] (52 patients) (%) | Hanson et al. [74] (41 patients) (%) | Cukiert et al. [70] (76 patients) (%) | Sunaga et al. [78] (75 patients) (%) | Tanriverdi et al. [79] (95 patients) (%) |
|---|---|---|---|---|---|---|
| Drop attacks | Cure | 80 | – | – | 84 | 44 |
| | >50% reduction | 92 | 80 | – | 93 | 99 |
| GTC | Cure | 12 | – | 57 | 27 | 50 |
| | >50% reduction | 61 | 50 | 57 | 56 | 94 |
| Atypical absences | Cure | 20 | – | 49 | 31 | 32 |
| | >50% reduction | 53 | – | 82 | 72 | 90 |
| CPS | Cure | 0 | – | – | 14 | 22 |
| | >50% reduction | 20 | 57 | – | 21 | 91 |
| Myoclonic seizures | Cure | 0 | – | 27 | – | 27 |
| | >50% reduction | 27 | – | 73 | – | 92 |

Consistently best results are reported in drop attacks and generalized tonic-clonic seizures
*GTC* generalized tonic-clonic seizures, *CPS* complex partial seizures
From Fauser and Zentner [126], with permission

## Outcome

With respect to the postoperative outcome, epileptological and functional results have to be considered. Seizure outcome depends on preoperative seizure types, the underlying pathology, the extent of callosal section, and the EEG features. Seizure semiology often changes after corpus callosotomy even when frequency does not or increases, with seizures sometimes becoming shorter in duration and less severe. Functional outcome refers to mood, emotional balance, memory functions, and self-care [91].

### Seizure Outcome

#### Overall Seizure Outcome

Several studies report long-term seizure outcomes after corpus callosotomy with observation periods ranging between 1 and 25 years [78, 79, 120–123]. All these studies agree that in the long run complete freedom from all seizure types after callosotomy is an absolute rarity, and only one patient has been documented [123]. Téllez-Zenteno et al. [122] noted in a meta-analysis comprising 3 series including 99 patients control of most disabling seizures in 35% of patients. In a survey of 563 patients, Berg et al. [124] reported a worthwhile improvement of seizures in 31.4% of cases. Overall, considerable improvement (≥50% seizure reduction), in particular of the most disabling seizure types, is consistently reported in 40–80% of patients [125]. The effect of CC on different seizure types is shown in Table 14.1.

- *Drop attacks.* Best responses to corpus callosotomy have been observed for drop attacks: According to larger series, 44–84% of patients were cured from tonic/atonic drop attacks, and 80–99% of patients (including cured individuals) were responders (seizure reduction ≥50%) [70, 74, 75, 78, 79]. In pediatric series, around 70% of children with atonic seizures became seizure free, and most of the remaining 30% were improved [56, 84, 85, 124, 127]. In the Dartmouth report [66], freedom from atonic seizures was achieved in 43%, a more than 80% reduction in 33%, and a 50–80% reduction in 10%, while 14% had no significant reduction in frequency of atonic seizures. Contrarily, in the Cleveland series of 19 children [128], freedom from atonic seizures was achieved in only one patient, and frequency of atonic seizures was reduced by 80% in 33% and by 50–80% in 44% of patients. For tonic seizures, a more than 80% reduction in seizure frequency has been reported in 50%, a 50–80% reduction in seizure frequency in 33%, and no reduction in 17% [128]. Overall, more than two-thirds of patients experience complete elimination or a substantial decrease of drop attacks in studies without prolonged follow-up [122]. However, long-term results suggest that only one-third of callosotomy patients remain free of drop attacks 5 years after surgery despite significant reduction in frequency [122, 129].

- *Secondarily generalized tonic-clonic seizures.* Favorable results were obtained in patients with secondarily generalized tonic-clonic seizures: In 12–57%, seizures were completely abolished, and 50–94% (including cured individuals) showed ≥50% reduction of seizure frequency [70, 74, 75, 78, 79].
- *Atypical absences.* Concerning atypical absences, satisfactory outcomes have been observed: In 20–49% of patients, atypical absences completely stopped, and 53–90% of patients (including cured cases) had ≥50% seizure reduction [70, 74, 75, 78, 79].
- *Complex partial seizures.* Less impressive results have been reported for complex partial seizures: 0–22% of patients were free from complex partial seizures, and 20–91% of patients (including cured individuals) had ≥50% seizure relief [70, 74, 75, 78, 79]. In patients with temporal lobe epilepsy, complex partial seizures were not influenced by anterior callosotomy [51, 125].
- *Myoclonic seizures.* Modest outcomes have been reported in myoclonic seizures: 0–27% of patients were seizure free, and 27–92% of patients (including cured individuals) had at least ≥50% seizure reduction [70, 74, 75, 78, 79].
- *Focal motor seizures.* Poor results have been reported in focal motor seizures: In the Dartmouth series, 22% of patients were free from focal motor seizures, and additional 14% had a more than 80% reduction in seizure frequency. However, 14% had an increase in the frequency, and 6% had de novo focal motor seizures following callosotomy [66]. Increased frequency of focal seizures after callosotomy has also been reported previously [32] hypothesizing loss of inhibitory function following callosal section [11, 32, 34, 35].

Pathology

Apart from the seizure type, the underlying pathology may play a role. Favorable surgical results have been reported in patients with bilateral malformations of cortical development (MCD) such as diffuse cortical dysplasia, tuberous sclerosis, and lissencephaly [79, 125].

Extent of Callosal Section

The extent of corpus callosum sectioning may influence the seizure outcome. Complete arrest of drop attacks was achieved in 90% of cases by total section of the callosum, but only in 67% by partial section in a series of 76 patients [125]. A meta-analysis restricted to children showed a 59% seizure reduction after anterior, compared to 88% after total corpus callosotomy [130]. Similarly, several other outcome analyses found that complete callosotomy was superior to anterior two-thirds callosal section, but the risk of peri- and postoperative complications was also slightly higher with complete callosotomy [62, 78–80, 123, 131–133]. Wyler [96] suggested that optimal outcome can be gained from the anterior 80–85% callosal sectioning leaving the splenium, and little may be gained from completing the callosal sectioning at a later time.

EEG Features

EEG features seem to have some prognostic significance concerning seizure outcome. Seizure onset with generalized slow spike-wave complexes, electrodecrement, or low-amplitude fast activity as well as interictal slow spike-wave activity were found to be associated with a favorable postoperative outcome. In contrast, interictal EEG recordings revealing bilateral independent spikes have been associated with poor outcome [74].

### Functional Outcome

Several studies report improvement in overall daily life functions after callosotomy [75, 123, 134]. Changes include reduction of hyperactivity, emotional balance, improvement of speech and memory functions, as well as improved attentiveness and self-care. Younger age (<18 years) at the time of surgery was an independent positive prognostic factor for functional outcome [75, 123], but not for seizure outcome [135]. The Cleveland experience in 19 children [128] suggests that according to parental assessment, the functional outcome may be even more important than the impact of callosotomy on seizure frequency: 76% of the patients had improvement in falls and injuries; alertness was improved in 82% of patients, unchanged in 6%, and worse in 12%; the need for special care was reduced in 47% of patients. These findings suggest that ≥50% reduction in targeted seizures after callosotomy along with improvement of functions constitutes a clinically favorable response [128]. Thus, not only seizure frequency but also the impact of seizures on daily life activities including injuries and the need for special care are important parameters in order to assess the value of callosotomy [91].

### Operative Sequelae

Operative sequelae include the acute disconnection syndrome, the spilt brain syndrome, and deficit reinstatement. Complications of callosotomy in the strict sense of the term are listed in the respective chapter.

#### Acute Disconnection Syndrome

The acute disconnection syndrome refers to a transitory, postoperative phenomenon characterized by mutism, apathy, hemineglect, urge incontinence, disinhibited bilateral grasp reflexes, Babinski reflexes, and increased focal seizures. The major finding is a decrease in spontaneity of speech [136].

##### Extent of Section

Acute disconnection syndrome seems to be related to the extent of section. In fact, none of the patients in the study of Provinciali et al. [137] revealed such symptoms after partial callosotomy, and one of them showed a disconnection syndrome when the callosotomy was completed. In contrast, nearly all patients undergoing single-stage total callosotomy in Wilson's early series expressed disconnection syndrome [44], while Van Wagenen and Herren [7] observed in their series of 10 single-stage complete callosotomies mutism in only one patient, and contralateral leg paresis in two individuals. Generally, incidence and severity of the acute disconnection syndrome have been found to be reduced when a two-stage callosotomy was performed [7, 28, 45, 138].

The posterior callosum is the major area for interhemispheric somatosensory, auditory, and visual transfer [138]. Thus, after section of the posterior callosum, somatosensory, auditory, and visual cortices of the nondominant hemisphere will be isolated from the language-dominant hemisphere. Patients will not be able to report verbally the somatosensory, auditory, and visual stimuli presented to the nondominant hemisphere for language [66, 91, 139]. These persistent sensory deficits, also termed interhemispheric sensory dissociation [91], have to be differentiated from the acute disconnection syndrome. They are usually well tolerated by the patients, and their verification requires sophisticated assessment [91]. All six patients undergoing splenial section as the second phase of a staged callosotomy reported by Ferguson et al. [140] exhibited deficits in the tactile and visual transfer.

##### Follow-Up

Obviously, the presence or absence of acute disconnection signs depends not only on the extent and the staging modality of callosotomy but also on the accuracy of neuropsychological assessment as well as the follow-up period. Levin et al. [141] found that even with partial callosal section some disconnection effect can occur when careful quantitative testing is carried out shortly after the operation. In 24 patients undergoing subtotal callosotomy, Purves et al. [64] noted acute disconnection signs in seven cases. Most important is the observation that the acute disconnection syndrome is usually temporary, lasting from days to weeks (mean duration 2–3 weeks), although a small number of patients may be disabled for months or longer [70, 136]. Makari et al. [142] found in a series of 20 subtotal callosotomies in most cases a transitory left-sided neglect and apraxia which cleared within 7–10 days postoperatively. However, no persistent neuropsychological deficits were observed [142].

#### Multiple Factors

It seems to be evident that section of the corpus callosum is not the only cause of the acute disconnection syndrome, because it does not exhibit a major problem in many patients [43, 54, 143–147]. Whether traction of the supplementary motor area alone or in combination with disconnecting the two callosally interconnected supplementary motor areas is the cause of mutism remains unclear [148]. As stated by Nakasu et al. [149], the acute disconnection syndrome may be a combined result of division of the corpus callosum, suppression of limbic system, lesions in the cingulate gyrus, the septum pellucidum, fornix, and impairment of the supplementary motor area, and the combination of these factors may differ from one case to the other [149].

### Split-Brain Syndrome

The split-brain syndrome is interindividually very differently pronounced. In its fullest expression it may represent a persistent disabling phenomenon which occurs in a subset of patients following either single or staged total callosotomy, rarely after partial sectioning [7, 140, 150]. Significant cognitive and behavioral alterations include language impairment, hemisphere competition, and a disorder of attention-memory sequencing. Of six patients undergoing two-stage total callosotomy reported by Ferguson et al. [140], three showed language impairment, two hemispheric competition, and four a disorder of attention-memory sequencing.

#### Language Impairment

Language impairment particularly refers to disordered speech initiation. Three distinct syndromes of language disturbance have been identified. The first, involving speech difficulty but sparing writing, is attributable to apraxia. The second involves speech and writing difficulties and occurs in right-hemisphere-dominant right-handed patients (crossed cerebral dominance). In this condition, the deficit can be disabling, and even anterior section alone may not avoid these deficits. The third involves dysgraphia with intact speech and occurs in left-hemisphere-dominant left-handed patients [86, 151].

#### Hemisphere Competition

Hemisphere competition means that the nondominant hand is unresponsive to verbal commands and acts antagonistically to the activities of the dominant hand (alien hand). Alien hand syndrome has been described both after sectioning the anterior portion of the corpus callosum as well as with procedures confined to the middle and posterior body of the corpus callosum [152]. This antagonism may be seen in basic manual tasks such as opening doors, turning on faucets, and eating. The dominant hemisphere tends to initiate these tasks following which the nondominant hemisphere will act contrary, e.g., "...pulling my dress on with the right and pulling it off with the left" [7]. As a rule, these antagonisms become less and less a problem within weeks to months. Their progressive amelioration is presumably the result of external cues. However, a small subset of patients may continue to be afflicted with this disorder on a permanent basis [34, 35, 150].

#### Disorder of Attention-Memory Sequencing

Disorder of attention-memory sequencing means that the patient is unable to pursue multiple strategies simultaneously. In addition, this syndrome is characterized by forgetfulness, inattention, and reduced dependability. These disorders may significantly impair performance of daily activities [139, 140].

### Deficit Reinstatement

Deficit reinstatement accounts for a selective decrement in performance IQ following complete callosotomy in patients with pre-existing but functionally compensated structural damage particularly of the right hemisphere. As suggested by Campbell et al. [153] who observed this syndrome in four patients with right hemispheric lesions, the corpus callosum actively facilitates recovery from early hemispheric injury ("transcallosal trophic support"). Thus, by interrupting callosal compensatory influences, the original deficit, clinically unrecognized before surgery, may reappear following callosotomy.

Patients at risk include those with (1) moderate right hemisphere injury, occurring later in childhood, in whom functionally recovery requires continuous transcallosal support of the injured by the normal hemisphere, (2) mixed hemispheric dominance, in whom language and handedness are localized in opposite hemispheres, (3) hemianopia contralateral to language, and (4) right-hemisphere language and left-hemisphere verbal memory following a partial left-hemisphere lesion [34, 35, 150, 154].

The possibility of deficit reinstatement after callosotomy highlights the necessity to evaluate callosotomy candidates for structural lesions and abnormalities of functional cerebral organization, particularly arising in response to early cerebral structural injury, e.g., by fMRI or amytal testing, to ensure that language, verbal memory, and handedness are localized ipsilaterally [139, 154].

#### 14.1.1.2 Multiple Subpial Transections (MST)

Multiple subpial transections (MST) were introduced in 1989 by Morrell as a disconnective procedure for patients with an epileptogenic zone localized in eloquent neocortex, such as the language, primary motor and sensory, and vision area [155]. This technique is based on the observation that a neuronal functional unit is organized vertically [156, 157], while the seizures spread horizontally [158, 159], and that a minimal contiguous cortical surface area is necessary for the maintenance of cortical activity [160, 161]. Thus, MST should theoretically preserve projection, commissural, and association fibers which are involved in important functions, but disrupt horizontally oriented cortico-cortical fibers which facilitate spreading of epileptic activity [155].

##### Selection of Surgical Candidates

MST can be used to treat epilepsies in critical brain areas where resection is not possible due to impending neurological deficits. In addition, MST have been found effective for patients with Landau–Kleffner syndrome [162–164]. However, as a stand-alone therapy, MST may only be indicated in highly selected cases. Nowadays, MST mainly are considered in conjunction with cortical resection or lesionectomy when the seizure focus encroaches on eloquent areas [165, 166].

##### Surgical Technique

MST are conducted according to the technique described by Morrell et al. [155]. Main steps include (Figs. 14.7 and 14.8):

- Using a sharp bipolar, almost avascular points spaced approximately 5 mm apart along a given gyrus are coagulated. Arachnoid and pia mater are incised with a sharp blade. Alternatively, arachnoid and pia mater can be incised in avascular areas without coagulation.
- The cortex is entered with the sharp hook through the incision, and the instrument sinks down by its own weight to a depth of approximately 2.0–2.5 cm perpendicular to the long axis of the gyrus. The instrument is gently drawn back along the subpial space on one side, and the tip of the hook is visualized through the pia mater.
- The procedure is continued by turning the tip of the hook, entering the cortex again at the same incision site and drawing the instrument back along the opposite pia mater of the gyrus.
- Serial MST are performed through the incised arachnoidal/pial points to the gyrus or multiple contiguous gyri in 5 mm distances.

With respect to the individual gyral-sulcal configuration, it is advantageous to have a set of hooks with different tip lengths (e.g., 0.5–1.0 cm) and angulations (e.g., 30–90°) available (Fig. 14.7). It is important that the handle of the instrument is relatively heavy, so that the hook sinks into the tissue by the own weight of the instrument. Care should be taken to avoid disrupting the pia mater or catching sulcal vessels during retraction of the instrument. With gentle retraction of the instrument leading the sharp hook along the pial border of the gyrus, damage to vascular structures is unlikely. At the end of surgery, a mild artificial subarachnoid hemorrhage is seen which is clinically irrelevant (Fig. 14.9). When MST are performed in multiple contiguous gyri in one or more lobes of the brain, intraoperative ultrasonography may be used at the end of the procedure to ensure that no underlying intracerebral hematoma was created. In addition, electrocorticography can be performed before and after MST to evaluate the interictal activity and response to surgery.

Ntsambi-Eba et al. [167] described a modification of the original technique using radiating MST of a gyrus with a single cortical incision. While the typical target for MST is the eloquent

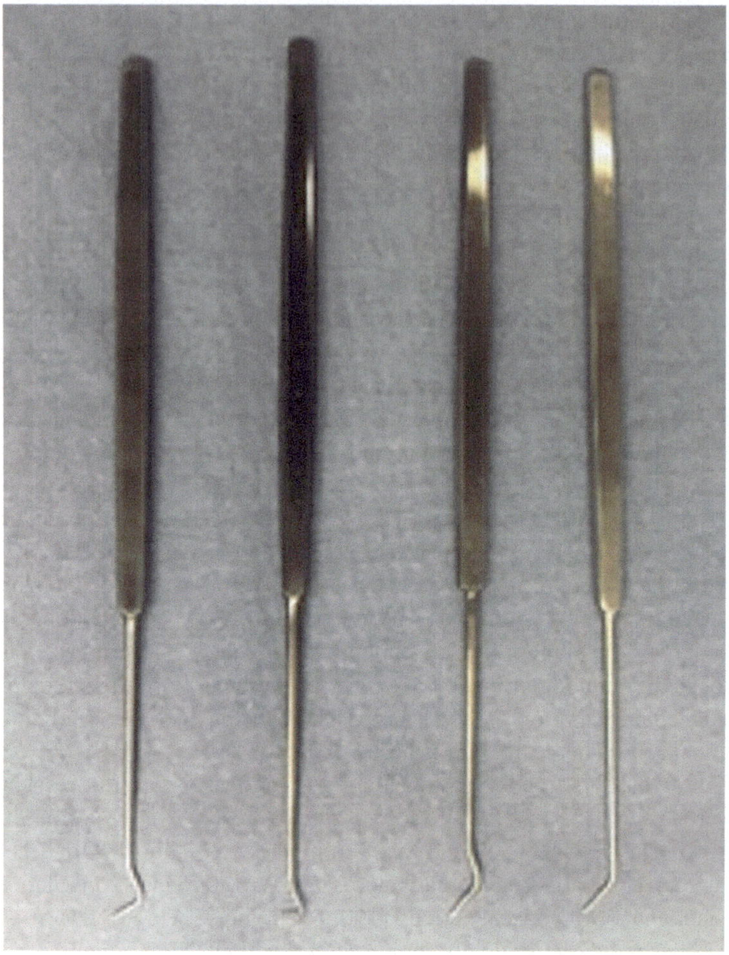

**Fig. 14.7** Transection hooks. Note different lengths and angulations of the tips. The handle of the instrument is relatively heavy; thus the hook sinks into the tissue by the own weight of the instrument (B. Braun, Tuttlingen, Germany, with permission)

neocortex, multiple hippocampal transections (MHT) have been proposed as a potentially verbal memory-preserving surgical approach for the treatment of MTLE on the dominant side [168] (see also Chap. 6).

## Seizure Outcome

### MST Alone

With MST alone, seizure-free outcome between 0% and 24% [122, 169–172] and a responder rate between 45% and 51% [169, 171, 172] have been reported. Téllez-Zenteno et al. [122] noted in a meta-analysis including 2 series and 74 patients seizure freedom in 16%. In another meta-analysis including 212 patients from 34 studies, Rolston et al. [170] observed 24% seizure-free patients, and 42% achieved Engel I–II outcome. Similarly, other series mainly including children and adolescents reported Engel class I–II outcome rates of 33–46% [165, 173, 174]. Behdad et al. [175]found Engel I–II outcomes in 4 of 6 children (67%) after MST of the Rolandic cortex. In contrast to most reports, Spencer et al. [176] analyzing 211 patients undergoing MST at six centers noted that 62% of patients with complex partial seizures and 71% of patients with generalized seizures had an "excellent" seizure outcome (>95% reduction in seizure frequency) with the use of MST alone. Overall, in most series, results of MST as standalone therapy are modest with 10–15% seizure-free patients and responder rates between 40% and 50%.

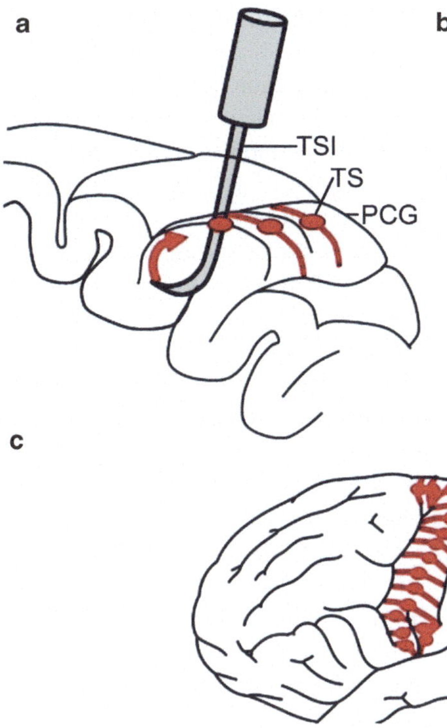


**Fig. 14.8** Illustration of multiple subpial transections (MST). (**a**) Transversal sectioning (TS) of the precentral gyrus (PCG) with the transection instrument (TSI). The PCG is entered through a point incision of the pia mater (red points). The instrument is gently drawn back along the subpial space (red arrow); (**b**) thereafter, TS is continued by turning the tip of the hook, entering the cortex again and drawing the instrument back along the opposite pia mater of the gyrus (red arrow); (**c**) parallel transections of the cortex are done in 5 mm distances (red lines). (With courtesy of T. Freimann, Dpt. of Neurosurgery, Freiburg)

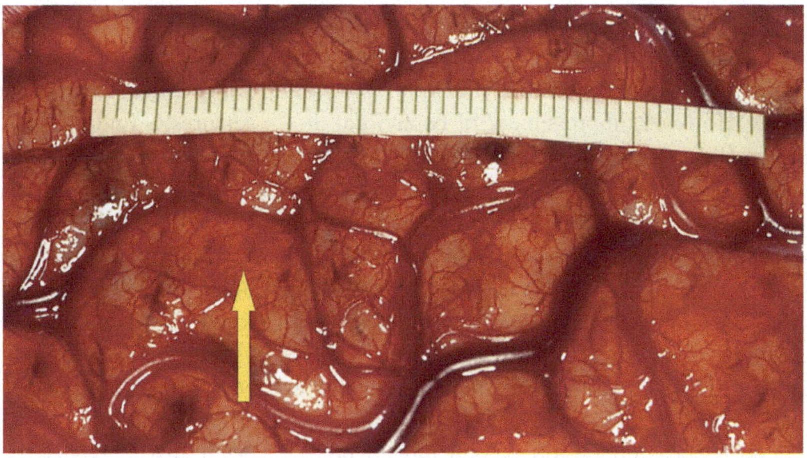

**Fig. 14.9** Intraoperative view on the transected cortical area. Note multiple incisions (arrow) of the cortex in 5 mm distances (distance between two long marks: 10 mm). There is a mild artificial subarachnoid hemorrhage

#### Resection Plus MST

When MST were performed in addition to cortical resection, reduction in seizure frequency >95% was found in 68% to 87% of cases in Spencer's meta-analysis. No significant response predictors were identified in this study [176]. The meta-analysis of Rolston et al. [170] showed seizure freedom in 55% of the individuals. Significant predictors for seizure freedom were a temporal lobe focus and partial resection of the focus [170]. In other series, 42–56% of patients became seizure-free, and in 80–88% (including seizure-free patients), seizure frequency was considerably (≥50%) reduced [165, 169, 172–174, 177]. However, in the long run (observation periods of 28–89 months after surgery), 19% of patients sustained an increase in seizure frequency several years after initial postoperative improvement [177]. In sum, seizure-free outcome rates between 40% and 60% and responder rates between 80% and 90% are achieved when MST are combined with resection.

#### Landau–Kleffner Syndrome (LKS)

Small patient series using MST in LKS have been reported. Morrell [164] reviewing experience with 14 patients observed marked improvement in speech and understanding in 79% after MST. Similar successful outcomes have been reported by Buelow et al. [162] and by Grote et al. [163]. Irwin et al. [178] presenting five children with LKS who underwent MST noted amelioration of seizures and improved language skills immediately after the intervention in all cases. However, improvement of behavioral disorders did not reach age-appropriate level in any case [178]. Cross and Neville [179] reporting a series of 10 patients found significant reduction of seizure frequency in 50% of individuals, and 70% showed improvement of language. In addition, significant behavioral improvement was noted in some cases. In contrast, Downes et al. [180] observed no differences in seizure status in patients with LKS who underwent MST targeting the posterior temporal lobe versus those who did not undergo intervention. Overall, mixed experience in single cases and small series has been reported. A large prospective study on the effect of MST in treating patients with LKS would be desirable [3].

### 14.1.2 Neurostimulation

Neurostimulation technologies can be used to replace lost functions, e.g., neuroprostheses such as cochlear implants [181], or to modulate the activity of the nervous system, e.g., by spinal cord stimulation for the treatment of chronic pain [182], or thalamic stimulation for Parkinson's disease [183]. Major efforts have been made during the last two decades to improve neuromodulation techniques for seizure control [184]. Today, three stimulation modalities are available that have proven to be useful in reducing seizure frequency: vagal nerve stimulation (VNS), deep brain stimulation (DBS), and responsive neurostimulation (RNS). Chronic subthreshold cortical stimulation (CSCS) is currently under investigation but is still in the experimental stage [185, 186]. Despite promising results, it has become obvious that from today's view stimulation techniques have a palliative character aiming at the reduction of most disabling seizures [186]. Reviews on neurostimulation have been provided by McGovern et al. [186], Hartshorn and Jobst [185], Kwon et al. [187], Kwaku et al. [188], Bigelow and Kouzani [189], and Schulze-Bonhage [190].

#### 14.1.2.1 Vagal Nerve Stimulation (VNS)

Already in the 1880s it has been observed that manual massage and compression of the carotid artery in the cervical region was able to mitigate seizures, a finding that was attributed to stimulation of the vagal nerve (cited after [188]). Early studies of Bailey and Bremer [191] and Dell and Olson [192] suggested that stimulation of the vagal nerve influences cortical activity by projections of the nucleus tractus solitarii. Zabara and Reese [193] developed the first generation of the vagal nerve stimulator through their incorporated company Cyberonics in 1987, now LivaNova. In 1988, Bell [194] implanted the first device, and preliminary experience with VNS has been reported by Penry and Dean [195]. VNS received Conformité Européenne (CE) approval in 1994 and approval by the United States Food and Drug Administration (U.S. FDA) in 1997. In addition, VNS has been approved by the U.S. FDA for the treatment of major depression, obesity, and episodic cluster headaches.

VNS has evolved to an established treatment for medically intractable epilepsy. In the meantime, more than 100.000 devices have been implanted worldwide [196]. The device consists of a pulse generator facilitating programmable cyclic stimulation of the vagal nerve by a lead that is wrapped around the nerve. VNS represents a unique non-resective modality to surgically treat a brain disease by stimulating a peripheral nerve [197]. To date, a large number of studies including controlled trials are available illustrating both benefits and limitations of VNS, thus facilitating to define the place of this treatment modality among other surgical options [198–202].

#### Mechanism of Action

The proposed mechanism of action of VNS is downregulation of excitatory pathways [185, 203]. The electrical pulse given by the pulse generator propagates up the tractus solitarius to the nucleus solitarius, which has widespread projections to numerous areas in the brainstem, forebrain, amygdala, and thalamus. The locus coeruleus and the raphe nuclei activated via the nucleus solitarius and projecting diffusely to the cortex play an important role, since both have been found to abolish VNS-induced seizure suppression when lesioned [204]. In addition, there are direct neural projections into serotonergic neurons and indirect ones into noradrenergic neurons involving the inhibitory neurotransmitter gamma-aminobutyric acid (GABA). Unilateral stimulation affects both cerebral hemispheres as demonstrated on functional imaging studies [205–207]. Although the mechanisms by which VNS decreases seizure activity are not entirely understood, it has been suggested that stimulation acts on the nucleus tractus solitarius by inducing desynchronization of cerebral electrical activity through modification of neurotransmitter concentrations and by changing distribution of cerebral blood flow in the thalamus [188, 208–211].

In addition to upward propagation, downward propagation of the electrical pulse should be kept in mind. The right versus left vagal cardiac innervation is quite different. The right vagal nerve innervates the atria and affects the sinoatrial (SA) node along with the right sympathetic nerves more than the atrioventricular (AV) node, whereas the left vagus nerve innervates the ventricles, and along with the left sympathetic nerves has more influence on the AV node than the SA node [188]. Therefore, the vagal nerve stimulator is implanted on the left side, since stimulation of the left vagal nerve is less likely to cause major cardiac adverse effects such as bradycardia and asystole [188, 212, 213].

#### Selection of Surgical Candidates

Indications for VNS therapy include focal and multifocal epilepsy, drop attacks (tonic/atonic seizures), Lennox–Gastaut syndrome, and tuberous sclerosis complex (TSC)-related multifocal epilepsy. Moreover, VNS may also be considered for other patients not amenable to resective procedures or in failed resective surgery [214, 215]. The main contraindication to VNS therapy is baseline cardiac conduction disorders, since efferent pulses may negatively influence cardiac conduction abilities. In addition, VNS therapy is also contraindicated in patients who have undergone bilateral or left cervical vagotomy procedures [188].

#### Surgical Procedure

##### First-Time Implantation

In order to select the adequate size of the helical electrode, it is important to consider the diameter of the vagal nerve. Vagal nerve diameters less than 2 mm have been found in 7 of 18 patients (39%) and more than 2 mm in 11 of 18 patients (61%) in the study of Santos [216]. Six of 13 patients (46%) reported by Shaw et al. [217] had a vagal nerve diameter of more than 2 mm. Thus, the human vagal nerve has a diameter of somewhat more than 2 mm on the average. The implantation procedure of the device for VNS is summarized in Fig. 14.10. First-time implantation includes the following main steps [218]:

- The patient is positioned supine with the head on a headrest, extended and turned slightly to the right side. A transverse skin incision is performed below the clavicle, and a subcutaneous pocket of around 6 × 6 cm is created by blunt dissection over the pectoralis muscle.

- A 4–5 cm transverse skin incision is made in the left neck, roughly halfway between the mastoid and the clavicle extending from the midline to medial border of the sternocleidomastoid muscle. The platysma is incised, and blunt dissection in continued until the common carotid artery and the jugular vein are reached. At this point, dissection should be continued using the operation microscope.
- The vagal nerve is found between the carotid artery and the internal jugular vein. It is mobilized using vessel loops and dissected for a length of 3–4 cm. With the skin incision performed as mentioned, the vagal nerve is exposed between the origin of the superior and inferior cervical cardiac branches and above the origin of the left recurrent laryngeal nerve. It is important to preserve as much of the nerve as possible because not all re-implantations can be performed at the original site, and a new section of vagal nerve may be necessary.
- The electrode is fixed to the vagal nerve. First, the tethering (inferior) anchor is secured. Thereafter, the positive (middle helical contact) and the negative (upper helical contact) electrodes are positioned.
- The lead is placed in the neck in a semicircular fashion and secured at two points with silicon sleeves at the deep cervical fascia. Thus, pulling at the electrode with movement of the head is avoided.
- Using a tunnelizer which is introduced from the subcutaneous thoracic pocket to the cervical incision, the lead is channeled to the thoracic site and connected to the generator. Impedance is tested.
- The generator is placed in the pocket that has been created and anchored to the fascia of the pectoralis muscle. Another loop of the lead is left at the thoracic site, allowing movement of the head and shoulder without stretching the lead.

The patient can be discharged one day after surgery. Stimulation is usually started 2 weeks after implantation. It is advisable to have continuous electrocardiogram monitoring and resuscitation equipment when the device is activated for the first time [219].

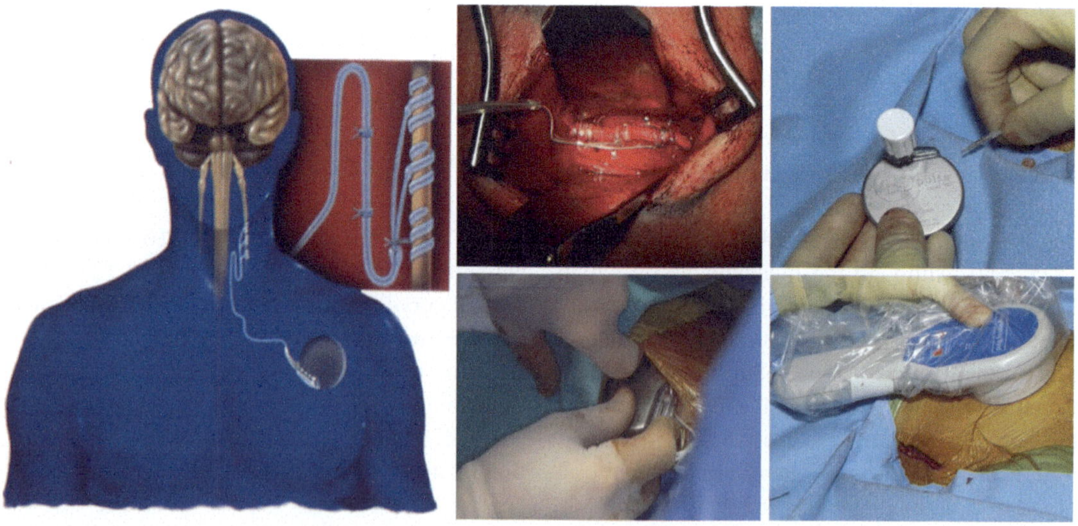

**Fig. 14.10** Implantation of the device for VNS. Left: Schematic illustration of placement of the generator and positioning of helical electrodes to the vagal nerve (magnification shows the nerve with electrodes). Right: Intraoperative aspects of surgery (from left above to right below): Fixation of electrodes to the vagal nerve, connection of the lead to the generator, placement of the generator in the pocket, and impedance testing

#### Surgical Revision

##### Indications and Incidence

With increasing use of VNS, revision of the device is more frequently necessary. Surgical revision is to be considered in case of device malfunction, failure of VNS therapy, intolerable side effects, infection, or because of patient's specific request " to get rid of all foreign material" or " to become as before" [220–232]. Couch et al. [222] reviewing 1144 consecutive VNS procedures between 1998 and 2012 noted that 644 of them were initial placements of the VNS device, and 46% of them required at least one revision surgery. The most common indications for revision surgery were generator battery depletion (27%), poor efficacy (9%), lead malfunction (8%), and infection (2%). Failure of the VNS device has been reported to occur in 4–16.8% of patients, and failure-related surgical revision followed in about one-half of those cases [220–230, 232].

##### Surgical Options

Revision procedures depend on the individual requirements. In principle, revision should focus at the part of the system that is affected. Of particular importance is the handling of electrodes when explantation of the device is planned. It seems to be advisable to leave the old electrodes in place whenever possible. However, there are situations when complete removal of the device with or without reimplantation is required. Some authors recommend to attempt to remove helical coils whenever the device is explanted to avoid lost foreign materials, especially in children, that could increase the risk of late infection and make high-field MRI impossible. This view is supported by literature data that do not report a significantly higher permanent morbidity after complete removal of the device and reimplantation as compared to the first-time implantation [197, 215, 220, 222–225, 227–230, 233].

##### Surgical Techniques

Surgical strategies for revision of VNS devices have been addressed in many reports [220, 222–225, 227–230]. Techniques for complete removal of the helical electrodes described in the literature include sharp and blunt dissection [220, 222–225, 227–231], or blunt dissection combined with ultrasharp low-voltage cautery dissection [233].

The procedure for removal and reimplantation of electrodes includes the following main steps:

- At first, the generator is removed from the subcutaneous pocket and disconnected from the lead to facilitate manipulation of the electrode lead.
- The transverse neck incision is reopened to expose the lead. The two fixation sleeves are removed.
- Under microscopic view, the lead is carefully dissected towards the helical contacts following the old scar into the neurovascular bundle using small scissors with blunt tips.
- Removal of the helical electrodes is done by sharp and blunt dissection or blunt dissection combined with ultrasharp low-voltage cautery dissection.
- After the old device is completely removed, the new electrodes can be positioned at the same segment of the vagal nerve or at an untouched segment cranial to the previous one.

In patients undergoing reimplantation of electrodes, previous electrodes can be left in place or removed completely. It has been shown that with reimplantation of electrodes at the same site or at another segment of the nerve, the effectiveness of seizure control can be expected to return to its pre-reimplantation level [223]. Alternatively, particularly in cases with extensive scarring or fibrosis of the nerve, the right vagal nerve can be used for reimplantation [197, 221, 222, 225, 226, 229–232, 234–241] (O'Neill et al. 2010).

### Seizure Outcome

##### Randomized Controlled Trials (RCTs)

There are seven RCTs assessing the efficacy of VNS in a total of 512 patients with refractory partial seizures with or without secondary generalization [199, 200, 242–246]. Five of them were blinded and tested low versus high intensity stimulation [199, 200, 242, 244, 247]. One of the non-blinded studies tested fast versus slow stimulation algorithms [246], and the other non-blinded study assessed three different duty cycles [243]. Six RCTs had a short duration of follow-up not exceeding 3 months [199, 200, 242, 243, 246] and 10 months [244], respectively. The seventh trial [245] tested whether VNS as an adjunct to best medical therapy is superior to best medical practice alone in improving long-term seizure status and health-related quality of life (HRQOL).

The randomized study of Ben-Menachem et al. [199] included 114 focal epilepsy patients who received either therapeutic or sham stimulation. The authors reported a significantly greater reduction in seizure frequency with therapeutic stimulation after 3 months of treatment (25% versus 6%), and 31% of patients receiving stimulation were responders (defined as ≥50% decrease in seizures). In a subsequent trial, Handforth et al. [200] randomized 196 patients with partial epilepsy to receive either therapeutic or sham stimulation. Patients with therapeutic stimulation achieved a 28% reduction in seizure frequency versus 15% with sham stimulation. At 3 months, responder rate in the therapeutic group was 23%. Amar et al. [242] achieved in a randomized controlled trial including 17 patients in 57% of cases ≥50% decrease in seizure frequency with therapeutic stimulation. In the trial of Scherrmann et al. [246], 28 patients were randomized to either a standard or rapid cycle stimulation (14 in each group). Six patients from the standard cycle group (43%) and 5 patients from the rapid cycle group (36%) experienced seizure response. Differences between the two groups were not significant [246]. DeGiorgio et al. [243] tested three different duty cycles in 61 patients. For the entire study group, the median reduction in seizures was 40% and responder rate 29%. There were no significant differences between the three subgroups. In a controlled trial for children, Klinkenberg et al. [244] randomized 35 patients with partial and 6 with generalized epilepsy to high or low stimulation for 20 weeks, followed by an add-on period of 19 weeks of high stimulation for all patients. At the end of the blinded period, responder rates were 16% in the high-stimulation and 21% in the low-stimulation cohort. After the add-on phase, 26% of patients experienced reduction of seizure frequency of at least 50%. Overall, these six randomized, controlled trials showed responder rates of 23–57% in the treatment groups versus 13–15% in the control groups at short-term follow-up [187, 248, 249].

The PuLsE (**P**rospective randomized **L**ong-term **E**ffectiveness) trial of Ryvlin et al. [245] analyzed 96 patients who either received VNS as an adjunct to best medical therapy or best medical therapy alone. At 12 months follow-up, seizure frequency was reduced by 22% in VNS patients compared to medical treatment alone, while responder rates did not differ significantly between both groups (32% versus 24%). HRQOL was significantly improved in the VNS group as compared to best medical practice alone. It was concluded that VNS is advantageous over medical therapy alone and that the benefits of VNS may extend beyond the sole reduction in seizure frequency [245].

#### Prospective Studies

As summarized by González et al. [248], 14 prospective observational studies, including more than 10 (between 15 and 195) patients with a follow-up of 3–64 months, are available [245, 247, 250–262]. The first large prospective long-term study of 114 patients [260] reported improvement of the median reduction in seizure frequency from 20% at 3 months to 32% at 12 months. DeGiorgio et al. [247], analyzing 195 patients, noted a mean seizure reduction of 45% and a responder rate of 35% at 12 months follow-up. The study of Vonck et al. [261] comprising 118 cases showed at >6 months follow-up a mean seizure reduction of 55% and a responder rate of 50%. Overall, these studies report a median seizure reduction rate between 17% and 55% and responder rates between 21% and 54% [248]. In addition, improved efficacy with increasing duration of VNS therapy has been shown to be a consistent finding, most likely due to long-term neuromodulatory effect on epileptogenic networks [190, 199, 247, 263–269].

### Retrospective Studies

Retrospective studies reported between 1999 and 2011 [173, 174, 265, 266, 270–278] demonstrated responder rates between 40% and 64%. In addition to reduction of seizure frequency, VNS may also stop or shorten seizures and clusters of seizures, or may improve postictal period [279].

### Meta-analyses

Morris et al. [201] showed in 454 patients enrolled in five studies that efficacy of stimulation tended to improve up to 1 year (from a median reduction of 35–44%), and then to level off at 1 and 2 years. In a meta-analysis of 16 studies including 1061 patients, Wang et al. [280] found an overall responder rate of 53.5%. Responder rates at 1–12 years after implantation increased from 43.4% to 82.9%. Analyzing 4483 patients of the device manufacturer's patient database, ≥50% reduction in seizure frequency was reached in 44% (1972 of 4483 patients) after 3 months of therapy, and in 56% (618 of 1104 Patients) after 24 months [281, 282]. A meta-analysis including 3321 patients from 77 reports [281, 282] demonstrated that 51% of patients treated with VNS obtained ≥50% reduction in seizure frequency as compared to the baseline. Seizure control rates rose as therapy duration increased [281, 282].

In the 2015 meta-analysis, Englot et al. [283] evaluated 5554 patients of the VNS Therapy Patient Outcome Registry and 2869 patients of a systematic literature review including 78 studies. From registry data, 49% of patients were responders, and 5.1% of patients were seizure-free at 4 months after implantation. Subsequently, at 24 months to 48 months, 63% of patients were responders with 8.2% achieving seizure freedom. From the literature review, 40% of patients were responders at 4 months and 2.6% were seizure-free. At last follow-up, 60.1% of patients responded to therapy and 8.0% achieved seizure freedom [3–5, 283].

Overall, long-term follow-up studies with VNS using various stimulation paradigms show response rates between 50% and 60%, and maximum seizure reduction may require 1-2 years of stimulation. Seizure-free outcome is achieved in up to 8% of patients [3–5].

### Stimulation Parameters

The optimum stimulation parameters were investigated in a multicenter trial comprising 113 patients [284]. Half of the patients were stimulated every 5 min for 30 s and the other half every 90 min for 30 s. The rest of the stimulation parameters were the same: 30 Hz frequency, 3.5 mA current, and pulse width of 500 ms. At 3 months, 31% in the high-stimulation group had a 50% reduction in seizure frequency compared to 13% in the low-stimulation group [284]. DeGiorgio et al. [247]. compared in a prospective study the efficacy of low- versus high-stimulation settings. After completion of the double-blind period, subjects originally randomized to low stimulation, were crossed to high stimulation, while individuals originally randomized to high stimulation were maintained on this setting throughout the 12-month period. In the high-stimulation group, the median reduction in seizures improved from 23% at the completion of the double-blind phase to 37% at 3 months, and to 46% at 12 months. For the low-stimulation group, the corresponding figures were 21%, 29%, and 40%. At 12 months, 35% of 195 patients had a ≥50% reduction in seizures, and 20% had a ≥75% reduction of seizure frequency.

### Lennox–Gastaut Syndrome

VNS has been reported to be effective in children with Lennox–Gastaut syndrome (Table 14.2). With this special syndrome, the responder rate was reported to range between 25% and 78% [262, 265, 271, 274, 285, 286]. The high variability may be related to different group sizes (between 7 and 30 patients) and different observation periods. In two studies comprising larger patient numbers [262, 285], effect of VNS on all seizure types has been demonstrated. Concerning tonic and atonic drop attacks, seizure freedom could be achieved in 8% and 24% of patients, and responder rates were 23% and 64%, respectively. Generalized tonic-clonic seizures were completely abolished in 0% and 15%, and 10% and

**Table 14.2** Seizure outcome per seizure type after VNS in Lennox–Gastaut syndrome

| Seizure type | Seizure outcome | Majoie et al. [262] (19 patients) (%) | Kostov et al. [285] 30 patients (%) |
|---|---|---|---|
| Drop attacks (or tonic/atonic seizures) | Cure | 8 | 24 |
| | >50% reduction | 23 | 64 |
| GTC | Cure | 0 | 15 |
| | >50% reduction | 10 | 55 |
| Atypical absences | Cure | 10 | 20 |
| | >50% reduction | 40 | 60 |
| CPS | Cure | 20 | 0 |
| | >50% reduction | 60 | 75 |
| Myoclonic seizures | Cure | 14 | 18 |
| | >50% reduction | 57 | 54 |

*GTC* generalized tonic-clonic seizures, *CPS* complex partial seizures
From Fauser and Zentner [126], with permission

55% of cases were responders. Atypical absences completely ceased in 10% and 20% of patients, and ≥50% seizure reduction was observed in 40% and 60%. Complex partial seizures were completely abolished in 0% and 20% of patients, responder rates were 60% and 75%. Myoclonic seizures were completely absent in 14% and 18% of patients, and 57% and 54% were responders [262, 285]. More favorable results in the study by Kostov et al. [285] may be related to a longer observation period.

#### Drop Attacks: VNS vs. Callosotomy

Englot et al. [281, 282] showed in a large, manufacturer's database a 43% reduction in drop attack frequency at 3 months after VNS implantation and a 75% reduction in patients receiving VNS treatment >2 years. Comparing the effect of VNS and callosotomy on drop attacks, Rolston et al. [287] demonstrated in a systematic review of 26 case series that patients were more likely to achieve ≥50% reduction in seizure frequency with callosotomy (86%) compared to VNS (58%).

#### Epilepsia Partialis Continua

In a prospective study comprising 39 patients including four children with epilepsia partialis continua (EPC), Marras et al. [288] observed a seizure reduction rate ≥50% or improvement of EPC in 74% of the patients. The authors concluded that VNS could also be considered as an effective procedure in this condition.

#### Poststroke Epilepsy

Kubota et al. [289] studied 10 patients who underwent VNS for drug-resistant poststroke epilepsy. Epilepsy was caused by hemorrhage and infarction. The duration from epilepsy onset to implantation of the VNS device was 70 months on average. At 2 years follow-up, 4 of the 10 patients (40%) remained seizure free, and in 6 cases (60%) seizures were reduced by ≥50%. No adverse events were reported [289].

#### Best Drug Treatment/Add-On VNS

Hoppe et al. [290] analyzed seizure outcome of 20 matched pairs of case and control patients in a retrospective study comparing best drug treatment alone with add-on VNS. At 2 years follow-up, more medically treated patients (12/20 or 60%) than VNS patients (4/20 or 20%) experienced a complete cessation of major seizures, whereas in non-seizure-free patients, VNS resulted in a better responder rate (12/19 or 63%) as compared to medical treatment alone (7/16 or 44%). Thus, no evidence for therapeutic benefits of adding VNS to best drug treatment was seen [290]. Similarly, Sherman et al. [291] found similar outcomes with VNS compared to best drug treatment, while Ryvlin et al. [245] reported in the PULSE study (see also above) superiority of VNS treatment 1 year after initiation.

#### Predictors

The following variables as predictors of improved response to VNS have been noted: temporal lobe epilepsy [277, 278], fewer failed AED [273], higher baseline seizure frequency [258], prior corpus callosotomy [265, 266], higher cognitive function at baseline [292], and focal rather than generalized seizures [266]. Contrarily, Englot et al. [281, 282] noted a greater reduction in seizure frequency in patients with generalized or multifocal epilepsy (58%) than focal epilepsy (43%). Neuronal migration disorders predicted a less favorable response to therapy in the study of Elliott et al. [277, 278].

Contradictory results have been reported as to patients' age at implantation [266, 270, 276], and duration of epilepsy [266, 273]. Englot et al. [3–5] identified across 5554 patients of the VNS Therapy Patient Outcome Registry and a systematic literature review of 78 studies including 2869 patients age at epilepsy onset as ≥12 years as a predictor for improved seizure outcome. A meta-analysis of Wang et al. [280] comprising 1061 patients identified shorter duration of epilepsy as a predictor for favorable seizure outcome, while age at implantation, age at seizure onset, seizure type, etiology, and history of previous epilepsy surgery did not significantly influence seizure outcome. Shorter duration of epilepsy has also been found by Arya et al. [293] to predict a favorable seizure outcome.

#### VNS After Failed Resective Surgery

Amar et al. [294] reported the effectiveness of vagus nerve stimulation (VNS) in patients who failed resective surgery. They compared seizure outcomes of 921 patients who had prior resective surgery with 3822 patients who had not. For the resective surgery cohort, the median reduction in seizure frequency was 42.5% after 3 months of VNS therapy, 42.9% at 6 months, 45.7% at 12 months, 52.0% at 18 months, and 50.5% at 24 months. Corresponding rates for the group without previous resective surgery were 47.0%, 52.9%, 60.0%, 62.7%, and 66.7%, respectively. Responder rate was 55% in the failed resective surgery group versus 62% in the group without previous surgery at last follow-up. Thus, patients who failed prior resective surgery did not respond quite as favorably as all other patients receiving VNS therapy [294].

A subgroup analysis reported by Ben-Menachem et al. [252] in 18 Swedish postsurgical patients showed decreased seizure frequency in six patients with reduction rates ranging from 20% to 75%. Similarly, Koutroumanidis et al. [295] analyzing 16 postsurgical patients observed no changes in seizure frequency after VNS in 10 of 16 patients (62.5%), and only 3 patients (18.8%) had an up to 50% reduction in frequency. Seizures of one patient had even increased after VNS placement [295]. Only marginal improvement in postoperative seizure burden with VNS has also been reported by Vale et al. [296]. In this study, 65% of patients had a less than 30% reduction in seizure frequency [296].

Overall, data suggest that individuals who have failed resective surgery may have less favorable VNS outcomes than patients without a history of resection [3, 4]. Therefore, the hypothesis of an increased efficacy of VNS due to reduced epileptogenic load by previous surgery [297] cannot be maintained [3, 4].

#### Post-traumatic Epilepsy

Englot et al. [298] showed in a retrospective study that VNS was more effective in patients with post-traumatic epilepsy as compared to patients with nontraumatic epilepsy. Reduction of seizure frequency at 3 months follow-up was 50% in post-traumatic cases versus 46% in nontraumatic epilepsies. Corresponding figures at 24 months follow-up were 73% and 57%, respectively. Furthermore, at 24 months, patients with post-traumatic epilepsy had an overall responder rate of 78% versus 61% in the nontraumatic group [298]. Lee et al. [299] studied the effect of VNS in 11 patients with post-traumatic epilepsy and failed epilepsy surgery. In the first 6 months, 11 patients showed an average of 74.3% seizure reduction. After 24 months, 7 patients had a 97.2% seizure reduction, and 6 patients were seizure free. In all, VNS may be a helpful treatment modality in patients with post-traumatic epilepsy as well as in post-traumatic epilepsy and failed surgery [299].

#### SUDEP

Ryvlin et al. [300] followed a total of 40,443 patients with VNS therapy up to 10 years postimplantation, accumulating 277,661 person-years, in the United States (1988–2012) to assess rates of sudden unexpected death in epilepsy patients (SUDEP). There were 3689 deaths, including 632 SUDEP (84% classified as possible and 16% as probable or definite). Age-adjusted SUDEP rates decreased significantly over time (by over 30%) from years 1 to 2 (2.47/1000 person-years) to years 3 to 10 (1.68/1000 person-years) of follow-up during VNS therapy [300].

#### Quality of Life (QOL)

No negative cognitive effects of VNS have been noted. Elger et al. [301] were the first to demonstrate that VNS therapy can cause improvement of mood and related symptoms in patients with epilepsy independent of whether or not seizures are reduced. These findings have been confirmed by others [302–305]. VNS therapy has been found to promote alertness and reduce daytime sleeping [305], to improve mood lowering depression [304], and to improve memory [302]. In the study of Amar et al. [294], analysis of QOL suggested a trend towards improvement with statistical significance for greater alertness with VNS. Ryvlin et al. [245] reported in the PULSE study (see above) a significantly superior quality of life in patients receiving adjunctive VNS on the long-term, while Hoppe et al. [290] did not find any clinically relevant effect of additional VNS treatment compared to best drug treatment alone on health-related quality of life (HRQOL) and mood at 2 years follow-up.

Englot et al. [306] examined 7 metrics related to QOL after VNS in over 5000 patients (including over 3000 with ≥12 months follow-up) based on the VNS Therapy Patient Outcome Registry. After VNS therapy, improvement of alertness was noted in 58–63% of patients (range over follow-up period). Specifically, the study reported improvements of postictal state (55–62%), cluster seizures (48–56%), mood (43–49%), verbal communication (38–45%), school/professional achievements (29–39%), and memory (29–38%). Overall, net improvement of QOL was observed in 74–77% of patients, worsening in 4–6% of individuals, and no overall change in 18–22% of patients. Net QOL improvement was more frequently found in seizure responders (81–84%) as compared to nonresponders (64–70%). Predictors of QOL improvement included shorter time to VNS implantation after diagnosis (<10 years versus ≥10 years), generalized seizure type, female gender, and Caucasian ethnicity [306].

Overall, in addition to the decrease in seizure frequency, VNS provides benefits in terms of QOL which represents an important treatment goal [302, 306]. Even with not satisfying epileptological results, patients on VNS are less likely to discontinue this therapy compared with those on medical therapy [221, 307]. In accordance, some individuals in the study of Koutroumanidis et al. [295] decided to continue stimulation for its positive psychotropic effect and stabilization of mood despite no change in seizure burden. Beneficial effects of VNS on QOL most likely reflect multiple connections of the vagal nerve with structures influencing psychic condition, e.g., the amygdala and the thalamus. On that basis, VNS has also been proposed for the treatment of major depression and Alzheimer's disease [215].

### Alternative VNS Techniques

#### Transcutaneous Vagal Nerve Stimulation (tVNS)

In 2000, Ventureyra [308] first reported the use of transcutaneous vagal nerve stimulation (tVNS) for the treatment of partial epilepsy. The system stimulates the auricular branch of the vagal nerve using an intra-auricular electrode (Fig. 14.11). In a proof-of-concept trial involving 10 patients with medically refractory epilepsy using 1-h treatments three times a day, Stefan et al. [309] found a reduction of seizure frequency of up to 48% after 9 months of treatment. Similarly, Aihua et al. [310] found that clinical effectiveness of tVNS was comparable with conventional VNS in the control of seizures. Transcutaneous VNS has received Conformité Européenne (CE) and the United States Food and Drug Administration (U.S. FDA) approval for the treatment of epilepsy.

##### Randomized Controlled Trial (RCT)

In 2016, Bauer et al. published a randomized, double-blind clinical trial to assess efficacy and safety of tVNS versus control stimulation [311]. A total

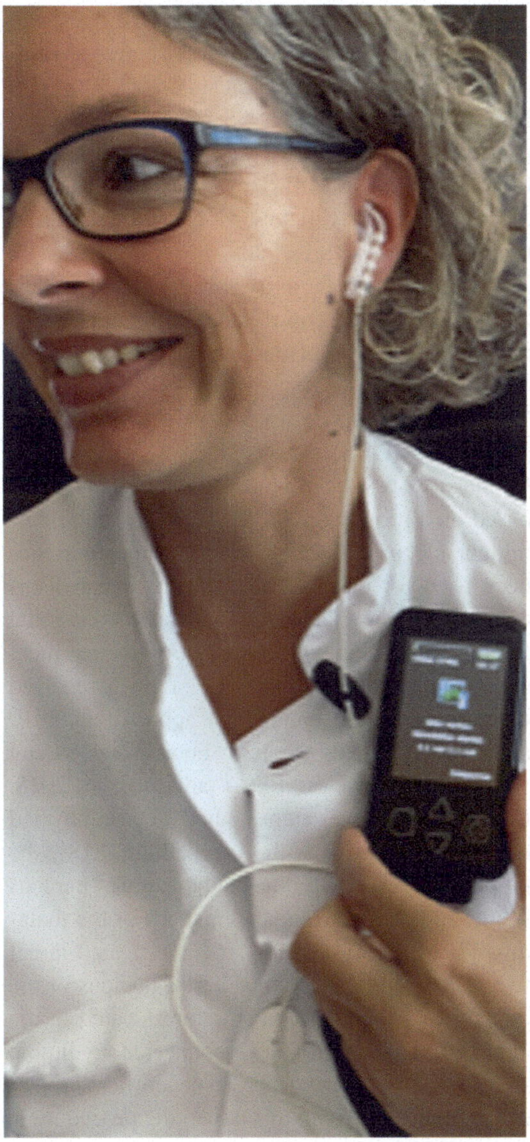

**Fig. 14.11** Placement of the device for transcutaneous vagal nerve stimulation (tVNS)

of 37 patients were randomized to high-level (active treatment, 25 Hz) t-VNS and 39 to low-level (active control, 1 Hz) stimulation. Eight patients of the 1 Hz group and 10 patients of the 25 Hz group prematurely discontinued the study. At 28 days, seizure reduction rate was 23.4% in the 25 Hz group, while seizure frequency increased by 2.9% in the control group. Differences did not reach statistical significance due to the very high variability in seizure frequencies in both groups. In particular, superiority of 25 Hz over 1 Hz tVNS could not be proven. However, seizure frequency decreased significantly by 34% in those patients who completed the intended 20 weeks of 25 Hz tVNS treatment [311].

Prospective Study

Efficacy and safety of tVNS were evaluated in a prospective study including 17 patients by Liu et al. [312]. After 3 months, seizure frequency was reduced by an average of 31.3% in 13 of 17 subjects, and by 64.4% in 16 of 17 patients after 6 months. Thus, the efficacy of tVNS improved with time. According to clinical and EEG findings, the frequency of the majority of generalized tonic-clonic seizures, simple partial seizures, and complex partial seizures could be reduced by tVNS. Moreover, treatment with tVNS also reduced anxiety and depression, and improved quality of life. No adverse events associated with tVNS treatment were observed [312].

In sum, tVNS seems to be efficient to reduce seizure frequency by approximately 50% and to improve QOL. However, the sparse data on tVNS available today are not conclusive. Long-term controlled trials are necessary to compare tVNS with conventional VNS and to prove its efficacy [189, 248].

**Responsive Vagal Nerve Stimulation (rVNS)**

The rationale of responsive vagal nerve stimulation (rVNS) is the observation that both focal and generalized seizures are associated with tachycardia in up to 82% of patients [313]. Furthermore, Eggleston et al. [313] noted that 64% of generalized seizures and 71% of partial-onset seizures were associated with significant heart rate changes. In addition, it has been shown that tachycardia frequently precedes electroencephalographic and clinical seizure patterns [314]. Change in heart rate triggering the stimulator in VNS systems is modifiable in the range from 20% to 70% [248]. To avoid too many false-positive results due to exercise, the stimulator is triggered by an increase from a baseline heart rate that is continually updated from a moving average. Moreover, the tachycardia detection can be turned on or off [185]. Closed-loop VNS has received Conformité Européenne (CE) and the United States Food and Drug Administration (U.S. FDA) approval in 2014.

Preliminary Studies

In 2015, Boon et al. [308] published the first prospective clinical trial testing cardiac-based seizure detection algorithms incorporated in a VNS device in 31 patients. This system provided combined stimulation of the vagal nerve in an open-loop mode as well as in a closed-loop fashion triggered by increase of heart rate of at least 20%. Evaluating 66 seizures, a ≥20% heart rate increase was found in 37 seizures, and 11 were associated with ictal tachycardia (≥100 beats per minute, bpm). In 10/17 seizures, where triggered VNS overlapped with an ongoing seizure, seizure activity stopped during stimulation. Based on a 20% increase of heart rate as a threshold to trigger VNS, sensitivity was high, while specificity was low with a false-positive rate of 7 stimulations/h. At 12 months follow-up, the responder rate was 30%, and quality of life showed significant improvement. It has been suggested that combined open- and closed-loop systems may be additive providing neuromodulatory effects and facilitating acute treatment of ictal events [253].

Fisher et al. [255] implanted a VNS system with tachycardia detection in 20 patients with known ictal tachycardia defined as a heart rate above 100 bpm during a seizure. At 1 year follow-up, 50% of patients were considered responders. In addition, seizures were found to be shorter due to less spatial propagation of ictal EEG activity [315]. Hamilton et al. [316] reported a study of 113 patients. Responder rate was 59% in 51 patients who had received a new VNS model and 53% in 62 cases with an existing system. After the generator was changed to the new device, 71% reported a further reduction of ≥50% in their seizure burden. It has been suggest that approximately 70% of patients with existing VNS insertions could have significant additional benefit from cardiac-based seizure detection achieving an overall responder rate of around 60% [316].

In sum, first experience suggests that ictal tachycardia-triggered VNS is as effective as standard open-loop VNS or even superior [248, 316]. Moreover, closed-loop VNS may provide some useful data on frequency and time-of-day variations of seizures [248]. However, the specificity of stimulation is still low, since with triggering the system at low thresholds, most duty cycles do not reflect seizure activity. Improvement of seizure detection and controlled trials is required to define the place of this technology.

#### 14.1.2.2 Deep Brain Stimulation (DBS)

Similar to VNS, deep brain stimulation (DBS) is based on a programmable device delivering intermittent electrical stimuli to brain nuclei. It has been used for the treatment of movement disorders, including Parkinson's disease, essential tremor, and dystonia [183, 317]. For the treatment of drug-resistant epilepsy, DBS received Conformité Européenne (CE) approval in 2010 and the United States Food and Drug Administration (U.S. FDA) approval in 2018. Many targets have been studied in uncontrolled clinical trials such as the cerebellum [318], the hippocampus [319], the subthalamic nucleus [320], and the centromedian nucleus of the thalamus [321]. However, the best investigated target for DBS in epilepsy is the anterior nucleus of the thalamus (ANT) [322], a structure located in the circuit of Papez intimately connected to limbic structures and with widespread neocortical projections [323–325]. With this target, the procedure is called ANT-DBS.

The implantation of the system has been described by Halpern et al. [326]. Experience from an international multicenter registry (MORE) supported the use of transventricular trajectories for placing contacts to the anterior thalamic nucleus [327]. Koeppen et al. [328] found best response rates to focal seizures with a center of stimulation 5 mm lateral to the wall of the third ventricle, and a lead tip 10 mm dorsal of the midcommissural plane. Schaper et al. [329] suggested that single-cell microelectrode recordings can aid targeting of the anterior thalamic nucleus during surgery.

Mirski et al. [330] demonstrated the anticonvulsant effect of anterior thalamic high-frequency stimulation in rats and postulated that the disruption of thalamocortical transmission prevents recruitment and synchronization of epileptic activity into a generalized seizure. Similarly, Laxpati et al. [320] suggested that high-frequency stimulation (>50 Hz) produces a reversible lesion mimicking ablation. However, the exact mechanisms remain unclear, and the gradual improvement in frequency and severity of seizures over time observed in human studies suggests that DBS may have a neuroprotective effect modulating neuronal network excitability through overriding pathological electrical activity [331, 332]. Figure 14.12 illustrates thalamic and hippocampal stimulation. Figure 14.13 demonstrates stimulation of the anterior thalamic nucleus in a single patient.

## Seizure Outcome

### Randomized Controlled Trials (RCTs)

There are five RCTs assessing the efficacy of DBS in patients with refractory epilepsy [333–337]. Velasco et al. [336] reported results of a pilot study based on bilateral superomedial cerebellar stimulation in five patients with medically refractory generalized tonic-clonic seizures. Patients were randomized to stimulation ($n = 3$) or non-stimulation ($n = 2$). Seizure frequency was reduced to 33% of the baseline values with stimulation, while no seizure reduction was observed without stimulation. Téllez-Zenteno et al. [335] performed a pilot study in four patients undergoing hippocampal stimulation which was turned on and off at random. Although not significant, results suggested a beneficial trend of stimulation. Fisher et al. [333] reported a

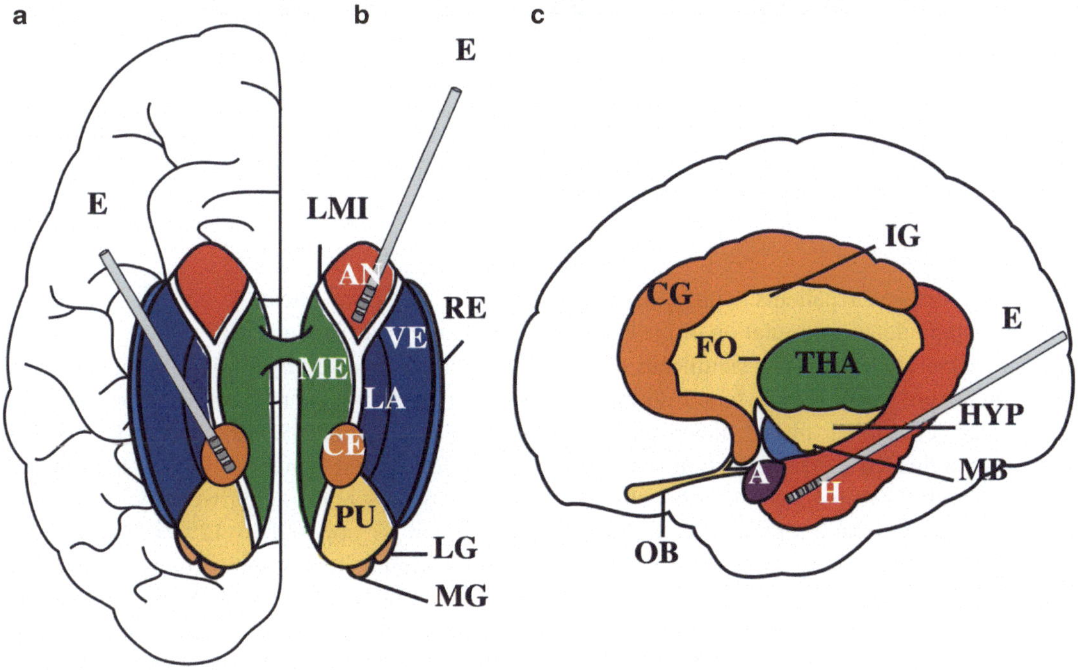


**Fig. 14.12** Schematic illustration of thalamic (left side, axial view) and hippocampal (right side, sagittal view) stimulation. Left side: Overview on the targets of the electrode (E) in thalamic stimulation. (**a**) Centromedian nucleus (CE); (**b**) anterior nucleus (AN). For anatomical orientation, other thalamic structures are marked: medial nucleus (ME), ventral nucleus (VE), lateral nucleus (LA), pulvinar (PU), lateral geniculate corpus (LG), medial geniculate corpus (MG), and lamina medullaris interna (LMI). (**c**) Electrode (E) placement for hippocampal (H) stimulation. *A* amygdala, *CG* cingulate gyrus, *FO* fornix, *HYP* hypothalamus, *IG* indusium griseum, *MB* mammillary body, *OB* olfactory bulb, *THA* thalamus. (From Fauser and Zentner [126], with permission)

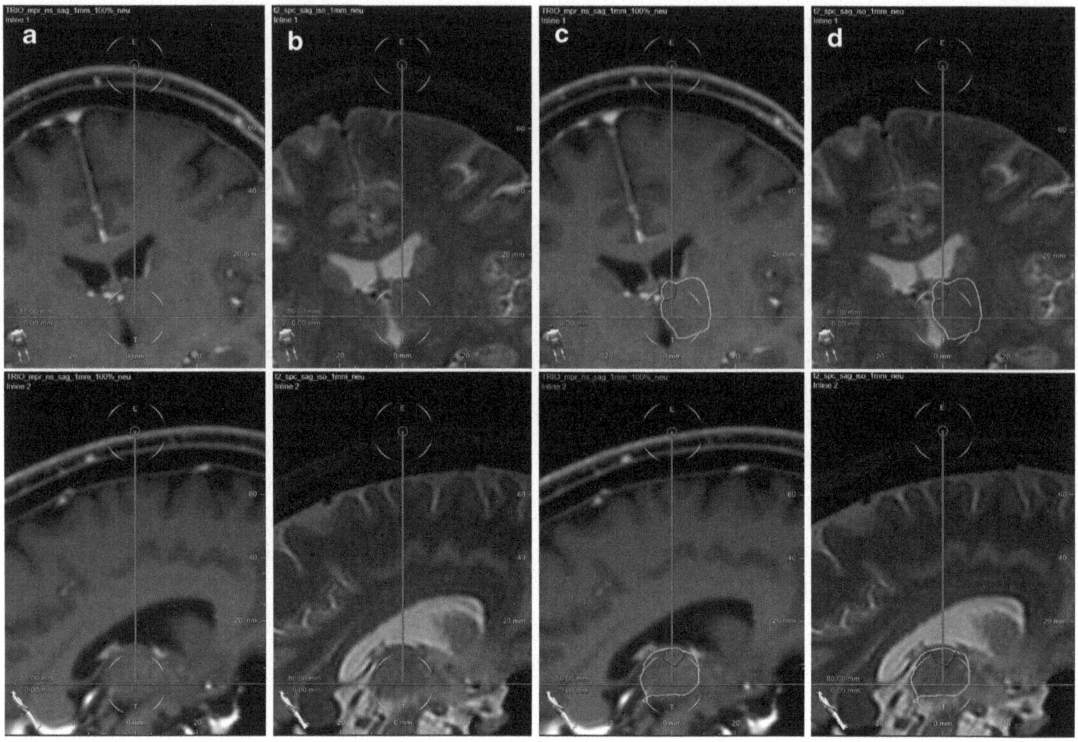


**Fig. 14.13** Stimulation of the anterior thalamic nucleus. Trajectory planning (in-line views) for electrode placement. (**a**) Contrast-enhanced T1-weighted MRI, (**b**) T2-weighted MRI (T2-SPACE), (**c**) Contrast-enhanced T1-weighted MRI including automatic anatomical segmentation of thalamus (blue) and anterior nucleus of the thalamus (pink), (**d**) T2-weighted MRI (T2-SPACE) including automatic anatomical segmentation of thalamus (blue) and anterior nucleus of the thalamus (pink). (With courtesy of P. Reinacher, Dpt. of Stereotactic and Functional Neurosurgery, Freiburg)

pilot study on seven patients with generalized seizures using bilateral stimulation of the centromedian thalamic nucleus. No significant differences in seizure control were found during the randomized controlled phase; however, three patients experienced a 50% reduction in seizure frequency on follow-up. Later on, Fisher changed to stimulation of the anterior thalamic nucleus.

In 2010, Fisher et al. [334] presented the *SANTE (Stimulation of the **A**nterior **N**ucleus of the **T**halamus for **E**pilepsy) trial* which was based on a prospective, randomized, double-blind, parallel-group design. This trial randomized 110 adult patients with medically refractory focal and secondarily generalizing epilepsy to either receive active stimulation or sham stimulation for 3 months. Electrodes were implanted bilaterally in the anterior nucleus of the thalamus. Stimulation was running with a cycle consisting of 1 min on followed by 5 min off, unresponsive to seizure activity (open loop). After the 3 months blind, all patients received stimulation (unblinded phase) for at least 9 months. During the blinded phase, focal seizures improved by 36% with stimulation as opposed to 12% in the control group, with the greatest improvement in patients with temporal seizure onset. At the end of the blinded phase, patients receiving stimulation had a 40% reduction in seizure frequency on average, compared to 15% in patients receiving sham stimulation. The differences were statistically significant. During the open-label phase, the mean seizure frequency decreased by 41% at 13 months with a responder rate of 43% [334].

Patients who carried the device for a longer period of time showed improved benefit with an average reduction in seizure frequency of 54% at 2 years. Long-term follow-up analysis of the SANTE trial at 5 years demonstrated a median seizure reduction of 69% and a responder rate of 68%. In the 5 years of follow-up, 16% of patients were seizure-free for at least 6 months [338].

In Norway, Herrman et al. [337] performed a single-center study with a prospective, randomized, double-blinded design including 18 patients. There was no significant difference in seizure frequency after the blinded period at 6 months between patients with or without stimulation. However, when considering all patients and comparing 6 months of stimulation with baseline, there was a 22% reduction in the frequency of all seizures. No increased effect over time was shown. Worse results compared to the SANTE trial were explained by the prevalence of more severe and refractory epilepsies. It has been concluded that the role of DBS treatment in refractory epilepsy still remains to be clarified [337].

Observational Studies

Similar to the SANTE trial, observational studies showed improved seizure outcome after DBS using the anterior thalamic nucleus as target. Oh et al. [339] reported a mean seizure reduction of 58% and Lee et al. [340] of 71%. Krishna et al. [341] noted response (≥50% seizure reduction) in 11 of 16 cases (69%). Analyzing 29 patients, Kim et al. [342] reported a median seizure reduction ranging from 62% to 80% after 3 to 11 years follow-up, and 14% of patients were seizure free at last follow-up. Improved seizure control over time suggests a neuromodulatory effect. Conversely, a Cochrane review [322] showed a limited effect of ANT-DBS after short-term (1–3 months) stimulation with a reduction in seizure frequency between 15% and 30%. Park et al. [343] reported 7 patients who failed VNS and underwent DBS. Postoperatively, 5 of the 7 patients (71%) experienced a ≥50% reduction of seizure frequency [343]. DBS has also been used in children and adolescents with seizure frequency reduction achieved in between 30% and 100% of cases [321, 344–346].

**Neuropsychological Outcome**

In the SANTE trial, postoperative depression was reported in 37.3%. However, two-thirds of them had a history of depression. Memory impairment was found in 27.3% of patients, and one half of those cases had a history of memory disturbances [331]. Follow-up testings showed a gradual improvement of attention, executive function, depression, tension anxiety, total mood disturbance, and subjective cognitive function [331]. Tröster et al. [347] reviewing neuropsychological outcome of the SANTE trial concluded that bilateral anterior thalamic nucleus stimulation was associated with subjective depression and memory adverse events during the blinded phase in a minority of patients that were not accompanied by objective, long-term neurobehavioral worsening. Similarly, psychiatric disorders and cognitive impairment were noted in some cases after thalamic stimulation by McGovern et al. [186]. Novais et al. [348] identified anterior thalamic stimulation for the treatment of MTLE as a risk factor for de novo psychopathology. Improvement of verbal fluency tasks and delayed verbal memory on follow-up after ANT-DBS was observed by Oh et al. [339].

#### 14.1.2.3 Responsive Neurostimulation (RNS)

Responsive neurostimulation (RNS) is based on the observation that cortical stimulation during functional mapping can abort epileptic afterdischarges which may evolve into clinical seizures [349]. The RNS device consists of an implanted stimulator connected to one or two subdural strips or depth leads, each containing four electrodes. To implant the pulse generator, a partial-thickness or full-thickness craniectomy is shaped. The generator is fixed to the skull using miniscrews. The electrodes are placed at the seizure foci with the aid of a frame-based system (Fig. 14.14). Tran et al. [350] as well as Chan et al. [351] proposed a robotic-assisted technique to implant the RNS system. Additional leads may be placed at the time of the initial procedure and connected to the neurostimulator at a future extradural surgery as needed [352, 353]. In a first step, implanted subdural and depth electrodes

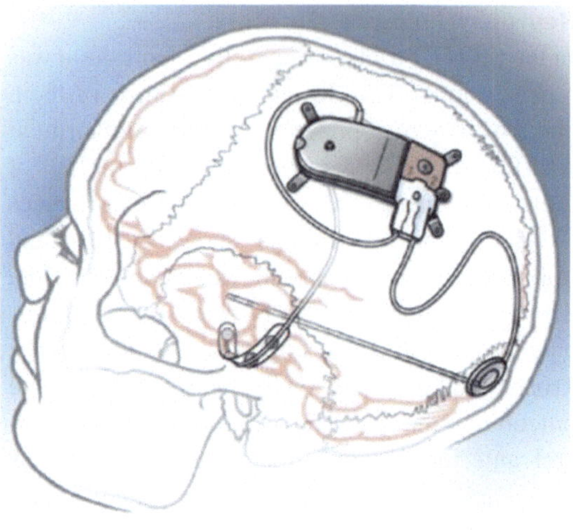

**Fig. 14.14** Schematic illustration of the technique of responsive stimulation (RNS). Placement of the stimulator in the skull which is connected to strip and depth electrodes placed at seizure foci. (From Hartshorn and Jobst [185], with permission)

record electrocorticographic activity during ictal events, and these data are analyzed for programming detection and stimulation settings of the device. Thereafter, the device provides responsive electrical stimulation when abnormal patterns indicative of an impending seizure according to its programmation are detected during continuous recordings at the seizure focus or foci. Thus, the device acts as a closed-loop system [354, 355].

RNS has been approved by the U.S. Food and Drug Administration (U.S. FDA) in 2013 for the treatment of focal epilepsy in adults, and it has been used off-label in children. Since then, over 2000 patients have been implanted [185]. RNS is restricted to patients whose seizure focus or foci clearly have been identified, but cannot be resected, e.g., patients with bitemporal epilepsy, or with a seizure focus in eloquent cortex [185, 353]. Different foci may be targeted one after the other to evaluate effects of stimulation [356]. In addition, chronic ECoG data can be used to identify patient-specific temporal dynamics in epileptiform activity in order to optimize detection and stimulation patterns. Thus, RNS may have the potential of providing a personalized therapy [357]. Moreover, ECoG data may be useful to evaluate epileptiform activity in response to new medications [353] or to identify patients who are likely to benefit in future from other surgical strategies [355].

### Seizure Outcome

#### The RNS System Pivotal Trial

After a 2-year open-label feasibility study including 65 patients, the efficacy of RNS was examined in a multicenter, randomized, double-blinded, controlled trial termed the RNS System Pivotal Trial [354]. In this study, 191 patients were included. About 50% of patients had mesial temporal lobe seizure onset, and seizure onset was bilateral in around 70% of them. Patients were randomized to receive either responsive stimulation or seizure detection without stimulation during a 12-week blinded period. After the blinded phase, patients of both groups received therapeutic stimulation (open study phase). During the 12-week blinded period, a 38% reduction in seizure frequency in the active group as compared to 17% in the control group was noted. By the end of the blinded phase, the average active stimulation patient had a 42% reduction in seizure frequency, as opposed to 9% for sham stimulation. In the open study phase, the median seizure reduction was 44% at 1 year and 53% at 2 years. Response rate was 55% at 1 and 2 years [358]. At 3 and 6 years follow-up, median seizure reduction was 48% and 66%, and responder rates were 59% and 61%, respectively [359]. At 9 years, the median seizure reduction was 75% [360]. No patient became completely seizure free, but 23% had at least one seizure-free period of 6 months or more and 12.9% of 1 year or longer [361].

#### Observational Studies

Favorable outcomes similar to the RNS System Pivotal Trial have been reported in noncontrolled studies. Geller et al. [362] reported on 111 patients with mesial temporal epilepsy, 72% with bilateral onset, and 28% with unilateral seizures. At mean follow-up of 6 years, a 70% median decrease in seizure frequency and a 64.6% responder rate were observed, with no differences seen between unilateral or bilateral patients

[362]. A study of 126 patients with neocortical epilepsy [363] showed an overall 58% median reduction of seizure frequency and a 55% responder rate at 6 years follow-up. On average, there was a 70% reduction in seizure frequency for patients with frontal and parietal seizure onset, 58% for those with temporal neocortical onset, and 51% for those with multilobar seizure onset. Seizure-free periods of at least 3, 6, and 12 months were reported in 37%, 26%, and 14% of cases, respectively [363]. Improved seizure control over time suggests a neuromodulatory effect of RNS [185]. Singhal et al. [364] reported the use of RNS in a 16-year-old patient with a left temporodorsal lesion suffering from daily seizures. By 6 months follow-up, the patient reported only auras but no seizures [364]. A non-randomized, observational, prospective study (post-approval study, PAS) is ongoing with planned enrollment of 300 patients across 30 centers. However, results have to be awaited [352].

#### Neuropsychological Outcome/Quality of Life (QOL)

Neuropsychological outcomes examined in the RNS trial patients [354] did not show any decline in cognitive functions [365] or mood [361]. In particular, no patients treated by responsive hippocampal stimulation had a memory decline under stimulation [357]. Patients with seizures beginning in a neocortical focus, especially in the frontal lobe, had statistically significant improvements in verbal fluency, and patients with seizures of mesial temporal lobe onset had a statistically significant improvement in learning, delayed free recall, and recognition [365]. In addition, increased quality of life (QOL) after RNS has been observed [358, 359]. Meador et al. [361] reported improvement in QOL at 2 years after RNS in 44% of patients, while 16% showed a decline. There was also a modest improvement in depression scores at 2 years follow-up. Patients with neocortical epilepsy did better than those with mesiotemporal epilepsy [361]. QOL improvements were not as high as for patients who achieve seizure freedom after resective surgery, but were higher than for medically intractable patients treated with best medical care [355].

### 14.1.2.4 Chronic Subthreshold Cortical Stimulation (CSCS)

Chronic subthreshold cortical stimulation (CSCS) is an open-loop continuous electrical stimulation approach. It provides constant, low-level stimulation to subdural electrodes located at or near the seizure onset zone [366]. The rationale of this technique is based on observations that continuous stimulation correlates with reduction of epileptiform spike rates [367–370]. CSCS delivers a continuous 0.2–0.4 mA stimulation (compared to 0.5–12 mA stimulation with RNS) [185]. The seizure focus has to be localized, and the proper stimulation location must be defined. Therefore, trial stimulation is required during invasive monitoring to optimize stimulation location and parameters before permanent implantation of the system is accomplished [366, 371]. Chronic subthreshold cortical stimulation is currently under clinical investigation, and only limited data are available assessing its efficacy.

#### Outcome

Lundstrom et al. [372] reported preliminary data with the use of CSCS in 13 patients. Results showed reduction in severity of epilepsy in 77% of the cases. In some patients, a reduction of interictal epileptiform discharges was noted. In addition, subjective improvement in life satisfaction has been observed [372]. In 2019, Lundstrom et al. [371] published a subsequent retrospective analysis of 21 patients. At 3 months follow-up, median reduction in seizure frequency was 93%, and the responder rate was 79%. At a median follow-up of 27 months, median percent reduction in seizure frequency of 100% and responder rate of 89% have been demonstrated. Seizure-free periods of at least 3 months were experienced by 63%, of at least 6 months by 50%, and of at least 12 months by 40% of patients. In addition, beneficial effects of CSCS on life satisfaction have been noted [371].

Overall, CSCS seems to be a feasible therapy [373]. Preliminary results in terms of seizure outcome are promising. However, further studies are needed to define the place of this novel modality among other techniques of neurostimulation. In addition, it has to be clarified whether continuous stimulation in eloquent cortex may induce unwanted side effects limiting its functionality [371, 373].

## 14.2 Curative Procedures

During the last decades a clear trend towards minimal and individually tailored surgical procedures is witnessed. This trend is mainly supported by improved MR imaging facilitating circumscribed approaches. In fact, minimal invasive interventions have proven to be successful, since the epileptogenic zone may be confined to the MRI visible lesion as it has been shown for some epilepsy-associated tumors [374–376], small bottom-of-sulcus FCD type IIb [377], and hypothalamic hamartomas [378–380]. With respect to the latter entity as well as other deep-seated pathologies such as periventricular nodular heterotopias, microsurgical resection is critical carrying high risks of neurological deficits despite sophisticated strategies including endoscopic-assisted techniques [381–387]. Therefore, both clinicians and patients may be reluctant towards resective surgery with those pathologies.

Stimulated by the limited accessibility of critically localized lesions for resective strategies, stereotactic procedures have evolved providing new chances for their treatment. Minimal invasiveness and high selectivity of stereotactic strategies imply that only limited volumes can be treated, and that exact localization and delineation of those volumes is required [186, 388]. Therefore, the critical key for the successful application of all stereotactic curative procedures is optimal presurgical MR imaging [388]. Today, two different stereotactic techniques are available: thermoablation and radiosurgery (Table 14.3). Reviews on these modalities have been provided by Quigg and Harden [389] and McGovern et al. [186].

**Table 14.3** Overview on curative stereotactic strategies

| Modality/technique | Mechanism of action/tool |
|---|---|
| Thermoablation | Denaturation of tissue proteins by heat (44–59 °C; RFTC 80 °C) |
| – Radiofrequency thermocoagulation (RFTC) | Electrical high-frequency current |
| – Laser-induced thermal therapy (LITT) | Laser light energy |
| – Focused ultrasound (FUS) | Ultrasound waves (230–1000 kHz) |
| Stereotactic radiosurgery | Ionizing radiation (20–25 Gy) |
| – Gamma Knife (GK) | Co-60 generated gamma radiation |
| – Linear Accelerator (LINAC) | Photon beams |

### 14.2.1 Thermoablation

The development of thermoablation for the treatment of epilepsy in the 1950s and 1960s was stimulated by stereotactic strategies to treat aggressive behavioral disorders, since some of those patients also suffering from epilepsy showed noticeably reduction of seizure frequency [390]. Spiegel and Wycis [391] recommended tissue ablation in the thalamus. In 1958, they changed their strategy to lesioning of the globus pallidus (pallidotomy) and the amygdala (amygdalotomy), mainly in combination (pallidoamygdalotomy) [392, 393]. Lesioning of the fornix (fornicotomy) and, if necessary, to create further lesions in the amygdala, hippocampus and globus pallidus was advocated by Umbach [394, 395]. In the pre-CT era, these procedures were guided by pneumoencephalographic X-ray studies and electrophysiological recordings. Narabayashi et al. [396] in Tokyo provided the first systematic report on amygdalotomy in 60 patients (46 with epilepsy, and 14 with EEG disturbances and behavioral symptoms). The target was ablated with an *oil-wax-lipiodol contrast dye mixture*. Substantial improvement was noted in 29 of 60 patients (48%). Complications included a temporary paresis and temporary behavioral disorders in each one patient, respectively [396]. Subsequent small trials in the 1960s achieved seizure freedom in 19–30% of patients [397, 398]. Heimburger et al. [397] used a *cryoprobe* for ablation of the amygdala.

During the 1970s, stereotactic ablation of the amygdala for the treatment of both epilepsy and behavioral disorders was widely used. Seizure freedom has been noted in up to 63% of patients [399, 400], and worthwhile reduction of seizure frequency in 50–100% [392, 394, 395, 400–409]. Summarizing four larger series including 124 patients, who were treated with unilateral or bilateral amygdalotomy both for behavioral disorders and epilepsy between 1963 and 1978, Parrent and Lozano [408] found seizure freedom in 15% and more than 50% reduction of seizure frequency in 43%. Mempel et al. [410] observed in their series of 70 patients who underwent amygdalotomy and anterior hippocampotomy seizure freedom in 11% of patients and reduction of seizure frequency in 75%. At this point it should be emphasized that the criteria for seizure freedom applied in the publications of the 1960s and 1970s, i.e., before the introduction of the Engel and ILAE classification, do not necessarily correspond to today's common outcome criteria, which somewhat limits comparability of those early results.

The use of ablation strategies for the treatment of epilepsies gained new interest with availability of MR imaging. Thermoablation (thermotherapy, thermocoagulation) applies heat (44–59 °C) in a focal manner to induce denaturation of tissue proteins (temperatures over 60 °C cause vaporization or carbonization of the tissue). Heating is achieved with three methods: (1) *radiofrequency thermocoagulation (RFTC)* induces heat by electrical current [388, 411, 412], (2) *laser-induced thermal therapy (LITT)* generates heat by absorption of interspersed laser light energy [413], and (3) *focused ultrasound (FUS)* produces heat by absorption of the interspersed ultrasound waves [414, 415]. With respect to the limited volume that can be treated, serial ablation in a segmental approach may be planned. Having ablated the best defined target, the patient is observed for a period of time. If seizure remission does not occur, repeated ablation can be performed [389, 416].

#### 14.2.1.1 Radiofrequency Thermocoagulation (RFTC)

Radiofrequency thermocoagulation (RFTC) for epilepsy was first used targeting the amygdalo-hippocampal complex in MTLE [417]. The probe is placed by a burr hole using a stereotactic frame. As suggested by Nádvorník and Šramka [418], the hippocampus is approached from an occipital trajectory along its longitudinal axis facilitating access to all mesiotemporal structures, while the inferior horn at the lateral aspect and the basal cisterns at the mesial aspect form a barrier preventing thermal injury to neighboring structures including nerves and vessels of the crural and ambient cisterns as well as the brainstem [419, 420]. In addition to its application in MTLE, RFTC has been used for the treatment of various pathologies such as neocortical seizure foci, periventricular heterotopias, hamartomas, and cavernomas [388, 421–424] (Fig. 14.15). Principles, development, and current applications of RFTC have been reviewed by Voges et al. [411] and Bourdillon et al. [425].

Two different approaches with RFTC are available: RFTC can be performed lesion guided and SEEG guided, and both techniques are complementary. SEEG-guided RFTC combines SEEG investigation with RFTC directly through the recording electrode. This technique was first reported in 2004 in a feasibility study [426]. SEEG-guided RFTC is of particular importance for non-lesional epilepsies as well as to confirm the suspected ictal onset zone in small lesions. When the seizure onset zone is small enough to be entirely covered by the coagulation volumes, SEEG-guided RFTC may be sufficient to cure the patient [425]. In other cases, when only a portion of the seizure onset zone can be targeted by the RFTC, the procedure may be a helpful tool predicting the success of subsequent resective surgery [427, 428]. In these cases, the electrodes may be left in place after the RFTC to continue SEEG recordings [425]. For SEEG-guided treatment of MTLE, Fan et al. [429] proposed implantation of a

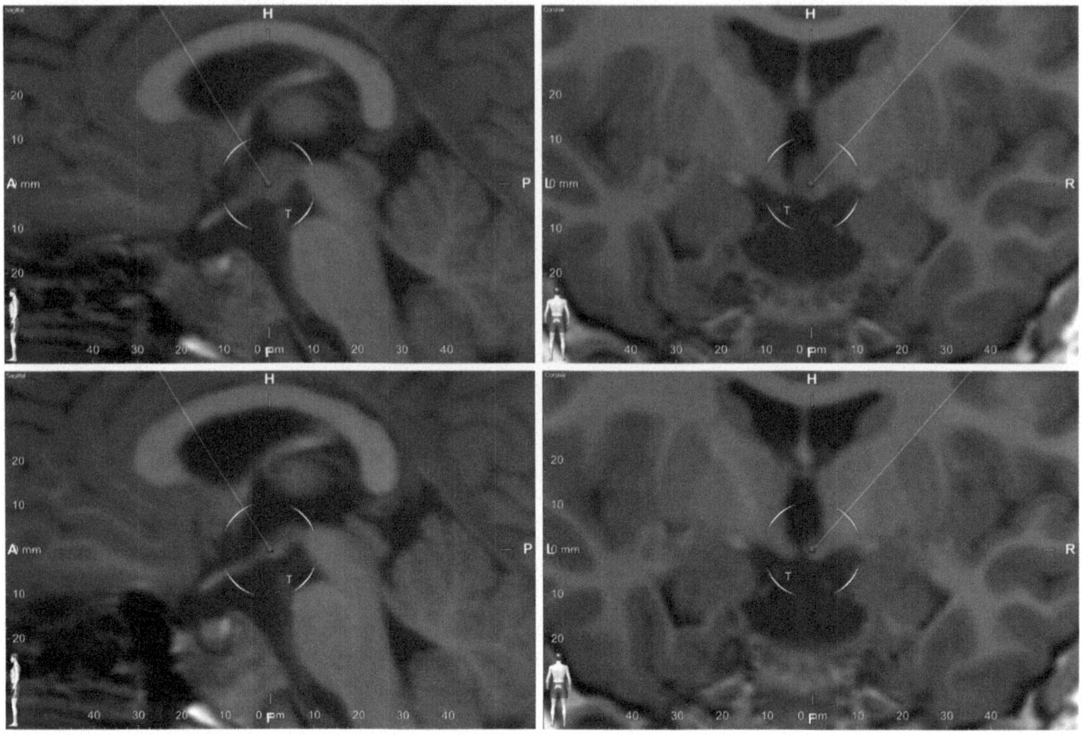


**Fig. 14.15** Hypothalamic hamartoma in a patient with gelastic seizures. Upper sequence: T1-MRI in sagittal (left) and coronal (right) view before RFTC; Lower sequence: T1-MRI in sagittal (left) and coronal (right) view after two RFTC therapies. Postoperatively, the patient was seizure free (with courtesy of P. Reinacher, Dep. Stereotactic and Functional Neurosurgery, Freiburg)

combination of SEEG electrodes to form a high-density focal stereo-array, including one electrode along the long axis of the amygdalohippocampal complex and three orthogonal electrodes to widely sample mesial temporal structures. This array facilitates coagulations between two contiguous contacts of the same electrode or between two adjacent contacts of different electrodes to produce larger lesions [429].

### Overall Outcome

Bourdillon et al. [430] reported a meta-analysis including 6 studies and a total of 296 patients with different pathologies. At 1 year after SEEG-guided RFTC, seizure-free rate was 23% and responder rate 58%. Although therapeutic efficacy was heterogeneous, two specific etiologies have been identified showing distinct results. With SEEG-guided lesioning of periventricular nodular heterotopias, 38% of patients were seizure free and 83% were responders. On the other hand, none of the patients who underwent SEEG-guided RFTC in TLE was seizure-free, and only 48% were responders at 1 year follow-up [430]. Dimova et al. [431] reported 23 patients (5 FCD, 1 heterotopia, 2 gliosis, 15 MR-negative) treated with SEEG-guided RFTC. At a mean follow-up of 32 months, eight patients (35%) experienced a ≥50% decrease of seizure frequency and one (4%) had a sustained seizure freedom [431]. In a pediatric population of 46 patients, Chipaux et al. [428] noted seizure freedom in 57% at 6 months and in 27% at 12 months after RFTC. Among 30 patients undergoing subsequent resective surgery, 73% became seizure free [428]. Overall, long-term seizure-free outcome after RFTC is mainly reported in 30–40% of cases and 50–70% experience ≥50% decrease of seizure frequency [426, 427, 430, 432].

#### MTLE

Variable results have been reported with RFTC in MTLE with seizure freedom rates between 2% and 75% [409, 433–436]. The Prague center achieved seizure freedom in 70–82% of patients, and combined seizure improvement or freedom in 80–100% of patients [434, 435, 437–439]. Moreover, Malikova et al. [440, 441] found significant improvements in global, verbal, semantic, and working memory, as well as in delayed recall and attention in both right-sided and left-sided lesions. These encouraging results have renewed interest in RFTC ablation [442, 443]. However, in her 2015 report, Malikova et al. [444] noted deterioration of verbal memory in left-sided patients. Analyzing seven patients who underwent RFTC for MTLE, Lee et al. [445] found that seizure frequency had decreased by a mean of 78% at 6 months follow-up. Overall, most studies found seizure-free outcomes in the range of 30–40% and improved patients between 40% and 60% [409, 426, 446, 447].

#### HH

Following early series [421, 422], Kameyama et al. [448] reported on a total of 140 RFTC procedures performed in 100 consecutive patients with hypothalamic hamartomas (HH). Freedom from gelastic seizures was achieved in 86% of the patients, and from all seizure types in 71% of cases. In addition, seizure freedom lead to improvement of behavioral disorders and cognitive functions. There were no differences in seizure outcome between patients with giant and non-giant hamartomas [448].

#### FCD

In 2014, Wellmer et al. [424] published RFTC of two eloquently located bottom-of-sulcus focal cortical dysplasias (FCD) type IIB with favorable outcomes in both cases (Engel Ia and Ib, respectively). Later on, the authors reported on 7 patients with bottom-of-sulcus FCD type IIb, and seizure freedom was achieved in 4 of 5 patients (80%) with complete lesion coagulation [377]. It has been shown that FCD type IIb is intrinsically epileptogenic [449], and that lesioning of the neocortical aspect of the malformation sparing the frequently associated MR hyperintense signal extending to the neighboring ventricle (transmantle sign) results in excellent seizure outcome [450]. Contrarily, none of the 11 patients in the series of Cossu et al. [451] with FCD (2 type I and 9 type II) became seizure free after RFTC.

#### Heterotopias

Schmitt et al. [452] reported a single patient with periventricular heterotopia who became seizure free (Engel Ib) after RFTC. Cossu et al. [442] achieved seizure freedom in 4 of 5 patients (80%) with nodular gray matter heterotopias who were treated with SEEG-guided RFCT. In their 2015 report, they noted seizure freedom in 8 of 12 patients (67%) with nodular heterotopias [451].

### 14.2.1.2 Laser-Induced Thermal Therapy (LITT)

Laser-induced thermal therapy (LITT), also named MR-guided LITT (MRgLITT), MR-guided thermal laser ablation (MTLA), or stereotactic laser ablation (SLA), constitutes an emerging minimally invasive procedure that consists of a fiber-optic catheter facilitating thermal ablation of specific anatomical structures [453]. Laser technology has been used in neurosurgery since the 1960s [454–457]. However, it gained increasing interest only years later when MR imaging was available [306, 458–465]. In parallel to epilepsy, LITT has been applied for the treatment of deep-seated brain tumors [462, 466–471] and for cingulotomy in chronic pain [472, 473].

The laser is introduced by a stereotactically implanted MRI-compatible probe. Li et al. [474] proposed a machine-learning approach for computer-assisted planning to predict entry and target points in order to optimize trajectories. At each point along the trajectory, a cylindrical lesion with an average total diameter of 15 mm can be created [475]. The ablation procedure is continuously monitored using a MR-based temperature control. Currently, two LITT platforms haven been approved: Visualase (Medtronic, USA) and NeuroBlate (Monteris Medical, USA), whereby for epilepsy mainly the Visualase system is used. Experience exists with the use of LITT for the treatment of MTLE, hypothalamic hamartomas, focal cortical dysplasia (FCD), heterotopias, and corpus callosotomy [458] [475]. Reviews on the use of LITT for epilepsy have been provided by LaRiviere and Gross [476], Gross et al. [477], Shimamoto et al. [475], Grewal and Tatum [453], and Hoppe et al. [478]. The largest increase with the use of LITT is noticed for the treatment of MTLE (Figs. 14.16 and 14.17).

### Overall Seizure Outcome

Evaluating 60 reports including 226 patients, Hoppe et al. [478, 479] suggested that seizure freedom achieved by LITT is only slightly worse than for resective surgery with differences between 10% and 20%. In 2018, Hoppe et al. [480] reviewed results of 25 uncontrolled pediatric series including 179 patients with different pathologies (64.2% hypothalamic hamartomas). Evaluating 127 patients, they noted seizure freedom (Engel I) in 57.5% of cases. Seizure control tended to decrease over time [480]. Others reported a seizure-free rate of 50% [461].

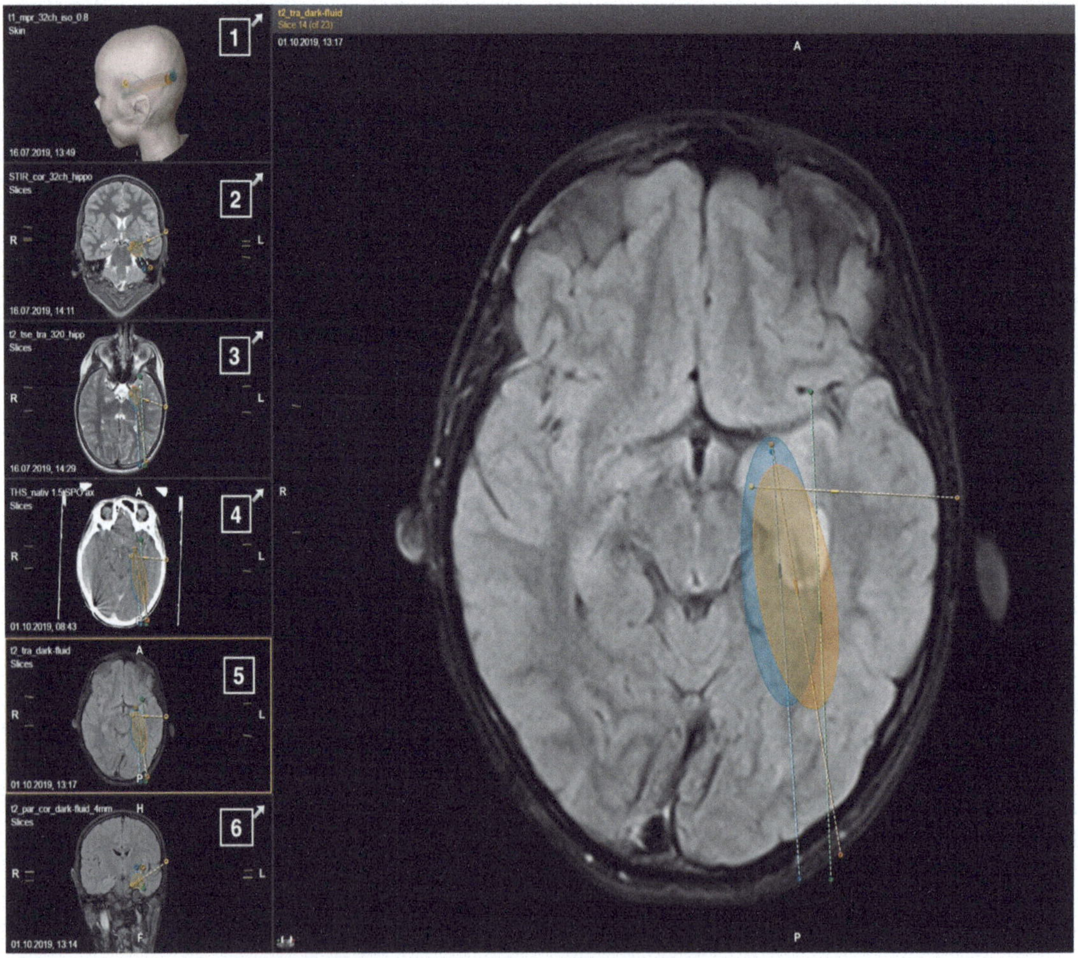


**Fig. 14.16** Stereotactic trajectory planning and targeting in a patient with a left temporomesial ganglioglioma. Images 1–3: Preoperative virtual planning with varying occipital trajectories and a temporal approach. Image 4: Stereotactic CT with attached stereotactic frame. Images 5 and 6: Intraoperative FLAIR sequence documenting the thermoablative effect. (With courtesy of T. Gasser, Beta Klinik, Bonn)

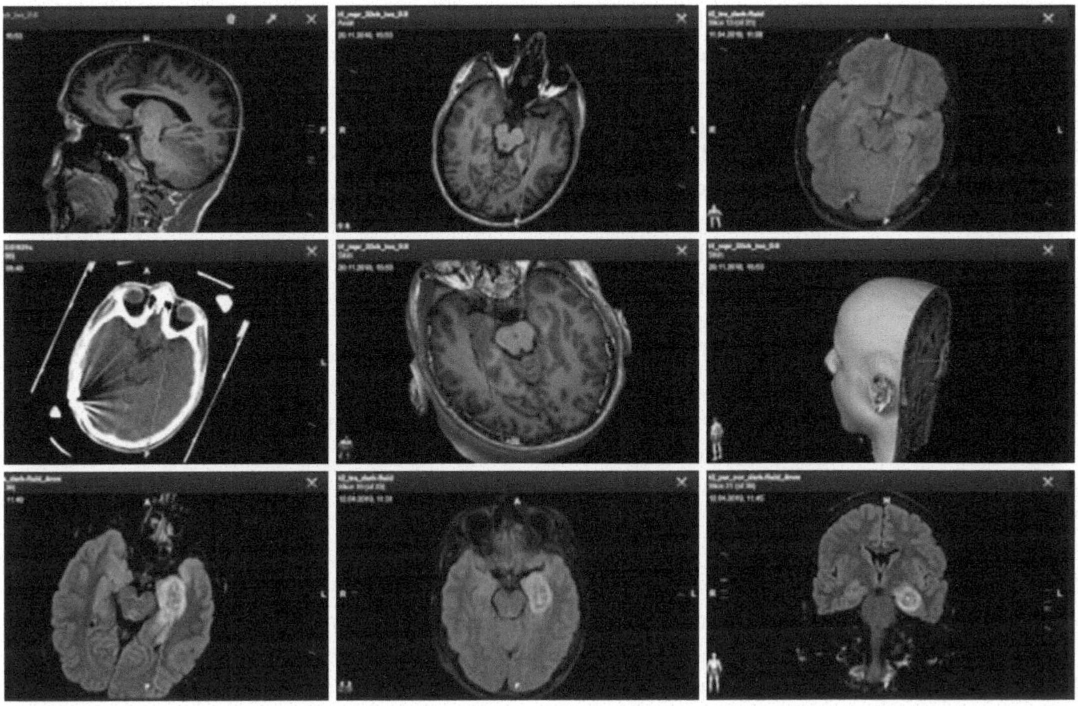

**Fig. 14.17** Stereotactic trajectory planning and targeting in a patient with a left hippocampal sclerosis. Upper sequence: Preoperative virtual planning with an occipital approach targeting the sclerotic hippocampus. Middle sequence: Stereotactic CT with attached stereotactic frame and 3D representation of the trajectory. Lower sequence: Early postoperative MRI (FLAIR sequence) documenting the thermoablative effect with superimposed trajectory. (With courtesy of T. Gasser, Beta Klinik, Bonn)

## MTLE

### Seizure Outcome

There are many reports mainly including small patient numbers on the application of LITT in mesial temporal lobe epilepsy (MTLE) [1, 420, 460, 481–491]. Seizure freedom has been found in 40–69%, mainly between 50% and 60% of patients [420, 461, 488, 491–493]. Drane et al. [483] observed seizure freedom in 52% of patients treated with LITT compared to 62% of those who received standard resection. Analyzing 43 patients undergoing LITT for MTLE, Donos et al. [494] achieved Engel I outcome in 79.5% at 6 months and in 67.4% at 20.3 months follow-up. Grewal et al. [495, 496] found seizure freedom in 43% of 23 patients at a median follow-up of 34 months. The largest case series including 58 MTLE patients has been reported by Gross et al. [477]. At a follow-up of at least 12 months, Engel I outcomes were 57.1% for all patients and 63.7% for patients with HS [477].

Shimamoto et al. [475] summarized results of 8 case series including a total of 243 MTLE patients. Seizure-free outcome was 58% for all patients and 62% on the average for cases with HS [488, 492–494, 497, 498]. Wu et al. [499] reported results of a retrospective multicenter study including 234 patients from 11 centers. In this study, all ablation cavities were manually traced on postoperative MRI, which were subsequently nonlinearly normalized to a common atlas to demonstrate most favorable ablation zones in a three-dimensional model. At 2 years after LITT, 58% achieved Engel I outcome, and 80% had only rare seizures (Engel I–II). Based on this model, ablations should prioritize the amygdala and include the hippocampal head, parahippocampal gyrus, and the entorhinal cortex to maximize chances of seizure freedom. A history of bilateral tonic-clonic seizures has been identified to predict lower changes for a seizure-free outcome, while MRI evidence of hippocampal sclerosis was not predictive [499]. Others described a shorter duration of epilepsy as a positive prognostic factor [500, 501]. LITT may also be used in combination with resective surgery [416, 482, 502].

In all, seizure-free outcome with LITT is in the range of 50–60%. LITT seems to be a particularly promising tool for the treatment of MTLE providing seizure outcomes approximating those achieved by resective surgery. Results of the ongoing SLATE (Stereotactic Laser Ablation for Temporal Lobe Epilepsy) study, a prospective single-arm clinical trial, have to be awaited [477, 503].

#### Neuropsychological Outcome

A study by Donos et al. [494] evaluated cognitive outcomes in 43 patients who underwent LITT for MTLE. They found relatively little postoperative cognitive decline for the most part. Patients with LITT in the dominant hemisphere showed small decrease in verbal long-term memory, whereas patients treated in the nondominant temporal lobe revealed decrease in one nonverbal long-term memory parameter. In line with the literature on conventional resective approaches, presurgical cognitive performance was the strongest predictor of postsurgical cognitive outcome [494]. Drane et al. [483] examined neuropsychological outcomes in 19 patients undergoing LITT for MTLE, compared to 39 individuals undergoing standard resection, using a prospective, non-randomized, parallel-group design. Compared to resective surgery, LITT was associated with significantly improved naming in patients with dominant hemisphere MTLE and better object recognition in individuals with MTLE of the non-dominant hemisphere. No patients showed decline in performance in naming and object recognition tasks after LITT [483]. Providing a review on TLE of various etiologies, Drane [504] concluded that the rate of cognitive decline following LITT in the dominant hemisphere may be smaller than with conventional resective surgery. Similar observations have been reported by Kang et al. [488] and Grewal et al. [495, 496]. Gross et al. [477] noted verbal memory decline in 4 of 49 (8.2%) patients overall, and in 7 of 49 (15%) cases treated on the dominant side. However, the research base is still limited in this area, and factors influencing the course of postoperative cognitive functioning, such as rates of seizure freedom, have to be considered in evaluating the neuropsychological outcomes.

### HH

Several reports address application of LITT for hypothalamic hamartomas (HH). LITT rather aims at the disconnection of the hamartoma from the hypothalamus which usually is sufficient to achieve total remission of gelastic seizures than at the coagulation of the complete lesion [381, 464, 465, 505–510]. In the series of Wilfong and Curry [508] comprising 14 children with HH, 86% were seizure free at a mean follow-up of 9 months. Others reported single cases and found seizure control in around half to two-thirds of the children [458, 464, 465]. Contrarily, Lewis et al. [461] did not note significant improvement after LITT. Summarizing 37 cases of the literature including one own case, Wright et al. [509] found seizure freedom in 37%. The largest series of HH comprising 71 patients treated with LITT has been published by Curry et al. [511]. After 1 year follow-up, 93% of patients were free from gelastic seizures with 23% requiring more than one ablation. At last follow-up, 12% of patients were free from all seizure types without medication. Memory deficit rate was 1.5% [511]. Xu et al. [512] reporting on 18 patients noted freedom from gelastic seizures in 80% and from all seizure types in 61% of cases at last follow-up (mean 17.4 months). It has been suggested that the combined use of MRgLITT technology and rs-fMRI (resting state fMRI) may improve focal ablation and disconnection of epileptic networks/pathways resulting in a higher rate of seizure freedom [513].

### Other Pathologies

LITT has been used for deep-seated cortical dysplasias [461, 502, 514, 515], periventricular nodular heterotopias [416, 516], tuberous sclerosis [517], and cavernomas [518]. In a series of 12 children with focal cortical dysplasias (FCD),

Lewis et al. [461] found seizure freedom in 42%. McCracken et al. [518] achieved seizure freedom in 4 of 5 patients (80%) with cavernomas. Regarding nodular periventricular heterotopias and tuberous sclerosis, only a few single cases have been reported, and in most cases LITT provided favorable results [416, 516]. Moreover, single cases of lesions in the insular cortex have been successfully treated with LITT [519, 520]. Cobourn et al. [521] felt that LITT based on SEEG data is best suited for patients with multiple, discrete, and widespread epileptic foci. Evaluating 4 children (2 tuberous sclerosis; 2 focal cortical dysplasia) with a total of 9 lesions, they noted that 3 patients were seizure free and 1 individual was significantly improved over a mean follow-up of 9.3 months [521].

**Reoperations**

In the study by Gross et al. [477], 9 patients underwent a second MRgLITT procedure, and seizure freedom was achieved in 7 cases (78%). Grewal et al. [495, 496] reported 3 repeated MRgLITT procedures with subsequent seizure freedom in all 3 individuals. Tao et al. [497] noted seizure control in 1 of 3 patients after a second MRgLITT. Although data are sparse, it seems that a second LITT procedure in case of failure may be effective. As an alternative to repeated LITT, resective surgery may be considered [495, 496].

#### 14.2.1.3 Focused Ultrasound (FUS)

Focused ultrasound (FUS) uses high-energy ultrasound waves of 230–1000 kHz, which are focused to a target point at which temperature can be modulated, thus to create a transient or permanent lesion [414, 522]. The location, volume, and change of temperature are monitored with simultaneous MRI (MR-guided FUS, MRgFUS). Thus, as with LITT, FUS ablation does not allow direct precise monitoring of the temperature. Originally, craniotomy was required for the application of ultrasound. However, current techniques allow reliable transcranial focusing of ultrasound without dispersion to deep-seated lesions; thus craniotomy is no longer necessary [389, 414]. Initial trials of MRI-guided FUS have been performed for the treatment of glioblastoma [523]. In addition to tumor therapy, MRgFUS has received Conformité Européenne (CE) approval for the treatment of essential tremor by lesioning the ventral intermediate nucleus of the thalamus [524, 525] and chronic neuropathic pain by medial thalamotomy [526], as well as the United States Food and Drug Administration (U.S. FDA) approval for the treatment of essential tremor.

**FUS for Ablation**

McDonell et al. [527] validated robotic-assisted MRgFUS in a swine model and found intraoperative and postoperative imaging to correlate with histological examination. In a theoretical modeling study, Parker et al. [528] developed a noninvasive MRgFUS ablation strategy for mesial temporal disconnection and provided the groundwork necessary for future clinical trials to apply this technique to patients with refractory MTLE. However, technological limitations still prohibit its application to limbic and neocortical epilepsies, since both targets are too close to the skull, and critical heating of the skull and structures outside the target region are feared. These well-known limitations [389, 414] are currently addressed. In open-label clinical trials, the role of MRgFUS is investigated for the ablation of subcortical epileptic lesions (NCT02804230) and for ablating the anterior thalamic nucleus in refractory focal onset seizures with secondary generalization (NCT03417297). Among those pioneers, the team at the Miami Children's Hospital successfully ablated a hypothalamic hamartoma with MRgFUS in an epilepsy patient (AES abstract 2017-2.344) [529].

**FUS for Modulation/Opening BBB**

It has been suggested that MRgFUS is able to modulate neurological functions without tissue damage [530]. Given that epilepsy is considered a network disease, MRgFUS may be used to interrupt or modulate those network structures [529]. Moreover, it has been demonstrated that FUS is able to precisely and spatially open the blood–brain barrier (BBB) [531]. Reversible opening of the BBB with MRgFUS could potentially offer novel therapeutic techniques such as targeted drug therapy [529].

In sum, FUS can be expected to be efficacious for targets in epilepsy. However, MRgFUS interventions for epilepsy are still in the experimental stage [529].

## 14.2.2 Stereotactic Radiosurgery (SRS)

Stereotactic radiosurgery (SRS) aims at the destruction of target tissue by ionizing radiation. SRS as a tool for functional neurosurgery has been pioneered by Leksell. It was first used for movement disorders and trigeminal neuralgia [532]. Later on, thalamotomies for tremor and for intractable pain, and capsulotomies for psychiatric disorders have been performed [533, 534]. Talairach applied SRS for the first time in epilepsy. Between 1955 and 1973, he implanted radioactive Yttrium into the amygdala and the hippocampus in 44 patients with MTLE [535]. Although first clinical results were promising, two patients experienced hemiparesis due to occlusion of the anterior choroid artery which was related to the use of the radionuclide [535]. Subsequently, this approach was abandoned.

Nowadays, SRS is mainly based on Gamma Knife (GK) and the linear accelerator (LINAC). Clinical experience with these modalities in arteriovenous malformations (AVM) and tumors (mostly metastases) revealed an anticonvulsive effect [536–539]. Of 247 patients treated for AVM between 1970 and 1984 in Stockholm, 59 had seizures, and 52 (88%) were seizure free after GK treatment [540]. The anticonvulsant effect of radiosurgery has also been shown by others [536, 541], and similar observations were made with the use of other radiotherapeutical modalities such as brachytherapy [538], conformal radiotherapy [537], and conventional radiotherapy [537]. The influence of radiotherapy on seizure activity was confirmed in animal experiments [542, 543], and a dose-dependent anticonvulsive effect has been described [544–546]. Consequently, the use of SRS has been promoted for epilepsy [547]. Although the exact mechanisms underlying the effect of radiosurgery on epilepsy are not fully understood, it is thought that both ischemic/necrotic and neuromodulatory effects are involved [548, 549]. Today, SRS is mainly used for the treatment of tumor-associated epilepsies (Fig. 14.18), MTLE, and HH. A literature review on radiosurgery for epilepsy has been given by McGonigal et al. [111] with the majority of existing data referring to Gamma Knife.

### 14.2.2.1 MTLE

Efficacy of SRS for the treatment of MTLE has been examined in two randomized controlled trials, one of them comparing high- and low-dose SRS [550] and the other comparing SRS with anterior temporal lobectomy (ATL) [551]. In addition, observational studies including one meta-analysis [552] and the European prospective multicenter study [553] evaluating SRS for MTLE are available. Another meta-analysis summarizing 19 observational studies [496] compared SRS with MRgLITT.

- *Randomized controlled trials (RCTs).* In a U.S. multicenter pilot study, Barbaro et al. [550] randomized 13 patients to high (24 Gy) and 17 patients to low (20 Gy) radiosurgery. At 36 months of follow-up, 77% of those who received a high-dose treatment (24 Gy), and 59% of those treated with a low dose (20 Gy) became seizure free. The overall seizure-free outcome rate was 67%. It has been suggested that MRI characteristics during the first year following SRS, specifically T2 hyperintensity 9 months after the procedure, are associated with seizure relief and were more pronounced in patients who received 24 Gy SRS compared to lower dose (20 Gy) treatment [550, 554]. Neuropsychological testing at 36 months revealed no decline in verbal memory in patients treated on the dominant side [555].

  The ROSE (**R**adiosurgery or **O**pen **S**urgery for **E**pilepsy) trial, a randomized single-blinded, controlled trial, was designed to compare Gamma Knife SRS with ATL for the treatment of MTLE [551]. Outcomes were seizure remission (absence of disabling sei-

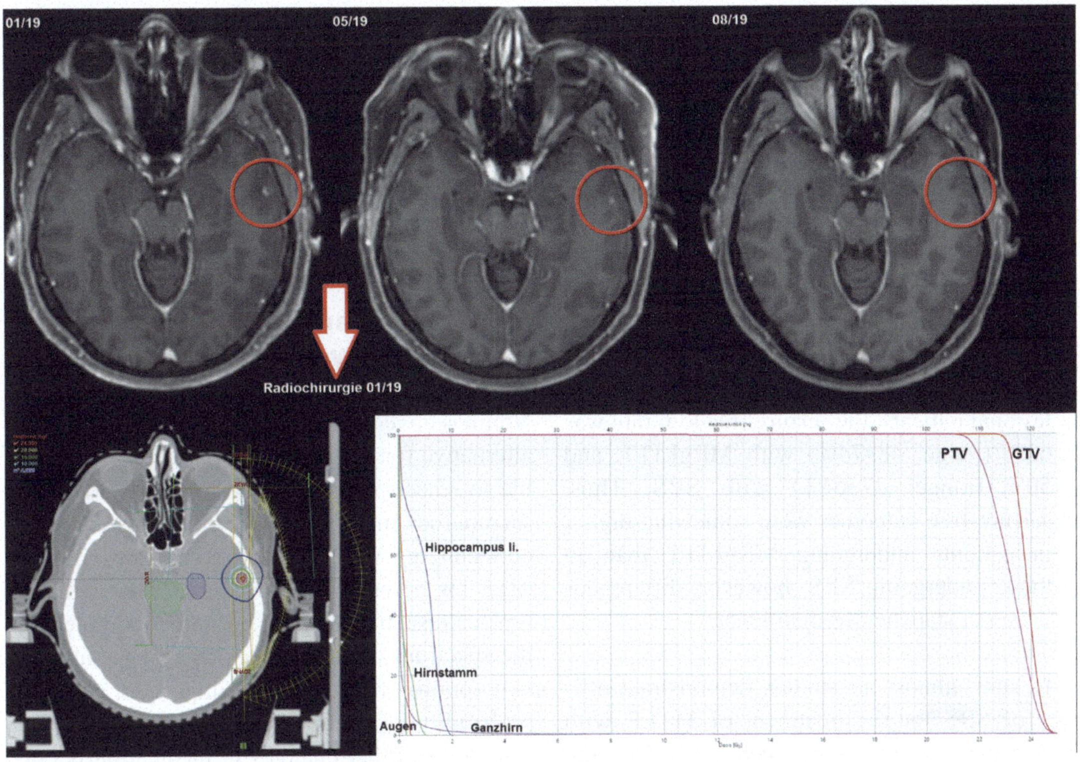


**Fig. 14.18** SRS for brain metastasis. 60-year-old female patient with focal seizures and known non-small cell bronchial carcinoma. A left temporal brain metastasis was diagnosed (top left). Radiosurgery with 20 Gy at the 80% isodose was performed. Illustration of the irradiation plan and dose distribution (bottom left). Dose-volume histogram (bottom right): average dose in the planning volume (PTV) 20 Gy, maximum dose in the lesion itself (GTV) 25 Gy, very low whole brain load and simultaneous protection of the risk organs (brain stem, eyes, hippocampus). Seizure control was achieved with complete remission of metastasis (top right). (With courtesy of A.L. Grosu, Dpt. of Radiotherapy, Freiburg)

zures), verbal memory, and quality of life (QOL) at 36 months follow-up. A total of 58 patients (31 in SRS, 27 in ATL) were treated. Sixteen (52%) SRS and 21 (78%) ATL patients achieved seizure control ($p = 0.82$). Mean verbal memory changes did not differ between groups. Worsening of verbal memory was observed in 36% of SRS and 57% of ATL patients. QOL improved with seizure remission. It has been concluded that ATL is superior to SRS and that resective surgery should be the treatment choice for MTLE [551].

- *Observational studies.* A meta-analysis including 13 articles and 168 patients of Feng et al. [552] reported seizure-free outcome (Engel I) in 51% of MTLE cases (range: 0–86%) at an average follow-up of 14 months (range: 6 months to 9 years) after SRS. In a European prospective multicenter study [553] evaluating 20 MTLE patients treated with GK radiosurgery (24 Gy), seizure-free outcome was shown in 65% at 2 years follow-up. Long-term follow-up (mean: 8 years) of 15 patients demonstrated seizure freedom in 73%. Seizure control has been found to increase over time, and the most effect occurred between 12 and 18 months after treatment [553, 556] coinciding with the development and resolution of maximal MRI changes [554]. Contrarily, Vojtech et al. [412] and Rheims et al. [557] documented seizure freedom in only 1 of 14 (7%) and 1 of 15 (7%) patients at a follow-up of 16 and 31 months, respectively, and Liang et al. [63] did not encounter any seizure-free patient at a follow-up of 24 months in a series of 7 cases after GK treatment.

- *SRS/MRgLITT.* Grewal et al. [496] pooled the data from 19 studies to compare seizure outcome in patients treated with MRgLITT and SRS, respectively, for MTLE. Of 19 studies including 415 patients, 9 studies (250 patients) were on MRgLITT, and 10 studies (165 patients) on SRS. Overall, seizure freedom was achieved in 50% of cases treated with MRgLITT (range: 44–56%), and in 42% treated with SRS (range: 27–59%). Among lesional patients, the seizure freedom rate was 62% (range: 48–74%) with MRgLITT, and 50% (range: 37–64%) with SRS. Thus, seizure-free outcomes were somewhat higher in patients undergoing MRgLITT than in those undergoing SRS; however, differences were not statistically significant.

In sum, almost all studies demonstrate efficacy of SRS for the treatment of MTLE with seizure-free outcome rates between 42% and 77%, mainly between 50% and 60%. Although not statistically significant, ATL has been found to be superior to SRS. Moreover, seizure-free outcome was somewhat higher with LITT as compared to SRS.

#### 14.2.2.2 HH

A single successfully treated case of a HH by GK has been reported by Arita et al. [558]. Régis et al. [559, 560] analyzed 10 HH cases from different centers. The median marginal dose was 15 Gy (range: 12–20 Gy). Two patients were treated twice. Overall, seizure control was observed in 50% of the patients and all were improved. The cumulated marginal dose was more than 17 Gy in the seizure-free group and below 13 Gy in the improved group. Behavior was clearly improved in 2 patients [559]. However, long-term studies have reported overall seizure remission rates of only 27% [389, 559]. In a series of 27 patients with HH who received doses between 13 and 26 Gy (median: 17 Gy), Régis et al. [561] observed 37% seizure-free and 22% improved patients. The authors noted dramatic behavioral and cognitive improvement [561]. As an alternative to GK and LINAC, brachytherapy by $^{125}$J-seeds is used in some centers. In a study of 24 patients, Engel I outcome was observed after 1 year in 38% of the patients [562]. Overall, seizure-free outcome after SRS in HH ranges between 30% and 50%.

## 14.3 Summary of Non-resective Surgery

Non-resective surgical strategies provide an alternative for drug-resistant patients not amenable to resective surgery due to poorly localized seizure foci, multiple foci, or epileptogenic zones co-localizing with eloquent areas carrying high risks for a resective procedure. They will not replace resective surgery, but rather complement the spectrum of surgical options. These alternative options are particularly important, since the probability of achieving a lasting seizure-free state with further changes in medication is only 5–10% [563–568]. In fact, non-resective strategies noticeably increase the number of patients who are candidates for surgery [3–5]. Moreover, they provide additional chances for patients after failed resective surgery. The following is a brief summary of conceptual considerations, data availability, patient selection, surgical aspects, and results including advantages and disadvantages of different non-resective surgical modalities. Complications of these strategies are summarized in the respective chapter.

### 14.3.1 Palliative Procedures

A generally accepted consensus on indications for the use of palliative procedures does not exist. Important aspects for selection of appropriate candidates include localization of the seizure focus, the most disabling seizure type that has to be controlled, intellectual performance, expected quality of life, patient's age, and the risks involved with the procedure. In principle, the major goal of all palliative procedures is to reduce or abolish most disabling seizure types. Efficacy of disconnective modalities (CC and MST) has been shown in long-term observational studies including meta-analyses. Effectiveness of stimulation procedures (VNS, ANT-DBS, RNS) was proven in randomized controlled and long-term observational trials. Reviewing the literature, however, questions arise at some points as to the significance of those data.

Although the extensive literature available particularly for VNS leaves no doubt as to its—albeit limited—effectiveness, it seems to be remarkable that two studies comparing the efficacy of VNS with the best medical treatment showed similar effects in terms of seizure outcome [290, 291], whereas only one study suggested superiority of VNS [245]. This calls for robust long-term outcome data to define the place of palliative surgical strategies and to provide patient selection criteria on a scientific basis. The situation is all the more complex because in addition to seizure reduction, some palliative procedures such as vagal nerve stimulation and callosotomy have beneficial effects on quality of life, positively influencing behavior and psychic condition. Thus, assessment of those modalities should not only be limited to seizure frequency but also include functional aspects.

The time-courses of seizure reduction of stimulation techniques (VNS, ANT-DBS, RNS) are similar [569]. Long-term assessment demonstrates continuously improving efficacy over many years suggesting a disease-modifying neuromodulation effect [190, 209]. Temporary or permanent seizure-free patients suggest that a subgroup of individuals can be expected to have a major benefit from those procedures. However, these subgroups have still to be characterized [190]. Neuromodulation seems to have a great potential to modify network abnormalities and thereby to reduce seizures and improve cognitive functions [570] Better understanding of brain networks and integration of artificial intelligence can be expected to promote those promising strategies [187].

Responsive neurostimulation offers new steps to a feedback-based stimulation for epilepsy. A critical issue with RNS and rVNS as actual available closed-loop systems refers to the low specificity of seizure detection inducing a high number of duty cycles without seizures when a high sensitivity of the system is desired. At this time, it may be speculated that efficacy of responsive systems rather reflects long-term neuromodulatory effects by frequent interventions than an acute seizure abolishing effect [190]. Advanced technologies and learning systems are required that can more reliably predict seizures, thus increasing specificity of those systems [571]. In parallel, stimulation paradigms including intensity, frequency, pulse width, pulse form, duty cycles, and timing need to be optimized to facilitate adequate responses [187, 190]. Chronic ECoG data delivered by RNS may be used to identify patient-specific temporal dynamics in epileptiform activity. Thus, by combining optimized seizure detection with individually most effective stimulation, responsive neurostimulation may have the potential of providing a personalized therapy [357].

#### 14.3.1.1 Disconnective Procedures

##### Conceptual Considerations

Disconnective procedures—corpus callosotomy (CC) and multiple subpial transections (MST)—aim at the prevention of seizure occurrence and propagation of seizure activity. Sectioning of the corpus callosum prevents seizure spread from one to the other hemisphere and synchrony of epileptiform discharges and is therefore best suited when rapid bihemispheric seizure propagation occurs. MST are based on the concept that neuronal functional units are organized vertically, while epileptic cortical activity spreads horizontally, and that development of a seizure requires a minimum volume of a neuronal network. Thus, by interrupting the horizontally oriented cortico-cortical fibers at 5 mm distances limiting synchronized volumes, development of a seizure and spread of epileptic activity may be prevented, while function mediated by vertically irradiating projection, commissural and association fibers should remain intact.

**Data Availability**

CC has been studied since the mid of the last century. Patient series with long follow-up periods and meta-analyses assessing in detail the effect of callosotomy on different seizure types are available. In addition, the extensive clinical and experimental research on CC in the mid of the last century provided important insights in the understanding of epileptogenesis and seizure spread. MST have been assessed during the last three decades in some larger observational studies with long-term follow-ups including a few meta-analyses. However, comprehensive data regarding special application fields, e.g., in Landau–Kleffner syndrome, are largely lacking. In addition, both for CC and MST, randomized controlled trials do not exist.

**Surgical Aspects**

CC remains a demanding procedure with a relatively high morbidity and a non-negligible mortality rate. Critical structures endangered include the supplementary motor cortex, the cingulate gyrus, septum pellucidum, and fornix. Postoperative disconnection syndrome may rather be related to these "extracallosal factors" than to proper sectioning of the callosum, since with increased surgical experience and a meticulous surgical technique, distinct disconnection signs have become rather unusual even after one-stage complete callosal section. Despite a significant temporary morbidity, MST of eloquent areas constitute an easy and safe procedure, and significant permanent adverse effects are rare.

**Patient Selection**

Although CC represented an integral part of the epilepsy surgery program in the 1960s and 1970s, it accounts only for a small number (around 2%) of all therapeutic interventions done for epilepsy in actual series. Callosotomy is mainly used in children and adolescents with severe tonic and atonic drop attacks in the absence of a locatable focus, but may also be considered in the adult age. MST can be used to treat epilepsies in eloquent brain areas, resection of which is not possible due to impending neurological deficits. In addition, MST have been found to be effective for patients with Landau–Kleffner syndrome. As a stand-alone therapy, MST may only be considered in highly selected cases. More frequently, MST are used in conjunction with cortical resection when the seizure focus encroaches on eloquent areas.

**Results**

Severe tonic or atonic drop attacks are reduced or abolished by CC in around 90% of patients. Responder rates for the most disabling seizure types range between 40% and 80%. Complete callosotomy has been shown to result in improved seizure outcome compared to partial callosal sectioning. However, nearly no patient becomes seizure free, and frequency of focal seizures may even increase [66, 75, 122, 124, 125]. As a stand-alone therapy, results of MST are modest with responder rates between 40% and 50%, and seizure-free outcome is observed in 10–15% of patients. More favorable results with seizure control between 40% and 60% and responder rates between 80% and 90% can be achieved when MST are combined with resection [122, 170, 173, 174, 176].

**Advantages/Disadvantages**

CC may positively influence functional outcome, i.e., by reduction of hyperactivity and improvement of speech, memory, attentiveness, and self-care. However, it represents the most invasive non-resective modality. Careful selection of appropriate candidates is necessary in order to avoid operative sequelae like the spit brain syndrome and deficit reinstatement. From a functional point of view, MST fulfill the requirements of the concept that no permanent neurological deficits have to be expected, while seizure outcomes do not meet conceptual expectations. The mild artificial subarachnoid hemorrhage as usually seen after MST is functionally not relevant. Accessibility of the cortex for MST is limited in some areas, e.g., at the mesial and basal aspects of the hemisphere and in the insula.

### 14.3.1.2 Neurostimulation

**Conceptual Considerations**

VNS and DBS are based on programmable devices delivering intermittent electrical stimuli.

In contrast, RNS and rVNS act as closed-loop systems on demand, triggered by early detection of epileptogenic activity from constant intracranial EEG recordings (RNS) and tachycardia (rVNS), respectively. It is suggested that VNS acts on the tractus solitarius inducing desynchronization of cerebral electrical activity through widespread modulation of noradrenaline and serotonin release and by changing distribution of cerebral blood flow in the thalamus. The anticonvulsant effect of anterior thalamic stimulation (ANT-DBS) is thought to be related to the disruption of thalamocortical transmission preventing recruitment and synchronization of extended brain areas as it occurs in bilateral tonic-clonic seizures. Gradual improvement of efficacy over time as observed with all neurostimulation modalities suggests a neuroprotective effect modulating neuronal network excitability through overriding electrical activity.

### Data Availability

VNS has been studied in several randomized controlled trials. In addition, large long-term observational studies and comprehensive meta-analyses are available. Efficacy of ANT-DBS and RNS has been shown in randomized controlled trials as well as in long-term observational studies.

### Surgical Aspects

VNS represents a very-low-risk procedure activating a peripheral nerve. The stimulation probe for ANT-DBS can be placed by burr hole trephination, while implantation of the RNS device requires a larger craniotomy/craniectomy. All procedures for implantation of stimulation devices are well tolerated.

### Patient Selection

In general, all neurostimulation modalities may be considered under various conditions for patients not amenable to resective procedures or in failed resective surgery. RNS is restricted to patients with no more than two seizure foci which have been clearly identified, but cannot be resected, e.g., patients with bitemporal epilepsy, or with seizure a focus/foci in eloquent cortex. Predominant involvement of the frontotemporal limbic areas in seizure activity may favor the use of ANT-DBS. VNS may be considered in multifocal epilepsy or in the presence of extended epileptogenic areas. However, evidence for these considerations is still lacking [190, 572].

### Results

Overall, long-term seizure outcomes of neurostimulation do not show major differences between the approaches available. With VNS, long-term responder rates range between 50% and 60%, and up to 8% of patients become seizure free [3–5, 201, 280–283]. Reliable long-term results of transcutaneous vagal nerve stimulation (tVNS) as well as of responsive vagal nerve stimulation (rVNS) have to be awaited. The SANTE trial for ANT-DBS showed a long-term responder rate of 68% [331, 334, 338, 344], in line with observational studies. The RNS System Pivotal Trial demonstrated a responder rate of 61% which favorably corresponds to observational studies [359, 362, 573]. Seizure-free periods of up to 6 months have been observed in around 20% of patients with ANT-DBS and RNS [248, 359, 362, 363, 573].

### Advantages/Disadvantages

VNS constitutes a unique modality and particularly low-risk procedure, since it activates a peripheral nerve for the treatment of a brain disease. Major cardiac side effects of VNS are extremely rare. Devices available for ANT-DBS and RNS have proven to be safe and are well tolerated. RNS requires exact localization of the seizure focus/foci. Optimization of seizure detection and stimulation patterns based on individual long-term EEG data provided by the RNS system may open the way to a personalized therapy. In addition, chronic EEG data may be used to identify patients who are likely to benefit from other surgical strategies. Even with not satisfying epileptological results, VNS is accepted by most patients as it shows beneficial effects on quality of life (QOL). Beneficial effects on the neurocognitive profile and improvement of QOL have also been shown for RNS. Contrarily, ANT-DBS can negatively influence the neurocognitive profile with respect to memory and depression at least in the short-term assessment.

### 14.3.2 Curative Procedures

Ablative modalities as well as radiosurgery pursue a curative goal. Along with minimal invasiveness they constitute desirable alternative options and promising non-resective tools for patients with lesions, the treatment of which on one hand is linked to favorable seizure outcome, but on the other hand carries significant risks with resective approaches. This is particularly true for patients with hypothalamic hamartomas, periventricular nodular heterotopias, or deep-seated focal cortical dysplasias. Due to the limited volume that can be treated, stereotactic techniques are only suitable for highly selected cases. Data comparing different stereotactic modalities in terms of effectiveness and neuropsychological outcomes on the long run are still lacking.

The efficacy of stereotactic techniques emphasizes that a circumscribed destruction may be sufficient to achieve seizure control, and this raises questions to conceptual considerations regarding the epileptogenic zone. It seems that the general validity of the classical concept of epilepsy surgery according to which the epileptogenic lesion is considered only one part of the epileptogenic zone and the resection volume categorically has to exceed lesion limits may be questioned [377]. This issue is particularly important with respect to the current discussion on the role of neuronal networks for epileptogenesis [3–5, 449, 574] as well as the perspective of minimal volume epilepsy surgery [377].

#### Conceptual Considerations

Radiofrequency thermocoagulation (RFTC) and laser-induced thermal therapy (LITT) aim at the denaturation of tissue proteins by heat (44–59 °C). Heat is generated by electrical current with RFTC and by absorption of interspersed laser light energy with LITT. Stereotactic radiosurgery (SRS) acts by ionizing radiation (20–25 Gy). The Gamma Knife (GK) system as most frequently used in epilepsy is based on gamma radiation generated by Co-60 sources, while the Linear Accelerator (LINAC) emits photon beams.

#### Data Availability

Efficacy of RFTC, LITT, and SRS on seizure control has been assessed by observational studies, some of them including larger numbers of patients. Randomized controlled trials are only available for SRS (U.S. multicenter pilot study [550]; ROSE (**R**adiosurgery or **O**pen **S**urgery for **E**pilepsy) trial comparing Gamma Knife SRS with ATL [551]).

#### Surgical Aspects

The guiding catheter for RFTC and the laser applicator for LITT can be inserted by burr hole trephination. The procedure is well tolerated. SRS does not require any surgical intervention.

#### Patient Selection

RFCT, LITT, and SRS have been used for the treatment of HH, MTLE, FCD, nodular heterotopias, and cavernomas. Although there are no clear indications, RFTC is preferred in patients requiring a SEEG data (SEEG-guided RFTC), e.g., for periventricular nodular heterotopias to determine the respective contribution of the heterotopia and neocortex in the epileptic network. Long-term SEEG data may also be useful to analyze the organization of the epileptogenic zone in order to predict the success of subsequent resective surgery [424]. LITT represents the system with the actually highest growth potential among non-resective curative procedures and has solidified its position, particularly for the treatment of MTLE, for which it may be considered as a minimally invasive alternative to resective surgery. SRS has proven to be effective for the treatment of HH and MTLE. The particular value of SRS lies in the treatment of small epilepsy-associated tumors including metastases pursuing both seizure and tumor control.

#### Results

Larger series demonstrated seizure freedom rates between 50% and 60% with LITT [448, 492, 499] and SRS [550, 552, 553, 555, 561], while seizure-free outcomes with RFTC are somewhat lower accounting for 30–40% [426, 430, 432, 448]. Freedom form gelastic seizures in hypothalamic hamartomas has been reported in between

80% and 90% of cases with different approaches [448, 511, 559, 560]. Overall, curative stereotactic approaches can be expected to become first-line treatment options for selected patients with circumscribed lesions such as hypothalamic hamartomas, periventricular nodular heterotopias, and deep-seated focal cortical dysplasia [424, 430, 453, 475, 476].

### Advantages/Disadvantages

The major advantage of RFTC is that the coagulation electrode can also be used for intraoperative mapping of the pyramidal tract and for SEEG recordings along the defined trajectory. RFTC allows online monitoring of tissue temperature with high accuracy. Although LITT does not allow direct precise monitoring of the temperature, MRgLITT facilitates intraoperative following the coagulation procedure. The size of an ablation created by the LITT probe is larger as compared to radiofrequency ablation. Neuropsychological outcome after LITT and SRS has been found to be superior to resective surgery, which, however, needs long-term confirmation. Due to the use of disposable material for every trajectory, costs of LITT are relatively high. SRS does not require trephination; however, tissue for pathological characterization is not available. With SRS, a latency of response of around 1 year has to be encountered. Dose-dependent MRI changes are observed after SRS suggesting edema or radionecrosis. The use of SRS in the pediatric population poses concerns for the risk of malignant tissue transformation.

## References


1. Chang EF, Englot DJ, Vadera S. Minimally invasive surgical approaches for temporal lobe epilepsy. Epilepsy Behav. 2015;47:24–33. https://doi.org/10.1016/j.yebeh.2015.04.033.
2. Englot DJ, Chang EF. Rates and predictors of seizure freedom in resective epilepsy surgery: an update. Neurosurg Rev. 2014;37:389–404; discussion 404–5. https://doi.org/10.1007/s10143-014-0527-9.
3. Englot DJ, Birk H, Chang EF. Seizure outcomes in nonresective epilepsy surgery: an update. Neurosurg Rev. 2016;40:181–92.
4. Englot DJ, Rolston JD, Wright CW, Hassnain KH, Chang EF. Rates and predictors of seizure freedom with vagus nerve stimulation for intractable epilepsy. Neurosurgery. 2016;79(3):345–53. https://doi.org/10.1227/NEU.0000000000001165.
5. Englot DJ, Konrad PE, Morgan VL. Regional and global connectivity disturbances in focal epilepsy, related neurocognitive sequelae, and potential mechanistic underpinnings. Epilepsia. 2016;57:1546–57.
6. Dandy WE. Operative experiences in cases of pineal tumors. Arch Surg. 1936;33:19–46.
7. Van Wagenen WP, Herren RY. Surgical division of commisural pathways in the corpus callosum: relation to spread of an epileptic attack. Arch Neurol Psychiatry. 1940;44:740–59.
8. Akelaitis AJE. A study of gnosis/praxis and language following section of the corpus callosum and anterior commissure. J Neurosurg. 1944;1:94–102.
9. Goldstein MN, Joynt RJ, Hartley RB. The long-term effects of callosal sectioning. Ann Neurol. 1975;32:52–3.
10. Sperry RW. Cerebral organization and behavior. Science. 1961;133:1749–57.
11. Blume WT. Corpus callosum section for seizure control: rational and review of experimental and clinical data. Cleve Clin Q. 1984;51:319–22.
12. Blume WT. Corrpus callosotomy: a critical review. In: Tuxhorn I, Holthausen H, Boenigk H, editors. Paediatric epilepsy syndromes and their surgical treatment. London: John Libbey; 1997. p. 815–29.
13. Bancaud J, Talairach J, Bonis A, Schaub D, Szikla G, Morel P, Bordas-Ferer M. La stereo-encephalographie dans lépilepsie. Paris: Masson; 1965.
14. Goldring S. The role of prefrontal cortex in grand mal convulsion. Arch Neurol. 1972;26:109–19.
15. Collins RC, Kennedy C, Sokoloff L, Plum F. Metabolic anatomy of focal motor seizures. Arch Neurol. 1976;33:536–42.
16. Engel J, Wolfson L, Brown L. Anatomical correlates of electrical and behavioral events related to amygdaloid kindling. Ann Neurol. 1978;3:538–44.
17. Fischer RS, Prince DA. Spike-wave rhythms in cat cortex induced by parenteral penicillin. Electroencephalographic features. Electroencephalogr Clin Neurophysiol. 1977;42:608–24.
18. Gloor P, Avoli M, Kostopoulos G. Thalamocortical relationships in generalized epilepsy with bilaterally synchronous spike-and-wave discharge. In: Avoli M, Gloor P, Kostopoulos G, Naquet R, editors. Generalized epilepsy, neurobiological approaches. Boston, MA: Birkhauser; 1990. p. 190–212.
19. Schwarzkroin PA, Mutani R, Prince DA. Orthodromic and antidromic effects of a cortical epileptoform focus on ventro-lateral nucleus of the cat. J Neurophysiol. 1975;38:795–811.
20. Aicardi J, Chevri JJ. Myoclonic epilepsies of childhood. Neuropaediatrie. 1971;3:177–90.
21. Blume WT, David RB, Gomez MR. Generalized sharp and slow wave complexes. Associated clinical features and long-term follow-up. Brain. 1973;96:289–306.

22. Gastaut H, Roger J, Soulayrol CA, Tassinari CA, Dravet C. Childhood epileptic encephalopathy with diffuse slow spike-waves (otherwise known as petit mal variant) or Lennox syndrome. Epilepsia. 1966;7:139–79.
23. Gloor P, Quesney LF, Zumstein H. Pathophysiology of generalized penicillin epilepsy in the cat: the role of cortical and subcortical structures. II. Topical application of penicillin to the cerebral cortex and to subcortical structures. Electroencephalogr Clin Neurophysiol. 1977;43:73–94.
24. Markand ON. Slow spike-wave activity in EEG and associated clinical features: often called Lennox or Lennox-Gastaut syndrome. Neurology. 1977;27:746–57.
25. Curtis HJ, Bard P. Intercortical connexions of the corpus callosum as indicated by evoked potentials. Am J Physiol. 1939;126:473.
26. Erickson TC. Spread of the epileptic discharge. An experimental study of the afterdischarge induced by electrical stimulation of cerebral cortex. Arch Neurol Psychiat. 1940;43:429–5.
27. Kopeleff N, Kennard MA, Pacella BL, Kopeleff LM, Chusid JG. Section of corpus callosum in experimental epilepsy in the monkey. Arch Neurol Psychiatry. 1950;63:719–27.
28. Marcus EM, Watson CW. Symmetrical epileptogenic foci in monkey cerebral cortex: mechanisms of interactions and regional variations in capacity for synchronous discharges. Arch Neurol. 1968;19:99–116.
29. Musgrave J, Gloor P. The role of corpus callosum in bilateral interhemispheric synchrony of spike and wave discharge in feline generalized penicillin epilepsy. Epilepsia. 1980;21:369–78.
30. Crowell RM, Marsan C. Topographical distribution and patterns of unit activity during electrically induced after-discharge. Electroencephalogr Clin Neurophysiol. 1972;31:59–73.
31. Schwarzkroin PA, Futamach KJ, Noebbels IL, Prince DA. Transcallosal effects of a cortical epileptiform focus. Brain Res. 1975;99:59–68.
32. Spencer SS, Spencer DD, Glaser GH. More intensive focal seizure types after callosal section: the role of inhibition. Ann Neurol. 1984;16:686–93.
33. Spiegel E. The central mechanism of generalized epileptic fits. Am J Psychiatry. 1931;88:595–609.
34. Spencer SS, Spencer DD, Sass KJ, Novelly RA, Williamson PD, Mattson RH. Partial vs. total callosotomy for epilepsy. Adv Epileptol. 1987;16:323–5.
35. Spencer SS, Gates JR, Reeves AG, Spencer DD, Maxwell RE, Roberts D. Corpus callosum section. In: Engel J, editor. Surgical treatment of the epilepsies. New York: Raven Press; 1987. p. 425–44.
36. Kusske JA, Rush JL. Corpus callosum and propagation of afterdischarge to contralateral cortex and thalamus. Neurology. 1978;28:905–12.
37. Ottino CA, Meglio M, Rossi GF, Tercero E. An experimental study of the structure mediating bilateral synchrony of epileptic discharges of cortical origin. Epilepsia. 1971;12:299–311.
38. Stavkry GW. Supersensitivity following lesions of the nervous system. Toronto: University of Toronto Press; 1961. p. 33–8.
39. Wada JA, Komai S. Effect of anterior two-thirds callosal bisection upon bisymmetrical and bisynchronous generalized convulsions kindled from amygdala in epileptic baboon. In: Reeves AG, editor. Epilepsy and the corpus callosum. New York: Plenum Press; 1985. p. 75–97.
40. Bogen J. Cerebral commissurotomy. A second case report. JAMA. 1965;194:1328–9.
41. Bogen J, Vogel PJ. Cerebral commisurotomy in man: preliminary case report. Bull Los Angeles Neurol Soc. 1962;27:139–72.
42. Bogen JE, Sperry RW, Vogel PJ. Commisural section and propagation of seizures. In: Jasper HH, Ward AA, Pope A, editors. Basic mechanisms or the epilepsies. Boston, MA: Little Brown; 1969. p. 439–40.
43. Wilson DH, Culver C, Waddington M, Gazzaniga M. Disconnection of the cerebral hemisphere. An alternative to hemispherectomy for the control of intractable seizures. Neurology. 1975;25:1149–53.
44. Wilson DH, Reeves A, Gazzaniga M, Culver C. Cerebral commissurotomy for control of intractable seizures. Neurology. 1977;27:708–15.
45. Wilson DH, Reeves A, Gazzaniga M. Division of the corpus callosum for uncontrollable epilepsy. Neurology. 1978;28:649–53.
46. Wilson DH, Reeves A, Gazzaniga M. "Central" commissurotomy for intractable generalized epilepsy: series two. Neurology. 1982;32:687–97.
47. Luessenhop AJ, dela Cruz TC, Fenichel GM. Surgical disconnection of the cerebral hemispheres for intractable seizures: results in infancy and childhood. JAMA. 1970;213:1630–6.
48. Reeves AG. Epilepsy and the corpus callosum. New York: Plenum Press; 1985.
49. Reeves AG, Roberts DW. Epilepsy and the corpus callosum. 2nd ed. New York: Plenum Press; 1995.
50. Gates JR. Corpus callosum candidacy. In: Lüders H, editor. Epilepsy surgery. New York: Raven Press; 1992. p. 119–25.
51. Purves SJ, Wada JA, Woodhurst WB. Corpus callosum section for complex partial seizures. In: Reeves AG, Roberts DW, editors. Epilepsy and the corpus callosum. 2nd ed. New York: Plenum Press; 1995. p. 175–82.
52. Engel J. Outcome with respect to epileptic seizures. In: Engel J, editor. Surgical treatment of the epilepsies. New York: Raven Press; 1987. p. 553–71.
53. Apuzzo MLJ. Surgery of the third ventricle. Baltimore, MD: Williams & Wilkins; 1987.
54. Apuzzo MLJ, Chikovani OK, Gott PS. Transcallosal, interfornical approaches for lesions affecting the third ventricle: surgical considerations and consequences. Neurosurgery. 1982;10:547–54.
55. Bogen JE. Some historical aspects of callosotomy for epilepsy. In: Reeves G, Roberts DW, editors. Epilepsy and the corpus callosum. 2nd ed. New York: Plenum Press; 1995. p. 107–21.

56. Reutens DC, Bye AM, Hopkins IL, Danks A, Sommerville E, Walsh J, Bleasel A, Ouvrier R, MacKenzie RA, Manson JL, Bladin PF, Berkovic SF. Corpus callosotomy for intractable epilepsy: seizure outcome and prognostic factors. Epilepsia. 1993;34:904–9.
57. Wyler AR. Corpus callosotomy. In: Wyllie E, editor. The treatment of epilepsy: principles and practice. 2nd ed. Baltimore, MD: Williams & Wilkins; 1997. p. 1097–102.
58. Fuiks KW, Wyler AR, Hermann BP, Sorres G. Seizure outcome from anterior and complete corpus callosotomy. J Neurosurg. 1991;74:573–8.
59. Gates JR, Maxwell R, Leppik IE, Gumnit RJ. Electroencephalographic and clinical effects of total corpus callosotomy. In: Reeves AG, editor. Epilepsia and the corpus callosum. New York: Plenum Press; 1985. p. 315–28.
60. Geoffroy G, Lassonde M, Delisle F, Decarie M. Corpus callosotomy for control of intractable epilepsy in children. Neurology. 1983;33:891–7.
61. Girvin JP. Operative techniques in epilepsy. Cham: Springer; 2015.
62. Kim DS, Yang KH, Kim TG, Chang JH, Chang JW, Choi JU, Lee BI. The surgical effect of callosotomy in the treatment of intractable seizures. Yonsei Med J. 2004;45:233–40.
63. Liang S, Li A, Jiang H, Meng X, Zhao M, Zhang J, Sun Y. Anterior corpus callosotomy in patients with intractable generaliszed epilepsy and mental retardation. Stereotact Funct Neurosurg. 2010;88:246–52.
64. Purves SJ, Wada JA, Woodhurst WB, Moyes PD, Strauss E, Kosaka B, Li D. Results of anterior corpus callosum section in 24 patients with medically intractable seizures. Neurology. 1988;38:1194–201.
65. Spencer SS, Spencer DD, Williamson PD, Sass K, Novelly RA, Mattson RH. Corpus callosotomy for epilepsy. I. Seizure effects. Neurology. 1988;38:19–24.
66. Roberts DW, Reeves AG, Nordgren RE. The role of posterior callosotomy in patients with suboptimal response to anterior callosotomy. In: Reeves AG, Roberts DW, editors. Epilepsy and the corpus callosum. 2nd ed. New York: Plenum Press; 1995. p. 183–90.
67. Madsen JR, Carmant L, Holmes GL, Black PM. Corpus callosotomy in children. Neurosurg Clin N Am. 1995;6(3):541–8.
68. Oguni H, Olivier A, Andermann F, Comair J. Anterior callosotomy in the treatment of medically intractable epilepsies: a study of 43 patients with a mean follow-up of 39 months. Ann Neurol. 1991;30(3):357–64.
69. Williamson PD. Corpus callosum section for intractable epilepsy. In: Reeves AG, editor. Epilepsy and the corpus callosum. New York: Plenum Press; 1985. p. 243–57.
70. Cukiert A, Burattini JA, Mariani PP, Câmara RB, Seda L, Baldauf CM, Argentoni M, Baise-Zung C, Forster CR, Mello VA. Extended, one-stage callosal section for treatment of refractory secondarily generalized epilepsy in patients with Lennox-Gastaut and Lennox-like syndromes. Epilepsia. 2006;47:371–4.
71. Cukiert A, Burattini JA, Mariani PP, Cukiert CM, Sárgentoni-Baldochi M, Baise-Zung C, Fortser CR, Mello VA. Outcome after extended callosal section in patients with primary idiopathic generalized epilepsy. Epilepsia. 2009;50(6):1377–80.
72. Gates JR, Leppik IE, Yap J, Gumnit RJ. Corpus callosotomy: clinical end electroencephalographic effects. Epilepsia. 1984;25:308–16.
73. Gates JR, Mireles R, Maxwell R, Sharbrough F, Forbes G. Nuclear magnetic resonance scan documentation of the extent of callosotomy. Epilepsia. 1984;25:650–1.
74. Hanson RR, Risinger M, Maxwell R. The ictal EEG as a predictive factor for outcome following corpus callosum section in adults. Epilepsy Res. 2002;49:89–97.
75. Maehara T, Shimizu H. Surgical outcome of corpus callosotomy in patients with drop attacks. Epilepsia. 2001;42:67–71.
76. Maehara T, Shimizu H, Oda M, Arai N. Surgical treatment of children with intractable epilepsy. Neurol Med Chir (Tokyo). 1996;36:306–9.
77. Mamelak AN, Barbaro NM, Walker JA, Laxer KD. Corpus callosotomy a quantitative study of extent of resection, seizure control, and neuropsychological outcome. J Neurosurg. 1993;79:688–95.
78. Sunaga S, Shimizu H, Sugano H. Long-term follow-up of seizure outcomes after corpus callosotomy. Seizure. 2009;18:124–8.
79. Tanriverdi T, Olivier A, Poulin N, Andermann F, Dubeau F. Long-term seizure outcome after corpus callosotomy: a retrospective analysis of 95 patients. J Neurosurg. 2009;110:332–42.
80. Jenssen S, Sperling MR, Tracy JI, Nei M, Joyce L, David G, O'Connor M. Corpus callosotomy in refractory idiopathic generalized epilepsy. Seizure. 2006;15:621–9.
81. Kwan SY, Lin JH, Wong TT, Chang KP, Yiu CH. A comparison of seizure outcome after callosotomy in patients with Lennox-Gastaut syndrome and positive or negative history of West syndrome. Seizure. 2006;15:552–7.
82. Pinard JM, Delalande O, Chiron C, Soufflet C, Plouin P, Kim Y, Dulac O. Callosotomy for epilepsy after West syndrome. Epilepsia. 1999;40:1727–34.
83. Wheless JW. Managing severe epilepsy syndromes of early childhood. J Child Neurol. 2009;24:24S–32S.
84. Gates JR, Rosenfeld WE, Maxwell RE. Response of multiple seizure types to corpus callosum section. Epilepsia. 1987;28:28–34.
85. Gates JR, Rosenfield WE, Maxwell RE, et al. Response of multiple seizure types to corpus callosum section. Epilepsia. 1987;28:28–38.
86. Sass KJ, Novelly RA, Spencer DD, Spencer SS. Postcallosotomy language impairments in patients with crossed cerebral dominance. J Neurosurg. 1990;72:85–90.

87. Englot DJ. A modern epilepsy surgery treatment algorithm: Incorporating traditional and emerging technologies. Epilepsy Behav. 2018;80:68–74.
88. Maxwell RE, Gates JR, Gumnit RJ. Corpus callosotomy at the University of Minnesota. In: Engel Jr J, editor. Surgical treatment of epilepsies. New York: Raven Press; 1986. p. 659–66.
89. Risse GL. Interhemispheric transfer in patients with incomplete section of the corpus callosum. Arch Neurol. 1989;46:437–43.
90. Roberts DW, Rayport M, Maxwell RE, Olivier A, Marino R. Corpus callosotomy. In: Engel J, editor. Surgical treatment of the epilepsies. New York: Raven Press; 1993. p. 519–26.
91. Villemure JG, Vernet O, Delalande O. Hemispheric disconnection: callsosotomy and hemispherectomy. Adv Tech Stand Neurosurg. 2000;26:25–78.
92. Yasargil MG. Microneurosurgery. Stuttgart, NY: Thieme; 1994.
93. Lang J, Ederer M. Über Form und Größe des Corpus Callosum und des Septum Pellucidum. Morph Jb (Leipzig). 1980;126:949–58.
94. Zentner J. Surgical aspects of corpus callosum section. In: Tuxhorn I, Holthausen H, Boenigk H, editors. Paediatric epilepsy syndromes and their surgical treatment. London: John Libbey; 1997. p. 830–49.
95. Seeger W, Zentner J. Neuronaviagation and neuroanatomy. Wien: Springer; 2002. p. 172–3.
96. Wyler AR. Corpus callosotomy in the treatment of epilepsy. Contemp Neurosurg. 1990;12:1–5.
97. Sood S, Marupudi NI, Asano E, Haridas A, Ham SD. Endoscopic corpus callosotomy and hemispherotomy. J Neurosurg Pediatr. 2015;16(6):681–6.
98. Luat AF, Asano E, Kumar A, et al. Corpus callosotomy for intractable epilepsy revisited: the Children's Hospital of Michigan Series. J Child Neurol. 2017;32(7):624–9.
99. Smyth MD, Vellimana AK, Asano E, et al. Corpus callosotomy—open and endoscopic surgical techniques. Epilepsia. 2017;58:73–9.
100. Avila JO, Radvany J, Huck FR, Pires de Camargo CH, Marino R, Ragazzo PC, Riva D. Anterior callosotomy as a substitute for hemispherectomy. Acta Neurochir. 1980;30:137–43.
101. Huck FR, Radvany J, Avila JO, Pires de Camargo CH, Marino R, Ragazzo PC, Riva D, Arlant P. Anterior callosotomy in epileptics with multiform seizures and bilateral synchronous spike and wave EEG pattern. Acta Neurochir. 1980;30:127–35.
102. Marino R, Ragazzo PC. Selection criteria and results of selective partial callosotomy. In: Reeves AG, editor. Epilepsy and the corpus callosum. New York: Plenum Press; 1985. p. 281–301.
103. Marino R, Radvany J, Huck F, de Camargo CHP, Gronich G. Selective EEG-guided microsurgical callosotomy for refractory generalized epilepsy. Surg Neurol. 1990;34:219–28.
104. Widjaja E, Zarei Mahmoodabadi S, Otsubo H, Snead OC, Holowka S, Bells S, Raybaud C. Subcortical alterations in tissue microstructure adjacent to focal cortical dysplasia: detection at diffusion-tensor MR imaging by using magnetoencephalographic dipole cluster localization. Radiology. 2009;251:206–15.
105. Raffelt D, Tournier JD, Rose S, et al. Apparent fibre density: a novel measure for the analysis of diffusion-weighted magnetic resonance images. Neuroimage. 2012;59(4):3976–94.
106. Bodaghabadi M, Bitaraf MA, Aran S, Alikhani M, Ashrafian H, Zahiri A, Alahverdi M. Corpus callosotomy with gamma knife radiosurgery for a case of intractable generalised epilepsy. Epileptic Disord. 2011;13:202–8.
107. Eder HG, Feichtinger M, Pieper T, Kurschel S, Schroettener O. Gamma knife radiosurgery for callosotomy in children with drug-resistant epilepsy. Childs Nerv Syst. 2006;22:1012–7.
108. Feichtinger M, Schröttner O, Eder H, Holthausen H, Pieper T, Unger F, Holl A, Gruber L, Körner E, Trinka E, Fazekas F, Ott E. Efficacy and safety of radiosurgical callosotomy: a retrospective analysis. Epilepsia. 2006;47:1184–91.
109. Pendl G, Eder HG, Schroettner O, Leber KA. Corpus callosotomy with radiosurgery. Neurosurgery. 1999;45(2):303–7.
110. Smyth MD, Klein EE, Dodson WE, Mansur DB. Radiosurgical posterior corpus callosotomy in a child with Lennox-Gastaut syndrome. Case report. J Neurosurg. 2007;106(4 Suppl):312–5.
111. McGonigal A, Sahgal A, De Salles A, et al. Radiosurgery for epilepsy: systematic review and International Stereotactic Radiosurgery Society (ISRS) practice guideline. Epilepsy Res. 2017;137:123–31.
112. Moreno-Jimenez S, San-Juan D, Larraga-Gutierrez JM, Celis MA, Alonso-Vanegas MA, Anschel DJ. Diffusion tensor imaging in radiosurgical callosotomy. Seizure. 2012;21:473–7.
113. Marino R, Gronich G. Corpus callosum stimulation and stereotactic callosotomy in the management of refractory generalized seizures. Arq Neuro-Psiquiat (Sao Paulo). 1989;47:320–5.
114. Marino R, Cukiert A, Gronich G. Open and stereotactic segmental callosotomy: effects on seizure frequency. In: Reeves AG, Roberts DW, editors. Epilepsy and the corpus callosum. 2nd ed. New York: Plenum Press; 1995. p. 209–15.
115. Ball T, Sharma M, White A, et al. Anterior corpus callosotomy using laser interstitial thermal therapy for refractory epilepsy. Stereotact Funct Neurosurg. 2019; https://doi.org/10.1159/000495414.
116. Ho AL, Miller KJ, Cartmell S, Inoyama K, Fisher RS, Halpern CH. Stereotactic laser ablation of the splenium for intractable epilepsy. Epilepsy Behav Case Rep. 2016;5:23–6.
117. Karsy M, Patel DM, Halvorson K, Mortimer V, Bollo RJ. Anterior two-thirds corpus callosotomy via stereotactic laser ablation. Neurosurg Focus. 2018;44(Video Suppl 2):V2.
118. Pruitt R, Gamble A, Black K, Schulder M, Mehta AD. Complication avoidance in laser interstitial thermal therapy: lessons learned. J Neurosurg. 2017;126(4):1238–45.

119. Tao JX, Satzer D, Issa NP, et al. Stereotactic laser anterior corpus callosotomy for Lennox-Gastaut syndrome. Epilepsia. 2020; https://doi.org/10.1111/epi.16535.
120. Jea A, Vachhrajani S, Johnson KK, Rutka JT. Corpus callosotomy in children with intractable epilepsy using frameless stereotactic neuronavigation: 12-year experience et the Hospital for sick children in Toronto. Neurosurg Focus. 2008;25:E7.
121. Jea A, Vachhrajani S, Widjaja E, Nilsson D, Raybaud C, Shroff M, Rutka JT. Corpus callosotomy in children and the disconnection syndromes: a review. Childs Nerv Syst. 2008;24:685–92.
122. Téllez-Zenteno JF, Dhar R, Wiebe S. Long-term seizure outcomes following epilepsy surgery: a systematic review and meta-analysis. Brain. 2005;128:1188–98. https://doi.org/10.1093/brain/awh449.
123. Turanli G, Yalnizoglu D, Genc-Acikgoz D, Akalan N, Topcu M. Outcome and longterm follow-up after corpus callosotomy in childhood onset intractable epilepsy. Childs Nerv Syst. 2006;22:1322–7.
124. Berg AT, Vickrey BG. Outcome measures. In: Engel J, Pedley TA, editors. Epilepsy: a comprehensive textbook. Philadelphia: Lippincott-Raven Publishers; 1998. p. 1891–9.
125. Shimizu H. Our experience with pediatric epilepsy surgery focusing on corpus callosotomy and hemispherectomy. Epilepsia. 2005;46(Suppl. 1):30–1.
126. Fauser S, Zentner J. Critical review of palliative surgical techniques for intractable epilepsy. In: Advances and technical standards in neurosurgery. Wien: Springer; 2013.
127. Cendes F, Ragazzo PC, da Costa V, Martins LF. Corpus callosotomy in treatment of medically resistant epilepsy: preliminary results in a pediatric population. Epilepsia. 1993;34(5):910–7.
128. Gilliam F, Wyllie E. Functional outcome of children following corpus callosum section. In: Tuxhorn I, Holthausen H, Boenigk H, editors. Paediatric epilepsy syndromes and their surgical treatment. London: John Libbey; 1997. p. 850–3.
129. Passamonti C, Zamponi N, Foschi N, Trignani R, Luzi M, Cesaroni E, Provinciali L, Scerrati M. Long-term seizure and behavioral outcomes after corpus callosotomy. Epilepsy Behav. 2014;41:23–9. https://doi.org/10.1016/j.yebeh.2014.08.130.
130. Graham D, Tisdall MM, Gill D. Corpus callosotomy outcomes in pediatric patients: a systematic review. Epilepsia. 2016;57(7):1053–68.
131. Jalilian L, Limbrick DD, Steger-May K, Johnston J, Powers AK, Smyth MD. Complete versus anterior two-third corpus callosotomy in children. Analysis of outcome. J Neurosurg Pediatr. 2010;6:257–66.
132. Rahimi SY, Park YD, Witcher MR, Lee KH, Marrufo M, Lee MR. Corpus callosotomy for treatment of pediatric epilepsy in the modern era. Pediatr Neurosurg. 2007;43:202–8.
133. Wong TT, Kwan SY, Chang KP, Hsiu-Mei W, Yang TF, Chen YS, Yi-Yen L. Corpus callosotomy in children. Childs Nerv Syst. 2006;22:999–1011.
134. Rathore C, Abraham M, Rao RM, George A, Sankara Sarma P, Radhakrishnan K. Outcome after corpus callosotomy in children with injurious drop attacks and severe mental retardation. Brain Dev. 2007;29:577–85.
135. Asadi-Pooya AA, Sharan A, Nei M, Sperling MR. Corpus callosotomy. Epilepsy Behav. 2008;13:271–8.
136. Ross MK, Reeves AG, Roberts DW. Post-commissurotomy mutism. Ann Neurol. 1984;16:114.
137. Provinciali L, Quattrini A, Papo I, del Pesce M, Mancini S. Neuropsychological changes after callosotomy in drug-resistant epilepsy: a study of the short-term evaluation. Acta Neurochir. 1988;94:15–22.
138. Roberts DW. Corpus callosotomy. In: Reeves AG, editor. Epilepsy and the corpus callosum. New York: Plenum Press; 1985. p. 259–67.
139. Pilcher WH, Ojemann GA. Complications of epilepsy surgery. In: Post KD, Friedman E, McCormick P, editors. Postoperative complications in intracranial neurosurgery. Stuttgart: Thieme; 1993. p. 157–65.
140. Ferguson SM, Rayport M, Corrie WS. Neuropsychiatric observations on behavioral consequences of corpus callosum section for seizure control. In: Reeves AR, editor. Epilepsy and the corpus callosum. New York: Plenum Press; 1985. p. 501–14.
141. Levin HS, Mattson AJ, Levander M, et al. Effects of transcallosal surgery on interhemispheric transfer of information. Surg Neurol. 1993;40:65–74.
142. Makari G, Holmes G, Murro A. Corpus callosotomy for the treatment of intractable epilepsy in children. J Epilepsy. 1989;2:1–7.
143. Bogen JE. Physiological consequences of complete and partial commissural section. In: Apuzzo MLJ, editor. Surgery of the third ventricle. Baltimore, MD: Williams & Wilkins; 1987. p. 175–94.
144. Gordon HW, Bogen JE, Sperry RW. Absence of deconnexion syndrome in two patients with partial section of the neocommissures. Brain. 1971;94:327–36.
145. Jeeves MA, Simpson DA, Geffen G. Functional consequences of the transcallosal removal of intraventricular tumours. J Neurol Neurosurg Psychiat. 1979;42:134–42.
146. Shucart WA, Stein BM. Transcallosal approach to the anterior ventricular system. Neurosurgery. 1978;3:339–43.
147. Winston KR, Cavazzuti V, Arkins T. Absence of neurological and behavioral abnormalities after anterior transcallosal operation for third ventricle lesions. Neurosurgery. 1979;4:386–93.
148. Reeves AG, Risse G. Neurological effects of callosotomy. In: Reeves AG, Roberts DW, editors. Epilepsy and the corpus callosoum 2. Advances in behavioral biology, vol. 45. New York: Plenum; 1995. p. 241–51.
149. Nakasu Y, Isozumi T, Nioka H, Handa J. Mechanism of mutism following transcallosal approach to the ventricles. Acta Neurochir. 1991;110:146–53.

150. Spencer SS. Corpus callosum section and other disconnection procedures for medically intractable epilepsy. Epilepsia. 1988;29:85–99.
151. Sass KJ, Spencer DD, Spencer SS, Novelly RA, Williamson PD, Mattson RH. Corpus callosotomy for epilepsy. II. Neurological and neuropsychological outcome. Neurology. 1988;38:24–8.
152. Geschwind DH, Jacobini M, Mega MS, Zaidel DW, Cloughesy T, Zaidel E. Alien hand syndrome: interhemispheric motor disconnection due to a lesion in the midbody of the corpus callosum. Neurology. 1995;45:802–8.
153. Campbell A, Bogen J, Smith A. Disorganization and reorganization of cognitive and sensorimotor functions in cerebral commissurotomy. Brain. 1981;104:493–511.
154. Sass KJ, Novelly R, Spencer DD, Spencer SS. Mnestic and attention impairments following corpus callosum section for epilepsy. J Epilepsy. 1988;1:61–6.
155. Morrell F, Whisler WW, Bleck TP. Multiple subpial transection. A new approach to the surgical treatment of focal epilepsy. J Neurosurg. 1989;70:231–9.
156. Mountcastle VB. The columnar organization of the neocortex. Brain. 1997;120:701–22.
157. Mountcastle VB. Modality and topographic properties of single neurons of cat's somatic cortex. J Neurophysiol. 1957;20:408–34.
158. Chervin RD, Pierce PA, Connors BW. Periodicity and directionality in the propagation of epileptiform discharces across neocortex. J Neurophysiol. 1988;60:1695–713.
159. Wadman WJ, Gutnick MJ. Non-uniform propagation of epileptiform discharge in brain slices of rat neocortex. Neurosience. 1993;52:255–62.
160. Lueders H, Bustamante LA, Zablow L, Goldensohn ES. The independence of closely spaced discrete experimental spike foci. Neurology. 1981;31:846–51.
161. Reichenthal E, Hocherman S. The critical cortical area for development of penicillin-induced epilepsy. Electrencephalogr Clin Neurophysiol. 1977;42:248–51.
162. Buelow JM, Aydelott P, Pierz DM, Heck B. Multiple subpial transection for Landau-Kleffner syndrome. AORN J. 1996;63:727–44.
163. Grote CL, Van Slyke P, Hoeppner JA. Language outcome following multiple subpial transections for Landau-Kleffner syndrome. Brain. 1999;122:561–6.
164. Morrell F, Whisler WW, Smith MC, Hoeppner TJ, de Toledo-Morrell L, Pierre-Louis SJ, Kanner AM, Buelow JM, Ristanovic R, Bergen D, et al. Landau-Kleffner syndrome. Treatment with subpial intracortical transection. Brain. 1995;118:1529–46.
165. Blount JP, Langburt W, Otsubo H, Chitoku S, Ochi A, Weiss S, Snead OC, Rutka JT. Multiple subpial transections in the treatment of pediatric epilepsy. J Neurosurg. 2004;100:118–24. https://doi.org/10.3171/ped.2004.100.2.0118.
166. Shimizu H, Maehara T. Neuronal disconnection for the surgical treatment of pediatric epilepsy. Epilepsia. 2000;41(Suppl 9):28–30.
167. Ntsambi-Eba G, Vaz G, Docquier MA, van Rijckevorsel K, Raftopoulos C. Patients with refractory epilepsy treated using a modified multiple subpial transection technique. Neurosurgery. 2013;72:890–7; discussion 897–8. https://doi.org/10.1227/NEU.0b013e31828ba750.
168. Patil AA, Andrews R. Long term follow-up after multiple hippocampal transection (MHT). Seizure J Br Epilepsy Assoc. 2013;22:731–4. https://doi.org/10.1016/j.seizure.2013.05.014.
169. Polkey CE. Multiple subpial transection: a clinical assessment. Int Rev Neurobiol. 2001;45:547–69.
170. Rolston JD, Deng H, Wang DD, Englot DJ, Chang EF. Multiple subpial transections for medically refractory epilepsy: a disaggregated review of patient-level data. Neurosurgery. 2017;82(5):613–20.
171. Schramm J, Aliashkevich AF, Grunwald T. Multiple subpial transections: outcome and complications in 20 patients who did not undergo resection. J Neurosurg. 2002;97:39–47.
172. Hufnagel A, Zentner J, Fernandez G, Wolf HK, Schramm J, Elger CE. Multiple subpial transection for control of epilleptic seizures: effectiveness and safety. Epilepsia. 1997;38:678–88.
173. Benifla M, Otsubo H, Ochi A, Snead OC 3rd, Rutka JT. Multiple subpial transection in pediatric epilepsy: indications and outcomes. Childs Nerv Syst. 2006;22:992–8.
174. Benifla M, Rutka JT, Logan W, Donner EJ. Vagal nerve stimulation for refractory epilepsy in children: indications and experience at the Hospital for Sick children. Childs Nerv Syst. 2006;22:1018–26.
175. Behdad A, Limbrick DD, Bertrand M, et al. Epilepsy surgery in children with seizures arising from the rolandic cortex. Epilepsia. 2009;50(6):1450–61.
176. Spencer SS, Schramm J, Wyler A, O'Connor M, Orbach D, Krauss G, Sperling M, Devinsky O, Elger C, Lesser R, Mulligan L, Westerveld M. Multiple subpial transection for intractable partial epilepsy: an international meta-analysis. Epilepsia. 2002;43:141–5.
177. Orbach D, Romanelli P, Devinsky O, Doyle W. Late seizure recurrence after multiple subpial transections. Epilepsia. 2001;42(9):1130–3.
178. Irwin K, Birch V, Lees J, Polkey C, Alarcon G, Binnie C, Smedley M, Baird G, Robinson RO. Multiple subpial transections in Landau-Kleffner syndrome. Dev Med Child Neurol. 2001;43:248–52.
179. Cross JH, Neville BG. The surgical treatment of Landau-Kleffner syndrome. Epilepsia. 2009;50(Suppl 7):63–7.
180. Downes M, Greenaway R, Clark M, Helen Cross J, Jolleff N, Harkness W, Kaliakatsos M, Boyd S, White S, Neville BG. Outcome following multiple subpial transection in Landau-Kleffner syndrome and related regression. Epilepsia. 2015;56(11):1760–6. https://doi.org/10.1111/epi.13132.
181. Gaylor JM, Raman G, Chung M, et al. Cochlear implantation in adults. A systematic review and meta-analysis. JAMA Otolaryngol Head Neck Surg. 2013;139(3):265–72.

182. North RB, et al. Spinal cord stimulation versus re-operation in patients with failed back surgery syndrome: an international multicenter randomised controlled trial (EVIDENCE Study). Neuromodulation. 2011;14:330–6.
183. Weaver FM, Follett K, Stern M, et al. Bilateral deep brain stimulation vs best medical therapy for patients with advanced Parkinson disease: a randomized controlled trial. JAMA. 2009;301(1):63–73.
184. Richardson RM, Abel TJ. A new era for surgical neurotherapeutics. Neurotherapeutics. 2019;16(1):1–2. https://doi.org/10.1007/s13311-019-00709-4.
185. Hartshorn A, Jobst B. Responsive brain stimulation in epilepsy. Ther Adv Chronic Dis. 2018;9(7):135–42.
186. McGovern RA, Banks GP, McKhann GM II. New techniques and progress in epilepsy surgery. Curr Neurol Neurosci Rep. 2016; https://doi.org/10.1007/s11910-016-0661-6.
187. Kwon C-S, Jetté N, Ghatan S. Perspectives on the current developments with neuromodulation for the treatment of epilepsy. Expert Rev Neurother. 2019; https://doi.org/10.1080/14737175.2020.1700795.
188. Kwaku K, Ohemeng BS, Parham K. Vagal nerve stimulation. Indications, implantation, and outcomes. Otolaryngol Clin N Am. 2020;53:127–43.
189. Bigelow MD, Kouzani AZ. Neural stimulation systems for the control of refractory epilepsy: a review. J Neuroeng Rehabil. 2019;16:126. https://doi.org/10.1186/s12984-019-0605-x.
190. Schulze-Bonhage A. Long-term outcome in neurostimulation of epilepsy. Epilepsy Behav. 2019;91:25–9.
191. Bailey P, Bremer F. A sensory cortical representation of the vagus nerve: with a note on the effects of low blood pressure on the cortical electrogram. J Neurophysiol. 1938;1(5):405–12.
192. Dell P, Olson R. Projections thalamiques, corticales et ce´re´belleuses des affe´rences visce´ rales vagales. Comptes rendus des se´ances de la Socie´te´ de biologie et de ses filiales. 1951;145(13-1):1084–8.
193. Zabara J. Inhibition of experimental seizures in canines by repetitive vagal stimulation. Epilepsia. 1992;33(6):1005–12.
194. Terry RS, Tarver WB, Zabara J. The implantable neurocybernetic prosthesis system. Pacing Clin Electrophysiol. 1991;14(1):86–93.
195. Penry JK, Dean C. Prevention of intractable seizures by intermittent vagal stimulation in humans: preliminary results. Epilepsia. 1990;31(Suppl 2):S40–3.
196. Browne G. Cyberonics announces 100,000th patient implant of VNS therapy. 2012.
197. Rychlicki F, Zamponi N, Cesaroni E, Corpaci L, Trignani R, Ducati A, et al. Complications of vagal nerve stimulation for epilepsy in children. Neurosurg Rev. 2006;29:103–7.
198. Ben-Menachem E. Vagus nerve stimulation for the treatment of epilepsy. Lancet Neurol. 2002;1(8):477–82.
199. Ben-Menachem E, Manon-Espaillat R, Ristanovic R, Wilder BJ, Stefan H, Mirza W, Tarver WB, Wernicke JF. Vagus nerve stimulation for treatment of partial seizures: 1. A controlled study of effect on seizures. First International Vagus Nerve Stimulation Study Group. Epilepsia. 1994;35:616–26.
200. Handforth A, DeGiorgio CM, Schachter SC, Uthman BM, Naritoku DK, Tecoma ES, Henry TR, Collins SD, Vaughn BV, Gilmartin RC, Labar DR, Morris GL 3rd, Salinsky MC, Osorio I, Ristanovic RK, Labiner DM, Jones JC, Murphy JV, Ney GC, Wheless JW. Vagus nerve stimulation therapy for partial-onset seizures: a randomized active-control trial. Neurology. 1998;51:48–55.
201. Morris GL, Mueller MW. Long-term treatment with vagus nerve stimulation in patients with refractory epilepsy. The vagus nerve stimulation study group E01-E05. Neurology. 1999;53:1731–5.
202. The Vagus Nerve Stimulation Study Group. A randomized controlled trial of chronic vagus nerve stimulation for treatment of medically intractable seizures. Neurology. 1995;45(2):224–30.
203. Alexander GM, Huang YZ, Soderblom EJ, et al. Vagal nerve stimulation modifies neuronal activity and the proteome of excitatory synapses of amygdala/piriform cortex. J Neurochem. 2017;140: 629–44.
204. Krahl SE, Clark KB. Vagus nerve stimulation for epilepsy: a review of central mechanisms. Neurol Int. 2012;3:S47–52. https://doi.org/10.4103/2152-7806.103015.
205. Henry TR, Bakay RAE, Votaw JR, et al. Brain blood flow alterations induced by therapeutic vagus nerve stimulation in partial epilepsy: I. Acute effects at high and low levels of stimulation. Epilepsia. 1998;39(9):983–90.
206. Van Laere K, Vonck K, Boon P, Versijpt J, Dierckx R. Perfusion SPECT changes after acute and chronic vagus nerve stimulation in relation to prestimulus condition and long-term clinical efficacy. J Nucl Med. 2002;43(6):733–44.
207. Vonck K, Van LK, Dedeurwaerdere S, Caemaert J, De RJ, Boon P. The mechanism of action of vagus nerve stimulation for refractory epilepsy: the current status. J Clin Neurophysiol. 2001;18:394–401.
208. Chase MH, Nakamura Y, Clemente CD, Sterman MB. Afferent vagal stimulation: neurographic correlates of induced EEG synchronization and desynchronization. Brain Res. 1967;5:236–49.
209. Ginn C, Patel B, Walker R. Existing and emerging applications for the neuromodulation of nerve activity through targeted delivery of electric stimuli. Int J Neurosci. 2019;129(10):1013–23.
210. Henry TR. Therapeutic mechanisms of vagus nerve stimulation. Neurology. 2002;59:S3–S14.
211. Koo B. EEG changes with vagus nerve stimulation. J Clin Neurophysiol. 2001;18:434–41.
212. Randall WC, Ardell JL, Becker DM. Differential responses accompanying sequential stimulation and ablation of vagal branches to dog heart. Am J Physiol. 1985;249:133–40.
213. Samadani U, Baltuch GH. Vagus nerve stimulation. In: Baltuch GH, Villemure JG, editors. Operative techniques in epilepsy surgery. New York: Thieme; 2009. p. 149–57.

214. De Oliveira T, Franciscco AN, Demartini Z, et al. The role of vagus nerve stimulation in refractory epilepsy. Arq Neuropsiquiatr. 2017;75(9):657–66.
215. Giordano F, Zicca A, Barba C, et al. Vagus nerve stimulation: surgical technique of implantation and revision and related morbidity. Epilepsia. 2017;58(Suppl. 1):85–90.
216. Santos PM. Evaluation of laryngeal function after implantation of the vagus nerve stimulation device. Otolaryngol Head Neck Surg. 2003;129(3):269–73.
217. Shaw GY, Sechtem P, Searl J, Dowdy ES. Predictors of laryngeal complications in patients implanted with the Cyberonics vagal nerve stimulator. Ann Otol Rhinol Laryngol. 2006;115(4):260–7.
218. Kumar R, Winston KR, Folzenlogen Z. Removal of vagus nerve stimulator leads and reuse of same site for reimplantation: technique and experience. World Neurosurg. 2016;91:190–4.
219. Ramani R. Vagus nerve stimulation therapy for seizures. J Neurosurg Anesthesiol. 2008;20(1):29–35.
220. Aalbers MW, Rijkers K, Klinkenberg S, et al. Vagus nerve stimulation lead removal or replacement: surgical technique, institutional experience, and literature overview. Acta Neurochir (Wien). 2015;157:1917–24.
221. Clark A, Kupermann RA, Auguste KI, et al. Intractable episodic bradycardia resulting from progressive lead traction in an epileptic child with a vagus nerve stimulator: a delayed complication. J Neurosurg Pediatr. 2012;9:389–93.
222. Couch JD, Gilman AM, Doyle WK. Long-term expectations of vagus nerve stimulation: a look at battery replacement and revision surgery. Neurosurgery. 2016;78:42–6.
223. Dlouhy BJ, Viljoen SV, Kung DK, et al. Vagus nerve stimulation after lead revision. Neurosurg Focus. 2012;32:E11.
224. Espinosa J, Aiello MT, Naritoku DK. Revision and removal of stimulating electrodes following long-term therapy with the vagus nerve stimulator. Surg Neurol. 1999;51:659–64.
225. Kahlow H, Olivecrona M. Complications of vagal nerve stimulation for drug-resistant epilepsy: a single center longitudinal study of 143 patients. Seizure. 2013;22:827–33.
226. Kalkanis JG, Krishna P, Espinosa JA, et al. Self-inflicted vocal cord paralysis in patients with vagus nerve stimulators. Report of two cases. J Neurosurg. 2002;96:949–51.
227. McDonald J, Couldwell WT. Revision of vagal nerve stimulator electrodes: technical approach. Acta Neurochir (Wien). 2004;146:567–70.
228. Ortler M, Unterhofer C, Dobesberger J, et al. Complete removal of vagus nerve stimulator generator and electrodes. J Neurosurg Pediatr. 2010;5:191–4.
229. Revesz D, Rydenhag B, Ben-Menachem E. Complications and safety of vagus nerve stimulation: 25 years of experience at a single center. J Neurosurg Pediatr. 2016;18:97–104.
230. Rijkers K, Berfelo MW, Cornips EM, et al. Hardware failure in vagus nerve stimulation therapy. Acta Neurochir (Wien). 2008;150:403–5.
231. Smyth MD, Tubbs RS, Bebin EM, Grabb PA, Blount JP. Complications of chronic of chronic vagus nerve stimulation for epilepsy in children. J Neurosurg. 2003;99:500–3.
232. Tran Y, Shah AK, Mittal S. Lead breakage and vocal cord paralysis following blunt neck trauma in a patient with vagal nerve stimulator. J Neurol Sci. 2011;304:132–5.
233. Ng WH, Donner E, Go C, et al. Revision of vagal nerve stimulation (VNS) electrodes: review and report on use of ultra-sharp monopolar tip. Childs Nerv Syst. 2010;26:1081–4.
234. Fahy BG. Intraoperative and perioperative complications with a vagus nerve stimulation device. J Clin Anesth. 2010;22:213–22.
235. Hatton KW, McLarney JT, Pittman T, et al. Vagal nerve stimulation: overview and implications for anesthesiologists. Anesth Analg. 2006;103:1241–9.
236. Horowitz G, Amit M, Fried I, et al. Vagal nerve stimulation for refractory epilepsy: the surgical procedure and complications in 100 implantations by a single medical center. Eur Arch Otorhinolaryngol. 2013;270:355–8.
237. Navas M, Navarrete EG, Pascual JM, et al. Treatment of refractory epilepsy in adult patients with right-sided vagus nerve stimulation. Epilepsy Res. 2010;90:1–7.
238. Spuck S, Tronnier V, Orosz I, Schönweiler R, Sepehrnia A, Nowak G, et al. Operative and technical complications of vagus nerve stimulator implantation. Neurosurgery. 2010;67:489–94.
239. Tatum WO, Moore DB, Stecker MM, et al. Ventricual asystole during vagus nerve stimulation for epilepsy in humans. Neurology. 1999;52:1267–9.
240. Zalvan C, Sulica L, Wolf S, et al. Laryngopharyngeal dysfunction from the implant vagal nerve stimulator. Laryngoscope. 2003;113:221–5.
241. O'Neill BR, Wilberger JE. Revision of vagal nerve stimulator electrodes through a posterior cervical triangle approach: technical note. Neurosurgery. 2010;67(2 Suppl Operative):457–60.
242. Amar AP, Heck CN, Levy ML, Smith T, DeGiorgio CM, Oviedo S, Apuzzo ML. An institutional experience with cervical vagus nerve trunk stimulation for medically refractory epilepsy: rationale, technique, and outcome. Neurosurgery. 1998;43:1265–76; discussion 1276–80.
243. DeGiorgio C, Heck C, Bunch S, Britton J, Green P, Lancman M, Murphy J, Olejniczak P, Shih J, Arrambide S, Soss J. Vagus nerve stimulation for epilepsy: randomized comparison of three stimulation paradigms. Neurology. 2005;65:317–9. https://doi.org/10.1212/01.wnl.0000168899.11598.00.
244. Klinkenberg S, Aalbers MW, Vles JS, et al. Vagus nerve stimulation in children with intractable epilepsy: a randomized controlled trial. Dev Med Child Neurol. 2012;54(9):855–61.

245. Ryvlin P, Gilliam FG, Nguyen DK, et al. The long-term effect of vagus nerve stimulation on quality of life in patients with pharmacoresistant focal epilepsy: the PuLsE (Open Prospective Randomized Long-term Effectiveness) trial. Epilepsia. 2014;55(6):893–900.
246. Scherrmann J, Hoppe C, Kral T, Schramm J, Elger CE. Vagus nerve stimulation: clinical experience in a large patient series. J Clin Neurophysiol. 2001;18:408–14.
247. DeGiorgio CM, Schachter SC, Handforth A, Salinsky M, Thompson J, Uthman B, Reed R, Collins S, Tecoma E, Morris GL, Vaughn B, Naritoku DK, Henry T, Labar D, Gilmartin R, Labiner D, Osorio I, Ristanovic R, Jones J, Murphy J, Ney G, Wheless J, Lewis P, Heck C. Prospective long-term study of vagus nerve stimulation for the treatment of refractory seizures. Epilepsia. 2000;41(9):1195–200.
248. González HFJ, Yengo-Kahn A, Englot DJ. Vagus nerve stimulation for the treatment of epilepsy. Neurosurg Clin N Am. 2019;30:219–30.
249. Wiebe S, Jette N. Randomized trials and collaborative research in epilepsy sugery: future directions. Can J Neurol Sci. 2006;33:365–71.
250. Ardesch JJ, Buschman HP, Wagener-Schimmel LJ, et al. Vagus nerve stimulation for medically refractory epilepsy: a long-term follow-up study. Seizure. 2007;16(7):579–85.
251. Ardesch JJ, Buschman HP, van der Burgh PH, Wagener-Schimmel LJ, van der Aa HE, Hageman G, et al. Cardiac responses of vagus nerve stimulation: intra-operative bradycardia and subsequent chronic stimulation. Clin Neurol Neurosurg. 2007;109:849–52.
252. Ben-Menachem E, Hellstrom K, Waldton C, Augustinson LE. Evaluation of refractory epilepsy treated with vagus nerve stimulation for up to 5 years. Neurology. 1999;52:1265–7.
253. Boon P, Vonck K, van Rijckevorsel K, et al. A prospective, multicenter study of cardiac-based seizure detection to activate vagus nerve stimulation. Seizure. 2015;32:52–61.
254. Chavel SM, Westerveld M, Spencer S. Long-term outcome of vagus nerve stimulation for refractory partial epilepsy. Epilepsy Behav. 2003;4(3):302–9.
255. Fisher RS, Afra P, Macken M, et al. Automatic vagus nerve stimulation triggered by ictal tachycardia: clinical outcomes and device performance—the U.S. E-37 trial. Neuromodulation. 2016;19:188–95.
256. Huf RL, Mamelak A, Kneedy-Cayem K. Vagus nerve stimulation therapy: 2-year prospective open-label study of 40 subjects with refractory epilepsy and low IQ who are living in long-term care facilities. Epilepsy Behav. 2005;6:417–23.
257. Kang HC, Hwang YS, Kim DS, Kim HD. Vagus nerve stimulation in pediatric intractable epilepsy: a Korean bicentric study. Acta Neurochir Suppl. 2006;99:93–6.
258. Labar D, Murphy J, Tecoma E. Vagus nerve stimulation for medication-resistant generalized epilepsy. E04 VNS Study Group. Neurology. 1999;52(7):1510–2.
259. Parker AP, Polkey CE, Binnie CD, et al. Vagal nerve stimulation in epileptic encephalopathies. Pediatrics. 1999;103(4):778–82.
260. Salinsky MC, Uthman BM, Ristanovic RK, et al. Vagus nerve stimulation for the treatment of medically intractable seizures. results of a 1-year open extension trial. Arch Neurol. 1996;53:1176–80.
261. Vonck K, Thadani V, Gilbert K, Dedeurwaerdere S, De Groote L, De Herdt V, et al. Vagus nerve stimulation for refractory epilepsy: a transatlantic experience. J Clin Neurophysiol. 2004;21:283–9.
262. Majoie HJ, Berfelo MW, Aldenkamp AP, Evers SM, Kessels AG, Renier WO. Vagus Nerve stimulation in children with therapy-resistant epilepsy diagnosed as Lennox-Gastaut syndrome. J Clin Neurophysiol. 2001;18:419–28.
263. Amar AP, Apuzzo ML, Liu CY. Vagus nerve stimulation therapy after failed cranial surgery for intractable epilepsy: results from the vagus nerve stimulation therapy patient outcome registry. Neurosurgery. 2004;55:1086–93.
264. George R, Salinsky M, Kuzniecky R, Rosenfeld W, Bergen D, Tarver WB, Wernicke JF, First International Vagus Nerve Stimulation Study Group. Vagus nerve stimulation for treatment of partial seizures: 3. Long-term follow-up on first 67 patients exiting a controlled study. Epilepsia. 1994;35:637–43.
265. Helmers SL, Whenless JW, Frost M, Gates J, Levisohn P, Tardo C, Conry JA, Yalnizoglou D, Madsen JR. Vagus nerve stimulation therapy in pediatric patients with refractory epilepsy: a retrospective study. J Child Neurol. 2001;16:843–8.
266. Labar D. Vagus nerve stimulation for 1 year in 269 patients on unchanged antiepileptic drugs. Seizure. 2004;13:392–8.
267. Murphy JV, Pediatric VNS Study Group. Left vagal nerve stimulation in children with medically refractory epilepsy. J Pediatr. 1999;134:563–6.
268. Patwardhan RV, Strong B, Bebin EM, Mathisen J, Grabb PA. Efficacy of vagal nerve stimulation in children with medically refractory epilepsy. Neurosurgery. 2000;47:1353–7; discussion 1357–8.
269. Spanaki MV, Allen LS, Mueller WM, et al. Vagus nerve stimulation therapy: 5-year of greater outcome at a university-based epilepsy center. Seizure. 2004;13:587–90.
270. Alexopoulos AV, Kotagal P, Loddenkemper T, Hammel J, Bingaman WE. Long-term results with vagus nerve stimulation in children with pharmacoresistant epilepsy. Seizure. 2006;15:491–503.
271. Frost M, Gates J, Helmers SL, Wheless JW, Levisohn P, Tardo C, Conry JA. Vagus nerve stimulation in children with refractory seizures associated with Lennox-Gastaut syndrome. Epilpesia. 2001;42:1148–52.
272. Murphy JV, Torkelson R, Dowler I, Simon S, Hudson S. Vagal nerve stimulation in refractory

epilepsy: the first 100 patients receiving vagal nerve stimulation at a pediatric center. Arch Adolesc Med. 2003;157:260–4.
273. Renfroe JB, Wheless JW. Earlier use of adjunctive nerve stimulation therapy for refractory epilepsy. Neurology. 2002;59:S26–30.
274. Shahwan A, Bailey C, Maxiner W, Harvey AS. Vagus nerve stimulation for refractory epilepsy in children: more to VNS than seizure frequency reduction. Epilepsia. 2009;50:1220–8.
275. Uthman BM, Reichl AM, Dean JC, Eisenschenk S, Gilmore R, Reid S, Roper SN, Wilder BJ. Effectiveness of vagus nerve stimulation in epilepsy patients: a 12-year observation. Neurology. 2004;63:1124–6.
276. De Herdt V, Boon P, Ceulemans B, Hauman H, Lagae L, Legros B, Sadzot B, Van Bogaert P, van Rijckevorsel K, Verhelst H, Vonck K. Vagus nerve stimulation for refractory epilepsy: a Belgian multicenter study. Eur J Paediatr Neurol. 2007;11:261–9.
277. Elliott RE, Morsi A, Kalhorn SP, Marcus J, Sellin J, Kang M, Silverberg A, Rivera E, Geller E, Carlson C, Devinsky O, Doyle WK. Vagus nerve stimulation in 436 consecutive patients with treatment-resistant epilepsy: long-term outcomes and predictors of response. Epilepsy Behav. 2011;20:57–63.
278. Elliott RE, Rodgers SD, Bassani L, et al. Vagus nerve stimulation for children with treatment-resistant epilepsy: a consecutive series of 141 cases. J Neurosurg Pediatr. 2011;7:491–500.
279. Tatum WOT, Helmers SL. Vagus nerve stimulation and magnet use: optimizing benefits. Epilepsy Behav. 2009;15:299–302.
280. Wang H-J, Zhu GTL, Chen D, et al. Predictors of seizure reduction outcome after vagus nerve stimulation in drug-resistant epilepsy. Eur J Epilepsy. 2019;66:53–60.
281. Englot DJ, Chang EF, Auguste KI. Vagus nerve stimulation for epilepsy: a meta-analysis of efficacy and predictors of response. J Neurosurg. 2011;115:1248–55.
282. Englot DJ, Chang EF, Auguste KI. Efficacy of vagus nerve stimulation for epilepsy by patient age, epilepsy duration, and seizure type. Neurosurg Clin N Am. 2011;22:443–8. https://doi.org/10.1016/j.nec.2011.07.002.
283. Englot DJ, Rolston JD, Wright CW, et al. Rates and predictors of seizure freedom with vagus nerve stimulation for intractable epilepsy. Neurosurgery. 2015;79(3):345–53.
284. Ben-Menachem E. Vagus nerve stimulation, side effects, and long-term safety. J Clin Neurophysiol. 2001;18:415–8.
285. Kostov K, Kostov H, Tauboll E. Longterm vagus nerve stimulation in the treatment of Lennox-Gastaut syndrome. Epilepsy Behav. 2009;16:321–4.
286. Rosenfeld WE, Roberts DW. Tonic and atonic seizures: what's next—VNS or callosotomy? Epilepsia. 2009;50(Suppl. 8):25–30.
287. Rolston JD, Englot DJ, Wang DD, Garcia PA, Chang EF. Corpus callosotomy versus vagus nerve stimulation for atonic seizures and drop attacks: a systematic review. Epilepsy Behav. 2015;51:13–7. https://doi.org/10.1016/j.yebeh.2015.06.001.
288. Marras CE, Chiesa V, et al. Vagus nerve stimulation in refractory epilepsy: new indications and outcome assessment. Epilepsy Behav. 2013; https://doi.org/10.1016/j.yebeh.2013.05.021.
289. Kubota Y, Nakamoto H, Miyao S, Kawamata T. Efficacy of vagal nerve stimulation for pharmacoresistant poststroke epilepsy. World Neurosurg. 2020;133:e448–51.
290. Hoppe C, Wagner L, Hoffmann JM, et al. Comprehensive long-term outcome of best drug treatment with or without add-on vagus nerve stimulation for epilepsy: a retrospective matched pairs case-control study. Seizure. 2013;22(2):109–15.
291. Sherman EM, Connolly MB, Slick DJ, Eyrl KL, Steinbok P, Farrell K. Quality of life and seizure outcome after vagus nerve stimulation in children with intractable epilepsy. J Child Neurol. 2008;23:991–8.
292. Aldenkamp AP, Majoie HJ, Berfelo MW, Evers SM, Kessels AG, Renier WO, Wilmink J. Long-term effects of 24-month treatment with vagus nerve stimulation on behavior in children with Lennox-Gastaut syndrome. Epilepsy Behav. 2002;3:475–9.
293. Arya R, Greiner HM, Lewis A, Horn PS, Mangano FT, Gonsalves C, et al. Predictors of response to vagus nerve stimulation in childhood-onset medically refractory epilepsy. J Child Neurol. 2014;29:1652–9.
294. Amar AP, Apuzzo ML, Liu CY. Vagus nerve stimulation therapy after failed cranial surgery for intractable epilepsy: results from the vagus nerve stimulation therapy patient outcome registry. Neurosurgery. 2008;62(Suppl 2):506–13.
295. Koutroumanidis M, Binnie CD, Hennessy MJ, Alarcon G, Elwes RDC, Toone BK, Chandler C, Selway R, Polkey C, O'Connor SA. VNS in patients with previous unsuccessful resective epilepsy surgery: antiepileptic and psychotropic effects. Acta Neurol Scand. 2003;107:117–21.
296. Vale FL, Ahmadian A, Youssef AS, Tatum WO, Benabis SR. Long-term outcome of vagus nerve stimulation therapy after failed epilepsy surgery. Seizure. 2011;20:244–8.
297. Lesser RP. Unexpected places. How did vagus nerve stimulation become a treatment for epilepsy? Neurology. 1999;52:1117–8.
298. Englot DJ, Rolston JD, Wang DD, Hassnain KH, Gordon CM, Chang EF. Efficacy of vagus nerve stimulation in posttraumatic versus nontraumatic epilepsy. J Neurosurg. 2012;117:970–7. https://doi.org/10.3171/2012.8.JNS122.
299. Lee HO, Koh EJ, Oh YM, Park SS, Kwon KH, Choi HY. Effect of vagus nerve stimulation in post-traumatic epilepsy and failed epilepsy surgery: preliminary report. J Korean Neurosurg Soc. 2008;44(4):196–8.
300. Ryvlin P, So EL, Gordon CM, et al. Long-term surveillance of SUDEP in drug-resistant epilepsy

patients treated with VNS therapy. Epilepsia. 2018;59(3):562–72.

301. Elger G, Hoppe C, Falkai P, et al. Vagus nerve stimulation is associated with mood improvements in epilepsy patients. Epilepsy Res. 2000;42(2–3):203–10.
302. Ergene E, Behr PK, Shih JJ. Quality-of-life assessment in patients treated with vagus nerve stimulation. Epilepsy Behav. 2001;2:284–7.
303. George MS, Rush AJ, Sackeim HA, et al. Vagus nerve stimulation (VNS): utility in neuropsychiatric disorders. Int J Neuropsychopharmacol. 2003;6(1):73–83.
304. Harden CL, Pulver MC, Radvin LD, Nikolov B, Halper JP, Labar DR. A pilot study of mood in epilepsy patients treated via vagus nerve stimulation. Epilepsy Behav. 2000;1:93–9.
305. Marlow BA, Edwards J, Marzec M, Sagher O, Ross D, Fromes G. Vagus nerve stimulation reduces daytime sleepiness in epilepsy patients. Neurology. 2001;57:879–84.
306. Englot DJ, Hassnain KH, Rolston JD, et al. Quality-of-life metrics with vagus nerve stimulation for epilepsy from provider survey data. Epilepsy Behav. 2017;66:4–9.
307. Cramer J. Exploration of changes in health related quality of life after 3 months of vagus nerve stimulation. Epilepsy Behav. 2001;2:460–5.
308. Ventureyra EC. Transcutaneous vagus nerve stimulation for partial onset seizure therapy. A new concept. Childs Nerv Syst. 2000;16(2):101–2.
309. Stefan H, Kreiselmeyer G, Kerling F, et al. Transcutaneous vagus nerve stimulation (tVNS) in pharmacoresistant epilepsies: a proof of concept trial. Epilepsia. 2012;53(7):115–8.
310. Aihua L, Lu S, Liping L, et al. A controlled trial of transcutaneous vagus nerve stimulation for the treatment of pharmacoresistant epilepsy. Epilepsy Behav. 2014;39:105–10.
311. Bauer S, Baier H, Baumgartner C, Bohlmann K, Fauser S, Graf W, et al. Transcutaneous vagus nerve stimulation (tVNS) for treatment of drug resistant epilepsy: a randomized, double-blind clinical trial (cMPsE02). Brain Stimul. 2016;9(3):356–63.
312. Liu A, Rong P, Gong L, et al. Efficacy and safety of treatment with transcutaneous vagus nerve stimulation in 17 patients with refractory epilepsy evaluated by electroencephalogram, seizure frequency, and quality of life. Med Sci Monit. 2018;24:8439–48.
313. Eggleston KS, Olin BD, Fisher RS. Ictal tachycardia: the head-heart connection. Seizure. 2014;23:496–505.
314. Chen W, Meng FG. Ictal heart rate changes and the effects of vagus nerve stimulation for patients with refractory epilepsy. Neuropsychiatr Dis Treat. 2017;13:2351–6.
315. Ravan M. Investigating the correlation between short-term effectiveness of VNS Therapy in reducing the severity of seizures and long-term responsiveness. Epilepsy Res. 2017;133:46–53.
316. Hamilton P, Soryal I, Dhahri P, Wimalachandra W, Leat A, Hughes D, et al. Clinical outcomes of VNS therapy with AspireSR® (including cardiac-based seizure detection) at a large complex epilepsy and surgery centre. Seizure. 2018;58:120–6.
317. Kringelbach ML, Jenkinson N, Owen SL, Aziz TZ. Translational principles of deep brain stimulation. Nat Rev Neurosci. 2007;8(8):623–35.
318. Moruzzi G. Effects at different frequencies of cerebellar stimulation upon postural tonus and myotatic reflexes. Electroencephalogr Clin Neurophysiol. 1950;2:463–9.
319. Tyrand R, Seeck M, Pollo C, Boex C. Effects of amygdala-hippocampal stimulation on synchronization. Epilepsy Res. 2014;108:327–30. https://doi.org/10.1016/j.eplepsyres.2013.11.024.
320. Laxpati NG, Kasoff WS, Gross RE. Deep brain stimulation for the treatment of epilepsy: circuits, targets, and trials. Neurotherapeutics. 2014;11:508–26. https://doi.org/10.1007/s13311-014-0279-9.
321. Velasco AL, Velasco F, Jimenez F, Velasco M, Castro G, Carrillo-Ruiz JD, Fanghänel G, Boleaga B. Neuromodulation of the centromedian thalamic nuclei in the treatment of generalized seizures and the improvement of quality of life in patients with Lennox-Gastaut syndrome. Epilepsia. 2006;47:1203–12.
322. Sprengers M, Vuncle K, Carrett E, et al. Deep brain and cortical stimulation for epilepsy. Cochrane Database Syst Rev. 2017;7:1–107.
323. Fridley J, Thomas JG, Navarro JC, Yoshor D. Brain stimulation for the treatment of epilepsy. Neurosurg Focus. 2012;32(3):E13. https://doi.org/10.3171/2012.
324. Rolston JD, Englot DJ, Wang DD, Shih T, Chang EF. Comparison of seizure control outcomes and the safety of vagus nerve, thalamic deep brain, and responsive neurostimulation: evidence from randomized controlled trials. Neurosurg Focus. 2012;32(3):E14. https://doi.org/10.3171/2012.1.
325. Rolston JD, Blevins LS Jr. Gamma knife radiosurgery for acromegaly. Int J Endocrinol. 2012; https://doi.org/10.1155/2012/821579. Epub 2012 Feb 13
326. Halpern CH, Samadani U, Litt B, Jaggi JL, Baltuch GH. Deep brain stimulation for epilepsy. Neurotherapeutics. 2008;5(1):59–67.
327. Lehtimäki K, Coenen VA, Ferreira AG, et al. The surgical approach to the anterior nucleus of thalamus in patients with refractory epilepsy: experience from the international multicenter registry (MORE). Neurosurgery. 2018; https://doi.org/10.1093/neuros/nyy023.
328. Koeppen JA, Nahravani F, Kramer M, et al. Electrical stimulation of the anterior thalamus for epilepsy: clinical outcome and analysis of efficient target. Neuromodulation. 2018; https://doi.org/10.1111/ner.12865.
329. Schaper FLWVJ, Zhao Y, Janssen MLF, et al. Single-cell recordings to target the anterior nucleus of the thalamus in deep brain stimulation for patients with refractory epilepsy. Int J Neural Syst. 2019;29(4):1850012. https://doi.org/10.1142/S0129065718500120.

330. Mirski MA, Rossell LA, Terry JB, Fisher RS. Anticonvulsant effect of anterior thalamic high frequency electrical stimulation in the rat. Epilepsy Res. 1997;28:89–100.
331. Salanova V. Deep brain stimulation for epilepsy. Epilepsy Behav. 2018; https://doi.org/10.1016/j.yebeh.2018.06041.
332. Van der Vils TAMB, Schijns OEMG, Schaper FLWVI, et al. Deep brain stimulation of the anterior nucleus of the thalamus for drug-resistant epilepsy. Neurosurg Rev. 2019;42(2):287–96.
333. Fisher RS, Uematsu S, Krauss G, Cysyk BJ, McPherson R, Lesser RP, Gordon B, Schwerdt P, Rise M. Placebo-controlled pilot study of centormedian thalamic stimulation in treatment of intractable seizures. Epilepsia. 1992;33:841–51.
334. Fisher R, Salanova V, Witt T, Worth R, Henry T, Gross R, Oommen K, Osorio I, Nazzaro J, Labar D, Kaplitt M, Sperling M, Sandok E, Neal J, Handforth A, Stern J, DeSalles A, Chung S, Shetter A, Bergen D, Bakay R, Henderson J, French J, Baltuch G, Rosenfeld W, Youkilis A, Marks W, Garcia P, Barbaro N, Fountain N, Bazil C, Goodman R, McKhann G, Babu Krishnamurthy K, Papavassiliou S, Epstein C, Pollard J, Tonder L, Grebin J, Coffey R, Graves N, SANTE Study Group. Electrical stimulation of the anterior nucleus of thalamus for treatment of refractory epilepsy. Epilepsia. 2010;51(5):899–908.
335. Téllez-Zenteno JF, McLachlan RS, Parrent A, Kubu CS, Wiebe S. Hippocampal electrical stimulation in mesial temporal lobe epilepsy. Neurology. 2006;66:1490–4.
336. Velasco F, Carrillo-Ruiz JD, Brito F, Velasco M, Velasco AL, Marquez I, Davis R. Double-blind, randomized controlled pilot study of bilateral cerebellar stimulation for treatment of intractable motor seizures. Epilepsia. 2005;46:1071–81.
337. Herrman H, Egge A, Konglund AE, Ramm-Pettersen J, Dietrichs E, Taubøll E. Anterior thalamic deep brain stimulation in refractory epilepsy: a randomized, double-blinded study. Acta Neurol Scand. 2019;139(3):294–304.
338. Salanova V, Witt T, Worth R, Henry TR, Gross RE, Nazzaro JM, Labar D, Sperling MR, Sharan A, Sandok E, Handforth A, Stern JM, Chung S, Henderson JM, French J, Baltuch G, Rosenfeld WE, Garcia P, Barbaro NM, Fountain NB, Elias WJ, Goodman RR, Pollard JR, Troster AI, Irwin CP, Lambrecht K, Graves N, Fisher R, Group SS. Long-term efficacy and safety of thalamic stimulation for drug-resistant partial epilepsy. Neurology. 2015;84:1017–25. https://doi.org/10.1212/WNL.0000000000001334.
339. Oh SY, Kim HJ, Lee JK, et al. Cognitive improvement after long-term electrical stimulation of bilateral anterior thalamic nucleus in refractory epilepsy patients. Seizure. 2012;21:183–7.
340. Lee KJ, Shon YM, Cho CB. Long-term outcome of anterior thalamic nucleus stimulation for intractable epilepsy. Stereotact Funct Neurosurg. 2012;90(6):379–85.
341. Krishna V, King NK, Sammartino F, Strauss I, Andrade DM, Wennberg RA, et al. Anterior nucleus deep brain stimulation for refractory epilepsy: insights into patterns of seizure control and efficacious target. Neurosurgery. 2016;78(6):802–11.
342. Kim SH, Lim SC, Kim J, Son BC, Lee KJ, Shon YM. Long-term follow-up of anterior thalamic deep brain stimulation in epilepsy: a 11-year, single center experience. Seizure. 2017;52:154–61.
343. Park HR, Choi SJ, Joo EY, et al. The role of anterior thalamic deep brain stimulation as an alternative therapy in patients with previously failed vagus nerve stimulation for refractory epilepsy. Stereotact Funct Neurosurg. 2019; https://doi.org/10.1159/000502344.
344. Kim SH, Lim SC, Yang DW, et al. Thalamo-cortical network underlying deep brain stimulation of centromedian thalamic nuclei in intractable epilepsy: a multimodal imaging analysis. Neuropsychiatr Dis Treat. 2017;13:2607–19.
345. Hachem LD, Yan H, Ibrahim GM. Invasive neuromodulation for the treatment of pediatric epilepsy. Neurotherapeutics. 2018; https://doi.org/10.1007/s13311-018-00685-1.
346. Valentin A, Garcia Navarrete E, Chelvarajah R, et al. Deep brain stimulation of the centromedian thalamic nucleus for the treatment of generalized and frontal epilepsies. Epilepsia. 2013;54(10):1823–33.
347. Tröster AI, Meador KJ, Irwin CP, et al. Memory and mood outcomes after anterior thalamic stimulation for refractory partial epilepsy. Seizure. 2017;45:133–41.
348. Novais F, Pestana LC, Loureiro S, et al. Predicting de novo psychopathology after epilepsy surgery: a 3-year cohort study. Epilepsy Behav. 2019;90:204–8. https://doi.org/10.1016/j.yebeh.2018.11.037.
349. Lesser RP, Luders H, Klem G, et al. Cortical afterdischarge and functional response thresholds: results of extraoperative testing. Epilepsia. 1984;25:615–21.
350. Tran DK, Paff M, Mnatsakanyan L, et al. A novel robotic-assisted technique to implant the responsive neurostimulation system. Oper Neurosurg. 2019; https://doi.org/10.1093/ons/opz226.
351. Chan AY, Tran DK, Paff MR, et al. Robotic orthogonal implantation of Responsive Neurostimulation (RNS) depth electrodes in the mesial temporal lobe: case series. Oper Neurosurg. 2019; https://doi.org/10.1093/ons/opz360.
352. Ma BB, Rao VR. Responsive neurostimulation: candidates and considerations. Epilepsy Behav. 2018;88:388–95.
353. Matias CM, Sharan AD, Wu C, et al. Responsive neurostimulation for the treatment of epilepsy. Neurosurg Clin N Am. 2018; https://doi.org/10.1016/j.nec.2018.12.006.
354. Morrell MJ, Group RNSSiES. Responsive cortical stimulation for the treatment of medically intractable partial epilepsy. Neurology. 2011;77:1295–304.

355. Skarpaas TL, Jarosiewicz B, Morrell MJ. Brain-responsive neurostimulation for epilepsy (RNS® System). Epilepsy Res. 2019;153:68–70.
356. Elder C, Friedman D, Devinsky O, Doyle W, Dugan P. Responsive neurostimulation targeting the anterior nucleus of the thalamus in 3 patients with treatmentresistant multifocal epilepsy. Epilepsia Open. 2019;4(1):187–92.
357. Sisterson ND, Wozny TA, Kokkinos V, et al. Closed-loop brain stimulation for drug-resistant epilepsy: towards an evidence-based approach to personalized medicine. Neurotherapeutics. 2018; https://doi.org/10.1007/s13311-018-00682-4.
358. Heck CN, King-Stephens D, Massey AD, Nair DR, Jobst BC, Barkley GL, Salanova V, Cole AJ, Smith MC, Gwinn RP, Skidmore C, Van Ness PC, Bergey GK, Park YD, Miller I, Geller E, Rutecki PA, Zimmerman R, Spencer DC, Goldman A, Edwards JC, Leiphart JW, Wharen RE, Fessler J, Fountain NB, Worrell GA, Gross RE, Eisenschenk S, Duckrow RB, Hirsch LJ, Bazil C, O'Donovan CA, Sun FT, Courtney TA, Seale CG, Morrell MJ. Two-year seizure reduction in adults with medically intractable partial onset epilepsy treated with responsive neurostimulation: final results of the RNS System Pivotal trial. Epilepsia. 2014;55:432–41. https://doi.org/10.1111/epi.12534.
359. Bergey GK, Morrell MJ, Mizrahi EM, Goldman A, King-Stephens D, Nair D, Srinivasan S, Jobst B, Gross RE, Shields DC, Barkley G, Salanova V, Olejniczak P, Cole A, Cash SS, Noe K, Wharen R, Worrell G, Murro AM, Edwards J, Duchowny M, Spencer D, Smith M, Geller E, Gwinn R, Skidmore C, Eisenschenk S, Berg M, Heck C, Van Ness P, Fountain N, Rutecki P, Massey A, O'Donovan C, Labar D, Duckrow RB, Hirsch LJ, Courtney T, Sun FT, Seale CG. Long-term treatment with responsive brain stimulation in adults with refractory partial seizures. Neurology. 2015;84:810–7.
360. Nair D, Morrell MJ, RNS System Investigators. Nine-year prospective safety and effectiveness outcomes from the long-term treatment trial of the RNS® system. In: AES. Annual Meeting Abstract Database. 2018. AESnet.org.
361. Meador KJ, Kapur R, Loring DW, et al. Quality of life and mood in patients with medically intractable epilepsy treated with targeted responsive neurostimulation. Epilepsy Behav. 2015;45:242–7.
362. Geller EB, Skarpaas TL, Gross RE, et al. Brain-responsive neurostimulation in patients with medically intractable mesial temporal lobe epilepsy. Epilepsia. 2017;58:994–1004.
363. Jobst BC, Kapur R, Barkley GL, et al. Brain-responsive neurostimulation in patients with medically intractable seizures arising from eloquent and other neocortical areas. Epilepsia. 2017;58:1005–14.
364. Singhal NS, Numis AL, Lee MB, et al. Responsive neurostimulation for treatment of pediatric drug-resistant epilepsy. Epilepsy Behav Case Rep. 2018;10:21–4.
365. Loring DW, Kapur R, Meador KJ, et al. Differential neuropsychological outcomes following targeted responsive neurostimulation for partial-onset epilepsy. Epilepsia. 2015;56:1836–44.
366. Lundstrom BN, Worrell GA, Stead M, et al. Chronic subthreshold cortical stimulation: a therapeutic and potentially restorative therapy for focal epilepsy. Expert Rev Neurother. 2017;17:661–6.
367. Child ND, Stead M, Wirrell EC, et al. Chronic subthreshold subdural cortical stimulation for the treatment of focal epilepsy originating from eloquent cortex. Epilepsia. 2014;55:e18–21.
368. Lundstrom BN, Meisel C, Van Gompel J, et al. Comparing spiking and slow wave activity from invasive electroencephalography in patients with and without seizures. Clin Neurophysiol. 2018;129:909–19.
369. Velasco M, Velasco F, Velasco AL, et al. Subacute electrical stimulation of the hippocampus blocks intractable temporal lobe seizures and paroxysmal EEG activities. Epilepsia. 2000;41:158–69.
370. Westin K, Lundstrom BN, Van Gompel J, et al. Neurophysiological effects of continuous cortical stimulation in epilepsy—spike and spontaneous ECoG activity. Clin Neurophysiol. 2019;130:38–45.
371. Lundstrom BN, Gompel JV, Khadjevand F, et al. Chronic subthreshold cortical stimulation and stimulation-related EEG biomarkers for focal epilepsy. Brain Commun. 2019; https://doi.org/10.1093/braincomms/fcz010.
372. Lundstrom BN, Gompel JV, Britton J, et al. Chronic subthreshold cortical stimulation to treat focal epilepsy. JAMA Neurol. 2016;73:1370–2.
373. Kerezoudis P, Grewal SS, Stead M, et al. Chronic subthreshold cortical stimulation for adult drug-resistant focal epilepsy: safety, feasibility, and technique. J Neurosurg. 2018;129:533–43.
374. Bourgeois M, Sainte-Rose C, Lellouch-Tubiana A, et al. Surgery of epilepsy associated with focal lesions in childhood. J Neurosurg. 1999;90:833–42.
375. Cascino GD, Kelly PJ, Sharbrough FW, Hulihan JF, Hirschorn KA, Trenerry MR. Long-term follow-up of stereotactic lesionectomy in partial epilepsy: predictive factors and electroencephalographic results. Epilepsia. 1992;33:639–44.
376. Pelliccia V, Deleo F, Gozzo F, et al. Early and late epilepsy surgery in focal epilepsies associated with long-term epilepsy-associated tumors. J Neurosurg. 2017;127(5):1147–52.
377. Wellmer J. Lesion focused radiofrequency thermocoagulation of bottom-of-sulcus focal cortical dysplasia type IIb: Conceptional considerations with regard to the epileptogenic zone. Epilepsy Res. 2018;142:143–8.
378. Fukuda M, Kameyama S, Wachi M, Tanaka R. Stereotaxy for hypothalamic hamartoma with intractable gelastic seizures: technical case report. Neurosurgery. 1999;44:1347–50.
379. Kuzniecky R, Guthrie B, Mountz J, Bebin M, Faught E, Gilliam F, et al. Intrinsic epileptogenesis of hypo-

thalamic hamartomas in gelastic epilepsy. Ann Neurol. 1997;42:60–7.
380. Munari C, Kahane P, Francione S, Hoffmann D, Tassi L, Cusmai R, et al. Role of the hypothalamic hamartoma in the genesis of gelastic fits (a video-stereo-EEG study). Electroencephalogr Clin Neurophysiol. 1995;95:154–60.
381. Calisto A, Dorfmuller G, Fohlen M, Bulteau C, Conti A, Delalande O. Endoscopic disconnection of hypothalamic hamartomas: safety and feasibility of robot-assisted, thulium laser-based procedures. J Neurosurg Pediatr. 2014;14:563–72.
382. Delalande O, Fohlen M. Disconnecting surgical treatment of hypothalamic hamartoma in children and adults with refractory epilepsy and proposal of a new classification. Neurol Med Chir (Tokyo). 2003;43:61–8.
383. Drees C, Chapman K, Prenger E, Baxter L, Maganti R, Rekate H, et al. Seizure outcome and complications following hypothalamic hamartoma treatment in adults: endoscopic, open, and Gamma Knife procedures. J Neurosurg. 2012;117:255–61.
384. Mittal S, Mittal M, Montes JL, Farmer JP, Andermann F. Hypothalamic hamartomas. Part 2. Surgical considerations and outcome. Neurosurg Focus. 2013;34(6):E7.
385. Pati S, Abla AA, Rekate HL, Ng YT. Repeat surgery for hypothalamic hamartoma in refractory epilepsy. Neurosurg Focus. 2011;30(2):E3.
386. Rekate HL, Feiz-Erfan I, Ng YT, Gonzalez LF, Kerrigan JF. Endoscopic surgery for hypothalamic hamartomas causing medically refractory gelastic epilepsy. Childs Nerv Syst. 2006;22:874–80.
387. Wait SD, Abla AA, Killory BD, Nakaji P, Rekate HL. Surgical approaches to hypothalamic hamartomas. Neurosurg Focus. 2011;30(2):E2.
388. Wellmer J, Parpaley Y, Rampp S, Popkirov S, Kugel H, Aydin Ü, Wolters CH, von Lehe M, Voges J. Lesion guided stereotactic radiofrequency thermocoagulation for palliative, in selected cases curative epilepsy surgery. Epilepsy Res. 2016;121:39–46.
389. Quigg M, Harden C. Minimally invasive techniques for epilepsy surgery: stereotactic radiosurgery and other technologies. J Neurosurg. 2014;121(Suppl):232–40.
390. Nádvorník P, Pogády J, Sramka M. Results of stereotaxic treatment in aggression syndrome. Cesk Psychiatry. 1973;69(6):357–62.
391. Spiegel EA, Wycis HT. Thalamic recordings in man with special reference to seizure discharges. EEG Clin Neurophysiol. 1950;2:23–7.
392. Flanigin HF, Nashold BS. Stereotactic lesions of the amygdala and hippocampus in epilepsy. Acta Neurochir. 1976;23:235–9.
393. Mundinger F, Becker P, Grolkner E. Late results of stereotactic surgery of epilepsy predominantly temporal lobe type. Acta Neurochir. 1976;23:177–82.
394. Umbach W. Long-term results of fornicotomy for temporal epilepsy. Confin Neurol. 1966;27:121–3. https://doi.org/10.1159/000103941.
395. Umbach W. Elektrophysiologische und vegetative Phänomene bei stereotaktischen Hirnoperationen. Heidelberg: Springer-Verlag; 1966.
396. Narabayashi H, Nagao T, Saito Y, Yoshida M, Nagahata M. Stereotaxic amygdalotomy for behavior disorders. Arch Neurol. 1963;9:1–16. https://doi.org/10.1001/archneur.1963.00460070011001.
397. Heimburger RF, Whitlock CC, Kalsbeck JE. Stereotaxic amygdalotomy for epilepsy with aggressive behavior. JAMA. 1966;198:741–5. https://doi.org/10.1001/jama.1966.03110200097026.
398. Schwab RS, Sweet WH, Mark VH, Kjellberg RN, Ervin FR. Treatment of intractable temporal lobe epilepsy by stereotactic amygdala lesions. Trans Am Neurol Assoc. 1965;90:12–9.
399. Nádvorník P, Šramka M. Anatomical considerations for the stereotaxic longitudinal hippocampectomy. Stereotact Funct Neurosurg. 1974;36:177–81. https://doi.org/10.1159/000102792.
400. Nádvorník P, Šramka M. Longitudinal hippocampectomy. A new stereotaxic approach to the gyrus hippocampi. Confin Neurol. 1975;37(1–3):245–8.
401. Bouchard G, Umbach W. Indications for open and stereotactic brain surgery in epilepsy. In: Present limits of neurosurgery. Amsterdam: Excerpta Medica; 1972. p. 403–6.
402. Heimburger RF, Small IF, Small JG, Milstein V, Moore D. Stereotactic amygdalotomy for convulsive and behavioral disorders. Stereotact Funct Neurosurg. 1978;41:43–51. https://doi.org/10.1159/000102399.
403. Kwan P, Schachter SC, Brodie MJ. Drug-resistant epilepsy. N Engl J Med. 2011;365:919–26. https://doi.org/10.1056/NEJMra1004418.
404. Narabayashi H, Mizutani T. Epileptic seizures and the stereotaxic amygdalotomy. Confin Neurol. 1970;32(2):289–97. https://doi.org/10.1159/000103429.
405. Schaltenbrand G, Spuler H, Nadjmi M, Hopf HC, Wahren W. Die stereotaktische Behandlung der Epilepsien. Stereotact Funct Neurosurg. 1966;27:111–3. https://doi.org/10.1159/000103939.
406. Talairach J, Szikla G. [Amygdalo-hippocampal partial destruction by yttrium-90 in the treatment of certain epilepsies of rhinencephalic manifestation]. Neurochirurgie. 1965;11:233–40.
407. Vaernet K. Stereotaxic amygdalotomy in temporal lobe epilepsy. Confin Neurol. 1972;34:4579788. https://doi.org/10.1159/000103055.
408. Parrent AG, Lozano AM. Stereotactic surgery for temporal lobe epilepsy. Can J Neurol Sci. 2000;27(Suppl 1):S79–84; discussion S92–6. https://doi.org/10.1017/S0317167100000718.
409. Parrent AG, Blume WT. Stereotactic amygdalohippocampotomy for the treatment of medial temporal lobe epilepsy. Epilepsia. 1999;40:1408–16. https://doi.org/10.1111/j.1528-1157.1999.tb02013.
410. Mempel E, Witkiewicz B, Stadnicki R, Luczywek E, Kuciński L, Pawłowski G, et al. The effect of medial amygdalotomy and anterior hippocampotomy on

behavior and seizures in epileptic patients. Acta Neurochir Suppl (Wien). 1980;30:161–7. https://doi.org/10.1007/978-3-7091-8592-6-20.
411. Voges J, Wellmer J, Büntjen L, Schmitt FC. Radiofrequency thermoablation—the neurosurgical perspective. Z Epileptol. 2017;30:98–104.
412. Vojtech Z, Malíková H, Krámská L, Liščák R, Vladyka V. MRI-guided stereotactic amygdalohippocampectomy: a single center experience. Neuropsychiatr Dis Treat. 2015;11:359–74.
413. Missios S, Bekelis K, Barnett GH. Renaissance of laser interstitial thermal ablation. Neurosurg Focus. 2015;38:E13.
414. Monteith S, Sheehan J, Medel R, Wintermark M, Eames M, Snell J, et al. Potential intracranial applications of magnetic resonance-guided focused ultrasound surgery. J Neurosurg. 2013;118:215–21.
415. Monteith S, Snell J, Eames M, Kassell NF, Kelly E, Gwinn R. Transcranial magnetic resonance-guided focused ultrasound for temporal lobe epilepsy: a laboratory feasibility study. J Neurosurg. 2016;125(6):1557–64.
416. Esquenazi Y, Kalamangalam GP, Slater JD, Knowlton RC, Friedman E, Morris SA, et al. Stereotactic laser ablation of epileptogenic periventricular nodular heterotopia. Epilepsy Res. 2014;108:547–54.
417. Patil AA, Andrews R, Torkelson R. Minimally invasive surgical approach for intractable seizure. Stereotact Funct Neurosurg. 1995;65:86–9. https://doi.org/10.1159/000098902.
418. Nadvornik P, Sramka M. Longitudinal hippocampectomy. A new stereotaxic approach to the gyrus hippocampi. Confin Neurol. 1975;37(1–3):245–8.
419. Gonzalez-Martinez J, Vadera S, Mullin J, Enatsu R, Alexopoulos AV, Patwardhan R, Bingaman W, Najm I. Robot-assisted stereotactic laser ablation in medically intractable epilepsy: operative technique. Neurosurgery. 2014;10(Suppl 2):167–72; discussion 172–3. https://doi.org/10.1227/NEU.0000000000000286.
420. Wu C, Boorman DW, Gorniak RJ, Farrell CJ, Evans JJ, Sharan AD. The effects of anatomic variations on stereotactic laser amygdalohippocampectomy and a proposed protocol for trajectory planning. Neurosurgery. 2015;11(Suppl. 2):345–56; discussion 356–7.
421. Homma J, Kameyama S, Masuda H, Ueno T, Fujimoto A, Oishi M, et al. Stereotactic radiofrequency thermocoagulation for hypothalamic hamartoma with intractable gelastic seizures. Epilepsy Res. 2007;76:15–21. https://doi.org/10.1016/j.eplepsyres.2007.06.007.
422. Kameyama S, Murakami H, Masuda H, Sugiyama I. Minimally invasive magnetic resonance imaging-guided stereotactic radiofrequency thermocoagulation for epileptogenic hypothalamic hamartomas. Neurosurgery. 2009;65:438–49.
423. Kuzniecky RI, Guthrie BL. Stereotactic surgical approach to hypothalamic hamartomas. Epileptic Disord. 2003;5:275–80.
424. Wellmer J, Kopitzki K, Voges J. Lesion focused stereotactic thermo-coagulation of focal cortical dysplasia IIB: A new approach to epilepsy surgery? Seizure. 2014;23:475–9.
425. Bourdillon P, Rheims S, Catenoix H, et al. Surgical techniques: stereoelectroencephalography-guided radiofrequency thermocoagulation (SEEG-guided RF-TC). Eur J Epilepsy. 2019; https://doi.org/10.1016/j.seizure.2019.01.021.
426. Guénot M, Isnard J, Ryvlvlin P, Fischer C, Mauguiere F, Sindou M. SEEG-guided RF thermocoagulation of epileptic foci: feasibility, safety, and preliminary results. Epilepsia. 2004;45:1368–74.
427. Bourdillon P, Isnard J, Catenoix H, Montavont A, Rheims S, Ryvlin P, et al. Stereo electroencephalography-guided radiofrequency thermocoagulation (SEEG-guided RF-TC) in drug-resistant focal epilepsy: results from a 10-year experience. Epilepsia. 2017;58:85–93. https://doi.org/10.1111/epi.13616.
428. Chipaux M, Taussig D, Dorfmuller G, Dorison N, Tisdall MM, Boyd SG, Thornton R, Eltze C, Fohlen M, Cross HJ, Ferrand-Sorbets S. SEEG-guided radiofrequency thermocoagulation of epileptic foci in the paediatric population: feasibility, safety and efficacy. Seizure. 2019;70:63–70. https://doi.org/10.1016/j.seizure.2019.07.004.
429. Fan X, Shan Y, Lu C, et al. Optimized SEEG-guided radiofrequency thermocoagulation for mesial temporal lobe epilepsy with hippocampal sclerosis. Eur J Epilepsy. 2019;71:304–11.
430. Bourdillon P, Cucherat M, Isnard J, Ostrowsky-Coste K, Catenoix H, Guénot M, et al. SEEG-guided radiofrequency thermocoagulations in patients with focal epilepsy: a systematic review and meta-analysis. Epilepsia. 2018;59(12):2296–304.
431. Dimova P, de Palma L, Job-Chapron AS, et al. Radiofrequency thermocoagulation of the seizure-onset zone during stereoelectroencephalography. Epilepsia. 2017;58(3):381–92.
432. Catenoix H, Bourdillon P, Guénot M, Isnard J. The combination of stereo-EEG and radiofrequency ablation. Epilepsy Res. 2018;142:117–20.
433. Kalina M, Lisck R, Vojtech Z, Adámková E, Procházka T, Marecková I, et al. Stereotactic amygdalohippocampectomy for temporal lobe epilepsy: promising results in 16 patients. Epileptic Disord. 2007;9(Suppl 1):S68–74. https://doi.org/10.1684/epd.2008.0158.
434. Liscak R, Malikova H, Kalina M, Vojtech Z, Prochazka T, Marusic P, et al. Stereotactic radiofrequency amygdalohippocampectomy in the treatment of mesial temporal lobe epilepsy. Acta Neurochir (Wien). 2010;152:1291–8.
435. Malikova H, Vojtech Z, Liscak R, Prochazka T, Vymazal J, Vladyka V, et al. Stereotactic radiofrequency amygdalohippocampectomy for the treatment of mesial temporal lobe epilepsy: correlation of MRI with clinical seizure outcome. Epilepsy Res. 2009;83:235–42. https://doi.org/10.1016/j.eplepsyres.2008.11.013.
436. Patil AA, Andrews R, Torkelson R. Stereotactic volumetric radiofrequency lesioning of intracra-

nial structures for control of intractable seizures. Stereotact Funct Neurosurg. 1995;64:123–33.
437. Malikova H, Liscak R, Vojtech Z, Prochazka T, Vymazal J, Vladyka V, et al. Stereotactic radiofrequency amygdalohippocampectomy: does reduction of entorhinal and perirhinal cortices influence good clinical seizure outcome? Epilepsia. 2011;52:932–40. https://doi.org/10.1111/j.1528-1167.2011.03048.
438. Vojtech Z, Kramska L, Malikova H, Seltenreichova K, Prochazka T, Kalina M, et al. Cognitive outcome after stereotactic amygdalohippocampectomy. Seizure. 2012;21:327–33. https://doi.org/10.1016/j.seizure.2012.02.008.
439. Vojtech Z, Malikova H, Kramska L, Anyz J, Syrucek M, Zamecnik J, et al. Long-term seizure outcome after stereotactic amygdalohippocampectomy. Acta Neurochir (Wien). 2014;156:1529–37. https://doi.org/10.1007/s00701-014-2126-5.
440. Malikova H, Kramska L, Liscak R, Vojtech Z, Prochazka T, Mareckova I, et al. Stereotactic radiofrequency amygdalohippocampectomy for the treatment of temporal lobe epilepsy: do good neuropsychological and seizure outcomes correlate with hippocampal volume reduction? Epilepsy Res. 2012;102:34–44. https://doi.org/10.1016/j.eplepsyres.2012.04.017.
441. Malikova H, Kramska L, Vojtech Z, Lukavsky J, Liscak R. Stereotactic radiofrequency amygdalohippocampectomy: two years of good neuro-psychological outcomes. Epilepsy Res. 2013;106:423–32. https://doi.org/10.1016/j.eplepsyres.2013.07.009.
442. Cossu M, Fuschillo D, Cardinale F, Castana L, Francione S, Nobili L, et al. Stereo-EEG-guided radio-frequency thermo-coagulations of epileptogenic grey-matter nodular heterotopy. J Neurol Neurosurg Psychiatry. 2014;85:611–7.
443. Wu Z, Zhao Q, Tian Z, Zhang J, Xiao X, Lin H, et al. Efficacy and safety of a new robot-assisted stereotactic system for radiofrequency thermocoagulation in patients with temporal lobe epilepsy. Exp Ther Med. 2014;7:1728–32. https://doi.org/10.3892/etm.2014.1620.
444. Malikova H, Kramska L, Vojtech Z, Sroubek J, Lukavsky J, Liscak R. Relationship between remnant hippocampus and amygdala and memory outcomes after stereotactic surgery for mesial temporal lobe epilepsy. Neuropsychiatr Dis Treat. 2015;11:2927–33. https://doi.org/10.2147/NDT.S95497.
445. Lee C-Y, Li H-T, Wu T, et al. Efficacy of limited hippocampal radiofrequency thermocoagulation for mesial temporal lobe epilepsy. J Neurosurg. 2018; https://doi.org/10.3171/2018.4.JNS184.
446. Blume WT, Parrent AG, Kaibara M. Stereotactic amygdalohippocampotomy and mesial temporal spikes. Epilepsia. 1997;38:930–6.
447. Yang W-D, Yu Q, Zhang J-N, Shen C-H, Wang F-L, Cui L-Y, et al. [Stereotactic combined amygdala and hippocampus lesions for treatment of medial temporal lobe epilepsy]. Zhonghua Wai Ke Za Zhi. 2005;43:616–9. https://doi.org/10.3760/j.issn.0529-5815.2005.09.019.
448. Kameyama S, Shirozu H, Masuda H, Ito Y, Sonoda M, Akazawa K. MRI-guided stereotactic radiofrequency thermocoagulation for 100 hypothalamic hamartomas. J Neurosurg. 2016;124:1503–12.
449. Gollwitzer S, Valente I, Rodionov R, Scott C, Ritter LM, Wehner T, Hamer HM, Bartolomei F, Diehl B. Visual and semiautomated evaluation of epileptogenicity in focal cortical dysplasias—an intracranial EEG study. Epilepsy Behav. 2016;58:69–75.
450. Wagner J, Urbach H, Niehusmann P, von Lehe M, Elger CE, Wellmer J. Focal cortical dysplasia type IIb: completeness of cortical, not subcortical, resection is necessary for seizure freedom. Epilepsia. 2011;52:1418–24.
451. Cossu M, Fuschillo D, Casaceli G, Pelliccia V, Castana L, Mai R, et al. Stereoelectroencephalography-guided radiofrequency thermocoagulation in the epileptogenic zone: a retrospective study on 89 cases. J Neurosurg. 2015;123:1358–67. https://doi.org/10.3171/2014.12.JNS141968.
452. Schmitt FC, Voges J, Buentjen L, Woermann F, Pannek HW, Skalej M, Heinze HJ, Ebner A. Radiofrequency lesioning for epileptogenic periventricular nodular heterotopia: a rational approach. Epilepsia. 2011;52:101–5.
453. Grewal SS, Tatum WO. Laser thermal ablation in epilepsy. Expert Rev Neurother. 2019; https://doi.org/10.1080/14737175.2019.1650642.
454. Heppner F. Experiences with the $CO_2$ laser in surgery of the nervous system. Zentralbl Neurochir. 1979;40:297–301, 303–4.
455. Rossomoff HL, Carroll F. Reaction of neoplasm and brain to laser. Arch Neurol. 1966;14(2):143–8.
456. Ryan RW, Spetzler RF, Preul MC. Aura of technology and the cutting edge: a history of lasers in neurosurgery. Neurosurg Focus. 2009;27(3):E6.
457. Stellar SPT, Bredemeier HC. Lasers in surgery. In: Wolbarsht ML, editor. Laser applications in medicine and biology, vol. 2. New York: Springer; 1974. p. 241–93.
458. Curry DJ, Gowda A, McNichols RJ, Wilfong AA. MR-guided stereotactic laser ablation of epileptogenic foci in children. Epilepsy Behav. 2012;24:408–14.
459. Karsy M, Guan J, Ducis K, Bollo RJ. Emerging surgical therapies in the treatment of pediatric epilepsy. Transl Pediatr. 2016;5:67–78.
460. Kelly PJ, Sharbrough FW, Kall BA, Goerss SJ. Magnetic resonance imaging-based computer-assisted stereotactic resection of the hippocampus and amygdala in patients with temporal lobe epilepsy. Mayo Clin Proc. 1987;62:103–8.
461. Lewis EC, Weil AG, Duchowny M, Bhatia S, Ragheb J, Miller I. MR-guided laser interstitial thermal therapy for pediatric drug-resistant lesional epilepsy. Epilepsia. 2015;56:1590–8.
462. Sugiyama K, Sakai T, Fujishima I, Ryu H, Uemura K, Yokoyama T. Stereotactic interstitial laser-hyperthermia using Nd-YAG laser. Stereotact Funct Neurosurg. 1990;55:501–5.

463. Tovar-Spinoza Z, Carter D, Ferrone D, Eksioglu Y, Huckins S. The use of MRI-guided laser-induced thermal ablation for epilepsy. Childs Nerv Syst. 2013;29:2089–94.
464. Buckley RT, Wang AC, Miller JW, Novotny EJ, Ojemann JG. Stereotactic laser ablation for hypothalamic and deep intraventricular lesions. Neurosurg Focus. 2016;41:E10. https://doi.org/10.3171/2016.7.FOCUS16236.
465. Buckley R, Estronza-Ojeda S, Ojemann JG. Laser ablation in pediatric epilepsy. Neurosurg Clin N Am. 2016;27:69–78.
466. Bettag M, Ulrich F, Schober R, Fürst G, Langen KJ, Sabel M, et al. Stereotactic laser therapy in cerebral gliomas. Acta Neurochir Suppl (Wien). 1991;52:81–3.
467. Fujishima I, Ryu H, Uemura K, Sakai T, Nakajima S, Sugiyama K, et al. Experimental study of deep brain radiation with the Nd-YAG laser: a possible new treatment for deep-seated brain tumor. Neurol Med Chir (Tokyo). 1986;26:621–7.
468. Kahn T, Bettag M, Ulrich F, Schwarzmaier HJ, Schober R, Furst G, et al. MRI-guided laser-induced interstitial thermotherapy of cerebral neoplasms. J Comput Assist Tomogr. 1994;18: 519–32.
469. Medvid R, Ruiz A, Komotar RJ, Jagid JR, Ivan ME, Quencer RM, et al. Current applications of MRI-guided laser interstitial thermal therapy in the treatment of brain neoplasms and epilepsy: a radiologic and neurosurgical overview. AJNR Am J Neuroradiol. 2015;36:1998–2006.
470. Sakai T, Fujishima I, Sugiyama K, Ryu H, Uemura K. Interstitial laserthermia in neurosurgery. J Clin Laser Med Surg. 1992;10:37–40.
471. Salem U, Kumar VA, Madewell JE, et al. Neurosurgical applications of MRI guided laser interstitial thermal therapy (LITT). Cancer Imaging. 2019;19:65. https://doi.org/10.1186/s40644-019-0250-4.
472. Patel P, Patel NV, Danish SF. Intracranial MR-guided laser-induced thermal therapy: single-center experience with the visualase thermal therapy system. J Neurosurg. 2016;125:853–60.
473. Sundararajan SH, Belani P, Danish S, Keller I. Early MRI characteristics after MRI-guided laser-assisted cingulotomy for intractable pain control. AJNR Am J Neuroradiol. 2015;36:1283–7.
474. Li K, Vakharia VN, Sparks R, et al. Optimizing trajectories for cranial laser interstitial thermal therapy using computer-assisted planning: a machine learning approach. Neurotherapeutics. 2019;16(2):182–91.
475. Shimamoto S, Wu C, Sperling MR. Laser interstitial thermal therapy in drug-resistant epilepsy. Curr Opin Neurol. 2019;32(2):237–45. https://doi.org/10.1097/WCO. PMID:30694919
476. LaRiviere MJ, Gross RE. Stereotactic laser ablation for medically intractable epilepsy: the next generation of minimally invasive epilepsy surgery. Front Surg. 2016; https://doi.org/10.3389/fsurg.2016.00064.
477. Gross RE, Stern MA, Willie JT, Fasano RE, Saindane AM, Soares BP, et al. Stereotactic laser amygdalohippocampotomy for mesial temporal lobe epilepsy. Ann Neurol. 2018;83:575–87.
478. Hoppe C, Witt J-A, Helmstaedter C, et al. Laser interstitial thermotherapy (LiTT) in epilepsy surgery. Seizure. 2017;48:45–52.
479. Hoppe C, Witt J-A, Helmstaedter C, Gasser T, Vatter H, Elger C-E. Stereotaktische Laserthermokoagulation in der Epilepsiechirurgie. Nervenarzt. 2017; https://doi.org/10.1007/s00115-017-0283-5.
480. Hoppe C, Helmstaedter C. Laser interstitial thermotherapy (LiTT) in pediatric epilepsy surgery. Seizure. 2018; https://doi.org/10.1016/j.seizure.2017.04.002.
481. Abel TJ, Kawasaki H, Barrash J. Naming and recognition after laser amygdalohippocampotomy: is the hippocampus involved? Epilepsia. 2015;56:1317.
482. Attiah MA, Paulo DL, Danish SF, Stein SC, Mani R. Anterior temporal lobectomy compared with laser thermal hippocampectomy for mesial temporal epilepsy: a threshold analysis study. Epilepsy Res. 2015;115:1–7.
483. Drane DL, Loring DW, Voets NL, Price M, Ojemann JG, Willie JT, et al. Better object recognition and naming outcome with MRI-guided stereotactic laser amygdalohippocampotomy for temporal lobe epilepsy. Epilepsia. 2015;56:101–13.
484. Dredla BK, Lucas JA, Wharen RE, Tatum WO. Neurocognitive outcome following stereotactic laser ablation in two patients with MRI-/PET+ mTLE. Epilepsy Behav. 2016;56:44–7.
485. Gross RE, Mahmoudi B, Riley JP. Less is more: novel less-invasive surgical techniques for mesial temporal lobe epilepsy that minimize cognitive impairment. Curr Opin Neurol. 2015;28:182–91.
486. Gross RE, Willie JT, Drane DL. The role of stereotactic laser amygdalohippocampotomy in mesial temporal lobe epilepsy. Neurosurg Clin N Am. 2016;27:37–50.
487. Jobst BC. Equal but different? MRI-guided stereotactic laser amygdalohippocampectomy and traditional temporal lobe surgery. Epilepsy Curr. 2015;15:250–2.
488. Kang JY, Wu C, Tracy J, Lorenzo M, Evans J, Nei M, et al. Laser interstitial thermal therapy for medically intractable mesial temporal lobe epilepsy. Epilepsia. 2016;57:325–34.
489. Meng Y, Suppiah S, Mansouri A. Journal club: real-time magnetic resonance-guided stereotactic laser amygdalohippocampotomy for mesial temporal lobe epilepsy. Neurosurgery. 2015;77:307–9.
490. Waseem H, Osborn KE, Schoenberg MR, Kelley V, Bozorg A, Cabello D, et al. Laser ablation therapy: an alternative treatment for medically resistant mesial temporal lobe epilepsy after age 50. Epilepsy Behav. 2015;51:152–7.
491. Willie JT, Laxpati NG, Drane DL, Gowda A, Appin C, Hao C, et al. Real-time magnetic resonance-guided stereotactic laser amygdalohippocampotomy for mesial temporal lobe epilepsy. Neurosurgery. 2014;74:569–84; discussion 584.

492. Jermakowicz WJ, Kanner AM, Sur S, Bermudez C, D'Haese PF, Kolcun JP, et al. Laser thermal ablation for mesiotemporal epilepsy: analysis of ablation volumes and trajectories. Epilepsia. 2017;58(5):801–10.
493. Youngerman BE, Oh JY, Anbarasan D, et al. Laser ablation is effective for temporal lobe epilepsy with and without mesial temporal sclerosis if hippocampal seizure onsets are localized by stereoelectroencephalography. Epilepsia. 2018;59:595–606.
494. Donos C, Breier J, Friedman E, et al. Laser ablation for mesial temporal lobe epilepsy: surgical and cognitive outcomes with and without mesial temporal sclerosis. Epilepsia. 2018;59:1421–32.
495. Grewal SS, Zimmerman RS, Worrell G, et al. Laser ablation for mesial temporal epilepsy: a multi-site, single institutional series. J Neurosurg. 2018; https://doi.org/10.3171/2018.2.JNS171873.
496. Grewal SS, Alvi MA, Lu VM, et al. Magnetic resonance-guided laser interstitial thermal therapy versus stereotactic radiosurgery for medically intractable temporal lobe epilepsy: a systematic review and meta-analysis of seizure outcomes and complications. World Neurosurg. 2018; https://doi.org/10.1016/j.wneu.2018.08.227.
497. Tao JX, Wu S, Lacy M, Rose S, Issa NP, Yang CW, et al. Stereotactic EEG-guided laser interstitial thermal therapy for mesial temporal lobe epilepsy. J Neurol Neurosurg Psychiatry. 2018;89:542–8.
498. Vakharia VN, Sparks R, Kuo L, et al. Automated trajectory planning for laser interstitial thermal therapy (LiTT) in mesial temporal lobe epilepsy. Epilepsia. 2018;59(4):814–24.
499. Wu C, Jermakovicz WJ, Chakravorti S, et al. Effects of surgical targeting in laser interstitial thermal therapy for mesial temporal lobe epilepsy: a multicenter study of 234 patients. Epilepsia. 2019;60(6):1171–83.
500. Radhakrishnan A, Menon R, Thomas SV, Abraham M, Vilanilam G, Kesavadas C, et al. "Time is Brain"—how early should surgery be done in drug-resistant TLE? Acta Neurol Scand. 2018;138:531–40.
501. Sun Z, Zuo H, Yuan D, Sun Y, Zhang K, Cui Z, et al. Predictors of prognosis in patients with temporal lobe epilepsy after anterior temporal lobectomy. Exp Ther Med. 2015;10:1896–902.
502. Ellis JA, Mejia Munne JC, Wang SH, McBrian DK, Akman CI, Feldstein NA, et al. Staged laser interstitial thermal therapy and topectomy for complete obliteration of complex focal cortical dysplasias. J Clin Neurosci. 2016;31:224–8.
503. Sperling MR, Gross RE, Alvarez GE, et al. Stereotactic laser ablation for mesial temporal lobe epilepsy: a prospective, multicenter, single-arm study. Epilepsia. 2020; https://doi.org/10.1111/epi.16529.
504. Drane DL. MRI-guided stereotactic laser ablation for epilepsy surgery: promising preliminary results for cognitive outcome. Epilepsy Res. 2018;142:170–5.
505. Brandmeir N, Acharya V, Sather M. Robot assisted stereotactic laser ablation for a radiosurgery resistant hypothalamic hamartoma. Cureus. 2016;8:e581.
506. Burrows AM, Marsh WR, Worrell G, Woodrum DA, Pollock BE, Gorny KR, et al. Magnetic resonance imaging-guided laser interstitial thermal therapy for previously treated hypothalamic hamartomas. Neurosurg Focus. 2016;41:E8.
507. Rolston JD, Chang EF. Stereotactic laser ablation for hypothalamic hamartoma. Neurosurg Clin N Am. 2016;27:59–67.
508. Wilfong AA, Curry DJ. Hypothalamic hamartomas: optimal approach to clinical evaluation and diagnosis. Epilepsia. 2013;54(Suppl. 9):109–14.
509. Wright JM, Staudt MD, Alonso A, et al. A novel use of the NeuroBlate SideFire probe for minimally invasive disconnection of a hypothalamic hamartoma in a child with gelastic seizures. J Neurosurg Pediatr. 2018;21:302–7.
510. Zubkov S, Del Bene VA, MacAllister WS, Shepherd TM. Disabling amnestic syndrome following stereotactic laser ablation of a hypothalamic hamartoma in a patient with a prior temporal lobectomy. Epilepsy Behav Case Rep. 2015;4:60–2.
511. Curry DJ, Raskin J, Ali I, Wilfong AA. MR-guided laser ablation for the treatment of hypothalamic hamartomas. Epilepsy Res. 2018;142:131–4.
512. Xu DS, Chen T, Hlubek RJ, et al. Magnetic resonance imaging-guided laser interstitial thermal therapy for the treatment of hypothalamic hamartomas: a retrospective review. Neurosurgery. 2018;83:1183–92.
513. Boerwinkle VL, Foldes ST, Torrisi SJ, et al. Subcentimeter epilepsy surgery targets by resting state functional magnetic resonance imaging can improve outcomes in hypothalamic hamartoma. Epilepsia. 2018;59(12):2284–95.
514. Clarke DF, Tindall K, Lee M, Patel B. Bilateral occipital dysplasia, seizure identification, and ablation: a novel surgical technique. Epileptic Disord. 2014;16:238–43.
515. Devine IM, Burrell CJ, Shih JJ. Curative laser thermoablation of epilepsy secondary to bottom-of-sulcus dysplasia near eloquent cortex. Seizure. 2016;34:35–7.
516. Thompson SA, Kalamangalam GP, Tandon N. Intracranial evaluation and laser ablation for epilepsy with periventricular nodular heterotopia. Seizure. 2016;41:211–6.
517. Dadey DY, Kamath AA, Leuthardt EC, Smyth MD. Laser interstitial thermal therapy for subependymal giant cell astrocytoma: technical case report. Neurosurg Focus. 2016;41:E9.
518. McCracken DJ, Willie J, Fernald BA, Saindane AM, Drane DL, Barrow DL, et al. Magnetic resonance thermometry-guided stereotactic laser ablation of cavernous malformations in drug-resistant epilepsy: imaging and clinical results. Oper Neurosurg. 2016;12:39–48.
519. Hawasli AH, Bagade S, Shimony JS, Miller-Thomas M, Leuthardt EC. Magnetic resonance imaging-guided focused laser interstitial thermal therapy for intracranial lesions: single-institution series. Neurosurgery. 2013;73:1007–17.

520. Hawasli AH, Bandt SK, Hogan RE, Werner N, Leuthardt EC. Laser ablation as treatment strategy for medically refractory dominant insular epilepsy: therapeutic and functional considerations. Stereotact Funct Neurosurg. 2014;92:397–404.
521. Cobourn K, Fayed I, Keating RF, Oluigbo CO. Early outcomes of stereoelectroencephalography followed by MR-guided laser interstitial thermal therapy: a paradigm for minimally invasive epilepsy surgery. Neurosurg Focus. 2018;45:1–9.
522. Jolesz FA, Hynynen K, McDannold N, Tempany C. MR imaging-controlled focused ultrasound ablation: a noninvasive image-guided surgery. Magn Reson Imaging Clin N Am. 2005;13(3): 545–60.
523. McDannold N, Clement GT, Black P, Jolesz F, Hynynen K. Transcranial magnetic resonance imaging-guided focused ultrasound surgery of brain tumors: initial findings in 3 patients. Neurosurgery. 2010;66:323–32.
524. Elias WJ, Huss D, Voss T, Loomba J, Khaled M, Zadicario E, et al. A pilot study of focused ultrasound thalamotomy for essential tremor. N Engl J Med. 2013;369:640–8.
525. Krishna V, Sammartino F, Cosgrove R, et al. Predictors of outcomes after focused ultrasound thalamotomy. Neurosurgery. 2019; https://doi.org/10.1093/neuros/nyz417.
526. Martin E, Jeanmonod D, Morel A, Zadicario E, Werner B. High-intensity focused ultrasound for noninvasive functional neurosurgery. Ann Neurol. 2009;66:858–61.
527. McDonell J, Patel N, Fischer G, et al. Robotic assisted MRI-guided interventional Interstitial MR guided focused ultrasound ablation in a swine model. Neurosurgery. 2018; https://doi.org/10.1093/neuros/nyy266.
528. Parker WE, Weidman EK, Chazen JL, et al. Magnetic resonance–guided focused ultrasound for ablation of mesial temporal epilepsy circuits: modeling and theoretical feasibility of a novel noninvasive approach. J Neurosurg. 2019; https://doi.org/10.3171/2019.4.JNS182694.
529. Ranjan M, Boutet A, Bhatia S, et al. Neuromodulation beyond neurostimulation for epilepsy: scope for focused ultrasound. Expert Rev Neurother. 2019; https://doi.org/10.1080/14737175.2019.1635013.
530. Foley JL, Little JW, Vaezy S. Effects of high-intensity focused ultrasound on nerve conduction. Muscle Nerve. 2008;37(2):241–50.
531. Lipsman N, Meng Y, Bethune AJ, et al. Blood-brain barrier opening in Alzheimer's disease using MR-guided focused ultrasound. Nat Commun. 2018;9(1):2336.
532. Leksell L. The stereotactic method and radiosurgery of the brain. Acta Chir Scand. 1951;102:316–9.
533. Leksell L. Stereotactic radiosurgery in trigeminal neuralgia. Acta Chir Scand. 1971;137:311–4.
534. Leksell L. Stereotaxis and radiosurgery. An operative system. Springfield, IL: Thomas CC; 1971.
535. Talairach J, Bancaud J, Szikla G, et al. Approche nouvelle de la neurochirurgie de l´épilepsie. Méthodologie stéréotaxique et résultants thérapeutiques. Neurochirurgie. 1974;20:92–8.
536. Heikkinen ER, Konnov B, Melnikow L. Relief of epilepsy by radiosurgery of cerebral arteriovenous malformations. Stereotact Funct Neurosurg. 1989;53:157–66.
537. Rogers L, Morris H, Lupica K. Effect of cranial irradiation on seizure frequency in adults with low-grad astrocytoma and medically intractable epilepsy. Neurology. 1993;43:1599–601.
538. Rossi G, Scerrati M, Roselli R. Epileptogenic cerebral low grade tumors: effect of interstitial stereotactic irradiation on seizures. Appl Neurophysiol. 1985;48:127–32.
539. Steiner L, Lindquist C, Adler J, Torner J, Alves W, Steiner M. Clinical outcome of radiosurgery for cerebral arteriovenous malformations. J Neurosurg. 1992;77:1–8.
540. Lindquist C, Kilström L, Hellstrand E. Functional neurosurgery—a future for the Gamma Knife? Stereotact Funct Neurosurg. 1991;57:72–81.
541. Whang CJ, Kwon Y. Long-term follow-up of stereotactic Gamma Knife radiosurgery in epilepsy. Stereotact Funct Neurosurg. 1996;66:349–56.
542. Barcia Salorio JL, Roldan P, Hernandez G, et al. Radiosurgery treatment of epilepsy. Appl Neurophysiol. 1985;48:400–3.
543. Gaffey CT, Monotoya V, Lyman J, et al. Restriction of the spread of epileptic discharges in cats by mean of Bragg Peak intracranial irradiation. Int J Appl Radiat Isot. 1981;32:779–87.
544. Chen ZF, Kamiryo T, Henson SL, et al. Anticonvulsant effects of gamma surgery in a model of chronic spontaneous limbic epilepsy in rats. J Neurosurg. 2000;94:270–80.
545. Maesawa S, Kondziolka D, Dixon C, et al. Subnecrotic stereotactic radiosurgery controlling epilepsy produced by kainic acid injection in rats. J Neurosurg. 2000;93:1033–40.
546. Mori Y, Kondziolka D, Balzer J, et al. Effects of stereotactic radiosurgery on an animal model of hippocampal epilepsy. Neurosurgery. 2000;46:157–65.
547. Boström JP, Delev D, Quesada C, Widman G, Vatter H, Elger CE, Surges R. Low-dose radiosurgery or hypofractionated stereotactic radiotherapy as treatment option in refractory epilepsy due to epileptogenic lesions in eloquent areas—preliminary report of feasibility and safety. Seizure. 2016;36:57–62.
548. Quigg M, Rolston J, Barbaro NM. Radiosurgery for epilepsy: clinical experience and potential antiepileptic mechanisms. Epilepsia. 2012;53(1):7–15.
549. Régis J, Carron R, Park M. Is radiosurgery a neuromodulation therapy? A 2009 Fabrikant award lecture. J Neurooncol. 2010;98(2):155–62.
550. Barbaro NM, Quigg M, Broshek DK, Ward MM, Lamborn KR, Laxer KD, Larson DA, Dillon W, Verhey L, Garcia P, Steiner L, Heck C, Kondziolka D, Beach R, Olivero W, Witt TC, Salanova V,

Goodman R. A multicenter, prospective pilot study of gamma knife radiosurgery for mesial temporal lobe epilepsy: seizure response, adverse events, and verbal memory. Ann Neurol. 2009;65:167–75. https://doi.org/10.1002/ana.21558.
551. Barbaro NM, Quigg M, Ward MM, et al. Radiosurgery versus open surgery for mesial temporal lobe epilepsy: The randomized, controlled ROSE trial. Epilepsia. 2018;59(6):1198–207.
552. Feng E-S, Sui C-B, Wang T-X, Sun G-L. Stereotactic radiosurgery for the treatment of mesial temporal lobe epilepsy. Acta Neurol Scand. 2016;134(6):442–51.
553. Régis J, Rey M, Bartolomei F, et al. Gamma knife surgery in mesial temporal lobe epilepsy: a prospective multicenter study. Epilepsia. 2004;45:504–15.
554. Chang EF, Quigg M, Oh MC, Dillon WP, Ward MM, Laxer KD, Broshek DK, Barbaro NM. Predictors of efficacy after stereotactic radiosurgery for medial temporal lobe epilepsy. Neurology. 2010;74:165–72. https://doi.org/10.1212/WNL.0b013e3181c9185d.
555. Quigg M, Broshek DK, Barbaro NM, Ward MM, Laxer KD, Yan G, et al. Neuropsychological outcomes after Gamma Knife radiosurgery for mesial temporal lobe epilepsy: a prospective multicenter study. Epilepsia. 2011;52:909–16.
556. Régis J, Bartolomei F, Chauvel P. Radiosurgery. In: Baltuch GH, Villemure J-G, editors. Operative techniques in epilepsy surgery. New York: Thieme; 2009. p. 187–96.
557. Rheims S, Didelot A, Guénot M, Régis J, Ryvlin P. Subcontinuous epileptiform activity after failed hippocampal radiosurgery. Epilepsia. 2011;52:1425–9.
558. Arita K, Kurusi K, Iida K, Hanaya R, Akimitsu T, Hibino S, Pant B, Hamasaki M, Shinagawa S. Subsidence of seizure induced by stereotactic radiation in a patient with hypothalamic hamartoma. J Neurosurg. 1998;89:645–8.
559. Régis J, Bartolomei F, de Toffol B, et al. Gamma knife surgery for epilepsy related to hypothalamic hamartomas. Neurosurgery. 2000;47:1343–51.
560. Régis J, Bartolomei F, Rey M, Hayashi M, Chauvel P, Peragut J. Gamma knife surgery for mesial temporal lobe epilepsy. J Neurosurg. 2000;93:141–6.
561. Régis J, Hayashi M, Eupierre LP, et al. Gamma knife surgery for epilepsy related to hypothalamic hamartomas. Acta Neurochir. 2004;91(Suppl):33–50.
562. Schulze-Bonhage A, Homberg V, Trippel M, et al. Interstitial radiosurgery in the treatment of gelastic epilepsy due to hypothalamic hamartomas. Neurology. 2004;62:644–7.
563. Gazzola DM, Balcer LJ, French JA. Seizure-free outcome in randomized add-on trials of the new antiepileptic drugs. Epilepsia. 2007;48:1303–7. https://doi.org/10.1111/j.1528-1167.2007.01136.x.
564. Kwan P, Brodie MJ. Early identification of refractory epilepsy. N Engl J Med. 2000;342:314–9. https://doi.org/10.1056/NEJM200002033420503.
565. Kwan P, Sperling MR. Refractory seizures: try additional antiepileptic drugs (after two have failed) or go directly to early surgery evaluation? Epilepsia. 2009;50(Suppl 8):57–62. https://doi.org/10.1111/j.1528-1167.2009.02237.x.
566. Thom M, Mathern GW, Cross JH, Bertram EH. Mesial temporal lobe epilepsy: how do we improve surgical outcome? Ann Neurol. 2010;68:424–34. https://doi.org/10.1002/ana.22142.
567. Wiebe S, Blume WT, Girvin JP, Eliasziw M. A randomized, controlled trial of surgery for temporal-lobe epilepsy. N Engl J Med. 2001;345:311–8. https://doi.org/10.1056/NEJM200108023450501.
568. Hauser WA. Status epilepticus: epidemiologic considerations. Neurology. 1990;40:9–13.
569. Dibué-Adjeia M, Kamp MA, Vonck K. 30 years of vagus nerve stimulation trials in epilepsy: do we need neuromodulation-specific trial designs? Epilepsy Res. 2019;153:71–5.
570. Suthana N, Haneef Z, Stern J, et al. Memory enhancement and deep-brain stimulation of the entorhinal area. N Engl J Med. 2012;366:502–10.
571. Elger CE, Mormann F. Seizure prediction and documentation—two important problems. Lancet Neurol. 2013;12:531–2.
572. Morris GL, Gloss D, Buchhalter J, Mack KJ, Nichels K, Harden C. Evidence-based guidline update: vagus nerve stimulation for the treatment of epilepsy. Neurology. 2013;81:1453–9.
573. Morrell M, Hirsch L, Bergey G, Barkley G, Wharen R, Murro A, Fisch B, Rossi M, Labar D, Duckrow R, Sirven J, Drazkowski J, Worrell G, Gwinn R. Long-term safety and efficacy of the RNS™ system in adults with medically intractable partial onset seizures. Epilepsia. 2008;49:480.
574. Grinenko O, Li J, Mosher JC, Wang IZ, Bulacio JC, Gonzalez-Martinez J, Nair D, Najm I, Leahy RM, Chauvel P. A fingerprint of the epileptogenic zone in human epilepsies. Brain. 2018;141(1):117–31.
575. Wolf A, Naylor K, Tam M. Risk of radiation-associated intracranial malignancy after stereotactic radiosurgery: a retrospective, multicentre, cohort study. Lancet Oncol. 2019;20(1):159–64.

# Complications 15

*Wise men learn by others' harms; fools by their own*

*Benjamin Franklin*

## Contents



Detailed and accurate knowledge of the potential complications is of paramount importance both for a counseling surgical candidate during the decision-making process as well as for development of strategies identifying and avoiding these risks. However, comparison between the reported complication rates is rendered difficult due to different surgical techniques, pathologies, and cohorts (children/adults) encountered in the respective series. Furthermore, some aspects of outcome like cognitive functions are not addressed at all in many publications [1].


J. Zentner, *Surgical Treatment of Epilepsies*, https://doi.org/10.1007/978-3-030-48748-5_15

Moreover, differences in complication rates may be related to the study methodology, e.g., whether data are obtained retrospectively or prospectively. In addition, data on adverse effects may differ between high- and low-volume epilepsy centers, thus depending on the data base used [2, 3]. The most obvious problem comparing different series, however, refers to the definition of a complication and the grading system used. In all, data provided on complications both for diagnostic and therapeutic procedures in epilepsy surgery noticeably vary between different institutions and do not necessarily reflect the objective outcome of the patients.

## 15.1 Definition

Although there is no generally accepted definition of complications after epilepsy surgery, most authors define a complication as an unexpected, unwanted, and uncommon event associated with either a diagnostic or therapeutic procedure [1, 4–6]. This definition includes that homonymous hemianopia after occipital lobe resection is not regarded as a complication since this event is expected and inevitable. Similarly, postoperative disturbances such as headaches, nausea, minor CSF leakage, and slightly increased temperatures after implantation of subdural electrodes should not be considered as complications but rather as side effects since all of them commonly occur after such procedures. However, it is still open for discussion, whether transient events like dysnomia, weakness, or numbness of an extremity or aseptic meningitis that resolve within the usual range of hospitalization should be counted as complications or as acceptable side effects.

Most authors differ between surgical (e.g., infection, pneumonia, deep vein thrombosis, etc.) and neurological (e.g., hemiparesis, aphasia, cranial nerve deficit, etc.) complications. However, a generally accepted grading system assessing the impact of complications on daily life in the short and long run does not exist. Different classifications have been suggested. Severity scales from 1 to 4 [7], or from 1 to 5 [8] have been used. Others use terms such as minor or major complications [6], which roughly correspond to the terms transient and permanent morbidity [4, 9]. However, the cutoff between minor and major complications, or transient and permanent morbidity (e.g., severity, duration) is individually defined by every author [1, 4–6, 10, 11].

## 15.2 Diagnostic Procedures

Invasive diagnostic procedures mainly include implantation of subdural strip, grid, and depth electrodes. The numbers of electrodes implanted vary noticeably, and frequently different electrode types are used in combination. Thus, different implantation schemes are used dependent on the requirements of the individual patient. Complications of diagnostic procedures are reported either in summary or regarding specific electrode types.

### 15.2.1 Overall Complication Rates

Using various combinations of strip, grid, and depth electrodes, complications rates between 3.6% and 23% have been reported mainly causing temporary morbidity [2, 3, 8, 12, 13], while permanent morbidity is low [14–16], and mortality is extremely rare [17, 18]. Behrens et al. [4] found in a series comprising 279 invasive diagnostic procedures a transient morbidity of 3.6% (2.9% surgical, and 0.7% neurological complications), and a permanent morbidity of 0.7%. Evaluating 242 patients of the Swedish National Epilepsy Register, Rydenhag and Silander [6] noted 6.3% minor complications (infection: 1.9%; hematoma: 3.4%; dislocation: 1.0%). Wellmer et al. [8] reported a total complication rate of 23%, and 9% required surgical revision, all without permanent morbidity. Evaluating extraoperative ECoG studies in 177 patients of the National Surgical Quality Improvement Program (NSQI) database, Rolston et al. [2] noted an overall complication rate of 11.9% (major complications 3.4%, minor complications 8.5%). Spencer [16] reported an incidence of 1% major complications. Comparing complications of subdural and depth electrodes in 260 procedures, Tandon et al. [19] found symptomatic hemorrhages in 5% and infections in 2.2% of 139 subdural electrode implantations, while no symptomatic adverse effect occurred in the 121 SEEG procedures.

#### 15.2.1.1 Hemorrhage

In a literature review, Pilcher et al. [12] reported a 2.5% hemorrhage rate in 1582 patients. Tebo et al. [13] found in a 32-year systematic review (1980–2012) and meta-analysis comprising 23 articles and 2467 patients bleeding complications in 3.2%. The complication rate rose from 1.9% in 1980–1995 to 4.2% in 1996–2012 [13]. Similar hemorrhage rates between 2% and 4% have been reported in other series [6, 12, 20–23].

#### 15.2.1.2 Infections

Infections have been reported to range between 0.8% and 12% [4, 5, 22, 24, 25]. Tebo et al. [13] found in his meta-analysis comprising 2467 patients infections in 3.4%. Infection rates increased from 2.3% in 1980–1995 to 4.3% in 1996–2012 [13]. In a literature review including 867 cases from 14 different institutions, van Buren [23] noted an infection rate of 1.3%. Some small studies reported no infections [20, 26]. Overall, infections vary between 1% and 5% in most series [12, 14, 15, 23, 26–31].

#### 15.2.1.3 Neurological Deficits

The meta-analysis of Tebo et al. [13] comprising 2467 patients reported neurological deficits in 4.3% of diagnostic procedures. Neurological complications decreased from 6.3% in 1980–1995 to 3.0% in 1996–2012. Persistent deficits were noted in 0.5% of patients [13].

### 15.2.2 Subdural Electrodes

#### 15.2.2.1 Mortality

Arya et al. [17] noted in their meta-analysis of 2542 patients receiving grid electrodes 5 deaths (0.2%). Reviewing the literature, there is no mortality attributable to invasive monitoring with subdural strip electrodes.

#### 15.2.2.2 Morbidity

Complications with subdural strip and grid electrodes reported range between 0% and 48.9% [7, 26, 32–34]. Morbidity referring to infection and hemorrhage mainly ranges between 2% and 5% for strip electrodes [2, 3, 35, 36] and between 10 and 15% for implantation of grids [8, 17].

**Strips and Grids**

In two publications, complication rates including transient and permanent morbidity of 26% [7] and 48.9% [33] have been reported. Hamer et al. [5] noted a complication rate of 26.3%, mainly related to infections. Others reported complication rates of 11% [37], 7.7% [38], 5.9% [36], 3.9% [35], 3.4% [2], and 0.85% [25]. Swartz et al. [39] noted in a prospective study only minor adverse effects without infections or hematomas, while others did not encounter any complications [26, 32, 34].

**Grids**

Grid electrodes carry a higher risk for complications compared to strip or depth electrodes [5, 8]. Hematomas were found in 16% in the series of Wellmer et al. [8], predominantly between dura and grid, and occasionally under the grid. Malow et al. [40] noted infections and epidural hematomas in 19%. Van Gompel et al. [41] documented in their cohort of 189 grid implantations major complications in 6.6%. In a meta-analysis comprising 21 studies and a total of 2542 patients with subdural grid electrodes, Arya et al. [17] noted the following complication rates: Infections (5.3%), hemorrhage (4.0%), and elevated intracranial pressure (2.4%). A total of 3.5% of complicated cases required surgical revision [17]. Figs. 15.1, 15.2, and 15.3 demonstrate typical hemorrhagic complications with subdural grids.

### 15.2.3 Depth Electrodes

#### 15.2.3.1 Mortality

In a meta-analysis comprising 33 studies including 2959 patients, Garcia-Lorenzo et al. [18] noted 6 deaths (0.2%). Two deaths (1.4%) from intracerebral hemorrhage have been reported by

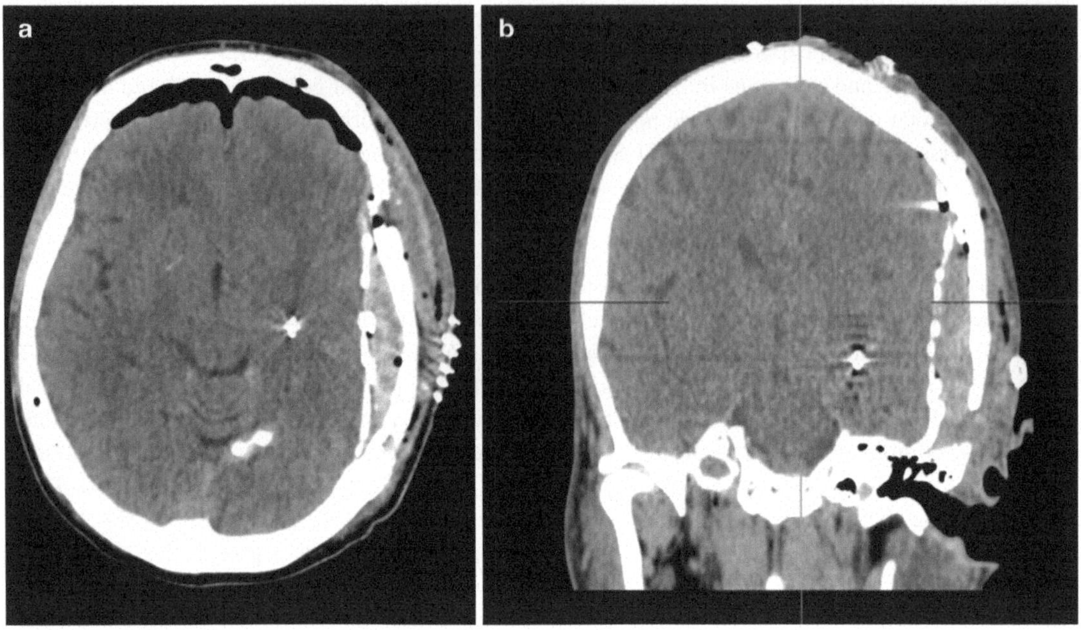


**Fig. 15.1** Implantation of a subdural grid electrode (8 × 8 cm) left temporo-parietal and a depth electrode to the long axis of the left hippocampus in a 55-year-old male patient. Axial (**a**) and coronal (**b**) CT scans at the first postoperative day show a space-occupying epidural hematoma which had been evacuated

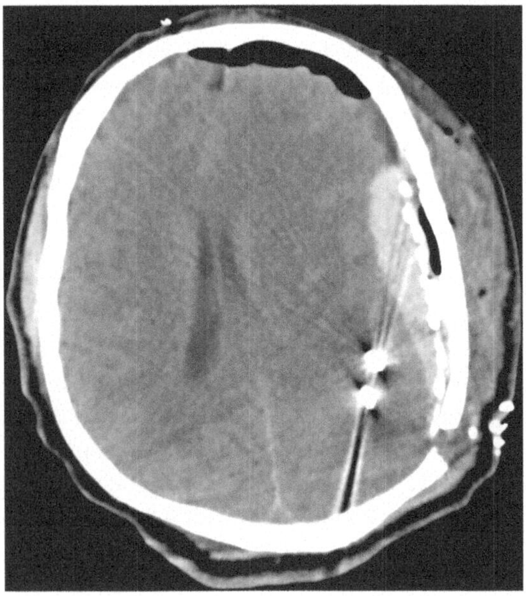

**Fig. 15.2** Implantation of a subdural grid electrode (8 × 8 cm) and depth electrode left temporo-parietal in a 42-year-old male. CT scan (axial view) at the first postoperative day shows a large subdural hematoma below the grid electrode which has been evacuated

Engel et al. [42] in a series of 140 patients. An exceptional report of two deaths from Creutzfeldt-Jakob disease acquired from reused depth electrodes has been provided by Bernoulli et al. [43] which caused exact regulations on sterilization procedures. Others noted mortality rates of 0.3% [44] and 0.13% [45]. The overall reported mortality with depth electrodes is far below 1% [18, 26–28, 44].

#### 15.2.3.2 Morbidity

Hemorrhage and infections are the most frequent complications with the use of depth electrodes and have been reported in most series between 1% and 3% [44–47]. Reviewing 57 articles including 2959 patients, Garcia-Lorenzo et al. [18] reported a permanent morbidity rate of 1.3%. Bottan et al. [48] did not encounter any morbidity in 50 patients who underwent robot-assisted insular depth electrode implantations.

##### Hemorrhage

The reported risk of hemorrhage following stereotactic placement of depth electrodes ranges from 0.5% to 4.4% [1, 12, 23, 30, 42, 47, 49–51]. Talairach et al. [30] noted 3 bleeding complications in 560 patients (0.5%). Pilcher et al. [12]

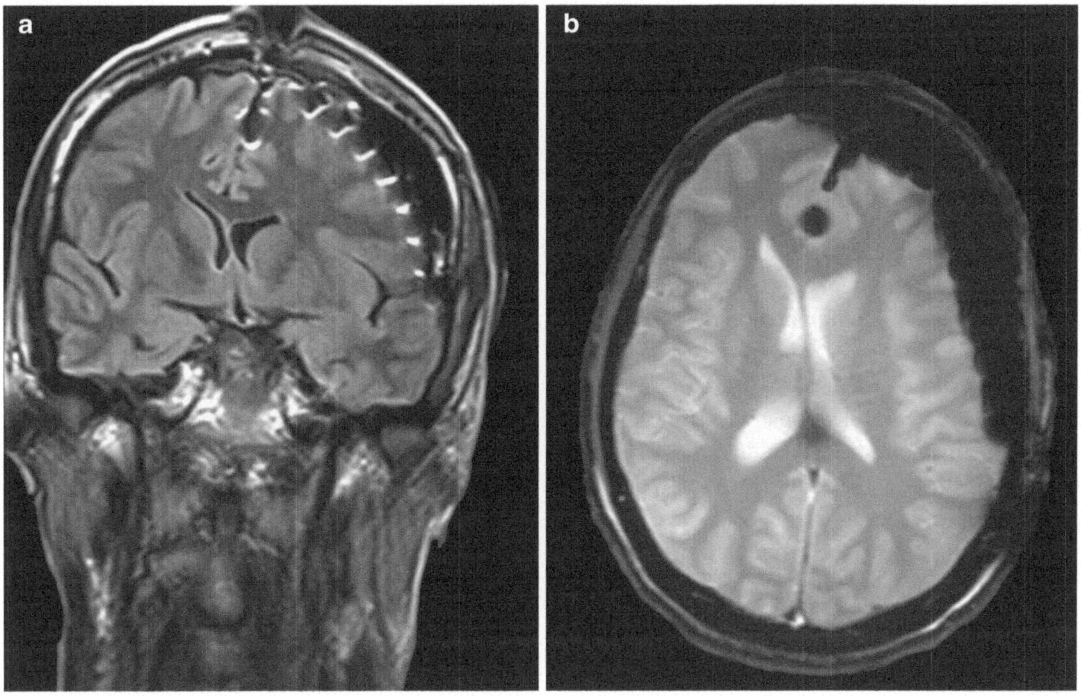


**Fig. 15.3** Implantation of a subdural grid electrode (8 × 8 cm) and multiple strip electrodes over the left frontal convexity and the interhemispheric fissure in a 21-year-old male. MRI scans in coronal (**a**) and axial (**b**) view show a left frontolateral subdural hematoma over the grid which has been evacuated

reported a 2.5% rate of hemorrhage in 1582 patients. Analyzing the MNI series, Tanriverdi et al. [1] found in 491 patients undergoing frameless stereotactic electrode placement hematomas in 0.8%. In van Buren's literature review comprising 879 depth electrode implantations, hemorrhage was observed in 2.7% [23]. Willems et al. [50] noted asymptomatic beedings in 2.8% in their own series and up to 4.4% in the literature. The authors emphasized systematic CT imaging after electrode explantation [50]. Others reported hemorrhage rates of 2.5% [42], 1.4% [49], and 1.0% [44]). Overall, hemorrhagic complications after depth electrode implantation are observed in the range of 1%–2%.

### Infections

Infections after depth electrode implantation have been found in 1–5% of patients. Meningitis was most common, while brain abscess rarely occurred [12, 14, 15, 23, 26–30, 49, 51]. In van Buren's literature review comprising 879 depth electrode implantations, infections were observed in 1.4% [23]. A total of 3022 depth electrode implantations in 217 patients reported by the MNI group encountered infections in 1.8% [27, 52]. Mullin et al. [44] noted an infection rate of 0.8%. In all, morbidity due to infections amounts to 1%–2%.

### Cognitive Function

Analyzing 16 patients, Ljung et al. [53] described significant loss in verbal memory after bilateral implantation of depth electrodes in the longitudinal axis of the hippocampus. Stimulated by this report, Helmstaedter et al. [54] studied the effect of this implantation scheme on cognitive functions in 31 patients. Memory was assessed before implantation, after explantation, and 3 months after left/right temporal lobe surgery. After explantation of depth electrodes, memory performance had significantly dropped in 60%–70% of the right temporal and in 52%–67% of the left temporal cases. After resective surgery, significant recovery from post-implantation impairment was found in right temporal patients, while left temporal resection patients stayed on the level seen after explantation and did not recover. Although surgery has its own effects in addition to the implantation, the results raise concerns as to the implantation of depth electrodes along the long axis in a functionally intact hippocampus. The authors suggest to either restrict implantation to the most likely affected hippocampus or to change to an orthogonal approach perpendicular to the long axis of the hippocampus [54].

#### Miscellaneous

Miscellaneous complications (electrodes pulled out, break of electrode lead, small areas of infarction, headaches, CSF leakage, urinary tract infection, etc.) were observed in 4.5% in a total of 3022 depth electrode implantations in 217 patients [27, 52].

### 15.2.4 Risk Factors

The following risk factors for complications with diagnostic procedures have been identified: The use of *grid electrodes,* the *total number of implanted electrode contacts*, the *number of burrholes and/or trephinations,* longer *duration of implantation*, *medication affecting blood coagulation* such as valproate, and *pediatric age* [1, 8, 17, 55]. Moreover, the *surgical technique*, the use of *antibiotics*, and *surveillance* of patients during the monitoring phase may influence the complication rate [6]. Others found that the *occipital/parieto-occipital* implantation site [8], and a *higher age* [6] are associated with an increased risk for complications.

#### 15.2.4.1 Grids

A study based on the Swedish National Epilepsy Register analyzing 271 patients showed complications in 4.8% with strips and depths, but in 7.4% with grids [55]. Similarly, higher complication rates with grids of up to 19% as compared to strips and depths have been reported by others [4, 5, 8, 40]. Arya et al. [17] noted in their meta-analysis 5 deaths (0.2%) with grid electrodes.

#### 15.2.4.2 Number of Electrodes and Electrode Contacts

Tanriverdi et al. [1] showed that risk of intracranial hemorrhage and infection increased with increasing number of electrodes per lobe and the number of lobes covered. In a prospective study, the infection rate was shown to increase if more than 100 electrode contacts were used, and if more than ten electrode cables were present [56].

#### 15.2.4.3 Duration of Implantation

Wiggins et al. [56] showed an increased infection rate if electrodes remained implanted for more than 14 days. Wellmer et al. [8] noted that the total number of complications decreased from 33% (1980–1991) to 19% (1992–1997). Pronounced decrease was seen in the rate of infections, which dropped from 18% to 6% over those time periods. Decrease of complications was thought to be correlated with a shorter monitoring period (median 13 versus 9 days) [8].

#### 15.2.4.4 Antibiotics

The low rate of infections as observed in many studies has been attributed to the use of antibiotics throughout the monitoring period [12, 14, 15, 23, 26–31, 49]. Wyler et al. [25] reported a prospective trial including 350 patients who received subdural strip electrodes. Patients were divided into two groups: one group received antibiotics intravenously during the entire period of implantation, while the other group received a single dose of antibiotics at the time of surgery. Overall infection rate was 0.9%. There were no significant differences between the two groups, and it was concluded that there was no benefit to continuing administration of antibiotics during the entire period of implantation [25]. In line with this report, most centers only use single shoot antibiosis at the time of surgery [4, 6, 12, 23, 57–60], while others do not recommend the use of antibiotics at all [1].

#### 15.2.4.5 Medication Affecting Blood Coagulation

Treatment with valproic acid may induce thrombocytopenia which seems to be dose-dependent with a negative correlation between valproic acid blood levels and platelet counts [61]. Although several studies have found no evidence that patients on valproate treatment are at an increased risk of surgical bleeding complications [62, 63], it has been recommended to stop medication with valproic acid prior to major invasive diagnostic interventions [1]. Hedegärd et al. [55] found that the ratio of subdural hematomas was slightly increased under valproate treatment. However, there was no permanent morbidity or mortality [55].

#### 15.2.4.6 Pediatric Age

Hader et al. [64] noted 7.7% minor complications, and 0.6% major complications with invasive monitoring in the pediatric age. Permanent morbidity was 0.3%. The rate of minor complications was higher in pediatric patients compared to adults (23.5% and 4.1%, respectively) [64].

**Concluding Remarks**

- ***Morbidity/mortality.*** *Extraoperative invasive EEG recordings are associated with complication rates of 1–3% with the use of depth electrodes, 2–5% with subdural strip electrodes, and 10–15% using grid electrodes, mainly referring to infections and hemorrhage. Mortality associated with grids and depths is far below 1%, and no mortality has been reported for strips. Depth electrode implantation along the long axis of a functionally intact hippocampus has been shown to cause decline of memory performance in approximately half of patients irrespective of the side of implantation.*
- ***Risk factors.*** *The use of grid electrodes, the total number of electrode contacts, and the number of burr holes and/or trephinations should be considered as risk factors when planning the implantation scheme. Cables of subdural electrodes should be tunneled away from the dural entrance point to avoid CSF leakage and infections. Skin incision for electrode placement should take into account the skin incision required for the expected therapeutic procedure. As practiced in most neurosurgical procedures, a single shoot antibiotic prophylaxis seems to be adequate. Weighing risks up to benefits, medication with valproic acid and aspirin should be stopped when extensive electrode implantations are planned.*
- ***Postoperative surveillance.*** *Patients should be adequately surveilled after implantation. Progressive tiredness and/or attenuation of EEG signals with subdural recordings are highly suspicious for bleeding complications.*

## 15.3 Resective Therapeutic Procedures

Resective therapeutic procedures include temporal, extratemporal, and insular resections, as well as reoperations. As with diagnostic interventions, complications are reported either in summary or in more detail considering specific procedures.

### 15.3.1 Overall Complication Rates

#### 15.3.1.1 Mortality

Mortality reported for temporal end extratemporal resective procedures ranges between 0% and 3.3% in different series [4, 6, 12, 23, 57, 58, 60, 65, 66]. Analyzing 475 adult patients of the US National Surgical Quality Improvement Program (NSQIP) providing a stringent surveillance including low-volume centers, Rolston et al. [3] found a mortality rate of 3.4%. Mortality rate in the report of Rydenhag and Silander [6] was 0.3%, while others did not encounter any fatality [4, 65, 66]. Overall, mortality in resective epilepsy surgery ranges between 1% and 3%.

When looking at surgical mortality, one must consider that patients with refractory epilepsy suffer from an increased risk of death, primarily due to seizure-related fatalities including sudden unexpected death (SUDEP). It has been suggested for temporal lobe epilepsy that successful surgery reduces the risk of death to that observed in the normal population [67, 68]. Thus, epilepsy surgery appears to have a positive impact on mortality, even when taking into account the risk of surgery-related fatalities [67]. However, others have failed to replicate these findings, or found no differences in the overall mortality and SUDEP rates between operated and medically treated patients [69, 70].

#### 15.3.1.2 Morbidity

The 2015 Cochrane review reported an overall complication rate of 7.3% for temporal end extra-temporal procedures [71]. Hader et al. [64] reviewing 76 articles noted minor surgical complications in 5.1%, and major surgical complications 1.5% of the patients. Minor neurological complications were encountered in 10.9% (children: 11.2%; adults: 5.5%), and major neurological complications in 4.7%. Overall, temporary morbidity caused by surgical and neurological complications amounted to 16.0%, and permanent morbidity to 6.2%. The complication rate was higher in extra-temporal as compared to temporal location as well as in children as compared to adults [64]. Rolston et al. [3] noted in 475 surgical procedures a complication rate of 17.9%. Presenting the national Swedish multicenter study comprising 449 therapeutic interventions, Rydenhag and Silander [6] reported minor complications in 6.3%, and major complications in 3.1% of patients. In a prospective Swedish study of 865 procedures, the rate of major adverse events was 3%, and that of minor adverse events 7.5% [72]. Gooneratne et al. [65] noted in a single institution study comprising 911 procedures an overall complication rate of 17%, with long-term new neurologic deficits in 3%, and Inoue et al. [73] reported a 5.1% rate of serious complications in 157 resective procedures. A retrospective analysis of a multi-institutional surgical registry including data between 2006 and 2014 demonstrated a noticeable reduction of morbidity for resective surgery over the years [74]. In sum complication rates of resective therapeutic procedures mainly range between 10% and 15% including a permanent morbidity of 3–6%.

##### Neurological Complications

At the MNI, neurological complications were encountered in 3.2% of 2449 surgical procedures, mainly related to hemiparesis and dysphasia [1]. Behrens et al. [4] found in 429 therapeutic procedures neurological complications in 5.4% (3.1% transient morbidity, and 2.3% permanent morbidity). Neurological morbidity reported from pediatric series range between 6.3% and 10% [59, 60]. Overall, in most series neurological complications range between 3% and 5% in adults and between 5% and 10% in children and adolescents [1, 4, 6, 23, 59, 60, 65].

##### Infections

Hader et al. [64] reviewing 76 articles found an infection rate of 3.0% (3.9% in children versus 1.9% in adults). In the MNI series comprising 2449 procedures in 1905 patients, infections were observed in 0.7% [75]. The Bonn group reported in a series of 708 procedures meningitis in 1.4% and bone flap infections in 3.5% [4]. In a Swedish multicenter study comprising 446 operations, infection rate was 5.3% [6]. Others reported infection rates of around 15% [7, 73], while Ventureyra and Higgins [60] did not find any infections in 47 pediatric patients. Overall, the infection rate in most larger series amounts to 3–4% [4, 6, 64].

##### Hemorrhage

In their review of 76 articles, Hader et al. [64] noted intracranial hematomas in 2.5% (4.0% in children versus 2.0% in adults). The MNI series comprising 2449 procedures encountered a hemorrhage rate of 0.9% [75]. Gooneratne et al. [65] found hematomas in 0.3%, while Ventureyra and Higgins [60] did not observe any hemorrhage in 47 children and adolescents.

##### Miscellaneous

The MNI report on 2449 patients includes CSF leak in 8.5% (14.3% in children, 4.3% in adults), aseptic meningitis in 3.6% (5.8% in children, 3.4% in adults), and deep vein thrombosis and pulmonary embolism in 3.6% [1]. Gooneratne et al. [65] found CSF leak in 1.2%, and hydrocephalus in 0.3%.

#### 15.3.1.3 Risk Factors

Gooneratne et al. [65] found a fourfold higher risk for infections (7.9%) with the use of *subdural EEG monitoring prior to resection*. The study of Hader et al. [64] reviewing 76 articles showed a higher complication rate in *children* as compared to adults both for infections (3.9% versus 1.9%) and hemorrhage (4.0% versus 2.0%). In contrast, dÓrio et al. [77] analyzing a cohort of 1282 patients operated in the pediatric and adult age, noted a severely complicated course in 7.8% for all cases, in 6.4% for children but in 8.6% for adult patients. While several authors have identified *older age* as a risk factor [3, 4, 6, 59, 60, 66, 72, 75, 78], others did not find differences in adverse events rates for individuals younger or older than 50 years [79, 80]. *ASA (American Society of Anesthesiologists) grades 2 and 3* of patients and the presence of *preoperative bleeding disorders* have been identified as risk factors by Rolston et al. [2, 3]. It should be emphasized that several studies have shown significantly higher mortality and morbidity rates in *low surgical volume hospitals* as compared to high-volume institutions, thus indicating a volume-outcome relationship [2, 3, 81, 82].

## 15.3.2 Temporal Resections

Specific complications with temporal resections refer to structures of the temporomesial area leading to *visual field deficits* by damage to Meyer's loop of the geniculocalcarine tract or the optic tract, *hemiparesis* due to manipulation of the anterior choroid artery or the lentriculostriate arteries, *oculomotor nerve palsy* with dissection of the crural cistern, and *neuropsychological deficits* caused by removal of limbic structures. In addition, *Wernicke's language area* may be endangered with temporodorsal resections.

A complication of supratentorial surgery, which in particular is known to occur after temporal resections for epilepsy is *cerebellar foliar hemorrhage*. This complication represents an increasingly recognized entity running a typical course (Fig. 15.4). The clinical symptoms are often mild and transient; however, even fatal outcomes have been described [83–85]. König et al. [84] were the first to mention that reduction of intracranial pressure enforced by a subgaleal suction drain may cause hemorrhage. Yoshida et al. [86] suggested a venous origin of hemorrhage since hematomas are mainly found bilaterally in the upper vermis and in the upper cerebellar folia facing the tentorium, where the draining veins of the cerebellar hemispheres are located. Angiography does not reveal any abnormalities [85, 86]. The crucial mechanism of postoperative cerebellar foliar hemorrhage may be a transtentorial pressure gradient. It is thought that the negative supratentorial pressure caused by a subgaleal suction drain reduces the pressure within tentorial and supratentorial veins, whereas the cerebellar venous pressure remains unchanged. Hence, by a suction effect blood is withdrawn from the infratentorial veins draining the upper cerebellum and vermis [87]. In all, postoperative suction drainage leading to major loss of CSF is the most likely cause of this complication.

### 15.3.2.1 Mortality

Rolston et al. [3] reported a mortality rate of 2.1% in 281 temporal lobectomies. The UCLA series noticed one death (0.8%) in 130 temporal resections [42], and in the NIH series 3 of 300 patients (1%) had died [23]. Hader et al. [64] reviewing 76 articles found a perioperative mortality of 0.4%. A large systematic review from Ontario noted mortality rates between 0.1% and 0.5% [88]. Pilcher and Ojemann [89] reported 1 death in 250 patients (0.4%). In a systematic review and meta-analysis of 25 studies including 2842 patients, Brotis et al. [90] reported a mortality rate of 1%. A 32-years systematic review (1980–2012) and meta-analysis comprising 21 articles and 2947 patients [13] did not note any deaths. No mortality was also reported in a previous MNI series of 526 patients [66], in a later MNI series of 1232 temporal patients [1], and in other studies [4, 68, 91, 92]. Overall, mortality in temporal resections is below 1% [4, 12, 13, 23, 42, 91].

### 15.3.2.2 Morbidity

Brotis et al. [90] reported a morbidity rate of 17% summarizing 25 studies including 2842 temporal patients. The complication rate reported by Rolston et al. [3] in 281 temporal lobectomies was 12.1%. Evaluating the relationships between hospital surgical volume and adverse events in US epilepsy centers, Englot et al. [81] found a rate of 6.1% for adverse events at high-volume epilepsy centers, and 12.9% at low-volume centers for temporal lobectomies. Tanriverdi et al. [1] reported a cumulative morbidity of 2.9% due

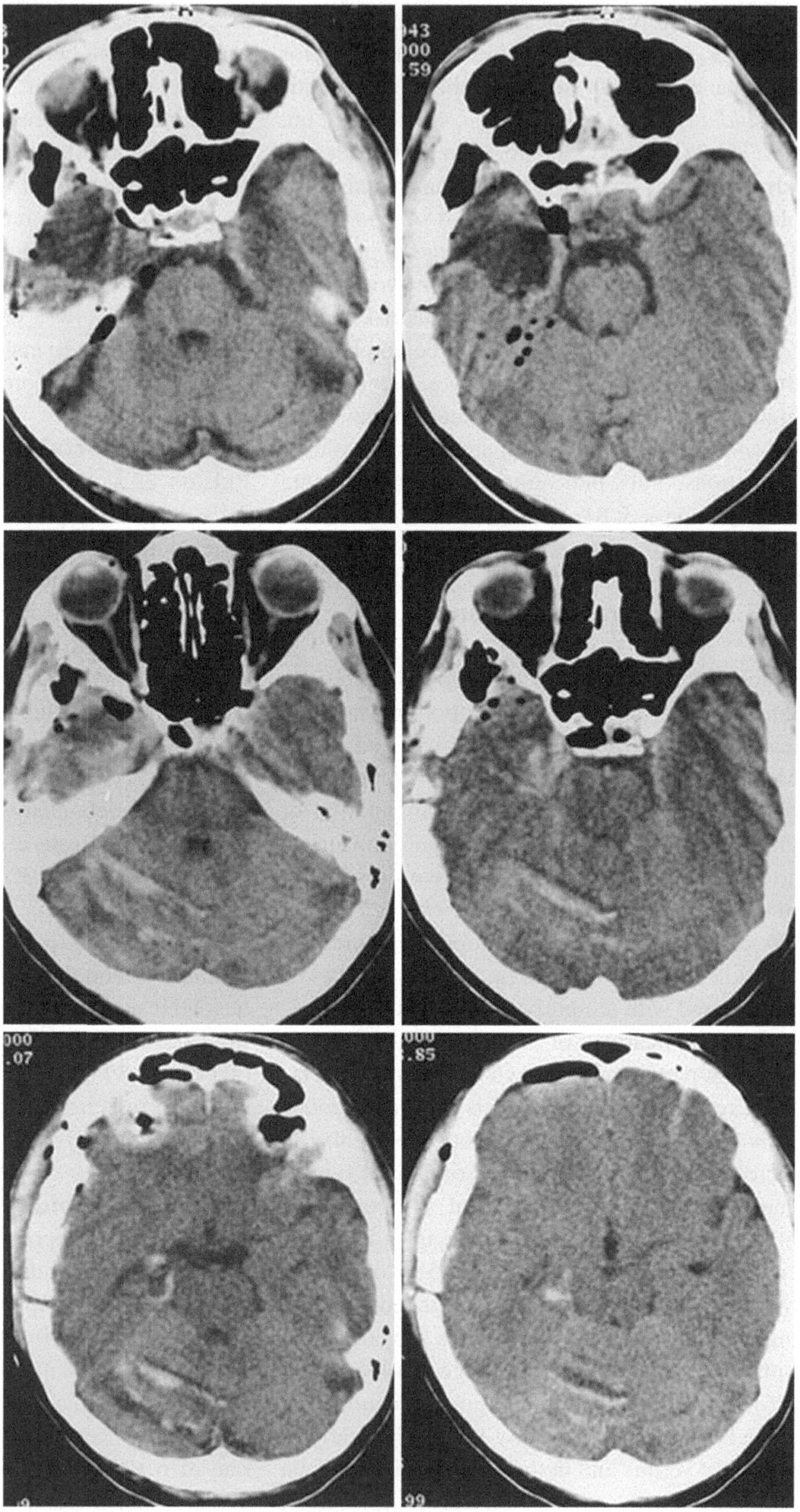

**Fig. 15.4** Cerebellar foliar hemorrhage. Postoperative CT scans after ATL in axial view are shown. Upper sequence (24 min post surgery): Right temporal defect after ATL. There is no evidence of cerebellar hemorrhage. Middle sequence (7 h post surgery): Hemorrhage is seen located within the upper vermis and right cerebellar folia. Lower sequence (27 h post surgery): There is no further increase in cerebellar hemorrhage (from Honneger et al. [87], with permission)

to surgical and neurological complications in the MNI series. The complication rate observed in the Mayo-Clinic accounts for 3.5% [93]. Rydenhag and Silander [6] noted 2.8% major (corresponding to permanent) deficits, and Behrens et al. [4] reported a 2.2% permanent morbidity in temporal resections. Georgiadis et al. [94] evaluated 58 epilepsy surgical reports from 1990 to 2013 including 6 pediatric series. The cumulative morbidity rates varied between 0% and 9.3% [59, 64, 95–100]. Evaluating 458 temporal patients, Schmeiser et al. [101] documented an overall permanent morbidity due to surgical and neurological complications of 4.4%. No statistically significant differences were found comparing different approaches (ATL, keyhole approach, extended lesionectomy, trans-sylvian SAHE, and subtemporal SAHE) [102]. Yasargil et al. [103] did not encounter any significant permanent morbidity in their transsylvian SAHE series. Reviewing a total of 2089 temporal resections in the pediatric age, Ormond et al. [104] noted a complication rate of 9.4% (except for visual field deficits). Similarly, the surgical morbidity in the Bonn pediatric series was 9.8% [104]. In all, the complication rate after temporal resections mainly amounts to 5%–10% at a permanent morbidity of 3%–5%.

#### Infections

The infection rate following temporal lobectomy was 1.4% in Olivier's series [66]. Tanriverdi et al. [1] reporting the later MNI series found infections in 0.5%. In a 32-year systematic review (1980–2012) and meta-analysis comprising 21 articles and 2947 patients with temporal resections, Tebo et al. [13] found wound infections/meningitis in 1.4%, decreasing from 2.5% to 1.1% over years. When implantation of electrodes was required to identify the epileptogenic area, the infection rate increased to 5.8% [13]. Wound infections and meningitis were observed between 1.5% and 8.5% in the literature review of Geogiadis et al. [94] comprising 58 temporal series. In the Freiburg cohort, infection rate was 3.0% [101] which is in line with others [92]. In the Bonn pediatric series, infections occurred in 4.4.% [104]. Brotis et al. [90] noted infections in 3% of 2842 patients. A review of 2089 pediatric temporal resections showed an infection rate of 3.7% [104]. In sum, the infection rate ranges in most series between 2% and 4%.

#### Hemorrhage

In a six-year nationwide survey comprising 182 patients, Koubeissi et al. [21, 105] found hemorrhagic complications in 0.6% after temporal lobectomy. Hemorrhage rate was 0.4% in Olivier's series [66], and 0.3% in the later MNI series[1]. Tebo et al. [13] noted hemorrhage in 1.2% of 2947 temporal patients, and the risk increased to 4.3%, when implantation of electrodes was required. The incidence of hemorrhage was 3% in the series of Sindou et al. [92]. Ormond et al. [104] noted hemorrhage in 1.2% in a series of 2089 pediatric cases, and Brotis et al. [90] in 2% of 2842 patients. Overall, hemorrhagic complications are seen in 1%–2% of temporal cases on the average.

#### Cerebellar Foliar Hemorrhage

After ATL, cerebellar foliar hemorrhage has been observed in 12.9% of patients which is much higher as compared to more limited temporal resections like SAHE [87]. However, most reports do not address this complication.

#### Neurological Complications

In a meta-analysis of 2947 temporal resections, Tebo et al. [13] found neurological complications in 19.3%. Complication rate decreased over time, from 41.8% in 1980–1995 to 5.2% in 1996–2012. Persistent neurological deficits occurred in 3.8%, decreasing from 9.7% to 0.8% between the two time periods [13]. Tanriverdi et al. [1] reporting the MNI series comprising 1232 patients found a neurological morbidity of 1.2%. Rydenhag and Silander [6] found major deficits in 2.8%, and Behrens et al. [4] documented a permanent neurological morbidity of 2.2%. In the pediatric series reviewed by Ormond et al. [104], permanent neurological complications were found in 1.9%. In sum, average permanent neurological morbidity amounts to 1%–2%.

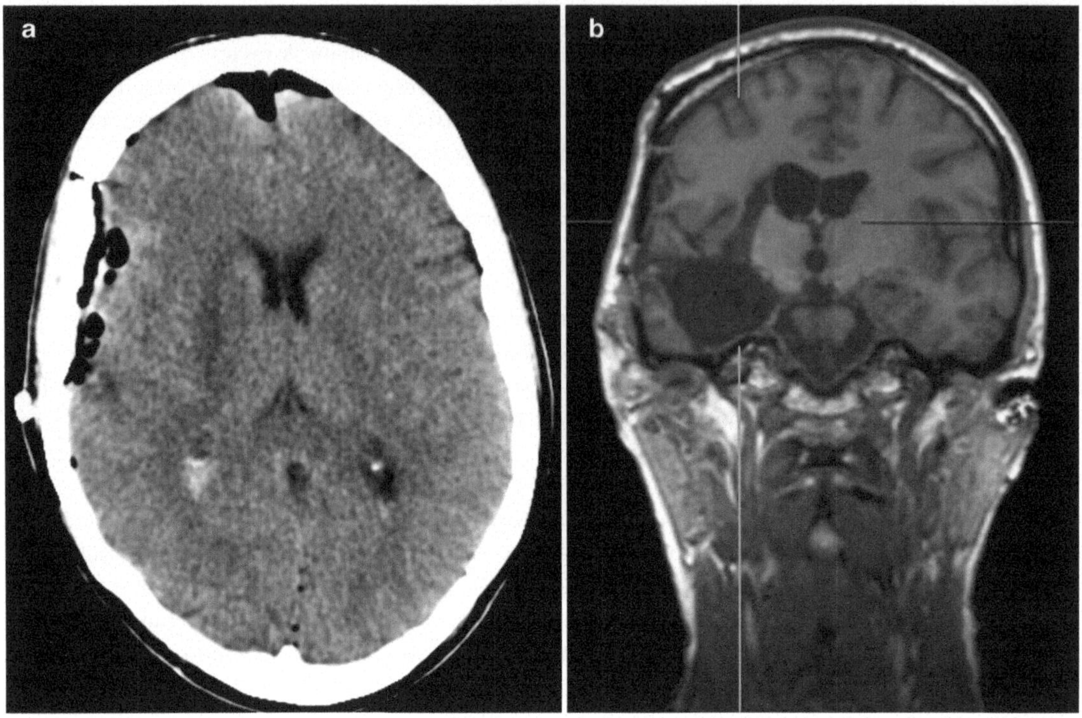


**Fig. 15.5** 50-year-old female patient with a pharmacoresistant epilepsy and a right temporomesial ganglioglioma that had been removed some years ago. Due to recurrent seizures, reoperation with ATL and removal of residual parts of the hippocampal formation has been performed. The postoperative course was complicated by a left hemiparesis. Axial CT scans at one day (**a**) and coronary T1-weighted MRI at 3 months after repeat surgery (**b**) show an infarction in the internal capsule. On follow-up, the patient was able to walk, however, a major hemiparesis persisted

*Hemiparesis*

Hemiparesis or hemiplegia has been reported in 5.7% of temporal resections along with a 2.5% incidence of serious disability in the early MNI era when resection of electrocorticographically abnormal insular cortex was felt to be advantageous [106, 107]. Penfield proposed as mechanisms either vascular manipulation ("manipulation hemiplegia") resulting in spasms or thrombosis of lenticulostriate arteries, or direct injury to the internal capsule during insular resection [106, 108]. Having abandoned insular resections, these complications have no longer been observed in a subsequent MNI series of 550 temporal lobectomies [109, 110]. Postoperative hemiparesis occurred in 8.5% in the series of Kim et al. [59], in 4.3% of patients reported by Erba et al. [95], in 3.1% of patients presented by Sinclair et al. [97], in 3% in the UCLA series [42], in 1.2% in the Freiburg series [101], in 0.9% in the cohort of Salanova et al. [68] and in 1.1% in a pediatric cohort reported by Ormond et al. [104]. Brotis et al. [90] noted in hemiparesis in 4% of 2842 patients. Overall, manipulation of the anterior choroid and lenticulostriate arteries has been thought as the main cause for postoperative hemiparesis [23, 66, 111] (Fig. 15.5).

*Visual Field Deficits (VFD)*

VFD can be divided in superior subquadrantic to quandrantic (minor) and incomplete to complete (major) deficits.

*Minor superior visual field deficits* are quite common. Usually, these deficits are not functionally disabling and not noticed by the patients themselves [112]. Superior subquadrantic or quadrant anopsia has been reported between 0% and 100% of patients [23, 59, 65, 97, 99, 100, 112–

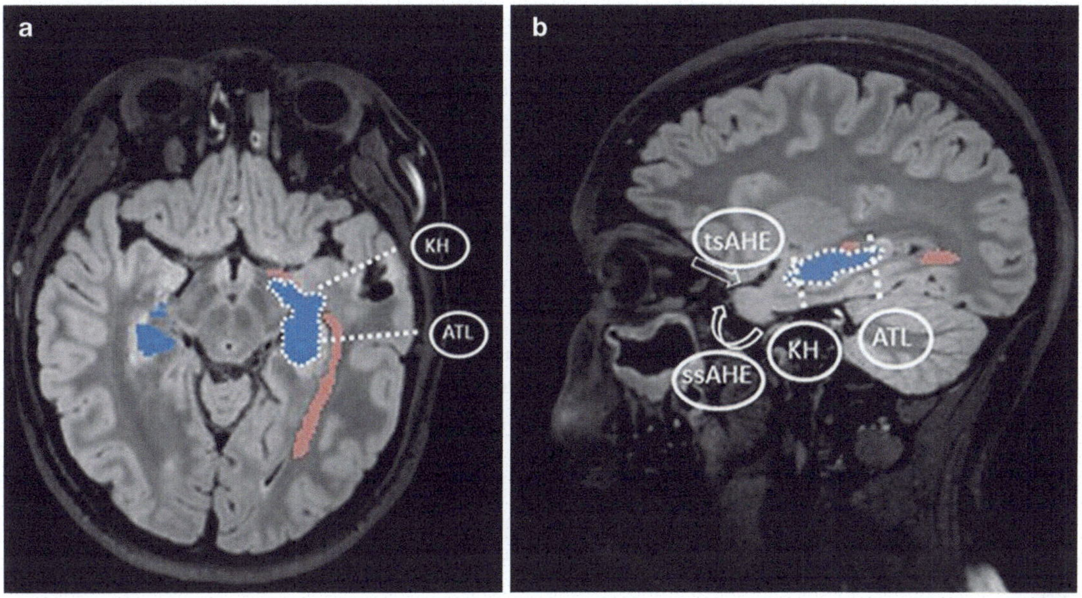


**Fig. 15.6** Depiction of the geniculocalcarine tract (red) in relation to the hippocampus (blue) in a single patient, and schematic representation of lateral resection limits of different approaches (dotted lines) in axial (**a**) and sagittal (**b**) view. ATL: anterior temporal lobectomy; KH: keyhole approach; tSAHE: transsylvian selective amygdalohippocampectomy; sSAHE: subtemporal selective amygdalohippocampectomy. Straight arrow (right image): approach for tSAHE; Bent arrow (right image): approach for sSAHE. According to lateral resection limits, Meyer's loop is most endangered with ATL. However, even with this procedure, visual field deficits may be avoided opening the inferior horn at its lateral and inferior aspects while leaving its proper roof intact (from Schmeiser et al. [140], with permission)

116]. This wide range of minor VFD rather reflects the different attitudes of authors to evaluate them as complications and the perimetry techniques used than their actual occurrence. In a review of 2089 pediatric temporal resections, VFD were noted in 14.4% [104]. In most reports, if noted at all, minor VFD occur in around 50% of temporal resections [4, 6, 12, 60, 89, 104]. Minor superior VFD can be attributed to the interference with Meyer's loop which shows a great variability, and may roughly correlate with extent of opening of the roof of the inferior horn at its superior rather than its lateral aspect [89, 110, 117] (Fig. 15.6).

*Major (incomplete to complete) visual deficits* have been reported in 0.7% in the Bonn cohort [4], in 0.7% in the Freiburg series [102], in 0.5% in van Buren's patients [23], in 0.4% in the Swedish series [6], in 0.4% in the MNI series [1], in 0.4% in Salanova's report [68], and in 0.2% of Gooneratne's patients [65]. Others observed major visual field deficits in 2–4% [12, 60, 95, 96, 112, 117–119]. Brotis et al. [90] found major VFD in 6% of 2842 patients. Similarly, Grivas et al. [78] reported such deficits in 5.8% of cases. In children, incomplete or complete hemianopia was observed in 6.4% by Ormond et al. [104], 4.3% by Erba et al. [95], and in 2.9% by Terra-Bustamente et al. [96]. In sum, major VFD are mainly in the range between 1% and 3% after temporal procedures. Major VFD have been thought to be correlated with larger temporal resections [117, 119] which, however, is not generally accepted [112]. Resection of the superior aspect of the roof of the inferior horn, damage to the optic tract, and ischemic damage to the lateral geniculate body following manipulation of the anterior choroid artery may all contribute to major visual field deficits [89, 111].

In rare cases, visual hallucinations without evidence of epileptic origin known as *Charles Bonnet syndrome* have been observed after resections affecting the optic radiation between the lateral geniculate body and the primary visual cortex. These hallucinations are thought to be generated in the visual association areas [120].

Schmeiser et al. [102] studied in a series of 366 temporal cases frequency and extent of VFD following different surgical approaches with respect to the ability to drive. Overall, postoperative VFD were found in 73% of patients (83% after ATL, 60% with the keyhole approach, 74% after transsylvian SAHE, and 56% after subtemporal SAHE). With respect to the German traffic regulations, driving-relevant VFD were noted in 48% of patients (58% after ATL, 43% with the keyhole approach, 48% with transsylvian SAHE, and 21% with subtemporal SAHE). Thus, the rate of VFD and particularly of driving-relevant VFD seems to be lower with subtemporal SAHE as compared to other approaches which is in line with other reports [121, 122]. However, data on frequency and extent of VFD with selective approaches, in particular with subtemporal SAHE, should be substantiated by higher numbers of cases investigated. Gooneratne et al. [65] noted driving-relevant VFD in only 9.4% of cases.

#### *III Nerve Palsy*

Brotis et al. [90] found III nerve deficits in 3% of 2842 patients, Erba et al. [95] in 2.1%, Tanriverdi et al. [1] in 0.2%, and Gooneratne et al. [65] in 0.1%. Van Buren [23] noted III nerve palsy in rare cases, and in most of them, deficits resolved completely.

#### *Language Disorders*

Language disorders following temporal lobectomy refer to anomic dysphasia. Studies of patients undergoing awake craniotomy with language mapping suggested considerable interpersonal variability of essential language sites [123–126]. However, already Penfield felt that persisting language disorders only occur when resection of the dominant temporal lobe exceeds 5–6 cm [127]. Minor and transient dysphasia was not uncommon in earlier series and has been reported in up to 30% of patients even when operations were performed under local anesthesia with language mapping [23, 128]. It may have been caused by intraoperative retraction of temporodorsal areas and postoperative edema. Minor dysphasia as also observed in a minority of temporal patients in more actual series which, however, resolves within the first postoperative days. Occasionally, patients may complain of a subtle word-finding difficulty persisting for some weeks [89]. Major dysphasia has been observed in 5.7% in the UCLA series [42], in 3.7% of Salanova's patients [68], in 0.8% in the early MNI series [66], in 0.7%, in the Freiburg series [101], in 0.7% of the patients reported by Lopez-Gonzalez et al. [100], and in 0.6% in the later MNI series [1]. Others noted major dysphasia to occur in rare cases [78, 129], while van Buren [23] did not encounter such deficits in any case of the NIH series.

### Neuropsychological Deficits

Neuropsychological impairment related to epilepsy can be caused by the underlying pathology, seizures, interictal epileptic discharges, anti-seizure drugs, and psychiatric comorbidities [130]. Surgery-related neuropsychological deficits mainly refer to deterioration of verbal memory following resection of the dominant temporal lobe, and to visual-spatial (nonverbal) memory after operations in the nondominant temporal lobe [130–135]. Postoperative neuropsychological deterioration has been reported in the range between 6% and 25% with higher risks in patients older than 50 years [78]. Brotis et al. [90] noted in their meta-analysis including 2842 patients postoperative cognitive deficits in 5–7% of cases. Contrarily, a meta-analysis of 22 studies [136] demonstrated a decline in verbal memory in 44% of patients with left temporal resections and in 20% with right temporal resections (see also Chap. 6). Although deficits in verbal memory may be mild, they may be important for patients with jobs dependent on a high functionality [137]. Global memory deficits following dominant temporal lobectomy were noted in 2.2% of patients in the early MNI series [132], in 0.6% in the later MNI series [1], and in 2% of the UCLA series [23].

#### Miscellaneous

Postoperative *hydrocephalus* requiring a shunting procedure occurred in 3.1% in the series of Sinclair et al. [97]. Similarly, Schmeiser et al. [101] observed hydrocephalus in 3.0%, and Sindou et al. [92] in 2% of cases. Although *vasospastic reactions* were observed in the postoperative course after transsylvian SAHE by transcranial doppler ultrasound, the course is usually benign and asymptomatic without the need of triple H-therapy [138]. However, also symptomatic vasospasms have been noted with different approaches [139].

## 15.3.3 Extratemporal Resections

Specific complications with extratemporal resections refer to *primary motor cortex*, the *supplementary motor area (SMA)*, *Broca's language area,* the *primary sensory cortex*, the *temporo-parieto-occipital transition area (angular and supramarginal gyri)*, and the *visual cortex.* Approximately two-thirds of all extratemporal interventions are lesionectomies or extended lesionectomies, while the remaining include lobectomies and multilobectomies.

### 15.3.3.1 Mortality

Rolston et al. [3] noted in 90 lobectomies a mortality rate of 8.9%. Reviewing 76 articles, Hader et al. [64] reported a perioperative mortality in 1.2% of extratemporal procedures. Tebo et al. [13] noted in a meta-analysis of 17 articles and 749 patients a mortality rate of 0.6%. Others did not encounter any mortality [4, 141]. Overall, the mortality rate in extratemporal procedures is in the range of 1%–2%.

### 15.3.3.2 Morbidity

The high variability of complications reported in extratemporal resections ranging between 3% and 55% reflects different topographical relationships of resection zones to eloquent areas and white matter tracts as well as different challenges depending on the type of intervention [4, 142–145]. Most studies report permanent morbidity rates between 10% and 15% for frontal and parietal resections [1, 3, 141, 146–149] and between 30% and 40% for Rolandic resections [142, 150, 151]. Intralobar occipital resections are followed by visual field deficits exceeding superior quadrantanopia in 40%–50% of cases [152–154].

#### Surgical complications

Reviewing 673 patients, Tanriverdi et al. [1] documented morbidity due to surgical complications in 5.4%. Tebo et al. [13] found in their meta-analysis wound infections/meningitis in 3.1%. The infection rate decreased from 5.3% in 1980–1995 to 1.9% in 1996–2012. Moreover, Tebo et al. [13] noted hydrocephalus in 1.6% of extratemporal procedures.

#### Neurological Complications

Neurological complications occurred in the MNI series in 5.6% of extratemporal resections [1]. Rydenhag and Silander [6] found 4.9% major (permanent) deficits. Similarly, Behrens et al. [4] noted a permanent morbidity of 4.3%. In a 32-year meta-analysis comprising 17 articles and 749 patients with extratemporal and multilobar resections, Tebo et al. [13] found neurological deficits in 23.8% of the patients. The total rate of neurological complications decreased over time from 30.2% in 1980–1995 to 19.5% in 1996–2012. Persistent neurological morbidity occurred in 5.2%, decreasing from 9.0% to 3.2% between the two time periods [13].

#### Frontal Resections

Frontal resections are followed by deficits (paresis, dysphasia, abulia, incontinence) in 15%–40% of patients with persistent deficits in 3%–5% [155–157].

#### Rolandic Resections (Fig. 15.7)

Resections in the Rolandic cortex caused postoperative deficits in 41% of patients reported by Pilcher et al. [158]. Van Offen et al. [142] noted additional postoperative deficits in 55% of the individuals. In line with these findings, Pondal-Sardo et al. [150] reporting on 52 cases observed additional deficits in 50%, and Behdad et al. [143] in 42% of their patients. In a review including 280 patients, Ostergard et al. [151] found immediate

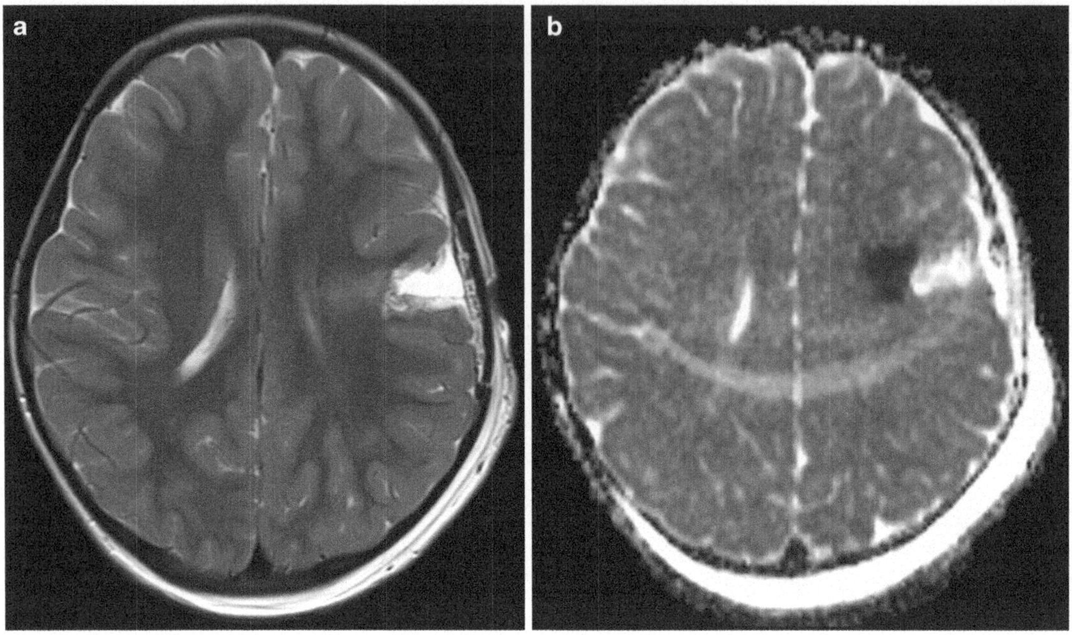


**Fig. 15.7** 6-year-old girl with a drug-resistant epilepsy caused by a glioneuronal tumor left frontolateral. Extended lesionectomy was performed. The neurological status immediately after surgery was intact. At the first postoperative day, a right hemiparesis was noted. (**a**) T2- and (**b**) diffusion-weighted MRI revealed ischemia mesial to the operation site. During the further course, hemiparesis was completely regredient, and the patient was seizure-free

postoperative deficits in 58% and long-term deficits in 23% of cases. In Lehman's study [159], 40% of cases had transient and 30% permanent deficits. Delev et al. [160] analyzing 66 patients documented a permanent neurological morbidity of 34%. Others reporting small series or single cases of Rolandic resections observed permanent neurological complications in 20% [161], 15% [162], 8% [163], and 7% [164], while Cukiert et al. [165, 166] and Otsubo et al. [167] did not encounter any permanent deficits.

#### Posterior Cortex Resections

Parietal resections may be followed by difficulties in spatial recognition (e.g., topographical orientation, face recognition). Resections affecting the angular and supramarginal gyri of the dominant hemisphere may result in Gerstmann's syndrome including dysgraphia, dyscalculia, agnosia, and apraxia. Of particular importance in posterior cortex resections are visual field deficits. Lesionectomies or extended lesionectomies in the occipital lobe were followed by new or aggravated visual field deficits after surgery in 42% of cases reported by Binder et al. [153]. Similarly, Heo et al. [154] analyzing visual function after surgery for occipital lobe epilepsy in 33 cases noted postoperative visual field deficits exceeding quadrantanopia in 42%, which is in line with others [168, 169]. In a meta-analysis comprising 584 occipital resections [152], postoperative visual decline was noted in 57% of patients. Pediatric series of posterior cortex resections revealed postoperative visual field deficits in 38%–81% of patients [153, 170, 171]. Liava et al. [172] noted that 32% of patients experienced de novo or aggravated postoperative visual field impairment.

### 15.3.4 Insular Resections

Complications after insular resections primarily refer to neurological deficits, in particular to hemiparesis and—if the dominant hemisphere is affected—to dysphasia. Data available mainly originate from tumor surgery, and only sparse information is available on complications of insular resections for epilepsy.

#### 15.3.4.1 Temporary Neurological Morbidity

Malak et al. [173] analyzing data from the 11 largest series of insular surgeries reported since 1988 found transient hemiparesis in 17% and transient dysphasia following surgery in the dominant hemisphere in 16% of cases. A similar temporary neurological morbidity rate of 17% (range: 0%–59%) has been reported in multicenter study including 635 patients by Ikegaya et al. [174]. Analyzing 25 patients undergoing operculo-insular corticectomy, Bouthillier and Nguyen [175] found temporary neurological deficits in 75% of their cases. Weil et al. [176] documented in 13 children undergoing opercular-insular corticectomy temporary hemiplegia in 2 cases (15%). Overall, temporary neurological morbidity after resection of insular tumors mainly referring to hemiparesis and dysphasia ranges between 20% and 40% in most series [145, 173, 177–182].

#### 15.3.4.2 Permanent Neurological Morbidity

Malak et al. [173] noted in their meta-analysis permanent motor deficits in 3%, and permanent dysphasia in 1.4%. In all complicated cases, permanent deficits were related to infarcts in the territory of the lenticulostriate arteries [173]. Similarly, Ikegaya et al. [174] found a permanent neurological morbidity in 4.6% (rangc: 0%–16.7%) in their analysis of 635 patients. In pediatric insulectomies, permanent hemiparesis has been reported in up to 20% [183]. Overall, permanent neurological morbidity after insular resections mainly ranges between 5% and 10% [145, 178, 180–182].

### 15.3.5 Reoperations

Reoperations as required in approximately 20% of very young children and in 10% of adults after failed resective surgery mainly refer to the extension of the first operation. Thus, the spectrum of inherent risks can be expected to be similar to that of the primary procedures while the absolute rate may be higher. Despite the relatively high volume, the literature on second surgical procedures is rather sparse, and most reports summarize temporal end extratemporal procedures.

#### 15.3.5.1 Surgical and Neurological Complications

Summarizing 15 adult case series of temporal and extratemporal reoperations including 402 patients, Surges and Elger [184] reported an overall complication rate of 13.5%. Krucoff et al. [185] noted in their meta-analysis including 36 repeat surgical studies neurological complication rates between 0% and 44%. The large variety of complications from 0% in reoperated temporal patients to 57.1% in patients reoperated for hypothalamic hamartomas as demonstrated in both meta-analyses mainly reflects the surgical spectrum offered with higher risks in reoperations affecting areas of high functionality [184, 185]. Grote et al. [186] noted surgical complications in 9%, neurological complications in another 9%, and visual field defects in 67% of repeat surgical cases, while Germano et al. [187] did not observe any complications in their series of 40 reoperations. Others reported hemiparesis in 7% [188], 5.1% [189], 1.9% [190], and 1.6% [191] of reoperations.

#### 15.3.5.2 Neuropsychological Complications

Neuropsychological evaluation as reported after second temporal resections demonstrated that repeat losses in the same cognitive domain were rare and that those losses after first surgery were followed by improvement rather than by decline [186]. Similarly, others observed neurocognitive decline after repeat surgery only in a few cases, usually followed by improvement in patients who ultimately achieved seizure freedom [192, 193].

## 15.4 Hemispherectomy/ Hemispherotomy

### 15.4.1 Anatomical Hemispherectomy

Anatomical hemispherectomy in the mid of the last century was associated with a hig rate of early and late complications.

#### 15.4.1.1 Early Complications

Early complications in the 1950s to 1970s included severe intraoperative bleeding, the need for large transfusions, hypotension, and intraoperative cardiac arrest [194–196]. Mortality rates of 5.9% [197], 8% [198, 199], and 5.1% [200] have been reported. In White's review of the world literature, the mortality due to early complications was estimated at 6.6% [201]. Falconer and Wilson [202] noted acute hydrocephalus and infection in 17% of patients, but did not observe any mortality.

#### 15.4.1.2 Late Complications

Anatomical hemispherectomy makes patients vulnerable to minor head trauma, leading to repeat microhemorrhage in regions of unsupported residual brain, resulting in blood accumulation, subdural hematomas, membrane formation, hemosiderosis, and hydrocephalus. Falconer and Wilson [202] reported delayed hemorrhage in 4 of 18 patients (22%), hydrocephalus in 1 of the 18 cases (5.6%), and loculation of the temporal horn in 2 of 18 cases (11.1%) requiring repeat surgery. In the long run, hemosiderosis and hydrocephalus occurred in 25% to 35% of patients [203, 204] which lead to death in 50% of individuals affected [198, 199, 203, 204] since in the pre-CT era the hydrocephalus mainly remained unrecognized [201, 202, 205–211].

In sum, early and late complications in the mid of the last century included a high mortality between 10% and 15% and a morbidity in the range of 30% to 50%. Although serious early complications such as metabolic derangement and cardiac arrest have become rarer during the following decades due andvanced surgical and-in particular-anesthesiological management, anatomical hemispherectomy is largely abandoned today. Sood et al. [212] re-advocated this procedure. Reporting 77 patients, mortality was 1.3% and serious morbidity 3.8%. Shunting was required in 21% of patients without and in 50% with previous surgery [212].

### 15.4.2 Modified Hemispherectomy/ Hemispherotomy Techniques

Modified hemispherectomy/hemispherotomy techniques as used in actual series, noticeably contribute to reduce surgical risks. In addition, development of hydrocephalus is easily recognized. However, even today, hemispheric procedures are associated with a high number of complications [213].

#### 15.4.2.1 Mortality

Mortality rates between 0.6% and 5.7% have been reported in more actual series [195, 196, 214–220]. Rolston et al. [3] noted one death in nine hemispherectomies (11.1%). A review including 13 centers and 323 cases showed a 1.5% mortality [221, 222]. The survey from the US database comprising 153 patients documented a mortality rate of 0.7% [21, 105]. In most studies, mortality with hemispherical procedures ranges between 2% and 4%, and there are no significant differences between the hemispherectomy/hemispherotomy techniques used [195, 196, 214–216, 218, 220].

#### 15.4.2.2 Morbidity

Rolston et al. [3] reported a morbidity of 55.6%. Similarly, the analysis of more than 1600 hemispherectomies performed between 1988 and 2010 showed a morbidity rate of 56% [223]. De Palma et al. [224] noted a morbidity of 23% including hemorrhage, ischemia, infection, hydrocephalus, and hygroma. There were no significant differences comparing vertical versus lateral approaches [224]. In sum, morbidity rates of hemispherical procedures mainly range between 30% and 50% with 10%–20% related to infections, hemorrhage, ischemia, hygroma, etc., and 20%–30% to hydrocephalus [195, 217, 218, 225].

## Morbidity

Morbidity following CC refers to surgical complications including hemorrhage, hydrocephalus, and infections, neurological deficits (hemiparesis), and memory disorders. Overall, temporary morbidity rate amounts to 10%–20%, and permanent morbidity to 5%–10% [1, 231, 247–251].

### *Surgical Complications*

Wyler [246] noted two epidural hematomas in 77 callosotomies (2.6%), and emphasized that the use of valproic acid may predispose to postoperative bleeding complications. In two small series, bleeding complications have been observed in up to 8% [245, 252]. Brain abscess requiring evacuation has been noted by Purves et al. [252] in 1 of 24 patients (4.2%). Wilson diagnosed bacterial meningitis in 3 of 8 patients (37.5%) in his early series [244], and in 3 of 12 cases (25%) in his later series [244]. Murro et al. [245] found superficial wound infection in 3 of 25 patients (12%). Overall, surgical complications including hemorrhage, hydrocephalus, and infections mainly range between 5% and 15% [1, 231, 247–251].

### *Neurological Complications*

Hemiparesis by hemorrhagic infarction of the frontal lobe was observed by Van Wagenen and Herren [253] in two of ten cases (20%) and by Wilson et al. [244, 254] in one of eight cases (12.5%). This complication can be attributed to the compromise of parasagittal bridging veins [89, 255, 256]. In later series, hemorrhagic infarction causing permanent neurological deficits has been noted in below 4% of patients [247, 249]. Tanriverdi et al. [1] reporting the MNI series found a neurological morbidity of 6.2%. Makari et al. [257] did not encounter any permanent neurological deficits in their series of 20 subtotal pediatric callosotomies. However, most of their patients experienced transitory left-sided neglect and ideomotor apraxia, altered mental status, and motor or sensory dysfunction, which have been thought to be caused in part by brain edema due to inadequate brain retraction. These symptoms cleared within 7–10 days postoperatively [257]. Murro et al. [245] found a mild hemiparesis in 1 of 25 patients (4%), and Luat et al. [258] noted permanent neurological deficits in 2 of 20 cases (10%). In sum, neurological complications mainly range between 5% and 10% [1, 245, 258].

### *Memory Deficits*

Permanent memory deficits are rarely observed, and may be related to damage to limbic structures, e.g., anterior commissure, hippocampal commissure, fornix, indusium griseum, and cingulum [248, 259].

## Multiple Subpial Transections (MST)

MST in areas of high functionality are frequently followed by minor and temporary deficits caused by local edema, while significant permanent deficits are rare [260]. Mild motor deficits have been reported in most series in approximately 50% of patients who underwent MST of the primary motor area. Similarly, mild dysphasia was found in around half of patients after transection of language areas [143, 260–263]. Temporary morbidity in Rolston's series was 20% [3]. Deficits usually resolve within some days to a few weeks, and only non-disabling subtle deficits may persist [2, 3, 143, 260–263].

## Concluding Remarks

- ***Callosotomy.*** *Operative sequelae such as the acute disconnection syndrome, the split-brain syndrome, and deficit reinstatement must be distinguished from proper surgical and neurological complications. Callosotomy represents the most invasive non-resective surgical procedure and is associated with a mortality rate of 1%–2%, a temporary morbidity in the range of 10%–20%, and a permanent morbidity of 5%–10%.*
- ***MST.*** *Although minor and temporary deficits after transection of eloquent areas may be expected in around one-half of patients, MST constitute a safe procedure since these deficits usually resolve almost completely, and only subtle but not disabling disorders may persist.*

### 15.5.1.2 Neurostimulation

#### Vagal Nerve Stimulation (VNS)

As with all neurostimulation techniques, complications of VNS therapy can be classified as early related to surgery, and late which can be ascribed to the device and to the stimulation. *Early or surgery-related complications* mainly refer to infections and vocal cord paralysis, while symptomatic hemorrhage is very rare. *Late or device/stimulation-related morbidity* includes malfunction of the device and laryngopharyngeal dysfunction during stimulation. Revesz et al. [264] reported in 497 procedures performed in 247 patients an overall complication rate of 12.4%, including surgical and device-related complications. In addition to complications of first-time implantation, morbidity due to surgical revision of devices which is not an infrequent procedure has to be addressed. In particular, removal of helical electrodes from the vagal nerve may pose some challenges.

*Surgery-Related Complications*

Surgery-related complications have been reported to range from 2.5% to 12.5% [264–276]. Qiabi et al. [277] noted a complication rate of 23.5%. In most series, however, surgery-related complications amount to 5–10%, mainly relating to infections and vocal cord palsy, and most of adverse events are temporary.

- *Infections* have been reported to occur in between 0% and 10.9% of the procedures [264, 265, 267, 269–272, 275–286]. The mean incidence of infections ranges between 4% and 6% [285, 287–290]. The infection rate seems not to be dependent on the site of positioning of the generator (thoracic versus axillary) [282]. In the series of Revesz et al. [264], infection rate in children was 4.5% as opposed to 2.6% in adults. Higher infections rates in children compared with adults have also been reported by others [291, 292]. Superficial infections can be treated by antibiotics, while in deep infections removal of the implant is necessary [281].
- *Vocal cord paralysis.* Vocal cord paralysis after first-time implantations of vagal nerve stimulators has been reported between 1% and 5.6% [264, 265, 272, 281, 283, 285, 286, 293–302]. Most studies note vocal cord paralysis in approximately 1% of patients [264, 265, 281, 283, 285, 297, 298, 303–305], and in the majority of cases, this complication is temporary. Permanent vocal cord paralysis is observed in <1% [283, 302, 306].

  In an analysis of 51,882 implantations in the USA from 1997 through 2012, Robinson et al. [293] found vocal cord paralysis in 193 patients (0.4%). In patients aged 18 years and older, the incidence of paralysis was 0.26% when the stimulator leads had coil diameters of 3 mm, and 0.51% when the leads had 2-mm-diameter coils. No statistically significant relationship between vocal cord paralysis and coil size was identified in patients younger than 18 years. Across all age groups, the incidence of vocal cord paralysis increased with age at implantation for leads having 2-mm-diameter coils [293]. Vocal cord paralysis has not been reported so far in children [282].
- *Miscellaneous.* There are three reports which mention a *Horner syndrome* [277, 283, 307]. *Scar related pain* has been observed in 4.7% of patients [282], and *cable discomfort* in 0.2% [264]. In the study of Elliott et al. [269, 275], there was 1 case of *pneumothorax.* Other anecdotal complications include *blunt trauma* to the neck ("twiddler's syndrome") causing vocal cord paralysis [304, 306], and *stretching of the nerve* [304, 308], which mainly occurs in mentally retarded patients. In addition, *dislodgement of the device* has been occasionally observed [264].

*Device-Related Complications*

Among device-related or hardware-related complications, lead fracture and malfunction are most common and have been reported in between 0% and 20.8% of implantations [265–269, 271–276, 281, 283, 284, 309]. In the Swedish series of 251 procedures in 143 patients [283], hardware-related complications were noted in 16.8%, mainly referring to lead fracture (12%). More anecdotal cases of device-related complications include lead disconnection, battery failure, material fatique with leakage current, and trauma-related malfunction [264, 281, 282, 310]. Overall, device-related complications have been mainly observed in the range of 5% [264, 265, 281, 295, 310].

*Stimulation-Related Complications*

Stimulation-related complications mainly refer to laryngeopharyngeal dysfunction (hoarseness, dyspnea, and coughing) which represents a side effect rather than a complication, while cardiac arrhythmias are unusual [264, 265, 272, 278, 281, 283, 297, 298, 304, 306, 308, 311–315].

- *Laryngopharyngeal dysfunction.* Temporary hoarseness, coughing, and changes of voice occur in up to two-thirds of patients, particularly in the initial phases of stimulation [264, 265, 272, 278, 281, 283, 297, 298, 304, 306, 308, 311–315]. However, in the long run, only a subset of patients (20%–30%) have been found to continue complaining of voice alteration and hoarseness during stimulation [281, 285, 292, 316–318].
- *Cardiac arrhythmias* can be observed sometimes, in particular at the beginning of stimulation. In rare cases also temporary atrial fibrillation, bradycardia, and asystole have been reported [311, 319, 320]. The estimated incidence of severe cardiac arrhythmias is 0.1% [319]. Kahlow and Olivecrona [283] reported one intraoperative episode of bradycardia (0.7%), and others noted asystole in the operating room in 0.1% [321]. In the long run, the effect of chronic stimulation on the variability of heart rate is low [322]. Spuck et al. [282] did not notice any cardiac symptoms in children.
- *Miscellaneous.* Some patients (<20%) complain symptoms such as local pain, paresthesia, dysphagia, obstructive sleep apnea, stimulation of the phrenic nerve, tonsillar pain mimicking glossopharyngeal neuralgia, sternocleidomastoid muscle contraction, and Horner's syndrome [264–266, 272, 281, 283, 285, 292, 294, 297, 298, 304, 306, 308, 311–318, 323]. In children, increased drooling and hyperactivity have been reported [310].

*Complications with Surgical Revision*

Khalow et al. [283] found a higher incidence of vocal cord palsy in patients receiving revision compared to first-time implantation (4.9% and 3.8%, respectively). Similarly, Aalbers et al. [302] noted that the incidence of vocal cord palsy was slightly higher after revision (3%) than for the primary procedure. Kumar et al. [324] reporting 31 procedures in 30 patients found that complete removal of the coils around the vagal nerve was achieved in all cases, and reimplantation followed immediately at the same location in 24 patients. Long-term vocal cord paralysis was noted in 2 of 9 (22%) surgeries performed with sharp dissection, but only in 1 of 22 (4.6%) surgeries in which electrocautery was used [324]. However, in the series of MacDonald and Couldwell [295], the lead has been removed completely using sharp dissection in seven patients without any complications which was followed by placing a new electrode just proximal to the original site in four cases. Similarly, others have reported successful removal and reimplantation of electrodes using different techniques without any complications [297, 300, 325–327]. Kahlow and Olivecrona [283] noted three cases of damage to the jugular vein, and two of them appeared while attempting to remove leads from the nerve.

**Deep Brain Stimulation (ANT-DBS)**

*Surgery-Related Complications*

In the series of Fisher et al. [328], the following complications were noted: Infection (9%), asymptomatic hemorrhage (5%), and pain at the implantation site (11%). The overall rate of serious adverse events was 1%–2% [328]. Kerrigan et al. [329] reported a 5% risk of infection and a 5–7.5% risk of intracerebral hemorrhage leading to clinical symptoms.

*Device-Related Complications*

Due to device-related complications, lead replacement was necessary in 9% of patients in the SANTE trial [328].

*Stimulation-Related Complications*

Paresthesias have been reported in 18.2% [328] and 16% [330] of cases. New seizure types were noted by Fisher et al. [328] in 6% of patients, and 9% had an increase in seizure frequency compared to the baseline. In 5% of patients, status epilepticus occurred, in each two cases following implantation and during stimulation, respectively, and in another case following discontinuation of stimulation [328]. In addition, both depression and memory complaints were significantly higher in the stimulation group as compared to the control group in the SANTE trial, that were, however, not associated with long-term neurobehavioral worsening [331]. Similarly, McGovern et al. [330] noted psychiatric disorders and cognitive impairment in some cases in the initial phase of thalamic stimulation.

#### Responsive Neurostimulation (RNS)

*Surgery-Related Complications*

Adverse events reported in the initial RNS trial include intracranial hemorrhage (5%) and infection (11%) [332–334]. In some cases, pain at the implantation site has been noted [334–336]. In another study, no surgery-related adverse events were observed [337].

*Device-Related Complications*

Hardware related complications noted in the initial RNS trial refer to lead damage (3.5%) and premature battery depletion (4.3%) [334].

*Stimulation-Related Complications*

Stimulation-related adverse effects reported in the initial RNS trial include paresthesias (6.3%), headaches (10.5%), increase in generalized (5.9%) or complex partial (7.8%) seizures, and the need for explantation of the device (5%) [332, 333]. No complications with respect to cognitive functions and mind have been observed [330, 332–334].

#### Concluding Remarks

- ***VNS.*** *Surgery-related complications are observed in the range of 5%–10%, mainly referring to infections and vocal cord paralysis (around 1% with first-time implantation and 3%–4% with electrode revision, mainly as a temporary deficit). It should be kept in mind that the diameter of the human vagal nerve lies somewhat over 2 mm on the average. With the use of helical electrodes with diameters <2.0 mm, the risk for damage to the nerve causing vocal paralysis is higher, particularly in elderly patients. Device-related complications are in the range of 5%. Severe stimulation-related cardiac adverse events are rare (approximately 0.1%). Laryngeal dysfunctions during stimulation that may be considered as side effects rather than as complications are initially observed in up to two-thirds of patients, but decrease over time, and are reported in the long run by 20%–30% of patients.*
- ***ANT-DBS/RNS.*** *Surgery and device-related complications are in the range of 10% with a permanent morbidity being encountered in approximately 2%–4% of patients. With both modalities, increased seizure frequency has been noted in 5%–10% of cases. While no adverse effects with respect to cognitive functions and mind have been observed with RNS, initial depression and memory decline have been noted with ANT-DBS, particularly in patients with preexistent disorders.*

## 15.5.2 Curative Procedures

Complications of non-resective curative procedures depend on the functionality of the target approached rather than on the technique used. Obviously, application of those strategies in hypothalamic hamartomas poses higher risks for adverse effects than their use in periventricular nodular heterotopias or in deep-seated dysplasias. Therefore, when assessing the complication rates of different technologies, the targets must be taken into account.

### 15.5.2.1 Thermoablation

#### Radiofrequency Thermocoagulation (RFTC)

*Hypothalamic Hamartomas (HH)*

Analyzing a total of 140 RFTC procedures in a series of 100 consecutive patients, Kameyama et al. [338] noted the following complications: *Horner's syndrome* (60%), *hyperphagia* (28%), *hyponatremia* (31%), *hyperthermia* (22%), short-term *memory disturbances* (9%), and prolonged *disturbance of consciousness* (0.7%). *Emotional facial paresis* as observed in 77% as a temporary symptom on the contralateral side was considered to be a syndrome of the supplementary motor area (SMA) by inactivation of the network between the mediodorsal nucleus of the thalamus and the hypothalamus. After twofold RFTC, two patients had postoperative *pituitary dysfunction.* Postoperative perifocal edema as observed in some cases, usually resolved within 3 months [338]. Vojtech et al. [339] reporting long-term data from 61 patients with HH treated with RFTC observed 4 hematomas (6.6%), one case of hydrocephalus (1.6%) requiring shunt placement, and 2 patients (3.3%) with meningitis. Three patients (4.9%) required open surgery, and 2 (3.3%) underwent repeat RFTC [339].

*Various Targets and Pathologies*

Bourdillon et al. [340] reported in a meta-analysis including 6 studies and a total of 296 patients a pooled complication rate with SEEG-guided RFTC of 2.5%, but only one (0.3%) complication had a minimal consequence on the patient's daily life. Others noted transient adverse events in around 3% [341–343]. Catenoix et al. [344] observed transient neurological adverse effects in 3 of 43 patients (7.0%), but no permanent neurological or cognitive impairment. Cossu et al. [342] noted syndrome of the angular gyrus and new seizure types after extensive coagulation in 1 of their 89 patients (1.1%). Malikova et al. [345] reported deterioration of verbal memory after RFTC of the left hippocampus, and Vojtech et al. [339]observed new psychiatric disorders including one suicide in 6 of 61 patient cases (9.8%).

**Laser-Induced Thermal Therapy (LITT)**

*Hypothalamic Hamartomas (HH)*

Curry et al. [346] noted in 71 patients with HH a persisting amnestic syndrome in 1 case (1.4%) due to lesioning the left mamillary body, disturbances of the electrolyte balance in 3 cases (4.2%), and a temporary increase of non-gelastic seizures in 9 individuals (12.7%). The authors concluded that the rate of memory deficits with LITT (1.4%) is much lower compared to the 15% rate with resective surgery [347] and the 7% rate with endoscopic resection [348]. In a series of 18 patients with HH, Xu et al. [349] found temporary neurological complications in 39%, and permanent adverse events in 22% (4 hemiparesis, 1 Horner's syndrome). In addition, 22% of individuals showed postoperative memory decline. Overall, 39% of the patients had a persistent neurological and/or neuropsychological deficit after LITT [349].

*Mesiotemporal Lobe Epilepsies (MTLE)*

Drane et al. [350] found in none of their 19 temporal LITT patients including 9 procedures in the dominant side deterioration of verbal or nonverbal memory. Others noted moderate [351] or significant [352–354] decline in verbal memory after LITT in the dominant temporal lobe. Evaluating 234 patients from 11 centers, Wu et al. [355] noted a complication rate of 15.0%, most of them causing permanent morbidity: visual field deficits (5.1%), worsening of a preexisting affective disorder (4.3%), hemorrhage (1.3%). The presence of a postoperative complication was associated with worse seizure outcome [355]. Grewal et al. [356] analyzed 9 studies including 250 patients. Overall complication rate was 20% (range: 14%–26%) and mainly referred to oculomotor and trochlear nerve palsies, hemorrhage, neuropsychologic complications, and gait abnormalities. In addition, visual field deficits were observed in 67% of patients [356].

*Various Targets and Pathologies*

Hoppe et al. [357] reviewed data from 60 studies including 226 cases. LITT was used for the treatment of mesial temporal lobe epilepsy (MTLE), hypothalamic hamartomas, focal cortical dysplasias, nodular periventricular heterotopias, tuberous sclerosis, and cavernomas. The following complications were noted in descending order: Hemorrhage, ipsilateral motor weakness, diplopia due to trochlear nerve palsy, short-term memory disturbance, transient aphasia, and homonymous hemianopsia. Moreover, headache, body weight loss/gain, impaired emotional wellbeing, and insomnia have been observed [357]. In a further review of 25 studies including 179 children, Hoppe et al. [358] found an overall complication rate of 23.5%, and a rate of severe complications of 3.4%. Contrarily, others did not note any complications with the use of LITT [359–363].

*Device-Related Complications*
With respect to device-related complications, misplacement of the catheter and malfunction of the cooling system have been reported [357, 364–366].

*Morphological Alterations*
LITT-induced structural alterations in the brain on MRI include T2-signal hyperintensity indicating perilesional edema, increased contrast uptake indicating necrosis [352, 357, 361, 367, 368], and increased FLAIR signal intensity indicating gliosis and cystic alterations [357, 368, 369]. In order to prevent edema, patients are treated after LITT with dexamethasone for some days [357].

#### 15.5.2.2 Stereotactic Radiosurgery (SRS)

*Hypothalamic Hamartomas (HH)*
Analyzing 48 SRS patients, Régis et al. [370] observed poikilothermia (6%), temporary increase of seizure frequency (17%), and deterioration of psychiatric comorbidities (8%). As noted by Wagner et al. [371], brachytherapy of HH with $^{125}$J-seeds in 24 patients caused noticeable increase of body weight in 17%. Detailed neuropsychological assessment revealed deterioration of partial cognitive functions in 20%–50% of the individuals [371].

*Mesiotemporal Lobe Epilepsies (MTLE)*
Hensley-Judge et al. [372] reported in the US multicenter study at 24 months after SRS visual field deficits (VFD) in 62.5% of patients, all with homonymous superior quadrantanopia. Verbal memory impairment was noted in 25% of dominant hemisphere patients and in 7% of nondominant hemisphere cases, but improvement in 16% and 7% of cases, respectively, with overall similar results at 24 and 36 months after SRS as compared to preoperative baselines [373]. Régis et al. [374] treating 20 MTLE patients with 20 Gy to 25 Gy at the 50% marginal isodose line and a target volume of 6500 mm$^3$ to 7000 mm$^3$ observed VFD in 36% of cases, of which one had a hemianopia due to damage to the optic tract. Barbarino et al. [375] noted VFD in 50% of their patients. Permanent neurological deficits were reported by Liang et al. [376] in 2 of 7 patients (29%). Barbaro et al. [377] noted adverse events (edema, infection, neurological deficits, exacerbation of seizures) in 12 of 31 patients (39%), one-third of them being serious. Analyzing 10 studies including 165 patients, Grewal et al. [356] reported a complication rate of 32% (range: 20%–46%), and most of them referred to VFD and neuropsychological deficits.

*Morphological Alterations*
Dose-dependent MRI changes have been described after Gamma Knife treatment for MTLE including a contrast enhanced ring and T2 signal changes inside the target volume at 6 months, followed by a contrast enhancing ring and a larger T2 signal outside the target volume at a median delay of 10.5 months [378]. These changes have been interpreted as radioinduced edema or radionecrosis [379, 380] and later on named radioinduced MR changes [378]. Chang et al. [381] found spectrographic evidence of necrosis in the target center in similar cases. Vojtech et al. [382] noted radionecrosis in all of his 14 MTLE cases after Gamma Knife treatment, in part with a progressive course, persisting as long as 16 years. These morphological alterations that may cause headache, nausea, vomiting, and depression [372, 375, 380] usually are successfully treated by methylprednisolone [380]. Edema, transient increase in focal seizures, and radionecrosis have also been noted by Usami et al. [383]. Histopathological evaluation of MTLE specimens obtained from patients who were operated because of poor outcome after SRS has shown various effects including edema, necrosis, chronic perivascular inflammation, microglial proliferation, reactive gliosis, and neuronal loss [382, 384–386].

*Oncogenesis*

Since SRS is mainly used for the treatment of tumors, it remains difficult to define its oncogenic potential due to the confounding overlap with the tumor course. A meta-analysis suggested three SRS-induced tumor cases in 200,000 applications (0.0015%) [387]. On the other hand, the cumulative rate of probably SRS-induced tumors in patients treated with SRS for arteriovenous malformations with a minimum of 10-years follow-up was 3 in 4692 person-years (0.064%) [388]. Thus, the real oncogenic potential of SRS may lie in between those numbers.

### Concluding Remarks

- ***Complications.*** *With all stereotactic strategies, treatment of HH shows the highest complication rates with a temporary morbidity in approximately two-thirds and a permanent morbidity in one-third of cases. Other targets can be treated with a permanent morbidity in the range of 3%–4%. In MTLE, minor VFD are noted in the range of 50% of patients. The expected superiority of minimal invasive techniques compared to resective strategies in terms of cognitive outcome has not yet been proven.*
- ***Morphological alterations/oncogenic potential.*** *Structural alterations after ablative procedures indicate perilesional edema, gliosis, and cystic alterations. Radionecrosis is observed in a high percentage after SRS. Although the oncogenic potential of SRS seems to be very low, this aspect should be considered when treatment of children is planned.*

## References

1. Tanriverdi T, Ajlan A, Poulin N, Olivier A. Morbidity in epilepsy surgery: an experience based on 2449 epilepsy surgery procedures from a single institution. J Neurosurg. 2009;110:1111–23.
2. Rolston JD, Englot DJ, Cornes S, Chang EF. Major and minor complications in extraoperative electrocorticography: a review of a national database. Epilepsy Res. 2016a;122:26–9.
3. Rolston JD, Englot DJ, Knowlton RC, Chang E. Rate and complications of adult epilepsy surgery in North America: analysis of multiple databases. Epilepsy Res. 2016b;124:55–62.
4. Behrens E, Schramm J, Zentner J, König R. Surgical and neurological complications in a series of 708 epilepsy surgery procedures. Neurosurgery. 1997;41:1–10.
5. Hamer HM, Morris HH, Mascha EJ, Karafa MT, Bingaman WE, Bej MD, Burgess RC, Dinner DS, Foldvary NR, Hahn JF, Kotagal P, Najm I, Wyllie E, Luders HO. Complications of invasive video-EEG monitoring with subdural grid electrodes. Neurology. 2002;58:97–103.
6. Rydenhag B, Silander HC. Complications of epilepsy surgery after 654 procedures in Sweden, September 1990-1995: A multicenter study based on the Swedish National Epilepsy Register. Neurosurgery. 2001;49:51–7.
7. Blauwblomme T, Ternier J, Romero C, Pier KS, D'Argenzio L, Pressler R, et al. Adverse events occurring during invasive electroencephalogram recordings in children. Neurosurgery. 2011;69:169–75.
8. Wellmer J, von der Groeben F, Klarmann U, Weber C, Elger CE, Urbach H, Clusmann H, von Lehe M. Risks and benefits of invasive epilepsy surgery workup with implanted subdural and depth electrodes. Epilepsia. 2012;53(8):1322–32.
9. Musleh W, Yassari R, Hecox K, et al. Low incidence of subdural grid-related complications in prolonged pediatric EEG monitoring. Pediatr Neurosurg. 2006;42:284–7.
10. Engel J Jr, Wiebe S, French J, Sperling M, Williamson P, Spencer D, et al. Practice parameter: temporal lobe and localized neocortical resections for epilepsy. Epilepsia. 2003;44:741–51.
11. Englot DJ, Ouyang D, Garcia PA, Barbaro NM, Chang EF. Epilepsy surgery trends in the United States, 1990-2008. Neurology. 2012;78:1200–6.
12. Pilcher WH, Roberts DW, Flanigin HF, Crandall PH, Wieser HG, Ojemann GA, et al. Complications of epilepsy surgery. In: Engel Jr J, editor. Surgical treatment of the epilepsies. 2nd ed. New York: Raven Press; 1993. p. 565–81.
13. Tebo CC, Evins AI, Christos PJ, et al. Evolution of cranial epilepsy surgery complication rates: a 32-year systematic review and meta-analysis. J Neurosurg. 2014;120:1415–27.
14. Bouvier G, Saint-Hilaire JM, Giard N, Lesage J, Cloutier I, Beique R. Depth electrode implantation at hospital Notre-Dame, Montreal. In: Engel Jr J, editor. Surgical treatment of the epilepsies. New York: Raven Press; 1987. p. 589–93.
15. Olivier A, Boling W. Stereotactic intracranial recording (stereoelectroencephalography). In: Schmidek HH, Sweet WH, editors. Operative neurosurgical techniques: indications, methods, and results. 4th ed. Philadelphia: WB Saunders; 2000. p. 1511–28.

16. Spencer S. Depth versus subdural electrode studies for unlocalized epilepsy. J Epilepsy. 1989;2:123–7.
17. Arya R, Mangano FT, Horn PS, Holland KD, et al. Adverse events related to extraoperative invasive EEG monitoring with subdural grid electrodes: A systematic review and meta-analysis. Epilepsia. 2013;54(5):828–39.
18. Garcia-Lorenzo B, del Pino-Sedeno T, Rocamora R, et al. Stereoelectroencephalography for refractory epileptic patients considered for surgery: systematic review, meta-analysis, and economic evaluation. Neurosurgery. 2019;84:326–38.
19. Tandon N, Tong BA, Friedman ER, et al. Analysis of morbidity and outcomes associated with use of subdural grids vs stereoelectroencephalography in patients with intractable epilepsy. JAMA Neurol. 2019; https://doi.org/10.1001/jamaneurol.2019.0098.
20. Burneo JG, Steven DA, McLachlan RS, Parrent AG. Morbidity associated with the use of intracranial electrodes for epilepsy surgery. Can J Neurol Sci. 2006;33:223–7.
21. Koubeissi MZ, Puwanat A, Jehi L, Alshekhlee A. In-hospital complications of epilepsy surgery: a six-year nationwide experience. Br J Neurosurg. 2009a;23(5):524–9.
22. Behrens E, Zentner J, van Roost D, Hufnagel A, Elger CE, Schramm J. Subdural and depth electrodes in the presurgical evaluation of epilepsy. Acta Neurochir. 1994;128:84–7.
23. Van Buren JM. Complications of surgical procedures in the diagnosis and treatment of epilepsy. In: Engel Jr J, editor. Surgical treatment of the epilepsies. New York: Raven Press; 1987. p. 465–75.
24. Onal C, Otsubo H, Araki T, Chitoku S, Ochi A, Weiss S, Elliott I, Snead OC 3rd, Rutka JT, Logan W. Complications of invasive subdural grid monitoring in children with epilepsy. J Neurosurg. 2003;98:1017–26.
25. Wyler AR, Walker G, Somes G. The morbidity of long-term seizure monitoring using subdural strip electrodes. J Neurosurg. 1991;74:734–7.
26. Ross D, Brunberg J, Drury I, Henry T. Intracerebral depth electrode monitoring in partial epilepsy: the morbidity and efficacy of placement using magnetic resonance image-guided stereotactic surgery. Neurosurgery. 1996;39:327–34.
27. De Almeida AN, Olivier A, Quesney F, Dubeau F, Savard G, Andermann F. Efficacy of and morbidity associated with stereoelectroencephalography using computerized tomography- or magnetic resonance imaging-guided electrode implantation. J Neurosurg. 2006b;104:483–7.
28. Espinosa J, Olivier A, Andermann F, Quesney F, Dubeau F, Savard G. Morbidity of chronic recording with intracranial depth electrodes in 170 patients. Stereotact Funct Neurosurg. 1994;63:63–5.
29. Olivier A, Marchand E, Peters TM, Tyler J. Depth electrodes implantation at the Montreal neurological institute and hospital. In: Engel Jr J, editor. Surgical treatment of the epilepsies. New York: Raven Press; 1987. p. 595–602.
30. Talairach J, Bancaud J, Szikla G, Bonis A, Gieger S, Vedrenne C. Approche nouvelle de la neurochirurgie de l'epilepsie: methodologie stereotaxique et resultants therapeutiques. 1. Introduction et historique. Neurochirurgie. 1974;20:1–240.
31. Spencer DD. Depth implantation at Yale University. In: Engel Jr J, editor. Surgical treatment of the epilepsies. New York: Raven Press; 1987. p. 603–7.
32. Blom S, Flink R, Hetta J, Hilton-Brown P, Hoffstedt C, Osterman PO, Spannare B. Interictal and ictal activity recorded with subdural electrodes during preoperative evaluation for surgical treatment of epilepsy. J Epilepsy. 1989;2:9–20.
33. Hitiris N, Suratman S, Kelly K, Stephen LJ, Sills GJ, Brodie MJ. Sudden unexpected death in epilepsy: a search for risk factors. Epilepsy Behav. 2007;10:138–41.
34. Rosenbaum TJ, Laxer KD, Vessely M, Brewster SW. Subdural electrodes for seizure focus localization. Neurosurgery. 1986;19:73–81.
35. Falowski SM, DiLorenzo DJ, Shannon LR, et al. Optimizations and nuances in neurosurgical technique for the minimization of complications in subdural electrode placement for epilepsy surgery. World Neurosurg. 2015;84:989–97.
36. Fountas KN, Smith JR. Subdural electrode-associated complications: a 20-year experience. Stereotact Funct Neurosurg. 2007;85:264–72.
37. Vale FL, Pollock G, Dionisio J, Benbadis SR, Tatum WO. Outcome and complications of chronically implanted subdural electrodes for the treatment of medically resistant epilepsy. Clin Neurol Neurosurg. 2013;115:985–90.
38. Placantonakis DG, Shariff S, Lafaille F, Labar D, Harden C, Hosain S, Kandula P, Schaul N, Kolesnik D, Schwartz TH. Bilateral intracranial electrodes for lateralizing intractable epilepsy: efficacy, risk, and outcome. Neurosurgery. 2010;66:274–83.
39. Swartz BE, Rich JR, Dwan PS, DeSalles A, et al. The safety and efficacy of chronically implanted subdural electrodes: a prospective study. Surg Neurol. 1996;46:87–93.
40. Malow BA, Sato S, Kufra CV, Blaxton TA, Figlozzi CM, Theodore WH. Haematoma-related seizures detected during subdural electrode monitoring. Epilepsia. 1995;36:733–5.
41. Van Gompel JJ, Worrell GA, Bell ML, Patrick TA, Cascino GD, Raffel C, Marsh WR, Meyer FB. Intracranial electroencephalography with subdural grid electrodes: techniques, complications, and outcomes. Neurosurgery. 2008;63:498–505.
42. Engel J, Crandall PH, Rausch R. The partial epilepsies. In: Rosenberg RN, Grossman RG, Schoceht S, et al., editors. The clinical neurosciences, vol. 2. New York: Churchill Livingstone; 1983. p. 1349–80.
43. Bernoulli C, Siegfried J, Baumgartner G, et al. Danger of accidental person-to-person transmission

of Creutzfeldt-Jakob disease by surgery. Lancet. 1977;1:478–9.
44. Mullin JP, Shriver M, Alomar S, Najm I, Bulacio J, Chauvel P, et al. Is SEEG safe? A systematic review and meta-analysis of stereo-electroencephalography-related complications. Epilepsia. 2016;57:386–401.
45. Cardinale F, Rizzi M, Vignati E, et al. Stereoelectroencephalography: retrospective analysis of 742 procedures in a single Centre. Brain. 2019; https://doi.org/10.1093/brain/awz196.
46. Mulligan L, Vives K, Spencer D. Placement of depth electrodes. In: Lüders H, editor. Textbook of epilepsy surgery: Informa Healthcare; 2008. p. 938–44.
47. Sansur C, Frysinger RC, Pouratian N, et al. Incidence of symptomatic hemorrhage after stereotactic electrode placement. J Neurosurg. 2007;107:998–1003.
48. Bottan JS, Rubino PA, Lau JC, et al. Robot-assisted insular depth electrode implantation through oblique trajectories: 3-dimensional anatomical nuances, technique, accuracy, and safety. Operat Neurosurg. 2019; https://doi.org/10.1093/ons/opz154.
49. Munari C. Depth electrode implantation at hospital Sainte Anne, Paris. In: Engel Jr J, editor. Surgical treatment of the epilepsies. New York: Raven Press; 1987. p. 583–8.
50. Willems LM, Reif PS, Spyrantis A, et al. Invasive EEG-electrodes in presurgical evaluation of epilepsies: systematic analysis of implantation-, video-EEG-monitoring- and explantation-related complications, and review of literature. Epilepsy Behav. 2018; https://doi.org/10.1016/j.yebeh.2018.05.012.
51. Cahan LD, Crandall PH. Neurosurgical aspects of epilepsy in children and adolescents. In: Youmans JR, editor. Neurological surgery. Philadelphia, PA: WB Sounders; 1990. p. 4271–87.
52. De Almeida AN, Marino R, Aguiar PH, Teixeira MJ. Hemispherectomy: a schematic review of the current techniques. Neurosurg Rev. 2006a;29:97–102.
53. Ljung H, Nordlund A, Strandberg M, et al. Verbal memory decline from hippocampal depth electrodes in temporal lobe surgery for epilepsy. Epilepsia. 2017;58:2143–52.
54. Helmstaedter C, Gielen GH, Witt JA. The immediate and short-term effects of bilateral intrahippocampal depth electrodes on verbal memory. Epilepsiy. 2018;59(6):78–84.
55. Hedegärd E, Bjellvi J, Edelvik A, Rydenhag B, Flink R, Malmgren K. Complications to invasive epilepsy surgery workup with subdural and depth electrodes: a prospective population-based observational study. J Neurol Neurosurg Psychiatry. 2014;85:716–20.
56. Wiggins GC, Elisevich K, Smith BJ. Morbidity and infection in combined subdural grid and strip electrode investigation for intractable epilepsy. Epilepsy Res. 1999;37:73–80.
57. Girvin JP. Complications of epilepsy surgery. In: Lüders H, editor. Epilepsy Surgery. New York, NY: Raven Press; 1991. p. 653–60.
58. Pilcher WH, Rusyniak WG. Complications of epilepsy surgery. Neurosurg Clin North Am. 1993;4:311–25.
59. Kim SK, Wang KC, Hwang YS, et al. Epilepsy surgery in children: outcomes and complications. J Neurosurg. 2008;1:277–83.
60. Ventureyra EC, Higgins MJ. Complications of epilepsy surgery in children and adolescents. Pediatr Neurosurg. 1993;19(1):40–56.
61. Nasreddine W, Beydoun A. Valproate-induced thrombocytopenia: a prospective monotherapy study. Epilepsia. 2008;49:438–45.
62. Anderson GD, Lin YX, Berge C, et al. Absence of bleeding complications in patients undergoing cortical surgery while receiving valproate treatment. J Neurosurg. 1997;87:252–6.
63. Ward MM, Barbaro NM, Laxer KD, et al. Preoperative valproate administration does not increase blood loss during temporal lobectomy. Epilepsia. 1996;37:98–101.
64. Hader WJ, Tellez Zenteno J, Metcalfe A, Hernandez-Ronquillo L, Wiebe S, Kwon C-S, Jette N. Complications of epilepsy surgery: A systematic review of focal surgical resections and invasive EEG monitoring. Epilepsia. 2013;54(5):840–7.
65. Gooneratne IK, Mannan S, de Tisi J, et al. Somatic complications of epilepsy surgery over 25 years at a single center. Epilepsy Res. 2017;132:70–7. https://doi.org/10.1016/j.eplepsyres.2017.02.016.
66. Olivier A. Risk and benefit of in the surgery of epilepsy: complications and positive results on seizures tendency and intellectual function. Acta Neurol Scand. 1988;117:114–21.
67. Ryvlin P, Montavont A, Kahane P. The impact of epilepsy surgery on mortality. Epileptic Disord. 2005;7(1):539–46.
68. Salanova V, Markand O, Worth R. Temporal lobe epilepsy surgery: complications, and late mortality rate in 215 patients. Epilepsia. 2002;43(2):170–4.
69. Hennessy MJ, Langan Y, Elwes RD, et al. A study of mortality after temporal lobe epilepsy surgery. Neurology. 1999;53:1276–83.
70. Nilsson L, Ahlbom A, Farahmand BY, et al. Mortality in a population-based cohort of epilepsy surgery patients. Epilepsia. 2003;44:575–81.
71. West S, Nolan SJ, Cotton J, et al. Surgery for epilepsy. Cochrane Database Syst Rev. 2015;7(7):CD010541.
72. Bjellvi J, Flink R, Rydenhag B, et al. Complications of epilepsy surgery in Sweden 1996-2010: a prospective, population-based study. J Neurosurg. 2015;122(3):519–25.
73. Inoue Y, Mihara T, Seino M. Timing of epilepsy surgery: its relevance for psychosocial rehabilitation. In: Tuxhorn J, Holthausen H, Boenigk H, editors. Pediatric epilepsy syndromes and their surgical treatment. London: John Libbey; 1997. p. 76–84.
74. Kerezoudis P, McCutcheon B, Murphy ME, et al. Thirty- day postoperative morbidity and mortality after temporal lobectomy for medically refractory epilepsy. J Neurosurg. 2017;23:1–7.

75. Olivier A, Boling WW, Tanriverdi T. Techniques in epilepsy surgery. The MNI approach. Cambridge, New York: Cambridge University Press; 2012.
76. Simon SL, Telfeian A, Duhaime AC. Complications of invasive monitoring used in intractable pediatric epilepsy. Pediatr Neurosurg. 2003;38:47–52.
77. dÓrio P, Rizzi M, Mariani V, et al. Surgery in patients with childhood-onset epilepsy: analysis of complications and predictive risk factors for a severely complicated course. J Neurol Neurosurg Psychiatry. 2018; https://doi.org/10.1136/jnnp-2018-318282.
78. Grivas A, Schramm J, Kral T, et al. Surgical treatment for refractory temporal lobe epilepsy in the elderly: seizure outcome and neuropsychological sequels compared with a younger cohort. Epilepsia. 2006;47(8):1364–72.
79. Patra S, Elisevich K, Podell K, et al. Influence of age and location of ictal onset on postoperative outcome in patients with localization-related epilepsy. Br J Neurosurg. 2014;28:61–7.
80. Murphy M, Smith PD, Wood M, et al. Surgery for temporal lobe epilepsy associated with mesial temporal sclerosis in the older patient: a longterm follow-up. Epilepsia. 2010;51:1024–9.
81. Englot DJ, Ouyang D, Wang DD, Rolston JD, Garcia PA, Chang EF. Relationship between hospital surgical volume, lobectomy rates, and adverse perioperative events at US epilepsy centers. J Neurosurg. 2013;118:169–74.
82. Lin Y, Harris DA, Curry DJ, Lam S. Trends in outcomes, complications, and hospitalization costs for hemispherectomy in the United States for the years 2000–2009. Epilepsia. 2014;56:139–46.
83. Brisman MH, Bederson JB, Sen CN, et al. Intracerebral hemorrhage occurring remote from the craniotomy site. Neurosurgery. 1996;39:1114–22.
84. König A, Laas R, Herrmann HD. Cerebellar haemorrhage as a complication after supratentorial craniotomy. Acta Neurochir. 1987;88:104–8.
85. Papanastassiou V, Kerr R, Adams C. Contralateral cerebellar hemorrhagic infarction after pterional craniotomy: report of five cases and review of the literature. Neurosurgery. 1996;39:841–52.
86. Yoshida S, Yonekawa Y, Yamashita K, et al. Cerebellar hemorrhage after supratentorial craniotomy—report of three cases. Neurol Med Chir. 1990;30:738–43.
87. Honegger J, Zentner J, Spreer J, et al. Cerebellar hemorrhage arising postoperatively as a complication of supratentorial surgery: a retrospective study. J Neurosurg. 2002;96:248–54.
88. Health Quality Ontario. Epilepsy surgery: an evidence summary. Ont Health Technol Assess Ser. 2012;12:1–28.
89. Pilcher WH, Ojemann GA. Complications of epilepsy surgery. In: Post KD, Friedman E, McCormick P, editors. Postoperative complications in intracranial surgery. New York: Thieme; 1993. p. 157–65.
90. Brotis AG, Giannis T, Kapsalaki E, et al. Complications after anterior temporal lobectomy for medically intractable epilepsy: A systematic review and meta-analysis. Stereotact Funct Neurosurg. 2019; https://doi.org/10.1159/000500136.
91. Guldvog B. Evaluation of epilepsy surgery in Norway 1949–1988. Oslo: University of Oslo; 1993. (dissertation)
92. Sindou M, Guenot M, Isnard J. Temporo-mesial epilepsy surgery: outcome and complications in 100 consecutive adult patients. Acta Neurochir. 2006;48(1):39–45.
93. Cohen-Gadol AA, Wilhelmi BG, Collignon F, et al. Long-term outcome of epilepsy surgery among 399 patients with nonlesional seizure foci including temporal lobe sclerosis. J Neurosurg. 2006;104:513–24.
94. Georgiadis I, Kapsalaki EZ, Fountas KN. Temporal lobe resective surgery for medically intractable epilepsy: a review of complications and side effects. Epilepsy Res Treat. 2013;2013:752195. https://doi.org/10.1155/2013/752195.
95. Erba G, Winston KR, Adler JR, et al. Temporal lobectomy for complex partial seizures that began in childhood. Surg Neurol. 1992;38(6):424–32.
96. Terra-Bustamente VC, Inuzuca LM, Fernandes RM, et al. Temporal lobe epilepsy surgery in children and adolescents: clinical characteristics and postsurgical outcome. Seizure. 2005;14(4):274–81.
97. Sinclair DB, Aronyk KE, Snyder TJ, et al. Pediatric epilepsy surgery at the University of Alberta: 1988–2000. Pediatr Neurol. 2003;29:302–11.
98. Clusmann H, Kral T, Fackeldey E, et al. Lesional mesial temporal lobe epilepsy and limited resections: prognostic factors and outcome. J Neurol Neurosurg Psychiatry. 2004;75:1589–96.
99. Vadera S, Kshettry VR, Klaas P, et al. Seizure-free and neuropsychological outcomes after temporal lobectomy with amygdalohippocampectomy in pediatric patients with hippocampal sclerosis. J Neurosurg. 2012;10:103–7.
100. Lopez-Gonzalez MA, Gonzalez-Martinez JA, Jehi L, et al. Epilepsy surgery of the temporal lobe in pediatric population: a prospective analysis. Neurosurgery. 2012;70:684–92.
101. Schmeiser B, Wagner K, Schulze-Bonhage A, et al. Surgical treatment of mesiotemporal lobe epilepsy: which approach is favorable? Neurosurgery. 2017; https://doi.org/10.1093/neuros/nyx138.
102. Schmeiser B, Moritz D, Evangelos K, et al. Visual filed defects following different resective procedures for mesiotemporal lobe epilepsy. Epilepsy Behav. 2017b;76:39–45.
103. Yasargil MG, Krayenbuhl N, Roth P, Hsu SP, Yasargil DC. The selective amygdalohippocampectomy for intractable temporal limbic seizures. J Neurosurg. 2010;112(1):168–85.
104. Ormond DR, Clusmann H, Sassen R, et al. Pediatric temporal lobe epilepsy surgery in Bonn and review of the literature. Neurosurgery. 2018; https://doi.org/10.1093/neuros/nyy125.
105. Koubeissi MZ, Syed TU, Syed I, Jordan J, Alshekhlee A, Kossoff EH. Hemispherectomy-

associated complications from the Kids'Inpatient database. Epilepsy Res. 2009b;87:47–53.
106. Penfield W, Lende R, Rasmussen T. Manipulation hemiplegia. J Neurosurg. 1961;18:760–76.
107. Crandall PH. Postoperative management and criteria for evaluation. In: Purpura DP, Penry JK, Walter RD, editors. Advances in neurology, vol. 8. New York: Raven Press; 1975. p. 265–79.
108. Lende R. Local spasm in cerebral arteries. J Neurosurg. 1978;17:90–103.
109. Rasmussen T. Surgery for epilepsy arising in regions other than the temporal and frontal lobes. In: Purpura DP, Penry JK, Walter RD, editors. Advances in neurology, vol. 8. New York: Raven Press; 1975a. p. 206–26.
110. Rasmussen T. Surgical treatment of patients with complex partial seizures. In: Penry JK, Daly DD, editors. Advances in neurology. New York, NY: Raven Press; 1975b. p. 415–49.
111. Helgason C, Caplan L, Goodwin J, Hedges T. Anterior choroidal artery-territory infarction. Arch Neurol. 1986;43:681–6.
112. Katz A, Awad I, Kong A, et al. Extent of resection in temporal lobectomy for epilepsy. II. Memory changes and neurological complications. Epilepsia. 1989;30:763–71.
113. Barton JJ, Hefter R, Chang B, et al. The field defects of anterior temporal lobectomy: a quantitative reassessment of Meyer's loop. Brain. 2005;128:2123–33.
114. Hughes TS, Abou-Khalil B, Lavin PJ, et al. Visual field defects after temporal lobe resection: a prospective quantitative analysis. Neurology. 1999;53(1):167–72.
115. Nilsson D, Malmgren K, Rydenhag B, et al. Visual field defects after temporal lobectomy – comparing methods and analyzing resection size. Acta Neurolo Scand. 2004;110(5):301–7.
116. Tecoma ES, Laxer KD, Barbaro NM, et al. Frequency and characteristics of visual field deficits after surgery for mesial temporal sclerosis. Neurology. 1993;43(6):1235–8.
117. Marino R, Rasmussen T. Visual field changes after temporal lobectomy in man. Neurology. 1968;18:825–35.
118. Heller AC, Padilla RV, Mamelak AN. Complications of epilepsy surgery in the first 8 years after neurosurgical training. Surg Neurol. 2009;71(6):631–7.
119. Falconer M, Wilson J. Visual field changes following anterior temporal lobectomy. Their significance in relation to "Myer's loop" of the optic radiation. Brain. 1958;81:1–14.
120. Freiman TM, Surges R, Vougioukas VI, et al. Complex visual hallucinations (Charles bonnet syndrome) in visual field defects following cerebral surgery. J Neurosurg. 2004;101:846–53.
121. Hori T, Yamane F, Ochiai T, et al. Selective subtemporal amygdalohippocampectomy for refractory temporal lobe epilepsy: operative and neuropsychological outcomes. J Neurosurg. 2007;106(1):134–41.
122. Thudium MO, Campos AR, Urbach H, et al. The basal temporal approach for mesial temporal surgery: sparing the Meyer loop with navigated diffusion tensor tractography. Neurosurgery. 2010;67:385–90.
123. Berger MS, Kincaid J, Ojemann G, et al. Brain mapping techniques to maximize resection, safety and seizure control in children with brain tumors. Neurosurgery. 1989;25:786–92.
124. Ojemann GA. Individual variability in cortical localization of language. J Neurosurg. 1979;50:164–9.
125. Ojemann GA. Brain organization for language from the perspective of electrical stimulation mapping. Behav Brain Sci J. 1983:189–230.
126. Ojemann GA, Ojemann J, Lettich E, et al. Cortical language localization in left, dominant hemisphere. J Neurosurg. 1989;71:316–26.
127. Penfield W, Jasper H. Epilepsy and the functional anatomy of the human brain. Boston: Little, Brown; 1954. p. 896.
128. Wyllie E, Lüders H, Morris HH, et al. Clinical outcome after complete or partial cortical resection for intractable epilepsy. Neurology. 1987;37:825–35.
129. Falowski SM, Wallace D, Kanner A, et al. Tailored temporal lobectomy for medically intractable epilepsy: evaluation of pathology and predictors of outcome. Neurosurgery. 2012;71(3):703–9; discussion 709
130. Helmstaedter C, Witt J-A. Clinical neuropsychology in epilepsy: theoretical and practical issues. Handb Clin Neurol. 2012;107:437–59.
131. Hermann BP, Wyler AR. Neuropsychological outcome of anterior temporal lobectomy. J Epilepsy. 1988;1:35–45.
132. Milner B. Psychological defects produced by temporal lobe excision. Res Publ Assoc Res Neur Ment Dis. 1958;36:244–57.
133. Milner B. Visually-guided maze learning in man: effects of bilateral hippocampal, bilateral frontal and unilateral cerebral lesions. Neuropsychologia. 1965;3:317–38.
134. Milner B. Visual recognition and recall after right temporal lobe excision in man. Neuropsychologia. 1968;6:191–209.
135. Rausch R, Crandall PH. Psychological status related to control of temporal lobe seizures. Epilepsia. 1982;23:191–202.
136. Sherman EM, Wiebe S, Fay-McClymont TB. Neuropsychological outcomes after epilepsy surgery: systematic review and pooled estimates. Epilepsia. 2011;52(5):857–69.
137. Delgado-Escueta A, Treiman D, Walsh G. The treatable epilepsies. N Engl J Med. 1983;308:1576–84.
138. Schaller C, Zentner J. Vasospastic reactions in response to the transsylvian 468. Approach. Surg Neurol. 1998;49(2):170–5.
139. Lackner P, Koppelstaetter F, Ploner P, et al. Cerebral vasospasm following temporal lobe epilepsy surgery. Neurology. 2012;78:1215–20.
140. Schmeiser B, Zentner J, Steinhoff BJ, Schulze-Bonhage A, Kogias E, Wendling A-S Hammen

T. Functional hemispherectomy is safe and effective in adult patients. Epilepsy Behav. 2017a;77:19–25.
141. Delev D, Oehl B, Steinhoff BJ. Surgical treatment of extratemporal epilepsy: results and prognostic factors. Neurosurgery. 2019;84(1):242–52.
142. Van Offen M, van Rijen PC, Leijten FS, et al. Central lobe epilepsy surgery – (functional) results and how to evaluate them. Epilepsy Res. 2017;130:37–46.
143. Behdad A, Limbrick DD, Bertrand M, et al. Epilepsy surgery in children with seizures arising from the rolandic cortex. Epilepsia. 2009;50(6):1450–61.
144. Benifla M, Sala F Jr, Jane J, et al. Neurosurgical management of intractable rolandic epilepsy in children: role of resection in eloquent cortex. Clinical article. J Neurosurg Pediatr. 2009;4(3):199–216.
145. von Lehe M, Wellmer J, Urbach H, Schramm J, Elger CE, Clusmann H. Insular lesionectomy for refractory epilepsy: management and outcome. Brain. 2009;132(Pt 4):1048–56.
146. Elsharkawy AE, Alabbasi AH, Pannek H, et al. Outcome of frontal lobe epilepsy surgery in adults. Epilepsy Res. 2008a;81:97–106.
147. Elsharkawy AE, Pannek H, Schulz R, et al. Outcome after extratemporal epilepsy surgery. Experience of a single center. Neurosurgery. 2008b;63:516–26.
148. Hanáková P, Brázdil M, Novák Z, et al. Long-term outcome and predictors of resective surgery prognosis in patients with refractory extratemporal epilepsy. Seizure. 2014;23(4):266–73.
149. Sarkis RA, Jehi L, Najm IM, Kotagal P, Bingaman WE. Seizure outcomes following multilobar epilepsy surgery. Epilepsia. 2012;53(1):44–50.
150. Pondal-Sordo M, Diosy D, Téllez-Zenteno JF, et al. Epilepsy surgery involving the sensory-motor cortex. Brain. 2006;129:3307–14.
151. Ostergard TA, Miller JP. Surgery for epilepsy in the primary motor cortex: A critical review. Epilepsy Behav. 2018; https://doi.org/10.1016/j.yebeh.2018.06.036.
152. Harward SC, Chen WC, Rolston JD, et al. Seizure outcomes in occipital lobe and posterior quadrant epilepsy surgery: A systematic review and meta-analysis. Neurosurgery. 2017; https://doi.org/10.1093/neuros/nyx158.
153. Binder DK, Lehe von M, Kral T, et al. Surgical treatment of occipital lobe epilepsy. J Neurosurg 2008;109(1):57-69.
154. Heo W, Kim JS, Chung CK, et al. Relationship between cortical resection and visual function after occipital lobe epilepsy surgery. J Neurosurg. 2017; https://doi.org/10.3171/2017.5.JNS162963.
155. Swartz BE, Gado-Escueta AV, Walsh GO, et al. Surgical outcomes in pure frontal lobe epilepsy and foci that mimic them. Epilepsy Res. 1998;29:97–108.
156. Schramm J, Kral T, Kurthen M, et al. Surgery to treat focal frontal lobe epilepsy in adults. Neurosurgery. 2002;51:644–54.
157. Kellinghaus C, Luders HO. Frontal lobe epilepsy. Epileptic Disord. 2004;6:223–39.
158. Pilcher C, Meacham WR, Holbrook TJ. Partial excision of the motor cortex in treatment of Jacksonian convulsions. Results of forty cases. Arch Surg. 1947;54:633–43.
159. Lehman R, Andermann F, Olivier A, Tandon PN, Quesney LF, Rasmussen TB. Seizures with onset in the sensorimotor face area: clinical patterns and results of surgical treatment in 20 patients. Epilepsia. 1994;35:1117–24.
160. Delev D, Send K, Wagner J, et al. Epilepsy surgery of the rolandic and immediate perirolandic cortex: surgical outcome and prognostic factors. Epilepsia. 2014;55:1585–93.
161. Cohen-Gadol AA, Britton JW, Collignon FP, et al. Nonlesional central lobule seizures: use of awake cortical mapping and subdural grid monitoring for resection of seizure focus. J Neurosurg. 2003;98:1255–62.
162. Kim YH, Kim CH, Kim JS, Lee SK, Han JH, Kim CY, et al. Topographical risk factor analysis of new neurological deficits following precentral gyrus resection. Neurosurgery. 2015;76:714–20. [discussion 20]
163. Devinsky O, Romanelli P, Orbach D, Pacia S, Doyle W. Surgical treatment of multifocal epilepsy involving eloquent cortex. Epilepsia. 2003;44:718–23.
164. Sandok EK, Cascino GD. Surgical treatment for perirolandic lesional epilepsy. Epilepsia. 1998;39(Suppl 4):S42–8.
165. Cukiert A, Buratini JA, Machado E, et al. Results of surgery in patients with refractory extratemporal epilepsy with normal or nonlocalizing magnetic resonance findings investigated with subdural grids. Epilepsia. 2001a;42:889–94.
166. Cukiert A, Buratini JA, Machado E, et al. Seizure's outcome after cortical resections including the face and tongue rolandic areas in patients with refractory epilepsy and normal MRI submitted to subdural grids' implantations. Arq Neuropsiquiatr. 2001b;59:717–21.
167. Otsubo H, Chitoku S, Ochi A, Jay V, Rutka JT, Smith ML, et al. Malignant rolandic-sylvian epilepsy in children: diagnosis, treatment, and outcomes. Neurology. 2001;57:590–6.
168. Blume WT, Wiebe S, Tapsell LM. Occipital epilepsy: lateral versus mesial. Brain. 2005;128(Pt 5):1209–25.
169. Kun Lee S, Young Lee S, Kim DW, Soo Lee D, Chung CK. Occipital lobe epilepsy: clinical characteristics, surgical outcome, and role of diagnostic modalities. Epilepsia. 2005;46:688–95.
170. Boesebeck F, Schulz R, May T, Ebner A. Lateralizing semiology predicts the seizure outcome after epilepsy surgery in the posterior cortex. Brain. 2002;125:2320–31.
171. Tandon N, Alexopoulos AV, Warbel A, Najm IM, Bingaman WE. Occipital epilepsy: spatial categorization and surgical management. J Neurosurg. 2009;110(2):306–18.

172. Liava A, Mai R, Tassi L, et al. Paediatric epilepsy surgery in the posterior cortex: a study of 62 cases. Epileptic Disord. 2014;16:141–64.
173. Malak R, Bouthillier A, Carmant L, et al. Microsurgery of epileptic foci in the insular region. J Neurosurg. 2009;110:1153–63.
174. Ikegaya N, Takahashi A, Kaido T, et al. Surgical strategy to avoid ischemic complications of the pyramidal tract in resective epilepsy surgery of the insula: technical case report. J Neurosurg. 2017; https://doi.org/10.3171/2017.1.JNS161278.
175. Bouthillier A, Nguyen DK. Epilepsy surgeries requiring an operculoinsular cortectomy: operative technique and results. Neurosurgery. 2017; https://doi.org/10.1093/neuros/nyx080.
176. Weil A, Minh N, Jayakar P, et al. Medically resistant pediatric insular-opercular/perisylvian epilepsy. Part 2: outcome following resective surgery. J Neurosurg Pediatr. 2016; https://doi.org/10.3171/2016.4.PEDS15618.
177. Lang FF, Olansen NE, DeMonte F, et al. Surgical resection of intrinsic insular tumors: complications avoidance. J Neurosurg. 2001;95:638–50.
178. Neuloh G, Pechstein U, Schramm J. Motor tract monitoring during insular glioma surgery. J Neurosurg. 2007;106:582–92.
179. Tamura A, Kasai T, Akazawa K, et al. Long insular artery infarction: characteristics of a previously unrecognized entity. Am J Neuroradiol. 2014;35:466–71.
180. Duffau H, Capelle L, Lopes M, Bitar A, Sichez JP, van Effenterre R. Medically intractable epilepsy from insular low-grade gliomas: improvement after an extended lesionectomy. Acta Neurochir. 2002;144:563–72; discussion 572–3
181. Simon M, Neuloh G, von Lehe M, Meyer B, Schramm J. Insular gliomas: the case for surgical management. J Neurosurg. 2009;110(4):685–95.
182. Zentner J, Meyer B, Stangl A, Schramm J. Intrinsic tumors of the insula: a prospective surgical study of 30 patients. J Neurosurg. 1996;85(2):263–71.
183. Dylgjeri S, Taussig D, Chipaux M, Lebas A, Fohlen M, Bulteau C, et al. Insular and insulo-opercular epilepsy in childhood: an SEEG study. Seizure. 2014;23:300–8.
184. Surges R, Elger CE. Reoperation after failed resective epilepsy surgery. Seizure. 2013;22:493–501.
185. Krucoff MO, Chan AY, Harward SC, et al. Rates and predictors of success and failure in repeat epilepsy surgery: A meta-analysis and systematic review. Epilepsia. 2017;58(12):2133–42.
186. Grote A, Witt JA, Surges R, von Lehe M, Pieper M, Elger CE, Helmstaedter C, Ormond DR, Schramm J, Delev D. A second chance—reoperation in patients with failed surgery for intractable epilepsy: long-term outcome, neuropsychology and complications. J Neurol Neurosurg Psychiatry. 2016;87:379–85.
187. Germano IM, Poulin N, Olivier A. Reoperation for recurrent temporal lobe epilepsy. J Neurosurg. 1994;81:31–6.
188. González-Martínez JA, Srikijvilaikul T, Nair D, Bingaman WE. Long-term seizure outcome in reoperation after failure of epilepsy surgery. Neurosurgery. 2007;60:873–80.
189. Salanova V, Quesney LF, Rasmussen T, Andermann F, Olivier A. Reevaluation of surgical failures and the role of reoperation in 39 patients with frontal lobe epilepsy. Epilepsia. 1994;35:70–80.
190. Wyler AR, Hermann BP, Richey ET. Results of reoperation for failed epilepsy surgery. J Neurosurg. 1989;71:815–9.
191. Siegel AM, Cascino GD, Meyer FB, McClelland RL, So EL, Marsh WR, et al. Resective reoperation for failed epilepsy surgery: seizure outcome in 64 patients. Neurology. 2004;63:2298–302.
192. Jung R, Aull-Watschinger S, Moser D, et al. Is reoperation an option for patients with temporal lobe epilepsy after failure of surgery? Seizure. 2013;22:502–6.
193. Pati S, Abla AA, Rekate HL, Ng YT. Repeat surgery for hypothalamic hamartoma in refractory epilepsy. Neurosurg Focus. 2011;30:E3.
194. Brian JE, Deshpande JK, McPherson RW. Management of cerebral hemispherectomy in children. J Clin Anesth. 1990;2:91–5.
195. Carson BS, Javedan SP, Freeman JM, Vining EP, Zuckerberg AL, Lauer JA, Guarnieri M. Hemispherectomy: a hemidecortication approach and review of 52 cases. J Neurosurg. 1996;84:903–11.
196. Peacock WJ, Wehby-Grant MC, Shields WD, Shewmon DA, Chugani HT, Sankar R, Vinters HV. Hemispherectomy for intractable seizures in children: a report of 58 cases. Childs Nerv Syst. 1996;12:376–84.
197. Hendrick EB, Hoffman HJ, Hudson AR. Hemispherectomy in children. Clin Neurosurg. 1969;16:315–27.
198. Wilson PJE. Cerebral hemispherectomy for infantile hemiplegia. A report of 50 cases. Brain. 1970a;93:147–80.
199. Wilson PJE. More "second thoughts" on hemispherectomy in infantile hemiplegia. Dev Med Child. 1970b;12:799–800.
200. Rasmussen T. Commentary: extratemporal cortical excisions and hemispherectomy. In: Engel J, editor. Surgical Treatment of the Epilepsies. New York: Raven Press; 1987. p. 417–24.
201. White HH. Cerebral hemispherectomy in the treatment of infantile hemiplegia. Review of the literature and report of two cases. Confin Neurol. 1961;21:1–50.
202. Falconer MA, Wilson PJE. Complications related to delayed hemorrhage after hemispherectomy. J Neurosurg. 1969;30:413–26.
203. Rasmussen T. Postoperative superficial cerebral hemosiderosis of the brain, its diagnosis, treatment and prevention. Am Neurol Assoc. 1973;98:133–7.
204. Wilson PJE. More "second thoughts" on hemispherectomy in infantile hemiplegia. Dev Med Child. 1980;12:799–800. (letter)

205. Carmichael EA. The current status of hemispherectomy for infantile hemiplegia. Clin Proc Child Hosp Dist Columbia. 1966;22:285–93.
206. Davies KG, Maxwell RE, French LA. Hemispherectomy for intractable seizures: long-term results in 17 patients followed for up to 38 years. J Neurosurg. 1993;78:733–40.
207. Griffith HB. Cerebral hemispherectomy for infantile hemiplegia in the light of the late results. Ann R Coll Surg. 1967;41:183–201.
208. Laine E, Pruvot P, Osson D. Resultats eloignes de l'hemispherectomie dans les cas d'hemiatrophie cerebrale infantile generatrice dépilepsie. Neurochirurgie. 1964;10:507–22.
209. Oppenheimer DR, Griffith HB. Persistent intracranial bleeding as a complication of hemispherectomy. J Neurol Neurosurg Psychiatry. 1966;9:229–40.
210. Villemure J-G. Hemispherectomy techniques. In: Tuxhorn I, Holthausen H, Boenigk H, editors. Paediatric epilepsy syndromes and their surgical treatment. London: John Libbey; 1997. p. 729–38.
211. Hoffman HJ, Hendrick EB, Dennis M, Armstrong D. Hemispherectomy for Sturge-Weber syndrome. Childs Brain. 1979;5:233–48.
212. Sood S, Ilyas M, Marapudi NI, et al. Anatomical hemispherectomy revisited—outcome, blood loss, hydrocephalus, and absence of chronic hemosiderosis. Childs Nerv Syst. 2019;35:1341–9.
213. Schramm J. Hemispherectomy techniques. Neurosurgery. 2002;37:113–34.
214. Freeman JM, Vining EPG, Pillas DJ, Uematsu S, Carson B, Brandt J, Boatman D, Pulsifer MB, Zuckerberg A. Seizure outcome after hemispherectomy: the John Hopkins experience. In: Tuxhorn I, Holthausen H, Boenigk H, editors. Paediatric epilepsy syndromes and their surgical treatment. London: John Libbey; 1997. p. 743–8.
215. Kossoff EH, Vining EP, Pillas DJ, Pyzik PL, Avellino AM, Carson BS, Freeman JM. Hemispherectomy for intractable unihemispheric epilepsy. Etiology versus outcome. Neurology. 2003;61:887–90.
216. Villemure JG. Hemispherectomy. In: Shorovon S, Dreifuss F, Fish D, Thomas D, editors. The treatment of epilepsy. Oxford: Blackwell Scientific Publications; 1996. p. 713–21.
217. Schramm J, Delev D, Wagner J, Elger CE, von Lehe M. Seizure outcome, functional outcome, and quality of life after hemispherectomy in adults. Acta Neurochir. 2012;154:1603–12.
218. Villemure JG, Vernet O, Delalande O. Hemispheric disconnection: Callosotomy and hemispherectomy. Adv Tech Stand Neurosurg. 2000;26:25–78.
219. Delalande O, Bulteau C, Dellatolas G, Fohlen M, Jalin C, Buret V, Viguier D, Dorfmuller G, Jambaque I. Vertical parasagittal hemispherectomy: surgical procedures and clinical long-term outcomes in a population of 83 children. Neurosurgery. 2007;60:19–32.
220. Terra-Bustamante VC, Inuzuka LM, Fernandes RM, et al. Outcome of hemispheric surgeries for refractory epilepsy in pediatric patients. Childs Nerv Syst. 2007;23(3):321–6.
221. Holthausen H, May TW, Adams CTB, Andermann F, Comair Y, Delalande O, Duchowny M, Freeman JM, Hoffman HJ, et al. Seizures post hemispherectomy. In: Tuxhorn I, Holthausen H, Boenigk H, editors. Paediatric epilepsy syndromes and their surgical treatment. London: John Libbey; 1997a. p. 749–73.
222. Holthausen H, Strobl K, Pieper T, Teixeira VA, Oppel F. Prediction of motor functions post hemispherectomy. In: Tuxhorn I, Holthausen H, Boenigk H, editors. Paediatric epilepsy syndromes and their surgical treatment. London: John Libbey; 1997b. p. 785–98.
223. Vadera S, Griffith SD, Rosenbaum BP, Seicean A, Kshettry VR, Kelly ML, Weil RJ, Bingaman W, Jehi L. National Trends and in-hospital complication rates in more than 1600 hemispherectomies from 1988–2010. Neurosurgery. 2015;77:185–91.
224. De Palma L, Pietrafusa N, Gozzo F, et al. Outcome after hemispherotomy in patients with intractable epilepsy: comparison of techniques in the Italian experience. Epilepsy Behav. 2019;93:22–8.
225. Di Rocco C, Iannelli A. Hemimegalencephaly and intractable epilepsy: complications of hemispherectomy and their correlations with the surgical technique. A report on 15 cases. Pediatr Neurosurg. 2000;33:198–207.
226. Rasmussen T, Andermann F. Hemispherectomy for seizures revisited. Can J Neurol Sci. 1983;10:71–8.
227. Tinuper P, Andermann F, Villemure JG, Rasmussen TB, Quesney LF. Functional hemispherectomy for the treatment of epilepsy associated with hemiplegia: rationale, indications, results, and comparison with callosotomy. Ann Neurol. 1988;24:27–34.
228. Cats EA, Kho KH, Van Nieuwenhuizen O, Van Veelen CW, Gosselaar PH, Van Rijen PC. Seizure freedom after functional hemispherectomy and a possible role for the insular cortex: the Dutch experience. J Neurosurg. 2007;107:275–80.
229. Kossoff EH, Buck C, Freeman JM. Outcomes of 32 hemispherectomies for Sturge-Weber syndrome worldwide. Neurology. 2002;59:1735–8.
230. Basheer SN, Connolly MB, Lautzenhiser A, Sherman EM, Hendson G, Steinbok P. Hemispheric surgery in children with refractory epilepsy: seizure outcome, complications, and adaptive function. Epilepsia. 2007;48:133–40.
231. Shimizu H. Our experience with pediatric epilepsy surgery focusing on corpus callosotomy and hemispherectomy. Epilepsia. 2005;46(Suppl 1):30–1.
232. Lam S, Mathern GW. Functional hemsispherectomy at UCLA. In: Cataltepe O, Jallo GI, editors. Pediatric Epilepsy. New York: Thieme; 2010. p. 230–40.
233. Binder DK, Schramm J. Transsylvian functional hemispherectomy. Childs Nerv Syst. 2006;22(8):960–6.
234. Shimizu H, Maehara T. Modification of peri-insular hemispherectomy and surgical results. Neurosurgery. 2000;47:367–72.

235. Villemure JG, Adams CB, Hoffman HJ, et al. Hemispherectomy. In: Engel J, editor. Surgical treatment of the epilepsies. New York: Raven Press; 1993. p. 511–8.
236. Vining EP, Freeman JM, Brandt J, et al. Progressive unilateral encephalopathy of childhood (Rasmussen´s syndrome): a reappraisal. Epilepsia. 1993;34:639–50.
237. Kestle J, Connolly M, Cochrane D. Pediatric peri-insular hemispherotomy. Pediatr Neurosurg. 2000;32:44–7.
238. Kwan A, Ng WH, Otsubo H, Ochi A, Snead OC, Tamber MS, Rutka JT. Hemispherectomy for the control of intractable epilepsy in childhood: comparison of 2 surgical techniques in a single institution. Neurosurgery. 2010;67:429–36.
239. Adams CBT. Hemispherectomy: a modification. J Neurol Neurosurg Psychiatry. 1983;46:617–9.
240. Villemure JG, Mascott CR. Peri-insular hemispherectomy: surgical principles and anatomy. Neurosurgery. 1995;37:975–81.
241. Gonzalez-Martinez JA, Gupta A, Kotagal P, Lachhwani D, Wyllie E, Luders HO, Bingaman WE. Hemispherectomy for catastrophic epilepsy in infants. Epilepsia. 2005;46:1518–25.
242. Gaubatz J, Ernst L, Prillwitz CC, et al. Pyramidal tract and alternate motor fibers complementarily mediate motor compensation in patients after hemispherotomy. Nature Sci Rep. 2020; https://doi.org/10.1038/s41598-020-57504-x.
243. Fujimoto A, Okanishi T, Sato K, et al. Hemispherotomy can cause post-operative strabismus. Brain Dev. 2019; https://doi.org/10.1016/j.braindev.2019.08.011.
244. Wilson DH, Reeves A, Gazzaniga M, Culver C. Cerebral commissurotomy for control of intractable seizures. Neurology. 1977;27:708–15.
245. Murro AM, Flanigan HF, Gallagher BB. Corpus callosotomy for the treatment of intractable epilepsy. Epilepsy Res. 1988;2:44–50.
246. Wyler AR. Corpus callosotomy in the treatment of epilepsy. Contemp Neurosurg. 1990;12:1–5.
247. Maerhara T, Shimizu H, Oda M, Arai N. Surgical treatment of children with intractable epilepsy. Neurol Med Chir (Tokyo). 1996;36:306–9.
248. Maehara T, Shimizu H. Surgical outcome of corpus callosotomy in patients with drop attacks. Epilepsia. 2001;42:67–71.
249. Nei M, O'Connor M, Liporace J, Sperling MR. Refractory generalized seizures: response to corpus callosotomy and vagal nerve stimulation. Epilepsia. 2006;47:115–22.
250. Jea A, Vachhrajani S, Johnson KK, Rutka JT. Corpus callosotomy in children with intractable epilepsy using frameless stereotactic neuronavigation: 12-year experience et the Hospital for sick children in Toronto. Neurosurg Focus. 2008;25:E7.
251. Sunaga S, Shimizu H, Sugano H. Long-term follow-up of seizure outcomes after corpus callosotomy. Seizure. 2009;18:124–8.
252. Purves SJ, Wada JA, Woodhurst WB, Moyes PD, Strauss E, Kosaka B, Li D. Results of anterior corpus callosum section in 24 patients with medically intractable seizures. Neurology. 1988;38:1194–201.
253. Van Wagenen WP, Herren RY. Surgical division of commisural pathways in the corpus callosum: relation to spread of an epileptic attack. Arch Neurol Psychiatry. 1940;44:740–59.
254. Wilson DH, Reeves A, Gazzaniga M. "Central" commissurotomy for intractable generalized epilepsy: series two. Neurology. 1982;32:687–97.
255. Spencer SS. Corpus callosum section and other disconnection procedures for medically intractable epilepsy. Epilepsia. 1988;29:85–99.
256. Spencer SS, Spencer DD, Williamson PD, Sass K, Novelly RA, Mattson RH. Corpus callosotomy for epilepsy. I Seizure effects. Neurology. 1988;38:19–24.
257. Makari G, Holmes G, Murro A. Corpus callosotomy for the treatment of intractable epilepsy in children. J Epilepsy. 1989;2:1–7.
258. Luat A, Asano F, Kumar A, et al. Corpus Callosotomy for intractable epilepsy revisited: the Children's Hospital of Michigan Series. J Child Neurol. 2017;32(7):624–9.
259. Reeves AG, Risse G. Neurological effects of callosotomy. In: Reeves AG, Roberts DW, editors. Epilepsy and the corpus callosoum 2. Advances in behavioral biology, vol. 45. New York: Plenum; 1995. p. 241–51.
260. Blount JP, Langburt W, Otsubo H, Chitoku S, Ochi A, Weiss S, Snead OC, Rutka JT. Multiple subpial transections in the treatment of pediatric epilepsy. J Neurosurg. 2004;100:118–24. https://doi.org/10.3171/ped.2004.100.2.0118.
261. Sawhney IM, Robertson IJ, Polkey CE, Binnie CD, Elwes RD. Multiple subpial transection: a review of 21 cases. J Neurol Neurosurg Psychiatry. 1995;58:344–9.
262. Rougier A, Sundstorm L, Claverie B, Saint-Hilaire JM, Labrecque R, Lurton D, Bouvier G. Multiple subpial transection: report of 7 cases. Epilepsy Res. 1996;24:57–63.
263. Mulligan LP, Spencer DD, Spencer SS. Multiple subpial transections: the Yale experience. Epilepsia. 2001;42:226–9.
264. Revesz D, Rydenhag B, Ben-Menachem E. Complications and safety of vagus nerve stimulation: 25 years of experience at a single center. J Neurosurg Pediatr. 2016;18:97–104.
265. Rychlicki F, Zamponi N, Cesaroni E, Corpaci L, Trignani R, Ducati A, Scerrati M. Complications of vagal nerve stimulation for epilepsy in children. Neurosurg Rev. 2006;29:103–7.
266. Murphy JV, Hornig GW, Schallert GS, Tilton CL. Adverse events in children receiving intermittent left vagal nerve stimulation. Pediatr Neurol. 1998;19:42–4.
267. Alexopoulos AV, Kotagal P, Loddenkemper T, Hammel J, Bingaman WE. Long-term results with

vagus nerve stimulation in children with pharmacoresistant epilepsy. Seizure. 2006;15:491–503.
268. Coykendall DS, Gauderer MW, Blouin BB, Morales A. Vagus nerve stimulation for the management of seizures in children: an 8 year experience. J Pediatr Surg. 2010;45:1479–83.
269. Elliott RE, Morsi A, Kalhorn SP, Marcus J, Sellin J, Kang M, Silverberg A, Rivera E, Geller E, Carlson C, Devinsky O, Doyle WK. Vagus nerve stimulation in 436 consecutive patients with treatment-resistant epilepsy: long-term outcomes and predictors of response. Epilepsy Behav. 2011a;20:57–63.
270. Hornig GW, Murphy JV, Schallert G, Tilton C. Left vagus nerve stimulation in children with refractory epilepsy: an update. South Med J. 1997;90:484–8.
271. Kang HC, Hwang YS, Kim DS, Kim HD. Vagus nerve stimulation in pediatric intractable epilepsy: a Korean bicentric study. Acta Neurochir Suppl. 2006;99:93–6.
272. Spuck S, Tronnier V, Orosz I, Schönweiler R, Sepehrnia A, Nowak G, et al. Operative and technical complications of vagus nerve stimulator implantation. Neurosurgery. 2010;67:489–94.
273. Tanganelli P, Ferrero S, Colotto P, Regesta G. Vagus nerve stimulation for treatment of medically intractable seizures. Evaluation of long-term outcome. Clin Neurol Neurosurg. 2002;105:9–13.
274. Ardesch JJ, Buschman HP, Wagener-Schimmel LJ, et al. Vagus nerve stimulation for medically refractory epilepsy: a long-term follow-up study. Seizure. 2007;16(7):579–85.
275. Elliott RE, Rodgers SD, Bassani L, et al. Vagus nerve stimulation for children with treatment-resistant epilepsy: a consecutive series of 141 cases. J Neurosurg Pediatr. 2011c;7:491–500.
276. Huf RL, Mamelak A, Kneedy-Cayem K. Vagus nerve stimulation therapy: 2-year prospective open-label study of 40 subjects with refractory epilepsy and low IQ who are living in long-term care facilities. Epilepsy Behav. 2005;6:417–23.
277. Qiabi M, Bouthillier A, Carmant L, Nguyen DK. Vagus nerve stimulation for epilepsy: the notre-dame hospital experience. Can J Neurol Sci. 2011;38:902–8.
278. Ben-Menachem E. Vagus nerve stimulation, side effects, and long-term safety. J Clin Neurophysiol. 2001;18:415–8.
279. Patel NC, Edwards MS. Vagal nerve stimulator pocket infections. Pediatr Infect Dis J. 2004;23:681–3.
280. Patwardhan RV, Stong B, Bebin EM, Mathisen J, Grabb PA. Efficacy of vagal nerve stimulation in children with medically refractory epilepsy. Neurosurgery. 2000;47:1353–7.
281. Smyth MD, Tubbs RS, Bebin EM, Grabb PA, Blount JP. Complications of chronic vagus nerve stimulation for epilepsy in children. J Neurosurg. 2003;99:500–3.
282. Spuck S, Nowak G, Sperner J. TronnierV. Implantation und Komplikationen der Vagusnervstimulation. J Neurol Neurosurg Psychiatry. 2007;8(4):16–20.
283. Kahlow H, Olivecrona M. Complications of vagal nerve stimulation for drug-resistant epilepsy: a single center longitudinal study of 143 patients. Seizure. 2013;22:827–33.
284. Kabir SM, Rajaraman C, Rittey C, Zaki HS, Kemeny AA, McMullan J. Vagus nerve stimulation in children with intractable epilepsy: indications, complications and outcome. Childs Nerv Syst. 2009;25:1097–100.
285. Handforth A, DeGiorgio CM, Schachter SC, Uthman BM, Naritoku DK, Tecoma ES, Henry TR, Collins SD, Vaughn BV, Gilmartin RC, Labar DR, Morris GL 3rd, Salinsky MC, Osorio I, Ristanovic RK, Labiner DM, Jones JC, Murphy JV, Ney GC, Wheless JW. Vagus nerve stimulation therapy for partial-onset seizures: a randomized active-control trial. Neurology. 1998;51:48–55.
286. Vonck K, Thadani V, Gilbert K, Dedeurwaerdere S, De Groote L, De Herdt V, et al. Vagus nerve stimulation for refractory epilepsy: a transatlantic experience. J Clin Neurophysiol. 2004;21:283–9.
287. Ben-Menachem E, Manon-Espaillat R, Ristanovic R, Wilder BJ, Stefan H, Mirza W, Tarver WB, Wernicke JF. Vagus nerve stimulation for treatment of partial seizures: 1. A controlled study of effect on seizures. First international Vagus nerve stimulation study group. Epilepsia. 1994;35:616–26.
288. DeGiorgio CM, Schachter SC, Handforth A, Salinsky M, Thompson J, Uthman B, Reed R, Collins S, Tecoma E, Morris GL, Vaughn B, Naritoku DK, Henry T, Labar D, Gilmartin R, Labiner D, Osorio I, Ristanovic R, Jones J, Murphy J, Ney G, Wheless J, Lewis P, Heck C. Prospective long-term study of vagus nerve stimulation for the treatment of refractory seizures. Epilepsia. 2000;41:1195–200.
289. Englot DJ, Chang EF, Auguste KI. Vagus nerve stimulation for epilepsy: a meta-analysis of efficacy and predictors of response. J Neurosurg. 2011a;115:1248–55.
290. Englot DJ, Chang EF, Auguste KI. Efficacy of vagus nerve stimulation for epilepsy by patient age, epilepsy duration, and seizure type. Neurosurg Clin N Am. 2011b;22:443–8. https://doi.org/10.1016/j.nec.2011.07.002.
291. Air EL, Ghomri YM, Tyagi R, Grande AW, Crone K, Mangano FT. Management of vagal nerve stimulator infections: do they need to be removed? J Neurosurg Pediatr. 2009;3(1):73–8.
292. Morris GL, Gloss D, Buchhalter J, Mack KJ, Nichels K, Harden C. Evidence-based guideline update: vagus nerve stimulation for the treatment of epilepsy. Neurology. 2013;81:1453–9.
293. Robinson LC, Pharm D, Winston KR. Relationship of vocal cord paralysis to the coil diameter of vagus nerve stimulator leads. Neurosurgery. 2015;122:532–5.
294. Ramsay RE, Uthman BM, Augustinsson LE, Upton AR, Naritoku D, Willis J, Treig T, Barolat G, Wernicke JF. Vagus nerve stimulation for treatment of partial seizures: 2. Safety, side effects, and tolerability. First international Vagus nerve stimulation study group. Epilepsia. 1994;35:627–36.

295. MacDonald J, Couldwell WT. Revision of vagal nerve stimulator electrodes: technical approach. Acta Neurochir. 2004;146:567–70.
296. Ben-Menachem E, Hellstrom K, Waldton C, Augustinson LE. Evaluation of refractory epilepsy treated with vagus nerve stimulation for up to 5 years. Neurology. 1999;52:1265–7.
297. Couch JD, Gilman AM, Doyle WK. Long-term expectations of vagus nerve stimulation: a look at battery replacement and revision surgery. Neurosurgery. 2016;78:42–6.
298. Rijkers K, Berfelo MW, Cornips EM, et al. Hardware failure in vagus nerve stimulation therapy. Acta Neurochir. 2008;150:403–5.
299. Dlouhy BJ, Viljoen SV, Kung DK, et al. Vagus nerve stimulation after lead revision. Neurosurg Focus. 2012;32:E11.
300. Espinosa J, Aiello MT, Naritoku DK. Revision and removal of stimulating electrodes following long-term therapy with the vagus nerve stimulator. Surg Neurol. 1999;51:659–64.
301. Ortler M, Unterhofer C, Dobesberger J, et al. Complete removal of vagus nerve stimulator generator and electrodes. J Neurosurg Pediatr. 2010;5:191–4.
302. Aalbers MW, Rijkers K, Klinkenberg S, et al. Vagus nerve stimulation lead removal or replacement: surgical technique, institutional experience, and literature overview. Acta Neurochir. 2015;157:1917–24.
303. Shaffer MJ, Jackson CE, Szabo CA, Simpson CB. Vagal nerve stimulation: clinical and electrophysiological effects on vocal fold function. Ann Otol Rhinol Laryngol. 2005;114:7–14.
304. Kalkanis JG, Krishna P, Espinosa JA, Naritoku DK. Self-inflicted vocal cord paralysis in patients with vagus nerve stimulators. Report of two cases. J Neurosurg. 2002;96:949–51.
305. Vagus Nerve Stimulation Study Group. A randomized controlled trial of chronic vagus nerve stimulation for treatment of medically intractable seizures. Neurology. 1995;45(2):224–30.
306. Tran Y, Shah AK, Mittal S. Lead breakage and vocal cord paralysis following blunt neck trauma in a patient with vagal nerve stimulator. J Neurol Sci. 2011;304:132–5.
307. Kim W, Clancy RR, Liu GT. Horner syndrome associated with implantation of a vagus nerve stimulator. Am J Ophthalmol. 2001;131:383–4.
308. Clark A, Kupermann RA, Auguste KI, et al. Intractable episodic bradycardia resulting from progressive lead traction in an epileptic child with a vagus nerve stimulator: a delayed complication. J Neurosurg Pediatr. 2012;9:389–93.
309. Landy HJ, Ramsay RE, Slater J, Casiano RR, Morgan R. Vagus nerve stimulation for complex partial seizures: surgical technique, safety, and efficacy. J Neurosurg. 1993;78:26–31.
310. Helmers SL, Whenless JW, Frost M, Gates J, Levisohn P, Tardo C, Conry JA, Yalnizoglou D, Madsen JR. Vagus nerve stimulation therapy in pediatric patients with refractory epilepsy: a retrospective study. J Child Neurol. 2001;16:843–8.
311. Tatum WO, Moore DB, Stecker MM, et al. Ventricual asystole during vagus nerve stimulation for epilepsy in humans. Neurology. 1999;52:1267–9.
312. Zalvan C, Sulica L, Wolf S, Cohen J, Gonzalez-Yanes O, Blitzer A. Laryngopharyngeal dysfunction from the implant vagal nerve stimulator. Laryngoscope. 2003;113:221–5.
313. Hatton KW, McLarney JT, Pittman T, et al. Vagal nerve stimulation: overview and implications for anesthesiologists. Anesth Analg. 2006;103:1241–9.
314. Fahy BG. Intraoperative and perioperative complications with a vagus nerve stimulation device. J Clin Anesth. 2010;22:213–22.
315. Horowitz G, Amit M, Fried I, et al. Vagal nerve stimulation for refractory epilepsy: the surgical procedure and complications in 100 implantations by a single medical center. Eur Arch Otorhinolaryngol. 2013;270:355–8.
316. Murphy JV, for the Pediatric VNS Study group. Left vagal nerve stimulation in children with medically refractory epilepsy. J Pediatr. 1999;134:563–6.
317. Charous SJ, Kempster G, Manders E, Ristanovic R. The effect of vagal nerve stimulation on Voice. Laryngoscope. 2001;111(11 Pt 1):2028–31.
318. Kirse DJ, Werle AH, Murphy JV, Eyen TP, Bruegger DE, Hornig GW, Torkelson RD. Vagus nerve stimulator implantation in children. Arch Otolaryngol Head Neck Surg. 2001;128:1263–8.
319. Asconape JJ, Moore DD, Zipes DP, Hartman LM, Duffell WH Jr. Bradycardia and asystole with the use of vagus nerve stimulation for the treatment of epilepsy: a rare complication of intraoperative device testing. Epilepsia. 1999;40:1452–4.
320. Srinivasan B, Awasthi A. Transient atrial fibrillation after the implantation of a vagus nerve stimulator. Epilepsia. 2004;45:1645.
321. Schlachter SC. Vagus nerve stimulation therapy. Five years after FDA approval. Neurology. 2002;59(Suppl 4):S15.
322. Ronkainen E, Korpelainen JT, Heikkinen E, Myllyla VV, Huikuri HV, Isojarvi JI. Cardiac autonomic control in patients with refractory epilepsy before and during vagus nerve stimulation treatment: a one-year follow-up study. Epilepsia. 2006;47:556–62.
323. Lundy DS, Casiano RR, Landy HJ, Gallo J, Gallo B, Ramsey RE. Effects of vagal nerve stimulation on laryngeal function. J Voice. 1993;7:359–64.
324. Kumar R, Winston KR, Folzenlogen Z. Removal of vagus nerve stimulator leads and reuse of same site for reimplantation: technique and experience. World Neurosurg. 2016;91:190–4.
325. Agarwal G, Wilfong AA, Edmonds JL. Surgical revision of vagus nerve stimulation electrodes in children. Otolaryngol Head Neck Surg. 2011;144(1):123–4.
326. Waseem H, Raffa SJ, Benbadis SR, et al. Lead revision surgery for vagus nerve stimulation in epilepsy: outcomes and efficacy. Epilepsy Behav. 2014;31:110–3.
327. Ng WH, Donner E, Go C, et al. Revision of vagal nerve stimulation (VNS) electrodes: review and

report on use of ultra-sharp monopolar tip. Childs Nerv Syst. 2010;26:1081–4.
328. Fisher R, Salanova V, Witt T, Worth R, Henry T, Gross R, Oommen K, Osorio I, Nazzaro J, Labar D, Kaplitt M, Sperling M, Sandok E, Neal J, Handforth A, Stern J, De Salles A, Chung S, Shetter A, Bergen D, Bakay R, Henderson J, French J, Baltuch G, Rosenfeld W, Youkilis A, Marks W, Garcia P, Barbaro N, Fountain N, Bazil C, Goodman R, McKhann G, Babu Krishnamurthy K, Papavassiliou S, Epstein C, Pollard J, Tonder L, Grebin J, Coffey R, Graves N, SANTE Study Group. Electrical stimulation of the anterior nucleus of thalamus for treatment of refractory epilepsy. Epilepsia. 2010;51(5):899–908.
329. Kerrigan JF, Litt B, Fisher RS, Cranstoun S, French JA, Blum DE, Dichter M, Shetter A, Baltuch G, Jaggi J, Krone S, Brodie M, Rise M, Graves N. Electrical stimulation of the anterior nucleus of the thalamus for the treatment of intractable epilepsy. Epilepsia. 2004;45:346–54.
330. McGovern RA, Banks GP, McKhann GM II. New techniques and progress in epilepsy surgery. Curr Neurol Neurosci Rep. 2016; https://doi.org/10.1007/s11910-016-0661-6.
331. Salanova V. Deep brain stimulation for epilepsy. Epilepsy Behav. 2018; https://doi.org/10.1016/j.yebeh.2018.06041.
332. Morrell MJ, Group RNSSiES. Responsive cortical stimulation for the treatment of medically intractable partial epilepsy. Neurology 2011;77:1295–1304.
333. Heck CN, King-Stephens D, Massey AD, et al. Two-year seizure reduction in adults with medically intractable partial onset epilepsy treated with responsive neurostimulation: final results of the RNS System Pivotal trial. Epilepsia. 2014;55:432–41. https://doi.org/10.1111/epi.12534.
334. Bergey GK, Morrell MJ, Mizrahi EM, et al. Long-term treatment with responsive brain stimulation in adults with refractory partial seizures. Neurology. 2015;84:810–7.
335. Geller EB, Skarpaas TL, Gross RE, et al. Brain-responsive neurostimulation in patients with medically intractable mesial temporal lobe epilepsy. Epilepsia. 2017;58:994–1004.
336. Jobst BC, Kapur R, Barkley GL, et al. Brain-responsive neurostimulation in patients with medically intractable seizures arising from eloquent and other neocortical areas. Epilepsia. 2017;58:1005–14.
337. Fountas KN, Smith JR, Murro AM, Politsky J, Park YD, Jenkins PD. Implantation of a closed-loop stimulation in the management of medically refractory focal epilepsy: a technical note. Stereotyct Funct Neurosurg. 2005;83:153–8.
338. Kameyama S, Shirozu H, Masuda H, Ito Y, Sonoda M, Akazawa K. MRI-guided stereotactic radiofrequency thermocoagulation for 100 hypothalamic hamartomas. J Neurosurg. 2016;124:1503–12.
339. Vojtech Z, Malikova H, Kramska L, Anyz J, Syrucek M, Zamecnik J, et al. Long-term seizure outcome after stereotactic amygdalohippocampectomy. Acta Neurochir. 2014;156:1529–37. https://doi.org/10.1007/s00701-014-2126-5.
340. Bourdillon P, Rheims S, Catenoix H, et al. Surgical techniques: Stereoelectroencephalography-guided radiofrequency thermocoagulation (SEEG-guided RF-TC). European Journal of Epilepsy. 2019; https://doi.org/10.1016/j.seizure.2019.01.021.
341. Bourdillon P, Isnard J, Catenoix H, Montavont A, Rheims S, Ryvlin P. Stereo-electroencephalography-guided radiofrequency Thermocoagulation (SEEG-guided RF-TC) in drug-resistant focal epilepsy: results from a 10-year experience. Epilepsia. 2017;58(1):85–93.
342. Cossu M, Fuschillo D, Casaceli G, Pelliccia V, Castana L, Mai R. Stereoelectroencephalography-guided radiofrequency thermocoagulation in the epileptogenic zone: a retrospective study on 89 cases. J Neurosurg. 2015;123(6):1358–67.
343. Guénot M, Isnard J, Ryvlin P, Fischer C, Mauguière F, Sindou M. SEEG-guided RF thermocoagulation of epileptic foci: feasibility, safety and preliminary results. Epilepsia. 2004;45:1368–74.
344. Catenoix H, Mauguière F, Guénot M, Ryvlin P, Bissery A, Sindou M, et al. SEEG- guided thermocoagulations: a palliative treatment of nonoperable partial epilepsies. Neurology. 2008;71:1719–26.
345. Malikova H, Kramska L, Vojtech Z, Sroubek J, Lukavsky J, Liscak R. Relationship between remnant hippocampus and amygdala and memory outcomes after stereotactic surgery for mesial temporal lobe epilepsy. Neuropsychiatr Dis Treat. 2015;11:2927–33. https://doi.org/10.2147/NDT.S95497.
346. Curry DJ, Raskin J, Ali I, Wilfong AA. MR guided laser ablation for the treatment of hypothalamic hamartomas. Epilepsy Res. 2018;142:131–4.
347. Harvey AS, Freeman JL, Berkovic SF, Rosenfeld JV. Transcallosal re-sectionof hypothalamic hamartomas in patients with intractable epilepsy. Epileptic Disord. 2003;5:257–65.
348. Ng YT, Rekate HL, Prenger EC, Wang NC, Chung SS, Feiz-Erfan I, Johnsonbaugh RE, Varland MR, Kerrigan JF. Endoscopic resection of hypothalamic hamartomas for refractory symptomatic epilepsy. Neurology. 2008;70(17):1543–8.
349. Xu DS, Chen T, Hlubek RJ, et al. Magnetic resonance imaging-guided laser interstitial thermal therapy for the treatment of hypothalamic hamartomas: a retrospective review. Neurosurgery. 2018;83:1183–92.
350. Drane DL, Loring DW, Voets NL, Price M, Ojemann JG, Willie JT, et al. Better object recognition and naming outcome with MRI-guided stereotactic laser amygdalohippocampotomy for temporal lobe epilepsy. Epilepsia 2015;56:101–113.
351. Donos C, Breier J, Friedman E, et al. Laser ablation for mesial temporal lobe epilepsy: surgical and cognitive outcomes with and without mesial temporal sclerosis. Epilepsia. 2018;59:1421–32.
352. Jermakowicz WJ, Kanner AM, Sur S, Bermudez C, D'Haese PF, Kolcun JP, et al. Laser thermal ablation for mesiotemporal epilepsy: analysis

of ablation volumes and trajectories. Epilepsia. 2017;58(5):801–10.
353. Kang JY, Wu C, Tracy J, Lorenzo M, Evans J, Nei M, et al. Laser interstitial thermal therapy for medically intractable mesial temporal lobe epilepsy. Epilepsia. 2016;57:325–34.
354. Gross R. The latest on lasers: improving the outcome of MRg-LITT amygdalohippocampectomy. Epilepsy Curr. 2018;18(6):382–6.
355. Wu C, Jermakovicz WJ, Chakravorti S, et al. Effects of surgical targeting in laser interstitial thermal therapy for mesial temporal lobe epilepsy: A multicenter study of 234 patients. Epilepsia. 2019;60(6):1171–83.
356. Grewal SS, Alvi MA, Lu VM, et al. Magnetic resonance-guided laser interstitial thermal therapy versus stereotactic radiosurgery for medically intractable temporal lobe epilepsy: A systematic review and meta-analysis of seizure outcomes and complications. World Neurosurg. 2018; https://doi.org/10.1016/j.wneu.2018.08.227.
357. Hoppe C, Witt J-A, Helmstaedter C, et al. Laser interstitial thermotherapy (LiTT) in epilepsy surgery. Seizure. 2017;48:45–52.
358. Hoppe C, Helmstaedter C. Laser interstitial thermotherapy (LiTT) in pediatric epilepsy surgery. Seizure. 2018; https://doi.org/10.1016/j.seizure.
359. Patel P, Patel NV, Danish SF. Intracranial MR-guided laser-induced thermal therapy: single-center experience with the Visualase thermal therapy system. J Neurosurg. 2016;125:853–60.
360. Devine IM, Burrell CJ, Shih JJ. Curative laser thermoablation of epilepsy secondary to bottom-of-sulcus dysplasia near eloquent cortex. Seizure. 2016;34:35–7.
361. McCracken DJ, Willie J, Fernald BA, Saindane AM, Drane DL, Barrow DL, et al. Magnetic resonance thermometry-guided stereotactic laser ablation of cavernous malformations in drug-resistant epilepsy: imaging and clinical results. Oper Neurosurg. 2016;12:39–48.
362. Hawasli AH, Bandt SK, Hogan RE, Werner N, Leuthardt EC. Laser ablation as treatment strategy for medically refractory dominant insular epilepsy: therapeutic and functional considerations. Stereotact Funct Neurosurg. 2014;92:397–404.
363. Cobourn K, Fayed I, Keating RF, Oluigbo CO. Early outcomes of stereoelectroencephalography followed by MR-guided laser interstitial thermal therapy: a paradigm for minimally invasive epilepsy surgery. Neurosurg Focus. 2018;45:1–9.
364. Lewis EC, Weil AG, Duchowny M, Bhatia S, Ragheb J, Miller I. MR-guided laser interstitial thermal therapy for pediatric drug-resistant lesional epilepsy. Epilepsia. 2015;56:1590–8.
365. Buckley RT, Wang AC, Miller JW, Novotny EJ, Ojemann JG. Stereotactic laser ablation for hypothalamic and deep intraventricular lesions. Neurosurg Focus. 2016;41:E10. https://doi.org/10.3171/2016.7.FOCUS16236.
366. Pruitt R, Gamble A, Black K, Schulder M, Mehta AD. Complication avoidance in laser interstitial thermal therapy: lessons learned. J Neurosurg. 2017;126(4):1238–45.
367. Hawasli AH, Bagade S, Shimony JS, Miller-Thomas M, Leuthardt EC. Magnetic resonance imaging-guided focused laser interstitial thermal therapy for intracranial lesions: single-institution series. Neurosurgery. 2013;73:1007–17.
368. Atsina KB, Sharan AD, Wu C, Evans JJ, Sperling MR, Skidmore CT, et al. Longitudinal qualitative characterization of MRI features after laser interstitial thermal therapy in drug-resistant epilepsy. AJR. 2016:1–8.
369. Curry DJ, Gowda A, McNichols RJ, Wilfong AA. MR-guided stereotactic laser ablation of epileptogenic foci in children. Epilepsy Behav. 2012;24:408–14.
370. Régis J, Lagmari M, Carron R, et al. Safety and efficacy of gamma knife radiosurgery in hypothalamic hamartomas with severe epilepsies: a prospective trial in 48 patients and review of the literature. Epilepsia. 2017;58:60–71.
371. Wagner K, Buschmann F, Zentner J, et al. Memory outcome one year after stereotactic interstitial radiosurgery in patients with epilepsy due to hypothalamic hamartomas. Epilepsy Behav. 2014;37:204–9.
372. Hensley-Judge H, Quigg M, Barbaro NM, Newman SA, Ward MM, Chang EF, et al. Visual field defects after radiosurgery for mesial temporal lobe epilepsy. Epilepsia. 2013;54:1376–80.
373. Quigg M, Broshek DK, Barbaro NM, Ward MM, Laxer KD, Yan G, et al. Neuropsychological outcomes after gamma knife radiosurgery for mesial temporal lobe epilepsy: a prospective multicenter study. Epilepsia. 2011;52:909–16.
374. Régis J, Rey M, Bartolomei F, et al. Gamma knife surgery in mesial temporal lobe epilepsy: a prospective multicenter study. Epilepsia. 2004;45:504–15.
375. Barbaro NM, Quigg M, Broshek DK, et al. A multicenter, prospective pilot study of gamma knife radiosurgery for mesial temporal lobe epilepsy: seizure response, adverse events, and verbal memory. Ann Neurol. 2009;65:167–75. https://doi.org/10.1002/ana.21558.
376. Liang S, Li A, Jiang H, Meng X, Zhao M, Zhang J, Sun Y. Anterior corpus callosotomy in patients with intractable generalized epilepsy and mental retardation. Stereotact Funct Neurosurg. 2010;88:246–52.
377. Barbaro NM, Quigg M, Ward MW, et al. Radiosurgery versus open surgery for mesial temporal lobe epilepsy: the randomized, controlled ROSE trial. Epilepsia. 2018; https://doi.org/10.1111/epi.14045.
378. Régis J, Bartolomei F, Hayashi M, Chauvel P. Gamma knife surgery, a neuromodulation therapy in epilepsy surgery! Acta Neurochir. 2002;84(Suppl):37–47.
379. Regis J, Peragut J, Rey M, et al. First selective amygdalohippocampic radiosurgery for mesial tem-

poral lobe epilepsy. Stereotact Funct Neurosurg. 1994;64:191–201.
380. Regis J, Semah F, Bryan R, Levrier O, Rey M, Samson Y, Peragut J. Early and delayed MR and PET changes after selective temporomesial radiosurgery in mesial temporal lobe epilepsy. AJNR. 1999;20:213–6.
381. Chang EF, Quigg M, Oh MC, Dillon WP, Ward MM, Laxer KD, Broshek DK, Barbaro NM. Predictors of efficacy after stereotactic radiosurgery for medial temporal lobe epilepsy. Neurology. 2010;74:165–72. https://doi.org/10.1212/WNL.0b013e3181c9185d.
382. Vojtech Z, Malíková H, Krámská L, Liščák R, Vladyka V. MRI-guided stereotactic amygdalohippocampectomy: a single center experience. Neuropsychiatr DisTreat. 2015;11:359–74.
383. Usami K, Kawai K, Koga T, et al. Delayed complication after gamma knife surgery for mesial temporal lobe epilepsy. J Neurosurg. 2012;116(6):1221–5.
384. Rheims S, Didelot A, Guenot M, Regis J, Ryvlin P. Subcontinuous epileptiform activity after failed hippocampal radiosurgery. Epilepsia. 2011;52:1425–9.
385. McGonigal A, Sahgal A, De Salles A, et al. Radiosurgery for epilepsy: systematic review and International Stereotactic Radiosurgery Society (ISRS) practice guideline. Epilepsy Res. 2017;137:123–31.
386. McGonigal A, Micoulaud-Franchi JA. Screening for anxiety and depression in epilepsy. Can J Neurol Sci. 2018;45(4):481–2.
387. Ganz JC. Gamma knife radiosurgery and its possible relationship to malignancy: a review. J Neurosurg. 2002;97(5 Suppl):644–52.
388. Starke RM, Yen CP, Chen CJ, Ding D, Mohila CA, Jensen ME, et al. An updated assessment of the risk of radiation-induced neoplasia after radiosurgery of arteriovenous malformations. World Neurosurg. 2014;82:395–401.

# Cost-Effectiveness of Epilepsy Surgery

# 16

*Economy is the wealth of the poor and the wisdom of the rich.*

*French Proverb*

## Contents



Economic considerations are particularly important for patients with medically refractory epilepsy accounting for approximately 30%–40% of all epilepsy patients [1–6]. Begley et al. [7] reported that the 20%–30% of children and adults with medically refractory epilepsy add to 38% of annual direct and 86% of indirect medical costs of epilepsy. In another analysis, Begley et al. [8] noted that the 15% of patients who are most refractory amount to >50% of the total costs of epilepsy. Direct costs result from physician consultations, emergency room visits, hospitalizations, medications, laboratory testings, imaging, etc. Indirect costs include lost productivity from unemployment, underemployment or lost work time, household expenditure, and lost work of relatives taking care of the patient [9]. In a prospective Danish cohort study, Jennum et al. [10] evaluated healthcare costs and socioeconomic data of 15,329 epilepsy patients with seizure onset before the age of 18 years compared with 31,414 controls. They concluded that epilepsy is associated with severe socioeconomic consequences including lower educational level and employment status. This holds particularly true, since - in contrast to other chronic diseases - epilepsy affects young patients


J. Zentner, *Surgical Treatment of Epilepsies*, https://doi.org/10.1007/978-3-030-48748-5_16

making them disabled during the most productive phase of their lives if not successfully treated.

Direct costs of medically intractable patients are much easier to assess than indirect ones and have been estimated to be four to nine times higher than those for controlled epilepsy patients [7, 11–14]. According to Italian [15] and Chinese studies [16], the highest costs refer to antiepileptic drugs (AED) accounting for about 50% of the total direct expenses. Jennum et al. [17] emphasized increasing direct costs with additional comorbidity in epilepsy patients as it has been stated by others [18]. In fact, pharmacoresistant epilepsy represents a substantial burden for the health care system. On the other hand, presurgical evaluation and surgical treatment are cost-intensive, too, requiring a highly specialized personnel and expensive equipment. In addition, there are high costs for implants when minimally invasive stereotactic procedures are used. High expenses of both pharmacoresistant epilepsy as well as epilepsy surgical programs emphasize the importance to evaluate of cost-effectiveness of epilepsy surgery.

## 16.1 Resective Surgery

### 16.1.1 Economic Studies in Adults

Most trials on economic evaluation of epilepsy surgery have been conducted in the United States, Canada, and Sweden. The majority of studies are retrospective and almost all refer to temporal lobe epilepsies. In addition, these studies reflect economic conditions of different health care systems [19–22]. Data from prospective and modeling trials are rare [9, 23, 24], and cost-effectiveness calculations addressing the major spectrum of resective and non-resective epilepsy surgery are even lacking. In addition, most studies consider only direct costs, and only sparse literature is available on the assessment of indirect ones.

#### 16.1.1.1 Direct costs

Wiebe et al. [22] concluded in his Canadian study that cumulated direct costs of continued medical versus surgical treatment were balanced after 9 years due to the decreased costs of AED in the surgical arm. Results of a US multicenter study showed that overall direct costs in seizure-free patients after temporal lobectomy had declined by 32% at 1-year follow-up. Most of the reduction was due to progressively lower expenses for AED and epilepsy-related hospitalizations [13, 14]. Picot et al. [23] found in a prospective study of 207 patients with a 5-years follow-up that direct costs became lower in surgical patients compared with medical patients 3 years after surgery, and that epilepsy surgery is cost-effective compared to medical treatment after a time interval between 9 and 10 years if all direct costs were taken into account. Based on the Danish National Patient Registry, Jennum et al. [25] compared in a matched case-control study 254 epilepsy patients treated by surgery and 989 controls in whom epilepsy was diagnosed but not surgically treated with a follow-up of 3 years between 1996 and 2000. Patients who underwent epilepsy surgery were more severely affected by their disease in terms of health care use before surgery, and they had significantly lower costs associated by medication, outpatient services, inpatient admissions, as well as accidents and emergency visits after surgery compared to the control group [25].

#### 16.1.1.2 Direct and indirect costs

Platt and Sperling [9] simulated in a modeling study direct and indirect costs based on a 70% probability for seizure freedom after surgery. The total costs—direct and indirect ones—were lower in the surgical group versus the medical one after 7.3 years, whereas direct costs of the two strategies balanced each other 14.4 years after surgery, and direct costs for medication after 35 years of treatment. The authors found at 10 years a reduction in indirect costs related to unemployment of 31% in the surgical group compared with the medical group [9]. Based on a similar US modeling study evaluating direct and indirect costs of temporal lobe epilepsy, Sheikh et al. [26] concluded that surgery becomes cost-effective within 3 years, and that there is an incremental cost-effectiveness at 5 years. In addition, presurgical evaluation has been found to be cost-effective in pharmacoresistant patients, even if the probability of being deemed a surgical candidate is only 5% to 10% [26].

## 16.1.2 Economic Studies in Children

Keene and Ventureyra [27] compared pediatric epilepsy surgery to medical management over 25 years. They found costs per patient 8% higher for the medical treatment group than for the surgical arm. Savings were realized 14 years after surgery. Since invasive recordings were not done in their patients, the costs of surgery may have been underestimated in this study. Cost-effectiveness in pediatric patients has also been evaluated in a decision tree analysis of Widjaja et al. [28] including 15 children in the surgical and in the medical arm, respectively. In this study, expenses for invasive intracranial monitoring was included. The authors found that the higher initial costs of surgery were offset within 1 year after surgical treatment [28]. In a Canadian study including children known to be suitable candidates for surgery, Bowen et al. [29] found that those undergoing surgery were less costly and revealed greater clinical benefit compared to continued medical management. Similarly, Oldham et al. [30] provided a US study comparing seizure frequency and costs of care for those children who were managed surgically versus those who, although eligible for surgery, chose to continue medical treatment. They found that for the 42% of surgical patients who achieved seizure freedom, annual follow-up costs were substantially lower than for patients treated medically. Contrarily, Catchpool et al. [31] concluded in an Australian study based on the data of 105 operated children followed over 7.6 years that surgery was more expensive than continued medical treatment, but resulted in a greater improvement in health-related quality of life (HRQL). However, differences in costs decreased over time, and the follow-up period may have been too short to reach balance.

## 16.1.3 Quality of Life, Psychosocial and Vocational Outcome, and Timing of Surgery

### 16.1.3.1 Quality of life

Using a decision analysis model to evaluate the cost-effectiveness of anterior temporal lobectomy, King et al. [19] found that surgical treatment was more costly but provided an average of 1.1 additional quality-adjusted life years (QUALYs). Reid et al. [32] retrospectively assessed psychosocial profile and quality of life (QOL) in patients who underwent epilepsy surgery between 1986 and 1994. Replicating the 1997 findings [33], they found significant differences between seizure-free and non-seizure-free patients with respect to anxiety, depression, self-esteem, mastery, stigma, affect balance, self-reported health, and QOL with better conditions in seizure-free cases. These results are in line with others [34] and support previous studies emphasizing the importance of seizure freedom on QOL [35–39]. However, as stated by Reid et al. [32], even of the 67 patients with persisting seizures, only 3 (4.5%) reported that they regretted having surgery.

### 16.1.3.2 Psychosocial and vocational outcome

Data on psychosocial and vocational outcome after epilepsy surgery are sparse and studies report inconsistent findings with increased, unchanged, or decreased employment opportunities after surgery [40]. Young age, presurgical work experience and employment, presurgical aims and expectations, postsurgical seizure freedom, an intact neuropsychological status, and further education after surgery have been found to be equally important and increase the likelihood of a favorable psychosocial and vocational outcome [34, 36, 41–45]. Evaluating 369 patients undergoing anterior temporal lobectomy with a mean follow-up of almost 10 years, psychosocial and vocational outcome were improved after surgery and correlated positively with seizure freedom [46, 47]. A Swedish study showed that a rehabilitation program after temporal lobe surgery improved employment status [48].

#### 16.1.3.3 Timing of surgery

It has been suggested that a major beneficial effect of surgery on social outcome and employment status may be limited by late surgical intervention [17, 49–52]. In the study of Jennum et al. [25], the surgical intervention had no significant effects on social status in terms of occupation and educational level, nor did Picot et al. [23] find a significant improvement in occupational activity in the surgical arm after 5 years of follow-up. Social effects of surgery may be stable or even decrease after a period exceeding 2 to 5 years [17, 25, 53, 54]. Puka et al. [55] provided a systematic review and meta-analysis of social outcomes for adults with a history of childhood-onset epilepsy. Among individuals, who had undergone epilepsy surgery in childhood, they found that 98% had completed high school, vocational training, college, or university, 75% were employed, and 29% lived independently. Seizure control has been found to be associated with better employment. Absence of cognitive problems constituted the most persistent predictor of better outcomes across most social domains [55]. These findings support early diagnosis and early surgical intervention to provide children and adolescents the best chances for a favorable cognitive development and psychosocial outcome.

## 16.2 Non-resective Surgery

Only a few cost-effectiveness studies have addressed non-resective surgical modalities. Economic analyses exist for vagal nerve stimulation (VNS), stereotactic radiosurgery (SRS), and MR-guided laser-induced thermal therapy (MRgLITT). Cost analyses of other non-resective surgical strategies are lacking [56].

### 16.2.1 VNS

Ben-Menachem et al. [57] retrospectively analyzed 43 patients receiving VNS for epilepsy and concluded that VNS results in an annual reduction of approximately 3000 dollars related to hospital costs per patient. Similarly, Helmers et al. [58] showed in a retrospective analysis based on US Medicaid Data that in children with intractable epilepsy, VNS is associated with cost savings and decreased use of health care resources as compared to medical therapy alone. De Kinderen et al. [59] studied the expected cost-utility and cost-effectiveness of the ketogenic diet, VNS, and care as usual, using a decision analytic model with a 5-year-time horizon. They concluded that ketogenic diet is more effective and less costly, and thus cost-effective after 12 months compared with VNS. However, compared to care as usual, neither ketogenic diet nor VNS have proven to be cost-effective options, they are both more effective but also more expensive [59].

### 16.2.2 SRS

Langfitt et al. [60] compared direct and indirect costs associated with the treatment of mesiotemporal lobe epilepsy (MTLE) either by stereotactic radiosurgery (SRS) or anterior temporal lobectomy (ATL) analyzing the ROSE (Radiosurgery or Open Surgery for Epilepsy) trial. The analysis showed that costs after ATL declined, but at a higher initial level. Costs following SRS showed a tendency to increase in the second year due to serious adverse events and hospitalizations associated with maximal radiation effect and then to decline. These higher costs eliminated initial savings, thus differences between SRS and ATL were offset. Over the course of the 3-years trial, total direct and indirect costs of ATL and SRS did not differ.

### 16.2.3 MRgLITT

In a model-based cost-effectiveness study, Widjaja et al. [61] compared MRgLITT with resective surgery in adults with MTLE. Outcomes of interest including direct health care costs and quality-adjusted life years (QALYs) were calculated on the basis of probabilities given by representative studies. The analysis suggested that MRgLITT resulted in more QALYs gained but also in higher costs compared to resective surgery. Major uncertainty of these conclusions has been attributed to the limited evidence of the long-term effectiveness of MRgLITT [61].

## 16.3 Limitations of Economic Studies

Major limitations of evaluating cost-effectiveness of epilepsy surgery refer to short periods of follow-up, different models used for cost calculation, and the lack of standardized measures assessing quality of life.

### 16.3.1 Follow-up Periods

As stated by Reid et al. [32], some follow-up studies have spanned only the first two postsurgical years. Wiebe et al. [62] felt that measurements at 1 or 2 years may be "biased or diluted", since these studies primarily rely on extrapolating short-term outcomes and cost data, as it has been stated by others [19, 34, 38, 63]. Since late seizure recurrence is not uncommon [64, 65], postsurgical health care costs that are based on short-term data might be underestimated [66]. Moreover, there is evidence that both medical and psychosocial postsurgical changes develop with time [67–69]. Markand et al. [37] identified time-contingent effects on social and cognitive function and overall quality of life including emotional status, attention/concentration, language, and social situation. They stated that changes might not be evident until at least 2 years after surgery [37]. Sperling et al. [44] noted that improvements in vocational status take as long as 6 years to occur. Assessing 39 patients after temporal resections, Coleman et al. [70] defined a common process of psychosocial development. Milestones included regaining of driving license, educational and vocational gains, and establishing long-term relationships and finally a family unit. Achieving those social milestones after surgery may take a span of 20 years [70]. In sum, larger sample sizes and long-term assessment are needed to create valid economic studies data [28].

### 16.3.2 Calculation of Costs

Indirect costs are not included in most analyses. While it is already difficult to evaluate indirect costs related to under- and unemployment and loss of productivity for the adult age, it poses much more challenges to calculate factors that are important for the pediatric age like cognitive functions and associated chances for professional achievement [71]. In a systematic review, Strzelczyk et al. [72] noted that indirect costs may contribute 12%–85% of the total costs of the disease, and Begley et al. [7] estimated indirect costs at 85% of total expenses. Given the enormous indirect cost implications of epilepsy beginning in childhood, restriction to only direct costs undoubtedly reduces the cost-effectiveness of surgical management [28]. Finally, direct costs noticeably differ both within the same and in particular between different health care systems [30, 73].

### 16.3.3 Standardized Measures

The value that patients place on quality of life improvements as a result of seizure freedom is an important non-monetary benefit that has been addressed by Langfitt et al. [74]. Besides socioeconomic consequences of the disease, patients and families may be concerned about the still existing social stigma [75]. Reviewing seven surgical studies, Rossi [76] emphasized the need for standardized measures assessing psychosocial well-being, overall disease burden, and value of health outcomes as has been stated by others [28, 77, 78]. Various measures may be useful such as the Quality-Adjusted Life Years (QUALYs) and the Disability-Adjusted Life Years (DALY) scores [79, 80].

**Concluding Remarks**

- ***Resective surgery****. Data available indicate that resective surgical treatment of drug-resistant epilepsy is cost-effective not only in the short term, but also in the long term, both for children and adults resulting in significant reduction of direct and indirect health care costs simulated over lifetime.*
- ***Non-resective surgery****. Only scarce reports on cost-effectiveness of non-resective surgical modalities (VNS, SRS, MRgLITT) are available, results of which are not conclusive.*
- ***Long-term data and standardized measures****. Long-term controlled trials and modeling studies assessing different surgical strategies including standardized psychosocial and health quality measures are necessary to provide valid data on the cost-effectiveness of epilepsy surgical programs.*

## References

1. Berg AT, Shinnar S, Levy SR, Testa FM, Smith-Rapaport S, Beckerman B. Early development of intractable epilepsy in children: a prospective study. Neurology. 2001;56:1445–52.
2. Farrell K, Wirrell E, Whiting S. The definition and prediction of intractable epilepsy in children. Adv Neurol. 2006;97:435–42.
3. Thijs RD, Surges R, O'Brien TJ, Sander LW. Epilepsy in adults. Lancet. 2019;393:689–701.
4. Kwan P, Brodie MJ. Early identification of refractory epilepsy. N Engl J Med. 2000;342(5):314–9.
5. Engel J Jr. What can we do for people with drug-resistant epilepsy? The 2016 Wartenberg Lecture. Neurology. 2016;87(23):2483–9.
6. Englot DJ. A modern epilepsy surgery treatment algorithm: incorporating traditional and emerging technologies. Epilepsy Behav. 2018;80:68–74.
7. Begley CE, Famulari M, Annegers JF, et al. The cost of epilepsy in the United States: an estimate from population-based clinical and survey data. Epilepsia. 2000;41:342–51.
8. Begley CE, Annegers JF, Lairson DR, Reynolds TF, Hauser WA. Cost of epilepsy in the United States: a model based on incidence and prognosis. Epilepsia. 1994;35:1230–43.
9. Platt M, Sperling MR. A comparison of surgical and medical costs for refractory epilepsy. Epilepsia. 2002;43:25–31.
10. Jennum P, Debes NMM, Ibsen R, Kjellberg J. Long-term employment, education, and healthcare costs of childhood and adolescent onset of epilepsy. Epilepsy Behav. 2020:107256. https://doi.org/10.1016/j.yebeh.2020.107256.
11. Begley CE, Durgin TL. The direct cost of epilepsy in the United States: a systematic review of estimates. Epilepsia. 2015;56:1376–87.
12. Jacoby A, Buck D, Baker G, McNamee P, Graham-Jones S, Chadwick D. Uptake and costs of care for epilepsy: findings from a U.K. regional study. Epilepsia. 1998;39:776–86.
13. Langfitt JT, Holloway RG, McDermott MP, Messing S, Sarosky K, Berg AT, Spencer SS, Vickrey BG, Sperling MR, Bazil CW, Shinnar S. Health care costs decline after successful epilepsy surgery. Neurology. 2007a;68:1290–8.
14. Langfitt JT, Holloway RG, McDermott MP, et al. Health care costs decline after successful epilepsy surgery. Neurology. 2007b;68:1290–8.
15. Luoni C, Canevini MP, Capovilla G, et al. A prospective study of direct medical costs in a large cohort of consecutively enrolled patients with refractory epilepsy in Italy. Epilepsia. 2015;56:1162–73.
16. Gao L, Xia L, Pan SQ, et al. Burden of epilepsy: a prevalence-based cost of illness study of direct, indirect and intangible costs for epilepsy. Epilepsy Res. 2015;110:146–56.
17. Jennum P, Gyllenborg J, Kjellberg J. The social and economic consequences of epilepsy: a controlled national study. Epilepsia. 2011;52:949–56.
18. Wilner AN, Sharma BK, Thompson A, et al. Diagnoses, procedures, drug utilization, comorbidities, and cost of health care for people with epilepsy in 2012. Epilepsy Behav. 2014;41:83–90.
19. King JT Jr, Sperling MR, Justice AC, et al. A cost-effectiveness analysis of anterior temporal lobectomy for intractable temporal lobe epilepsy. J Neurosurg. 1997;87:20–8.
20. Langfitt JT. Cost-effectiveness of anterotemporal lobectomy in medically intractable complex partial epilepsy. Epilepsia. 1997;2:154–63.
21. Malmgren K, Hedstrom A, Granqvist R, et al. Cost analysis of epilepsy surgery and of vigabatrin treatment in patients with refractory partial epilepsy. Epilepsy Res. 1996;25:199–207.
22. Wiebe S, Gafni A, Blume WT, et al. An economic evaluation of temporal lobe epilepsy. Epilepsy. 1995;8:227–35.
23. Picot M-C, Jaussent A, Neveu D, Kahane P, Crespelle A, et al. Cost-effectiveness analysis of epilepsy surgery in a controlled cohort of adult patients with intractable partial epilepsy: a 5-year follow-up study. Epilepsia. 2016; https://doi.org/10.1111/epi.13492.
24. Jennum P, Christensen J, Ibsen R, Kjellberg J. Long-term socioeconomic consequences and health care costs of childhood and adolescent-onset epilepsy. Epilepsia. 2016;57(7):1078–85.
25. Jennum P, Sabers A, Christensen J, Ibsen R, Kjellberg J. Socioeconomic outcome of epilepsy surgery: a controlled national study. Seizure. 2016;42:52–6.
26. Sheikh SR, Steinmetz MP, Kattan MW, et al. The cost-effectiveness of epilepsy surgery and surgical

evaluation in the United States. Neurosurgery. 2019; https://doi.org/10.1093/neuros/nyz310_165.
27. Keene D, Ventureyra EC. Epilepsy surgery for 5- to 18-year old patients with medically refractory epilepsy—is it cost efficient? Childs Nerv Syst. 1999;15(1):52–4. discussion 55
28. Widjaja E, Li B, Schinkel CD, Ritchie LP, Weaver J, Snead OC, Rutka JT, Coyte PC. Cost-effectiveness of pediatric epilepsy surgery compared to medical treatment in children with intractable epilepsy. Epilepsy Res. 2011;94:61–8.
29. Bowen JM, Snead OC, Chandra K, Blackhouse G, Goeree R. Epilepsy Care in Ontario: an economic analysis of increasing access to epilepsy surgery. Ont. Health Technol. Assess. Ser. 2012;12(18):1–41.
30. Oldham MS, Horn P, Tsevat J, Standridge S. Costs and clinical outcomes of epilepsy surgery in children with drug-resistant epilepsy. Pediatr Neurol. 2015. Doi: 10.10.16/j
31. Catchpool M, Dalziel K, Mahardya RTK, et al. Cost-effectiveness of epileptic surgery compared with medical treatment in children with drug-resistant epilepsy. Epilepsy Behav. 2019;97:253–9.
32. Reid K, Herbert A, Baker G. Epilepsy surgery: patient-perceived long-term costs and benefits. Epilepsy Behav. 2004;5:81–7.
33. Kellet MW, Smith DF, Baker GA, Chadwick DW. Quality of life after epilepsy surgery. J Neurol Neurosurg Psychiatry. 1997;63:52–8.
34. Wheelock I, Peterson C, Buchtel HA. Presurgery expectations, postsurgery satisfaction, and psychosocial adjustment after epilepsy surgery. Epilepsia. 1998;39:487–94.
35. Berto P. Quality of life in patients with epilepsy and impact of treatments. PharmacoEconomics. 2000;20:1039–59.
36. Derry PA, McLachlan RS. Causal attributions for seizures: relation to preoperative psychological adjustment and postoperative psychosocial function in temporal lobe epilepsy. J Epilepsy. 1995;8:74–8.
37. Markand ON, Salanova V, Whelihan E, Emsley CL. Health- related quality of life outcome in medically refractory epilepsy treated with anterior temporal lobectomy. Epilepsia. 2000;41:749–59.
38. McLachlan RS, Rose KJ, Derry PA, Bonnar C, Blume WT, Girvin JP. Health related quality of life and seizure control in temporal lobe epilepsy. Ann Neurol. 1997;41:482–91.
39. Vickery BG, Hays RD, Rausch R, Engel J, Visscher BR, Ary CM. Quality of life of epilepsy surgery patients as compared with outpatients with hypertension, diabetes, heart disease, and/or depressive symptoms. Epilepsia. 1995;35:597–607.
40. Malmgren K, Edelvik A. Long-term outcomes of surgical treatment for epilepsy in adults with regard to seizures, antiepileptic drug treatment and employment. Seizure. 2017;44:217–24.
41. Lendt M, Helmstaedter C, Elger CE. Pre- and postoperative socioeconomic development of 151 patients with focal epilepsies. Epilepsia. 1997;38:1330–7.
42. Derry P, Wiebe S. Psychological adjustment to success and to failure following epilepsy surgery. Can J Neurol Sci. 2000;27(Suppl):116–20.
43. Taylor DC. Patients´ aims for epilepsy surgery: desires beyond seizure freedom. Epilepsia. 2001;42:629–33.
44. Sperling MR, Saykin AJ, Roberts FD, et al. Occupational outcome after temporal lobectomy for refractory epilepsy. Neurology. 1995;45(5):970–7.
45. Vakharia VN, Duncan JS, Witt JA, et al. Getting the best outcomes from epilepsy surgery. Ann Neurol. 2018;83(4):676–90.
46. Hamiwka L, Macrodimitris S, Tellez-Zenteno JF, et al. Social out-comes after temporal or extratemporal epilepsy surgery: a systematic review. Epilepsia. 2011;52:870–9.
47. Zarroli K, Tracy JI, Nei M, et al. Employment after anterior temporal lobectomy. Epilepsia. 2011;52:925–31.
48. Thorbecke R, May TW, Koch-Stoecker S, Ebner A, Bien CG, Specht U. Effects of an inpatient rehabilitation program after temporal lobe epilepsy surgery and other factors on employment 2 years after epilepsy surgery. Epilepsia. 2014;55:725–33.
49. Alonso NB, Mazetto L, de Araujo Filho GM, Vidal-Dourado M, Yacubian EM, Centeno RS. Psychosocial factors associated with in postsurgical prognosis of temporal lobe epilepsy related to hippocampal sclerosis. Epilepsy Behav. 2015;53:66–72.
50. Andersson-Roswall L, Engman E, Samuelsson H, Malmgren K. Psychosocial status 10 years after temporal lobe resection for epilepsy, a longitudinal controlled study. Epilepsy Behav. 2013;28:127–31.
51. Dupont S, Tanguy ML, Clemenceau S, Adam C, Hazemann P, Baulac M. Long-term prognosis and psychosocial outcomes after surgery for MTLE. Epilepsia. 2006;47:2115–24.
52. Elsharkawy AE, May T, Thorbecke R, Koch-Stoecker S, Villagran A, Urak L, Pfafflin M, Pannek H, Pietila TA, Ebner A. Long-term outcome and determinants of quality of life after temporal lobe epilepsy surgery in adults. Epilepsy Res. 2009;86:191–9.
53. Jennum P, Ibsen R, Kjellberg J. Social consequences of sleep disordered breathing on patients and their partners: a controlled national study. Eur Respir J. 2014;43:134–44.
54. Bendix T, Kjellberg J, Ibsen R, Jennum PJ. Whiplash(–like) injury diagnoses and co- morbidities - both before and after the injury: a national registry-based study. BMC Musculoskelet Disord. 2016;17:24.
55. Puka K, Tavares T, Speechley K. Social outcomes for adults with a history of childhood-onset epilepsy: a systematic review and meta-analysis. Epilepsy Behav. 2019;92:297–305.
56. Englot D, Birk H, Chang EF. Seizure outcomes in nonresective epilepsy surgery: an update. Neurosurg Rev. 2016;40(2):181–94.
57. Ben-Menachem E, Hellstrom K, Verstappen D. Analysis of direct hospital costs before and 18 months after treatment with vagus nerve stimulation therapy in 43 patients. Neurology. 2002;59:S44–7.

58. Helmers SL, Duh MS, Guerin A, Sarda SP, Samuelson TM, Bunker MT, Olin BD, Jackson SD, Faught E. Clinical outcomes, quality of life, and costs associated with implantation of vagus nerve stimulation therapy in pediatric patients with drug- resistant epilepsy. Eur J Paediatr Neurol. 2012;16:449–58. https://doi.org/10.1016/j.ejpn.2012.01.001.
59. De Kinderen RJA, Postulart D, et al. Cost-effectiveness of the ketogenic diet and vagus nerve stimulation for the treatment of children with intractable epilepsy. Epilepsy Res. 2015;110:119–31.
60. Langfitt JT, Quigg M, Yan G, et al. Direct and indirect costs associated with stereotactic radiosurgery or open surgery for medial temporal lobe epilepsy: results from the ROSE trial. Epilepsia. 2019;60:1453–61.
61. Widjaja E, Papastavros T, Sander B, et al. Early economic evaluation of MRI-guided laser interstitial thermal therapy (MRgLITT) and epilepsy surgery for mesial temporal lobe epilepsy. PLoS One. 2019;14(11):e0224571. https://doi.org/10.1371/journal.pone.0224571.
62. Wiebe S, Rose K, Derry P, McLachlan R. Outcome assessment in epilepsy: comparative responsiveness of quality of life and psychosocial instruments. Epilepsia. 1997;38(4):430–8.
63. Choi H, Sell RL, Lenert L, et al. Epilepsy surgery for pharmacoresistant temporal lobe epilepsy: a decision analysis. JAMA. 2008;300:2497–505.
64. De Tisi J, Bell GS, Peacock JL, et al. The long-term outcome of adult epilepsy surgery, patterns of seizure remission, and relapse: a cohort study. Lancet. 2011;378:1388–95.
65. Tellez-Zenteno JF, Dhar R, Wiebe S. Long-term seizure outcomes following epilepsy surgery: a systematic review and meta-analysis. Brain. 2005;128:1188–98.
66. Schiltz NK, Kaiboriboon K, Koroukian SM, Singer MR, Love TE. Long-term reduction of health costs and utilization after epilepsy surgery. Epilepsia. 2016;57(2):316–24.
67. Eliashiv S, Dewar S, Wainwright I, Engel J, Fried I. Long-term follow up after temporal lobe resection for lesions associated with chronic seizures. Neurology. 1997;48:621–6.
68. Ewes RDC, Dunn G, Binnie CD, Polkey CE. Outcome following resective surgery for temporal lobe epilepsy: a prospective follow up study of 102 consecutive cases. J Neurol Neurosurg Psychiatry. 1991;54:949–52.
69. Spencer S. Long-term outcome after epilepsy surgery. Epilepsia. 1996;37:807–13.
70. Coleman H, McIntosh A, Wilson SJ. Identifying the trajectory of social milestones 15-20 years after epilepsy surgery: realistic timelines for postsurgical expectations. Epilepsiy. 2019; https://doi.org/10.1002/epi4.12341.
71. Dlugos DJ. The early identification of candidates for epilepsy surgery. Arch Neurol. 2001;58:1543–6.
72. Strzelczyk A, Reese JP, Dodel R, Hamer HM. Cost of epilepsy: a systematic review. Pharmaceconomics. 2008;26(6):463–76.
73. Redelmeier D, Fuchs V. Hospital expenditures in the United States and Canada. N Engl J Med. 1993;328:772–8.
74. Langfitt JT, Vickrey BG, McDermott M, et al. Validity & responsiveness of generic preference-based HRQOL instruments in chronic epilepsy. Qual Life Res. 2006;15:899–914.
75. Jacoby A, Austin JK. Social stigma for adults and children with epilepsy. Epilepsia. 2007;48:6–9.
76. Rossi GF. Evaluation of surgical treatment outcome in epilepsy. Crit Rev Neurosurg. 1998;8:282–9.
77. Sadanand V. Economics of epilepsy surgery. Ann Indian Acad Neurol. 2014;17(Suppl. 1):S120–3.
78. Sheikh SR, Thompson N, Frech F, et al. Quantifying the burden of generalized tonic-clonic seizures in patients with drug-resistant epilepsy. Epilepsia. 2020; https://doi.org/10.1111/epi.16603.
79. Ashenfelter O. Measuring the value of statistical life: problems and prospects. Econ. 2006;116:10–23.
80. Viscusi WK, Aldy JE. The value of a statistical life: a critical review of market estimates throughout the world. J Risk Uncert. 2003;27:5–76.

# The Current Place of Epilepsy Surgery

# 17

*Our knowledge is for today, the truth is for eternity*

*Ramon Y Cajal*

## Contents



Over the last decades, surgical options for the treatment of pharmacoresistant epilepsies have found increasing acceptance [1]. This development is reflected by increased establishment and performance of epilepsy surgical centers worldwide. According to a review of the US National Association of Epilepsy Centers, the number of surgical centers for epilepsy rose from 37 to 189 between 2003 and 2012 [2]. Zelano et al. [3] evaluated the status of epilepsy surgery in 33 European countries after 2000 based on the European Epilepsy Services Inventory (EESI) form as used 17 years ago to assess epilepsy surgical care before 2000 [4]. Comparing data they concluded: (1) The number of specialists involved in epilepsy surgery had increased for all investigated disciplines, with the exception of pediatric neurologists, the number of which was unchanged between the surveys; (2) the gap between the least and the best provided areas had diminished; (3) the capacity of multidisciplinary teams with epilepsy surgery programs had extended while their regional density remained almost stable with one team per 9 million inhabitants for all



J. Zentner, *Surgical Treatment of Epilepsies*, https://doi.org/10.1007/978-3-030-48748-5_17

ILAE chapters (range: no team to one team per 1 million inhabitants) and one team per 5.48 million inhabitants for EU countries (range: no team to one team per 1 million inhabitants). However, 6 out of 33 (18%) countries reported no comprehensive multidisciplinary teams at all, including 5 out of 23 EU countries (22%).

The efficacy of resective epilepsy surgery in terms of seizure control has been confirmed by randomized controlled trials [5–7]. Analyzing 182 studies, the 2019 Cochrane Review [8] evaluated worldwide seizure outcome data. Of the 16,756 patients who underwent a surgical procedure, 10,696 (64%) achieved seizure-free outcome (Engel class I) (range: 13.5–92.5%). Assessing 120 studies, the following prognostic factors associated with a better seizure outcome were identified: Abnormal preoperative MRI, presence of a tumor, presence of mesial temporal sclerosis, history of febrile seizures, absence of focal cortical dysplasia/malformation of cortical development, concordance of preoperative MRI and EEG, presence of unilateral interictal spikes, no use of intracranial recordings, complete lesion resection, and right-sided resection [8]. The success rates of resective epilepsy surgery have been found to have increased from 43% to 85% during the period from 1986 to 1999 [9, 10]. Thus, there is a general consensus today that surgery is a valuable option for the treatment of medically intractable epilepsy [8, 10, 11]. In addition, the importance of early surgical intervention on the psychosocial development of children and adolescents suffering from drug-resistant epilepsy is increasingly recognized, and pediatric programs have largely expanded both in Europe [12] and in North America [13, 14] to afford the need to mitigate long-term cognitive disabilities [15–19].

Despite some differences in treatment algorithms and decision-making processes influenced by institutional philosophies, available technologies, and experiences, there is a high-level consensus between epilepsy surgical centers and an encouraging global trend to follow guidelines and recommendations leading to a more harmonized approach in epilepsy care [1, 20]. According to Engel [13], the current status of epilepsy surgery may be summarized by the following statements.

## 17.1 Epilepsy Surgery Is Still Underused

The percentage of people with drug-resistant epilepsies who can be considered candidates for surgery is thought to range between 10% and 25%. However, less than 1% of drug-resistant epilepsy patients are referred to full-service epilepsy centers, where multidisciplinary epilepsy specialists can decide whether surgery is appropriate [13, 21]. Thus, only a fraction of potential surgical candidates actually receives surgery [2, 13, 20, 22–24]. The underuse of epilepsy surgery in the pediatric population is particularly noticeable [25]. Applying results of a community-based cohort study to the general population of children in the USA, the incidence of drug-resistant focal epilepsy has been estimated at 12.7 per 100,000 per year, the incidence of presurgical evaluation at 5.2 per 100,000 per year, and the incidence of surgical interventions at 2.7 per 100,000 per year [26]. This treatment gap in childhood and adolescence has been confirmed in studies in both North American and European cohorts [14, 27].

The probability of achieving a lasting seizure-free state with further changes in medication is only 5%–10% for patients who fail to respond to the first two antiepileptic drugs that are tried [28–30]. There is a general consensus that these individuals should be referred to a full-service epilepsy center [13, 31, 32]. The reluctance to refer patients to epilepsy centers may be caused by ignorance of surgical options, misunderstandings, misconceptions, ambiguous views on pharmacoresistance, reservation about benefits, and the fear of surgical complications and personality changes [13, 22, 27, 33–36]. For these reasons, Engel [21] proposed that recommendations should focus on referral to an epilepsy center and not on referral for epilepsy surgery. In fact, every patient with drug-resistant epilepsy deserves assessment by a multidisciplinary team of epilepsy specialists in a full-service epilepsy center with respect to different treatment options, including consideration of surgery [21]. In a screening process based on outpatient visits, patients can be selected for non-invasive evaluation (MRI, fMRI, neuropsychological and neuropsychiatric assessment, scalp video-EEG), and psychogenic non-epileptic seizures (PNES) which are not infrequent and easily misdiagnosed as pharmacoresistant epilepsy can be identified. It may be expected that half of those patients undergoing non-invasive assessment will not proceed further, 25%–40% may be recommended for surgery without further investigation, and 10%–25% will require intracranial EEG [37]. In addition to treating seizures, full-service epilepsy centers can support patients in everyday problems encountered with epilepsy, independent of whether they are surgical candidates or not [13].

## 17.2 Epilepsy Surgery Is Considered Too Late

The incidence of epilepsy shows a peak in the first year of life [38]. Despite the high incidence of pharmacoresistant epilepsies in infancy and the proven efficacy of surgical treatment in selected cases, the latency between epilepsy onset and referral for presurgical evaluation and, eventually, surgical intervention remains steadily high [39], and most patients undergo surgery only in the young adult age. In accordance, the 2004 ILAE survey comprising data of 20 epilepsy centers, and 401 children and adolescents [40] found that although two-thirds of children suffered from seizures in the first 2 years of life, only one-third of these children had undergone surgery within 2 years of the onset of epilepsy, in particular children with catastrophic epilepsies. The average delay from the onset of epilepsy to surgical referral in general, however, is 15–20 years [41]. A European survey comparing a mixed population of 562 pediatric and adult patients from 16 tertiary centers operated between 1997 and 1998 with 736 cases operated between 2012 and 2013 showed that duration of epilepsy decreased between the 1990s and the 2010s by 5.2 years on average, with significant shortening in both children and adults. However, others felt that the delay has not significantly changed during the last decade [22, 33, 42].

Epilepsy in the first years of life often refers to lesional epilepsy with a predominance of malformations of cortical development [40]. Early surgical intervention was identified as a positive predictor not only for the postoperative seizure outcome but also for the cognitive, developmental, and adaptive outcome based on the superior compensatory capacity of young children who benefit from the plasticity of the brain [13, 16–18]. Similarly, Bjellvi et al. [43] reported in a systematic review and meta-analysis of 12 studies including 3746 patients (children and adults) that patients with shorter epilepsy duration are more likely to be seizure-free at follow-up which holded also true for cases with very long epilepsy durations. The study could not clarify whether the duration of drug-resistant phase of epilepsy is a more important predictor or the total epilepsy duration [43]. The positive association between shorter epilepsy duration and seizure freedom is particularly important since timing of surgery is the only modifiable factor to effectively improve long-term prognosis. Therefore, presurgical investigations should be suggested and planned in appropriate surgical candidates without delay. Conversely, surgery is often too late to reverse the psychological and social comorbidity responsible for dependency on family and society [13, 16–18, 43].

## 17.3 Resective Epilepsy Surgery Decreases in Adults and in Temporal Location

Cloppenborg et al. [44] evaluated the referral of surgical candidates for preoperative evaluation between 1990 and 2011 in Germany. Although the number of patient referrals increased over time, they noted a decline in resective surgery after 2009. Similarly, the US National Association of Epilepsy Centers analyzing data from 2003 to 2012 found an increase in patients with drug-resistant epilepsy who underwent resective surgery up to 2009 from 0.35% to 0.63% per year, but a decrease in subsequent years [2]. Stable or declining rates of epilepsy surgery despite increased referrals to large epilepsy centers have also been reported in a nationwide study by Schiltz et al. [45]. The development of major epilepsy centers between 1991 and 2011, including seven centers in the USA, one in Germany and one in Australia, was analyzed by Jehi et al. [46]. Eight of the nine centers reported a reduction in the treatment of hippocampal sclerosis, and only one center reported an increase. In addition, the 2018 European survey demonstrated that resections for hippocampal sclerosis decreased by half between the 1990s and 2010s [1].

Several hypotheses have been discussed to explain the decrease in temporal resections as reported in most studies [1, 46]: (1) Decreasing temporal surgery is a purely artificial finding due to increasing numbers of extratemporal surgeries, particularly in children, leading to a relative drop in the proportion of temporal procedures [12, 13, 47]; (2) more and more patients with temporal epilepsy are operated on in community hospitals that are not included in the corresponding analyses [2, 13]; (3) the decline of temporal resections mainly refers to the continuously decreasing prevalence of classical temporomesial epilepsy [12, 14, 36, 44, 47, 48]. In fact, Jehi et al. [46] demonstrated in their analysis a reduction of absolute numbers of hippocampal sclerosis-related resective surgeries. This may be attributed to better treatment of risk factors predisposing to hippocampal sclerosis such as infections and complex febrile seizures with anti-inflammatory medications [49–51]. In addition, the reduction in resective treatment of temporomesial epilepsies in adults may be related to the increasing use of minimal-invasive non-resective surgical techniques.

## 17.4 There is a Shift to Pediatric Epilepsy Surgery and More Complex Extratemporal Resections

A nationwide Italian study comprising data of nine pediatric epilepsy surgery centers [47] and a study of the Dutch Collaborative Epilepsy Surgery Programme [12] that feature a higher prevalence of cortical malformations and a lower prevalence of hippocampal sclerosis and tumors as the underlying etiology presented decreasing temporal and increasing extratemporal surgeries. A stable volume of surgeries over time with a decrease of temporal lobectomies and an increase of extratemporal resections and invasive EEG recordings has also been observed by others [33, 44]. The European survey [1] demonstrated an increase of extratemporal resections for focal cortical dysplasia by four times between the 1990s and 2010s. In contrast, Rolston et al. [24] evaluating rates of adult epilepsy surgery in North America using two independent databases found that the rate of temporal end extratemporal surgeries remained overall stable, and that 59% of the procedures still refer to the temporal lobe.

The key to optimal outcome is early identification of possible surgical candidates and their timely referral to epilepsy surgical centers [52, 53]. In accordance, most studies note a shift toward pediatric epilepsy surgery as well as to extratemporal resections [1, 18, 33, 44, 47]. It seems to be remarkable that even though more complex cases are evaluated and operated over time, success rates regarding seizure freedom remain stable or even improved as it has been shown in pediatric series [12, 54]. Similarly, the European survey [1] found that overall postsurgical seizure-freedom rates slightly improved from 66.7% in the 1990s to 70.9% in the 2010s despite of more complex cases. Improvement was most pronounced for surgical subgroups, including MRI-negative temporal lobe epilepsies (from 48% to 68%) and lesional extratemporal epilepsies (from 54% to 68%). Despite increasing surgical complexity, the overall complication rate remained stable at around 5% [1] and has decreased comparing actual with significantly longer periods back data. Of note, the European cohort encompassed only one perisurgical death but five seizure-related deaths in patients who were not seizure-free after surgery, highlighting that the surgical risks have to be balanced with the cumulative lifetime risks of continued seizures [1, 55].

## 17.5 There are Promising Developments in the Epilepsy Surgical Program

### 17.5.1 Diagnostics

#### 17.5.1.1 Selection of Surgical Candidates

Previous recommendations to guide selection of surgical candidates were kept rather general and mainly referred to severity of seizures and their interference with daily life activities [10, 56]. In 2003, the ILAE

Pediatric Epilepsy Surgery Subcommission proposed that the following individuals should be considered as possible surgical candidates: (1) Those who have failed two appropriate AED; (2) those who are disabled by medication side effects; (3) those with seizures that do not fit into a definite electroclinical epilepsy syndrome based on the ILAE classification; and (4) those who have an identified lesion seen on neuroimaging [31]. Similarly, the American Epilepsy Society consensus conference underlined in 2009 the importance of criteria selecting patients for presurgical assessment [57].

Kwon et al. [58] reviewed 384 articles to evaluate changes in selection criteria over time (before 2000 versus after 2000). With increasing evidence that earlier surgery is associated with better outcomes, the major change over the years was recommending to evaluate patients as soon as they have failed medical treatment [58] corresponding to the definition of drug-resistant epilepsy by the ILAE Commission on Classification and Terminology published in 2009 [59]. Thus, Kwon et al. [58] concluded that everyone who fails adequate trials of two tolerated and appropriately chosen and used AED schedules (whether as monotherapies or in combination) to achieve sustained seizure freedom should be promptly evaluated for possible surgery, regardless of seizure frequency. Conte et al. [60] advocated the use of an epilepsy surgical grading scale for the prognostic stratification of patients with drug-resistant focal epilepsy undergoing presurgical evaluation. Finally, biomarkers are under investigation including genetic, molecular, cellular, imaging, and electrophysiological measures that might predict the development or progression of an epileptic condition, the effects of anti-epileptogenic treatment, and outcome after surgery [61].

#### 17.5.1.2 MR Imaging

MR imaging constitutes the most important tool of presurgical evaluation, and evidence of a structural abnormality pointing to the epileptogenic zone has proven to be the best prognostic factor for seizure control. In addition, detection of small lesions frequently causing devastating epilepsy is the essential basis for the successful application of stereotactic treatment strategies. The actual mainstay is high-quality structural 3T MRI, and possibly 7T imaging may be additionally used in future [53]. Epilepsy-specific imaging protocols as suggested by the ILAE in 1997 have been provided by Wellmer et al. [62]. Innovative post-acquisition processing of MRI increases detection of subtle abnormalities although reducing specificity [63–65], and diffusion tensor imaging (DTI) facilitates delineation of white matter tracts [66]. If the planned resection borders close to eloquent cortex, functional mapping such as by language and motor fMRI may be helpful [67]. Tractography derived from diffusion-weighted MRI sequences can localize major white matter tracts such as the corticospinal tract and optic radiation [68]. In addition, fMRI has gained increasing interest to study neuronal networks responsible for epileptogenesis [69, 70]. Actually, the technique of resting fMRI (rs-fMRI) is applied to identify functional disturbances associated with the epileptic activity [53]. In addition, magnetic resonance spectroscopy (MRS) may provide useful information to localize disturbances in a variety of metabolic processes [71].

#### 17.5.1.3 Radionuclide Imaging and Combined Techniques

A trend to more frequently use radionuclide imaging and to combine different diagnostic modalities has been noted in a European survey [1]. Radionuclide imaging including FDG-PET and ictal SPECT provides valuable information for localizing the epileptogenic area particularly in MRI-negative cases or in the presence of multiple or diffuse lesions such as tuberous sclerosis, schizencephaly, or polymicrogyria, where only one of several lesions, or a part of a diffuse lesion, is epileptogenic [72–74]. Diagnostic significance of combined techniques, e.g., MRI/PET fusion for delineation of focal cortical dysplasias, EEG/fMRI for localizing BOLD signals associated with epileptiform discharges, and MEG with MRI and EEG for non-invasive recording of pathological high-frequency oscillations (pHFOs) are areas of actual research [75–77]. In addition, optical imaging [78] measuring alterations in light passing through the brain has been used to visualize the onset and propagation of ictal activity along the neocortex [53].

#### 17.5.1.4 Electrophysiology

There is a clear trend in Europe from the use of subdural strip and grid electrodes toward implantation of depth electrodes for invasive recordings, which seems to become also apparent in the United States [37, 53, 79, 80]. According to the European multicenter study [1], the frequency of invasive recordings remained unchanged between the 1990s and 2010s, encompassing around one-third of all cases, with an increasing proportion of stereo-EEG facilitating a better spatial resolution of epileptic activity as compared to subdural electrodes [81]. High degree co-localization of automated MRI lesion detection and stereo-EEG has been shown [37]. Source localization techniques can noticeably contribute to the delineation of the epileptogenic zone [37]. In addition, pathological high-frequency oscillations (pHFOs) which as biomarkers characterize brain tissue capable of generating spontaneous seizures provide a promising diagnostic tool for a more exact localization of the epileptogenic area [82–85]. Novel markers such as very-fast ripples of up to 2000 Hz and more advanced analyses considering the network properties of HFOs constitute promising research areas [86].

#### 17.5.1.5 Epilepsy as a Network Disease

There is an increasing tendency to appreciate epilepsy as a network disease. Even focal seizures may depend on widely distributed disturbances of connectivity. Network alterations co-localized with the irritative zone may trigger secondary bilateral synchrony as demonstrated by diffusion tensor imaging [87]. Dynamical computational models are being constructed in order to identify areas of high epileptogenicity, resection or disruption of which can be expected to provide seizure control [88–90]. Functional connectivity studies can be combined with structural connectivity data using DTI techniques to decide for the most appropriate intervention strategy [13]. Interictal HFOs recorded from suspected epileptogenic regions have been found to be organized in networks [91]. Moreover, it has been suggested that evidence of a thalamic network (thalamic hubness) may serve as a biomarker indicating seizure recurrence after temporal resections [92]. Those networks could also contribute to the understanding of the impact of focal epilepsy on epilepsy-related cognitive disturbances [93]. Kini et al. [94] suggested that surgical outcome can be accurately predicted using a network model of synchronizability of EEG. Stacey et al. [95] summarized the current state-of-the-art in applying network analyses to EEG data emphasizing the tremendous potential of those research activities. Foit et al. [96] concluded that epilepsy is increasingly defined as a disorder of large-scale networks, and that connectome-based biomarkers have the potential to improve surgical treatment.

### 17.5.2 Surgical Treatment

#### 17.5.2.1 Minimal Volume Epilepsy Surgery

Aided by advances in structural and functional imaging, there is a general trend toward smaller resections and minimal volume epilepsy surgery. Temporal resections have been modified from standard temporal lobectomy (ATL) to selective amygdalohippocampectomy (SAHE). In extratemporal location, resective surgery continues to be primarily lesionally guided [13]. Resections in or around eloquent areas as well as in the insula are facilitated by neuronaviation and techniques of functional topographic mapping and monitoring [97].

Of note, risks of epilepsy surgery have noticeably decreased over the last decades, and it has been suggested that morbidity and mortality from drug-resistant seizures are higher than from surgical complications [34]. In fact, surgery appears to reduce mortality of those epilepsy patients who experience a significant postoperative decrease in generalized tonic–clonic seizure frequency and, therefore, are less susceptible to sudden unexpected death in epilepsy (SUDEP), even when taking into account the risk of surgery-related fatalities [13, 34, 98].

#### 17.5.2.2 Cost-Effectiveness of Resective Surgery

Data available confirm that resective surgical treatment of drug-resistant epilepsy is cost-effective in the long-term both in children and adults [99]. It has been shown that surgery may become cost-effective within 3 years, and that there may be an incremental cost-effectiveness at 5 years [100]. In addition, presurgical evaluation has been found to be cost-effective in pharmacoresistant patients, even if the probability of being deemed a surgical candidate is only 5% to 10% [100].

#### 17.5.2.3 Non-Resective Surgical Strategies

Non-resective surgical strategies including neurostimulation techniques (VNS, DBS, RNS) [101–104], thermoablation procedures (RFTC, LITT) [105–110] , as well as radiosurgery (SRS) [111–113] noticeably widen the surgical spectrum. Curative stereotactic approaches (RFTC, LITT, SRS) can be expected to become first-line treatment options for selected patients with circumscribed lesions such as hypothalamic hamartomas, periventricular nodular heterotopias, and deep-seated focal cortical dysplasia [110]. In addition, LITT may be considered as an alternative to resective surgery in temporomesial epilepsies [114, 115]. The place of focused ultrasound ablation (FUS) [116] has to be awaited. Other future approaches could make use of currently experimental novel technologies such as optogenetic manipulation of discreet neuronal cell populations [53, 117]. The success of these minimally invasive strategies raises questions as to the validity of the classical hypothesis on epileptogenicity according to which the lesion constitutes only part of the epileptogenic area.

#### 17.5.2.4 Closed-Loop Intervention Systems

Responsive neurostimulation (RNS) [118] and responsive vagal nerve stimulation (rVNS) [119] constitute first steps toward closed-loop systems triggered by electrocorticographic patterns (RNS) and increase of heart rate (rVNS), respectively, indicative of an impending seizure. Improved algorithms for seizure detection [120–122] may increase specificity of those systems and facilitate development of other implantable devices acting on demand by local release of potent anticonvulsants. With respect to the latter option, Altenmüller et al. [123] demonstrated in a pilot study antiepileptic effects of cortically applied valproate. Moreover, chronic ECoG data delivered by responsive systems may be used to identify patient-specific temporal dynamics in epileptiform activity, thus providing a personalized therapy [124].

#### 17.5.2.5 Clinical trials

Evidence for efficacy and safety of different surgical treatment options is best documented in randomized controlled trials (RCTs). It seems to be important to perform such RCTs at an early stage when the therapeutic modality to be assessed is not available outside a study. If the treatment modality has been approved and patients can decide for the respective option without participating in a study, recruitment processes may be rendered difficult. For example, the Early Randomized Surgical Epilepsy Trial (ERSET) that intended to randomize 200 MTLE patients to ATL or continued pharmacotherapy [125] had to be terminated after only 38 patients were enrolled over 2 years despite the participation of 16 centers. In such circumstances, appropriately designed prospective single-arm observational studies may be preferred providing valuable data [126].

#### 17.5.2.6 Novel Therapeutic Approaches

Novel strategies that are currently in the experimental stage may open new therapeutic options [127]. *Gene therapy* for the treatment of drug-resistant epilepsy aims to induce local release of anticonvulsants, e.g., by altering the expression of some therapeutic genes such as GABA-A receptor [128]. In addition to gene replacement, *gene editing* transferring exogenous genes into the desired sequence of target cells seems to be a promising approach [129]. *Stem cell therapy* has been considered to overcome the intrinsic inability of the nervous tissue to induce efficient self-repairing processes [130]. *Exosome therapy* means the use of vesicles secreted by cells of the nervous system as vehicles for delivering anti-seizure agents [131]. Finally, *molecular networks* such as mTOR and Wnt/β-catenin signaling pathways are considered as favorable anti-epileptogenic targets for future therapeutic approaches [132].

### 17.5.3 Postoperative Care

#### 17.5.3.1 Clinical Assessment

With respect to the possibility of both recurrent and remitted seizure activity during postoperative years, long-term outcome data with follow-ups of 10–20 years are desired [37, 133]. In addition to the seizure and neuropsychological outcome, postoperative clinical assessment should include standardized health-related quality of life (HRQOL) measures that evaluate psychosocial and vocational outcome data and overall disease burden in order to get comprehensive information on the impact of epilepsy and surgical procedures on patients' life situation [34, 37, 74, 134].

#### 17.5.3.2 Pathological Substrates

Analysis of pathological substrates contributes to the understanding of epileptogenesis and facilitates clinicopathological correlation [135]. In addition to well-known epilepsy-specific pathological substrates, there may be histopathological entities that have still to be characterized such as oligodendroglial hyperplasia in white matter and hyaline protoplasmic astrocytopathy [136, 137]. The relatively high rate of seizure-free outcome in patients without specific histopathological findings questions the concept of epileptogenesis based on specific structural abnormalities indicating successful surgical interruption of functional epileptogenic networks.

#### 17.5.3.3 Rehabilitation

Even after successful epilepsy surgery, young patients often suffer from cognitive deficits related to epilepsy, medication, and/or surgery that hinder their social and professional development. Rehabilitation measures particularly addressing cognitive functioning have been shown to improve psychosocial development and the employment status after surgery [138]. Therefore, adequate rehabilitation programs are needed to provide young patients the best possible chance to live an independent life [37].

## 17.6 The Bare Essentials

Analyzing the current state of epilepsy surgery, the most urgent tasks of epilepsy surgery can be summarized as follows [13, 37]: (1) All epilepsy patients who fail to gain seizure control with two appropriate AED schedules should get access to a full-service epilepsy center for assessment by a multidisciplinary team of epilepsy specialists, (2) as soon as drug resistance of epilepsy is evident, a screening process based on non-invasive diagnostic facilities, particularly high-resolution 3T MRI, should be offered to select patients who can be expected to benefit from surgery and to refer others to appropriate conservative therapeutic modalities, (3) the right time for surgical intervention including in the first years of life has to be defined in pediatric epilepsy syndromes, in order to facilitate young children an undisturbed development at sensitive windows of brain maturation, (4) minimal-invasive surgical strategies including closed-loop intervention systems should be refined and evaluated in the context of the entire surgical spectrum, thus defining selection criteria to offer patients the individually most suitable resective or non-resective treatment modality, and (5) rehabilitation programs particularly addressing cognitive functioning are needed to support the process toward the best possible psychosocial development and an independent life.

In sum, epilepsy surgery has proven to be very successful. In addition to patients' care, it offers a unique chance for scientific research as a "window to the brain" to learn more about functioning and diseases of the brain. However, large investments and a highly specialized personnel are required to efficiently run this program. Therefore, it seems to be advisable to concentrate epilepsy surgery to selected centers where all competences necessary are available, and where sufficient experience with more complicated cases exists in order to ensure high-quality care by high-volume centers and to take advantage of its scientific potential. Given the favorable results of epilepsy surgery and its cost-effectiveness, adequate resources should be made available to provide patients the chance to become seizure-free by a surgical intervention, and, particularly, to enable children the start into a life without the burden of epilepsy.

## References

1. Baud MO, Perneger T, Rácz A, et al. European trends in epilepsy surgery. Neurology. 2018;91(2):e96–e106. https://doi.org/10.1212/WNL.0000000000005776.
2. Kaiboriboon K, Malkhachroum AM, Zrik A, et al. Epilepsy surgery in the United States: analysis of data from the National Association of epilepsy centers. Epilepsy Res. 2015;116:105–9.

3. Zelano J, Klecki J, Christensen J, et al. The provision of epilepsy care across Europe 2017: a 17 years follow-up survey. Epilepsia. 2019;4(1):144–52. https://doi.org/10.1002/epi4.12306.
4. Malmgren K, Flink R, Guekht AB, et al. ILAE Commission of European Affairs Subcommission on European guidelines 1998-2001: the provision of epilepsy care across Europe. Epilepsia. 2003;44:727–31.
5. Dwivedi R, Ramanujam B, Chandra PS, et al. Surgery for drug-resistant epilepsy in children. N Engl J Med. 2017;377:1639–47.
6. Engel J Jr, McDermott MP, Wiebe S, et al. Early surgical therapy for drugresistant temporal lobe epilepsy: a randomized trial. JAMA. 2012;307:922–30.
7. Wiebe S, Blume WT, Girvin JP, Eliasziw M. A randomized, controlled trial of surgery for temporal lobe epilepsy. N Engl J Med. 2001;345:311–8.
8. West S, Nevitt SJ, Cotton J, et al. Sugery for epilepsy (review). Cochrane Database Syst Rev. 2019;6 https://doi.org/10.1002/14651858.CD010541.pub3.
9. Engel J Jr, Shewmon DA. Overview. Who should be considered a surgical candidate? In: Surgical treatment of the epilepsies. 2nd ed. New York: Raven Press; 1993. p. 23–34.
10. Engel J Jr, Wiebe S, French J, Sperling M, Williamson P, Spencer D, Gumnit R, Zahn C, Westbrook E, Enos B. Quality standards Subcommittee of the American Academy of neurology, American Epilepsy Society, American Association of Neurological Surgeons. Neurology. 2003;60:538–47.
11. Engel J, Van Ness PC, Rasmussen TB, Ojemann LM. Outcome with respect to epileptic seizures. In: Engel Jr J, editor. Surgical treatment of the epilepsies. 2nd ed. New York: Raven Press; 1993. p. 609–21.
12. Lamberink HJ, Boshuisen K, van Rijen PC, Gosselaar PH, Braun KPJ. Dutch Collaborative Epilepsy Surgery Program (DCESP). Changing profiles of pediatric epilepsy surgery candidates over time: a nationwide single-center experience from 1990 to 2011. Epilepsia. 2015;56(5):717–25.
13. Engel J. The current place of epilepsy surgery. Curr Opin Neurol. 2017;30 https://doi.org/10.1097/WCO.0000000000000528.
14. Pestana Knight EM, Schiltz NK, Bakaki PM, Koroukian SM, Lhatoo SD, Kaiboriboon K. Increasing utilization of pediatric epilepsy surgery in the United States between 1997 and 2009. Epilepsia. 2015;56:375–81.
15. Jenny B, Smoll N, Hassani El Y, et al. Pediatric epilepsy surgery: could age be a predictor of outcomes? J Neurosurg Pediatr. 2016;18:235–41.
16. Jonas R, Asarnow RF, LoPresti C, et al. Surgery for symptomatic infant- onset epileptic encephalopathy with and without infantile spasms. Neurology. 2005;64(4):746–50.
17. Loddenkemper T, Holland KD, Stanford LD, et al. Developmental outcome after epilepsy surgery in infancy. Pediatrics. 2007;119:930e5.
18. Ramantani G, Kadish NE, Anastasopoulos C, et al. Frontal lobe epilepsy surgery in childhood and adolescence: predictors of long-term seizure freedom, overall cognitive and adaptive functioning. Neurosurgery. 2017; https://doi.org/10.1093/neuros/nyx340.
19. Skirrow C, Cross JH, Cormack F, Harkness W, Vargha-Khadem F, Baldeweg T. Long- term intellectual outcome after temporal lobe surgery in childhood. Neurology. 2011;76:1330–7.
20. Englot DJ. A modern epilepsy surgery treatment algorithm: incorporating traditional and emerging technologies. Epilepsy Behav. 2018;80:68–74.
21. Engel J Jr. What can we do for people with drug-resistant epilepsy? The 2016 Wartenberg lecture. Neurology. 2016;87:2483–9.
22. Haneef Z, Stern J, Dewar S, Engel JJ. Referral pattern for epilepsy surgery after evidence-based recommendations: a retrospective study. Neurology. 2010;75(8):699–704.
23. Lhatoo SF, Solomon JK, McEvoy AW, et al. A prospective study of the requirement for and the provision of epilepsy surgery in the United Kingdom. Epilepsia. 2003;44(5):673–6.
24. Rolston JD, Englot DJ, Knowlton RC, Chang EF. Rate and complications of adult epilepsy surgery in North America: analysis of multiple databases. Epilepsy Res. 2016;124:55–62.
25. Cross JH, Jayakar P, Nordli D, et al. International League against Epilepsy, Subcommission for Paediatric Epilepsy Surgery; Commissions of Neurosurgery and Paediatrics. Proposed criteria for referral and evaluation of children for epilepsy surgery: recommendations of the Subcommission for Pediatric Epilepsy Surgery. Epilepsia. 2006;47(6):952–9.
26. Berg AT, Mathern GW, Bronen RA, Fulbright RK, DiMario F, Testa FM, et al. Frequency, prognosis and surgical treatment of structural abnormalities seen with magnetic resonance imaging in childhood epilepsy. Brain J Neurol. 2009;132(Pt 10):2785–97.
27. Neligan A, Haliasos N, Pettorini B, Harkness WFJ, Solomon JK. A survey of adult and pediatric epilepsy surgery in the United Kingdom. Epilepsia. 2013;54(5):e62–5.
28. Hauser WA. Status epilepticus: epidemiologic considerations. Neurology. 1990;40:9–13.
29. Kwan P, Brodie MJ. Early identification of refractory epilepsy. N Engl J Med. 2000;342:314–9.
30. Pohlen MS, Jin J, Tobias RS, Maheshwari A. Pharmacoresistance with newer anti- epileptic drugs in mesial temporal lobe epilepsy with hippocampal sclerosis. Epilepsy Res. 2017;137:56–60.
31. Cross JH, Jayakar P, Nordli D, et al. Proposed criteria for referral and evaluation of children for epilepsy surgery: recommendations of the subcommission for pediatric epilepsy surgery. Epilepsia. 2006;47(6):952–9.
32. Labiner DM, Bagic AI, Herman ST, Fountain NB, Walczak TS, Gumnit RJ, et al. Essential services, personnel, and facilities in specialized epilepsy centers—revised 2010 guidelines. Epilepsia. 2010;51:2322–33.

33. Englot DJ, Ouyang D, Garcia PA, et al. Epilepsy surgery trends in the United States, 1990-2008. Neurology. 2012;78:1200–6.
34. Sperling MR, Barshow S, Nei M, Asadi-Pooya AA. A reappraisal of mortality after epilepsy surgery. Neurology. 2016;86:1938–44.
35. Dewar SR, Pieters HC. Perceptions of epilepsy surgery: a systematic review and an explanatory model of decision making. Epilepsy Behav. 2015;44:171–8.
36. Jetté N, Sander JW, Keezer MR. Surgical treatment for epilepsy: the potential gap between evidence and practice. Lancet Neuro. 2016;15:982–94.
37. Vakharia VN, Duncan JS, Witt JA, et al. Getting the best outcomes from epilepsy surgery. Ann Neurol. 2018;83(4):676–90.
38. Hauser WA, Annegers JF, Kurland LT. Incidence of epilepsy and unprovoked seizures in Rochester, Minnesota: 1935–1984. Epilepsia. 1993;34(3):453–68.
39. Ryvlin P, Cross JH, Rheims S. Epilepsy surgery in children and adults. Lancet Neurol. 2014;13:1114–26.
40. Harvey AS, Cross JH, Shinnar S, Mathern GW, ILAE Pediatric Epilepsy Surgery Survey Taskforce. Defining the spectrum of international practice in pediatric epilepsy Sur- gery patients. Epilepsia. 2008;49:146–55.
41. Berg AT, Langfitt J, Shinnar S, et al. How long does it take for partial epilepsy to become intractable? Neurology. 2003;60:186–90.
42. Choi H, Carlino R, Heiman G, et al. Evaluation of duration of epilepsy prior to temporal lobe epilepsy surgery during the past two decades. Epilepsy Res. 2009;86:224–7.
43. Bjellvi J, Olsson I, Malmgren K, et al. Epilepsy duration and seizure outcome in epilepsy surgery. Neurology. 2019;93:e159–66. https://doi.org/10.1212/WNL.0000000000007753.
44. Cloppenborg T, May TW, Blümcke I, et al. Trends in epilepsy surgery: stable surgical numbers despite increasing presurgical volumes. J Neurol Neurosurg Psychiatry. 2016;87:1322–9.
45. Schiltz NK, Koroukian SM, Lhatoo SD, Kaiboriboon K. Temporal trends in pre-surgical evaluations and epilepsy surgery in the U.S. from 1998 to 2009. Epilepsy Res. 2013;103(2–3):270–8.
46. Jehi L, Friedman D, Carlson C, et al. The evolution of epilepsy surgery between 1991 and 2011 in nine major epilepsy centers across the United States, Germany, and Australia. Epilepsia. 2015;56:1526–33.
47. Barba C, Specchio N, Guerrini R. Increasing volume and complexity of pediatric epilepsy surgery with stable seizure outcome between 2008 and 2014: a nationwide multicenter study. Epilepsy Behav. 2017;75:151–7.
48. Ramantani G, Holthausen H. Epilepsy after cerebral infection: review of the literature and the potential for surgery. Epileptic Disord. 2017;19(2):117–36.
49. Choy M, Dube CM, Ehrengruber M, et al. Inflammatory processes, febrile seizures, and subsequent epileptogenesis. Epilepsy Curr. 2014;14:15–22.
50. Dube CM, Ravizza T, Hamamura M, et al. Epileptogenesis provoked by prolonged experimental febrile seizures: mechanisms and biomark- ers. J Neurosci. 2010;30:7484–94.
51. Helmstaedter C, May TW, von Lehe M, et al. Temporal lobe surgery in Germany from 1988 to 2008: diverse trends in etiological subgroups. Eur J Neurol. 2014;21:827–34.
52. Arzimanoglou A, Cross JH, Gaillard WD, Holthausen H, Jayakar P, Kahane P, Gaillard G. Pediatric epilepsy surgery. Paris: John Libbey Eurotext; 2016.
53. Engel J Jr. Evolution of concepts in epilepsy surgery. Epileptic Disord. 2019;21(5):391–409.
54. Barba C, Cross JH, Braun K, Cossu M, et al. Trends in pediatric epilepsy surgery in Europe between 2008 and 2015: country-, center-, and age-specific variation. Epilepsia. 2020;61(2):216–27.
55. Tomson T, Nashef L, Ryvlin P. Sudden unexpected death in epilepsy: current knowledge and future directions. Lancet Neurol. 2008;7:1021–31.
56. Jones MW, Andermann F. Temporal lobe epilepsy surgery: definition of candidacy. Can J Neurol Sci. 2000;27(Suppl. 1):S11–3. discussion S20-1
57. Duncan JS. Selecting patients for epilepsy surgery: synthesis of data. Epilepsy Behav. 2011;20: 230–2.
58. Kwon C-S, Neal J, Telléz-Zenteno J, et al. Resective focal epilepsy surgery – has selection of candidates changed? A systematic review. Epilepsy Res. 2016;122:37–43.
59. Kwan P, Arzimanoglou A, Berg AT, Brodie MJ, Hauser WA, Mathern G, Moshé SL, Perucca E, Wiebe S, French J. Definition of drug resistant epilepsy: consensus proposal by the ad hoc Task Force of the ILAE Commission on Therapeutic Strategies. Epilepsia. 2010;51:1069–77.
60. Conte F, Paesschen WV, Legros B, et al. The epilepsy surgery grading scale: validation in an independent population with drug-resistant focal epilepsy. Epilepsia. 2019; https://doi.org/10.1111/epi.16096.
61. Engel J, Pitkänen A. Biomarkers for Epileptogenesis and its treatment. Neuropharmacology. 2019; https://doi.org/10.1016/j.neuropharm.2019.107735.
62. Wellmer J, Quesada CM, Rothe L, Elger CE, Bien CG, Urbach H. Proposal for a magnetic resonance imaging protocol for the detection of epileptogenic lesions at early outpatient stages. Epilepsia. 2013;44:1977–87.
63. Bernasconi A, Cendes F, Theodore WH, et al. Recommendations for the use of structural magnetic resonance imaging in the care of patients with epilepsy: a consensus report from the international league against epilepsy neuroimaging task force. Epilepsia. 2019;60:1054–68.
64. Hong S-J, Kim H, Schrader D, et al. Automated detection of cortical dysplasia type II in MRI-negative epilepsy. Neurology. 2014;83(1): 48–55.

65. Wagner J, Weber B, Urbach H, et al. Morphometric MRI analysis improves detection of focal cortical dysplasia type II. Brain. 2011;134(Pt 10):2844–54.
66. Smith SM, Jenkinson M, Johansen-Berg H, et al. Tract-based spatial statistics: Voxelwise analysis of multi-subject diffusion data. NeuroImage. 2006;31(4):1487–505.
67. Bauer PR, Reitsma JB, Houweling BM, et al. Can fMRI safely replace the Wada test for preoperative assessment of language lateralisation? A meta-analysis and systematic review. J Neurol Neurosurg Psychiatry. 2014;85(5):581–8.
68. Nowell M, Vos SB, Sidhu M, et al. Meyer's loop asymmetry and language lateralisation in epilepsy. J Neurol Neurosurg Psychiatry. 2016;87(8):836–42.
69. Engel J Jr, Thompson PM, Stern JM, Staba RJ, Bragin A, Mody I. Connectomics and epilepsy. Curr Opin Neurol. 2013;26:186–94.
70. Tavakol S, Royer J, Lowe AJ, et al. Neuroimaging and connectomics of drug-resistant epilepsy at multiple scales: from focal lesions to macroscale networks. Epilepsia. 2019;60:593–604.
71. Petroff OA, Duncan JS. Magnetic resonance spectroscopy. In: Engel Jr J, Pedley TA, editors. Epilepsy:AComprehensive textbook. 2nd ed. Lippincott Williams & Wilkins: Philadelphia; 2008. p. 975–88.
72. Duncan JS, Winston GP, Koepp MJ, Ourselin S. Brain imaging in the assessment for epilepsy surgery. Lancet Neurol. 2016;15:420–33.
73. Muhlhofer W, Tan YL, Mueller SG, Knowlton R. MRI-negative temporal lobe epilepsy – what do we know? Epilepsia. 2017;58:727–42.
74. Ryvlin P, Rheims S. Predicting epilepsy surgery outcome. Curr Opin Neurol. 2016;29:182–8.
75. Andrade-Valenca LP, Dubeau F, Mari F, Zelmann R, Gotman J. Interictal scalp fast oscillations as a marker of the seizure onset zone. Neurology. 2011;77(6):524–31.
76. Tamilia E, Madsen JR, Grant PE, et al. Current and emerging potential of magnetoencephalography in the detection and localization of high-frequency oscillations in epilepsy. Front Neurol. 2017;8:14. https://doi.org/10.3389/fneur.2017.00014.
77. Van Klink N, van Rosmalen F, Nenonen J, et al. Automatic detection and visualization of MEG ripple oscillations in epilepsy. Neuroimage Clin. 2017;15:689–701.
78. Haglund MM, Hochman D, Toga AW. Optical imaging of seizure activity. In: Engel Jr J, Pedley TA, editors. Epilepsy: a comprehensive textbook. 2nd ed. Lippincott-Raven: Philadelphia; 2008. p. 1025–30.
79. Valentin A, Hernando-Quintana N, Moles-Herbera J, et al. Depth versus subdural temporal electrodes revisited: impact on surgical outcome after resective surgery for epilepsy. Clin Neurophysiol. 2017;128:418–23.
80. Yang M, Ma Y, Li W, et al. A retrospective analysis of stereoelectroencephalography and subdural electroencephalography for preoperative evaluation of intractable epilepsy. Stereotact Funct Neurosurg. 2017;95:13–20.
81. Wagstyl K, Adler S, Pimpel B, et al. Planning stereoelectroencephalography using automated lesion detection: Retrospective feasibility study. Epilepsia. 2020; https://doi.org/10.1111/epi.16574.
82. Bragin A, Engel J Jr, Wilson CL, et al. Hippocampal and entorhinal cortex high frequency oscillations (100-500 Hz) in kainic acid-treated rats with chronic seizures and human epileptic brain. Epilepsia. 1999;40:127–37.
83. Frauscher B, Bartolomei F, Kobayashi K, et al. High-frequency oscillations: the state of clinical research. Epilepsia. 2017;58:1316–29.
84. Jiruska P, Alvarado-Rojas C, Schevon CA, et al. Update on the mechanisms and roles of high-frequency oscillations in seizures and epileptic disorders. Epilepsia. 2017;58:1330–9.
85. Zijmans M, Worrell GA, D€umpelmann M, et al. How to record highfrequency oscillations in epilepsy: a practical guideline. Epilepsia. 2017;58:1305–15.
86. Thomschewski A, Hincapié A-S, Frauscher B. Localization of the epileptogenic zone using high frequency oscillations. Front Neurol. 2019; https://doi.org/10.3389/fneur.2019.00094.
87. Hammen T, Reisert M, Juschkat W, et al. Alterations of intracerebral connectivity in epilepsy patients with secondary bilateral synchrony. Epilepsy Res. 2020; https://doi.org/10.1016/j.eplepsyres.2020.106402.
88. Bartolomei F, Lagarde S, Wendling F, et al. Defining epileptogenic networks: contribution of SEEG and signal analysis. Epilepsia. 2017;58:1131–47.
89. Lopes MA, Richardson MP, Abela E, et al. An optimal strategy for epilepsy surgery: disruption of the rich-club? PLoS Comput Biol. 2017;13:e1005637.
90. Sinha N, Dauwels J, Kaiser M, et al. Predicting neurosurgical outcomes in focal epilepsy patients using computational modelling. Brain. 2017;140:319–32.
91. González Otárula KA, von Ellenrieder N, Cuello-Oderiz C, et al. High-frequency oscillation networks and surgical outcome in adult focal epilepsy. Ann Neurol. 2019;85:485–94.
92. He X, Doucet GE, Pustina D, et al. Presurgical thalamic "hubness" predicts surgical outcome in temporal lobe epilepsy. Neurology. 2017;88(24):2285–93.
93. Gil F, Padilla N, Soria-Pastor S, et al. Beyond the epileptic focus: functional epileptic networks in focal epilepsy. Cerebral Cortex. 2019; https://doi.org/10.1093/cercor/bhz243.
94. Kini LG, Bernabei JM, Mikhail F, et al. Virtual resection predicts surgical outcome for drug-resistant epilepsy. Brain. 2019; https://doi.org/10.1093/brain/awz303.
95. Stacey W, Kramer M, Gunnarsdottir K, et al. Emerging roles of network analysis for epilepsy. Epilepsy Res. 2019; https://doi.org/10.1016/j.eplepsyres.2019.106255.
96. Foit N, Bernasconi A, Bernasconi N. Functional networks in epilepsy presurgical evaluation. Neurosurg Clin N Am. 2020; https://doi.org/10.1016/j.nec.2020.03.004.
97. Nguyen DK. Topical issue: insular cortex epilepsy. J Clin Neurophysiol. 2017;34:300–39.

98. Ryvlin P, Montavont A, Kahane P. The impact of epilepsy surgery on mortality. Epileptic Disord. 2005;7(1):539–46.
99. Widjaja E, Li B, Schinkel CD, Ritchie LP, Weaver J, Snead OC, Rutka JT, Coyte PC. Cost-effectiveness of pediatric epilepsy surgery compared to medical treatment in children with intractable epilepsy. Epilepsy Res. 2011;94:61–8.
100. Sheikh SR, Steinmetz MP, Kattan MW, et al. The cost-effectiveness of epilepsy surgery and surgical evaluation in the United States. Neurosurgery. 2019; https://doi.org/10.1093/neuros/nyz310_165.
101. Geller EB, Skarpaas TL, Gross RE, et al. Brain-responsive neurostimulation in patients with medically intractable mesial temporal lobe epilepsy. Epilepsia. 2017;58:994–1004.
102. Jobst BC, Kapur R, Barkley GL, et al. Brain-responsive neurostimulation in patients with medically intractable seizures arising from eloquent and other neocortical areas. Epilepsia. 2017;58: 1005–14.
103. Papageorgiou PN, Deschner J, Papageorgiou SN. Effectiveness and adverse effects of deep brain stimulation: umbrella review of meta-analyses. J Neurol Surg A Cent Eur Neurosurg. 2017;78:180–90.
104. Sprengers M, Vonck K, Carrette E, et al. Deep brain and cortical stimulation for epilepsy. Cochrane Database Syst Rev. 2017;7:CD008497.
105. Cossu M, Cardinale F, Casaceli G, et al. Stereo-EEG-guided radiofrequency thermocoagulations. Epilepsia. 2017;58:66–72.
106. Dimova P, de Palma L, Job-Chapron AS, et al. Radiofrequency thermocoagulation of the seizure-onset zone during stereoelectroencephalography. Epilepsia. 2017;58:381–92.
107. Jermakowicz WJ, Kanner AM, Sur S, et al. Laser thermal ablation for mesiotemporal epilepsy: analysis of ablation volumes and trajectories. Epilepsia. 2017;58:801–10.
108. Kang JY, Sperling MR. Epileptologist's view: laser interstitial thermal ablation for treatment of temporal lobe epilepsy. Epilepsy Res. 2017; https://doi.org/10.1016/j.epilepsyres.2017.07.007.
109. Wicks RT, Jermakowicz WJ, Jagid JR, et al. Laser interstitial thermal therapy for mesial temporal lobe epilepsy. Neurosurgery. 2016;79:S83–91.
110. Wellmer J, Parpaley Y, Rampp S, Popkirov S, Kugel H, Aydin Ü, Wolters CH, von Lehe M, Voges J. Lesion guided stereotactic radiofrequency thermocoagulation for palliative, in selected cases curative epilepsy surgery. Epilepsy Res. 2016;121:39–46.
111. Régis J, Rey M, Bartolomei F, et al. Gamma knife surgery in mesial temporal lobe epilepsy: a prospective multicenter study. Epilepsia. 2004;45:504–15.
112. Régis J, Hayashi M, Eupierre LP, et al. Gamma knife surgery for epilepsy related to hypothalamic hamartomas. Acta Neurochir. 2004;91:33–50.
113. Barbaro NM, Quigg M, Ward MW, et al. Radiosurgery versus open surgery for mesial temporal lobe epilepsy: the randomized, controlled ROSE trial. Epilepsia. 2018; https://doi.org/10.1111/epi.14045.
114. Gross R. The latest on lasers: improving the outcome of MRg-LITT amygdalohippocampectomy. Epilepsy Curr. 2018;18(6):382–6.
115. Wu C, Jermakovicz WJ, Chakravorti S, et al. Effects of surgical targeting in laser interstitial thermal therapy for mesial temporal lobe epilepsy: a multicenter study of 234 patients. Epilepsia. 2019;60(6):1171–83.
116. Krishna V, Sammartino F, Cosgrove R, et al. Predictors of outcomes after focused ultrasound thalamotomy. Neurosurgery. 2019; https://doi.org/10.1093/neuros/nyz417.
117. Camporeze B, Manica BA, Bonafé GA, et al. Optogenetics: the new molecular approach to control functions of neural cells in epilepsy, depression and tumors of the central nervous system. Am J Cancer Res. 2018;8(10):1900–18.
118. Hartshorn A, Jobst B. Responsive brain stimulation in epilepsy. Ther Adv Chronic Dis. 2018;9(7):135–42.
119. Boon P, Vonck K, van Rijckevorsel K, et al. A prospective, multicenter study of cardiac-based seizure detection to activate vagus nerve stimulation. Seizure. 2015;32:52–61.
120. Elger CE, Mormann F. Seizure prediction and documentation–two important problems. Lancet Neurol. 2013;12:531–2.
121. Schulze-Bonhage A. Long-term outcome in neurostimulation of epilepsy. Epilepsy Behav. 2019;91:25–9.
122. Usman SM, Khalid S, Akhtar R, et al. Using scalp EEG and intracranial EEG signals for predicting epileptic seizures: review of available methodologies. Europ J Epilep. 2019;71:258–69.
123. Altenmüller D-M, Hebel JM, Deniz C, et al. Electrocorticographic and neurochemical findings after local cortical valproate application in patients with pharmacoresistant focal epilepsy. Epilepsia. 2020; https://doi.org/10.1111/epi.16523.
124. Sisterson ND, Wozny TA, Kokkinos V, et al. Closed-loop brain stimulation for drug-resistant epilepsy: towards an evidence-based approach to personalized medicine. Neurotherapeutics. 2018; https://doi.org/10.1007/s13311-018-00682-4.
125. Engel J Jr, McDermott MP, Wiebe S, et al. Design considerations for a multicenter randomized controlled trial of early surgery for mesial temporal lobe epilepsy. Epilepsia. 2010;51(10):1978–86.
126. Sperling MR, Gross RE, Alvarez GE, et al. Stereotactic laser ablation for mesial temporal lobe epilepsy: A prospective, multicenter, single-arm study. Epilepsia. 2020; https://doi.org/10.1111/epi.16529.
127. Mehdizadeh A, Barzegar M, Negargar S, et al. The current and emerging therapeutic approaches in drug-resistant epilepsy management. Acta Neurol Belgica. 2019; https://doi.org/10.1007/s13760-019-01120-8.
128. Raol YH, Lund IV, Bandyopadhyay S, Zhang G, Roberts DS, Wolfe JH, Russek SJ, Brooks-Kayal

AR. Enhancing GABAA receptor α1 subunit levels in hippocampal dentate gyrus inhibits epilepsy development in an animal model of temporal lobe epilepsy. J Neurosci. 2006;26(44):11342–6.
129. Mollanoori H, Teimourian S. Therapeutic applications of CRISPR/Cas9 system in gene therapy. Biotechnol Lett. 2018;40:907–14.
130. Rao G, Mashkouri S, Aum D, Marcet P, Borlongan CV. Contemplating stem cell therapy for epilepsy-induced neuropsychiatric symptoms. Neuropsychiatr Dis Treat. 2017;13:585–96.
131. Tiwari D, Peariso K, Gross C. MicroRNA-induced silencing in epilepsy: opportunities and challenges for clinical application. Dev Dyn. 2018;247(1):94–110.
132. Hodges SL, Lugo JN. Wnt/β-catenin signaling as a potential target for novel epilepsy therapies. Epilepsy Res. 2018;146:9–16.
133. Bell GS, de Tisi J, Gonzalez-Fraile JC, et al. Factors affecting seizure outcome after epilepsy surgery; an observational series. J Neurol Neurosurg Psychiatry. 2017;88(11):933–40.
134. Ramos-Perdigués S, Baillés E, Mané A, et al. A prospective study contrasting the psychiatric outcome in drug-resistant epilepsy between patients who underwent surgery and a control group. Epilepsia. 2016;57:1680–90.
135. Blümcke I, Spreafico R, Haaker G, et al. Histopathological findings in brain tissue obtained during epilepsy surgery. N Engl J Med. 2017;377:1648–56.
136. Schurr J, Coras R, Rössler K, et al. Mild malformation of cortical develop ment with oligodendroglial hyperplasia in frontal lobe epilepsy: a new clinico-pathological entity. Brain Pathol. 2017;27:26–35.
137. Hedley-Whyte ET, Goldman JE, Nedergaard M. Hyaline protoplasmic astrocytopathy of neocortex. J Pathol Exp Neurol. 2009;68(2):136–47.
138. Thorbecke R, May TW, Koch-Stoecker S, Ebner A, Bien CG, Specht U. Effects of an inpatient rehabilitation program after temporal lobe epilepsy surgery and other factors on employment 2 years after epilepsy surgery. Epilepsia. 2014;55:725–33.

# A Personal View 18

*If we knew what it is we are doing, it would not be called science, would it?*

*Albert Einstein*

## Contents



Medicine is often understood as a scientific discipline. It prides itself on the scientific methodology of its findings and its actions on the basis of reliable and reproducible data as well as the general validity and transferability of its results. In fact, medicine had achieved its greatest successes when, in the middle of the nineteenth century, it broke away from the humanistic tradition, from holistic thinking, turned to the rational consideration of scientific phenomena, and tried to master its tasks with the means of modern natural science. These successes were so impressive that the whole field of medicine was regarded as a branch of the natural sciences, as applied natural science. And so one was convinced that knowledge of the scientific facts and laws was sufficient to gain insight into what is useful and helpful for the sick person [1, 2].

After initial euphoria, it has been recognized that it is an inadmissible reduction to interpret medicine only as applied natural science because this overlooks the fact that medicine, although applying scientific findings, does not relate its self-image to material reality [2]. Thus, the former president of the German Medical Association, Jörg Dietrich Hoppe, came to the conclusion: “Medicine is not a natural science.” In contrast to the natural sciences, medicine does not seek knowledge for the sake of recognition, but to be able to help. Medicine differs from the natural sciences because of its very own purpose. It is only constituted through the sick person who needs to be treated [2]. The doctor must therefore act to satisfy the needs of sick people. Medical action goes beyond what is scientifically justified and justifiable [3]. In order that the knowledge gained from research can actually have a healing effect, it is necessary to link natural science with an insight into the needs of individual people. The Austrian philosopher Ludwig Wittgenstein (1889–1951) formulated this in his Tractatus logico-philosophicus in 1918 ([4], quoted after [2]): “We feel that even when all sorts of scientific questions have been answered, our life problems are still not touched.” Medicine must go beyond the understanding of natural science; it needs the reference to human nature [2, 5].



J. Zentner, *Surgical Treatment of Epilepsies*, https://doi.org/10.1007/978-3-030-48748-5_18

In medicine, therefore, it must be about combining knowledge from the natural science with action for the benefit of the sick person. One could say with Hartmann [3]: "Medicine aims at scientifically founded action." However, different requirements are associated with knowledge and action. Knowledge claims to be exact, generally valid and repeatable. Action, on the other hand, is always directed at an individual person, binding and definitive. In view of these fundamental differences between natural science and the obligation of a physician to act in individual cases, the question inevitably arises as to how the two areas can be combined [5].

In order to make the abstract knowledge usable for medical practice, medical standards are defined, which essentially consist of the two elements: Scientific knowledge and medical experience. Standardization enables the dissemination of medical knowledge and experience [6]. Standards and the resulting guidelines are scientifically based and practice-oriented aids for an appropriate medical approach to specific health problems. Standards and guidelines mean safety in the decision-making processes, but they also imply a certain amount of obligation. This is particularly true for the "gold standard," a term that is used to describe the highest level of evidence-based medicine as a result of randomized controlled trials. The practice of evidence-based medicine thus means combining the best possible external evidence from systematic research with individual clinical action [6].

The Austro-British philosopher Karl Popper (quoted after [7]) turns away in his philosophy of science from irrefutable and universally valid truths, which in anyway no longer exist since Newton's view of the world was replaced by relativity and quantum mechanics. For him, scientificity rather means the willingness to subject conjectures and hypotheses to constant critical evaluation. Similarly, Max Weber already in 1914 had demanded the strict distinction between facts and valuations as the essential postulate for science. This philosophy of science can be applied well to medicine. According to K.D. Bock (quoted after [7]), medicine is an action science that selects and modifies methods and theories of the natural sciences from the viewpoint of their usefulness for the diagnosis, treatment, and prevention of diseases and empirically develops rules for their application in practice [7]. The ability to adequately translate theoretical knowledge into action, at the end of which a therapy recommendation is made that meets the needs of the individual patient, is also known as healing arts [2, 5, 8].

What is the point of these statements? If we look at epilepsy surgery under the scientific understanding of medicine, it quickly becomes clear how thin the basis of that everyday activity which we call scientific is in fact. Although resective epilepsy surgery is now about 100 years old, its efficiency compared to drug therapy alone is verified by only three prospective randomized studies, which have an extremely simple design that allows only limited scientific conclusions. Indeed, there is a large body of observational studies emphasizing the advantages of surgery over medical epilepsy therapy. However, the vast majority of these studies are hardly or not at all robust due to shortcomings in terms of relevance, focusing, study design, and methods regarding variability of populations, definition of outcomes, observation periods, and analysis as well as reporting of results. Even seemingly simple data such as the seizure outcome are only comparable to a limited extent, while valid data on the neuropsychological and psychosocial outcomes and patients' quality of life are almost completely missing. The definition of the epileptogenic area is only a vague hypothesis, and it remains unclear whether it is based more on structural principles or on network properties of the tissue. Accordingly, there is a great uncertainty as to estimating the correct extent of the resection. Decisions for therapeutic procedures such as lesionectomy, extended lesionectomy, or tailored resection are based on gut feeling rather than on scientific evidence. If a surgical intervention does not lead to seizure freedom, it remains open whether the epileptogenic area has been resected marginally too scarce or whether it has been missed completely. Conversely, if the patient is seizure-free, the question remains open as to how much not epileptic tissue has been removed.

Similarly, questions remain unanswered about the best timing of a surgical intervention in childhood, taking into account clinical, electrophysiological, cognitive, and morphological criteria.

Evaluating 182 studies including 16,855 participants that document overall reported outcomes of epilepsy surgery, the 2019 Cochrane Review [9] stated as follows: "Most studies included in this review were of poor quality and had a retrospective design (whereby individuals are recruited after the result of surgery has been recorded, which looks back for the existence of factors related to the results of surgery). Researchers used variable surgical approaches for different sites of the brain, different processes to select candidates for surgery, and different definitions of freedom from seizures after surgery, and they measured these outcomes at varying points. Fewer than half the studies gave details of complications and deaths associated with surgery." The authors continue as follows: "Study design issues and limited information presented in the included studies mean that our results provide limited evidence to aid patient selection for surgery and prediction of likely surgical outcomes." With respect to the randomized controlled trials (RCTs) assessed in the review, West et al. [9] stated: "We judged evidence from the nine RCTs to be of moderate to very low quality due to lack of information reported about the randomized trial design and the restricted study populations."

Reflecting this analysis and taking a sober view on the clinical routine in epilepsy surgery, the lack of scientific evidence to support medical practices cannot be ignored. And yet, epilepsy surgery is extremely successful. To remain successful, however, medicine needs knowledge as the basis for therapeutic actions. The importance of medical research, the results of which affect people more directly than those of other sciences, is undisputed and enjoys broad public recognition [10]. The findings of research are of outstanding importance for the progress of medicine. As the British philosopher and statesman Francis Bacon (Bacon, around 1600, quoted after [10, 11]) already put it: "At last I would like to remind everyone once and for all to keep in mind the true aims of science. One should not strive for them for the sake of the mind, not to quarrel, not to despise others, not for the sake of advantage or fame and power or other base intentions, but to serve and benefit life." Precisely because epilepsy surgery successfully aims to serve and benefit life, and because excellent perspectives for further progress in the surgical treatment of epilepsies are apparent, it is time to think about, or—better said—to remember, criteria for sound medical research.

In fact, such criteria already exist. The recommendations published by the German Research Foundation to ensure good scientific practice [12] and the "Guidelines for the Conduct of Scientific Research within the Public Health Service" of the Office of Research Integrity (ORI), an institution of the US Department of Health and Human Services [13], may be mentioned as good examples [10]. According to Bauer [14], these recommendations and guidelines are not easily measurable "brute facts" but rather "soft institutional facts" that have to be implemented in a sensitive way [10]. In line, the Cochrane Review 2019 [9] concluded the following: "We encourage researchers that future studies should have a prospective design (a design whereby individuals are recruited before surgery has taken place, which identifies factors of interest before surgery and follows up with individuals after surgery to record outcomes). Studies should use appropriate statistical methods to examine the collective effect of factors that may predict the outcome of surgery," furthermore: "Journal editors should not accept papers for which study authors did not record adverse events from a medical intervention. Researchers have achieved improvements in cancer care over the past three to four decades by answering well-defined questions through the conduct of focused RCTs in a step-wise fashion. The same approach to surgery for epilepsy is required."

The philosopher Karl Jaspers ([15], quoted after [10]) even saw in scientific action a fundamental attitude, when he formulated in 1950: "There is no more truthfulness, no reason and no human dignity without genuine scientificity, if this is possible for people through tradition and situation. If science is lost, the gloamings, the twilight, the unclearly edifying feelings and the fanatical decisions awaken in self-imposed blindness." This philosophical attitude will not only contribute to the continued success of epilepsy surgery but it also likely to promote the well-being of society.

## References

1. Fiedler H. Ist die Medizin eine Wissenschaft? Die Zeit. 1961;29
2. Maio G. Mittelpunkt Mensch: Ethik in der Medizin. Stuttgart: Schattauer; 2012. p. 1–9.
3. Hartmann F. In der Heilkunde wirksame Begriffe von Wissenschaft und die Frage nach einem möglichen Wissenschaftsbegriff in der Medizin. Sonderheft 5, Wiesbaden: Studia Leibnitiana; 1975. p. 57–84.
4. Wittgenstein L. Tractatus logico-philosphicus. Frankfurt: Suhrkamp; 1999.
5. Wiesing U. Medizin zwischen Wissenschaft, Technologie und Kunst. Zeitschr Med Ethik. 1993;39:121–30.
6. Jansen C. Der Medizinische Standard, Kölner Schriften zum Medizinrecht 25. Heidelberg: Springer; 2019. https://doi.org/10.1007/978-3-662-59997-6_2.
7. Köbberling J. Der Begriff der Wissenschaft in der Medizin. Düsseldorf: Arbeitsgemeinschaft der Wissenschaftlichen Medizinischen Fachgesellschaften (AWMF); 2005.
8. Toellner R. Über das Verhältnis von Wissenschaftsanspruch, Bildungsprogramm und Praxis in der Medizin. Ber Wiss. 1988;11:193–205.
9. West S, Nevitt SJ, Cotton J, et al. Sugery for epilepsy (review). Cochrane Database Syst Rev. 2019;6 https://doi.org/10.1002/14651858.CD010541.pub3.
10. Haux R. Kriterien für gute medizinische Forschung. Vortrag im Rahmen des Kolloquiums „Wissenschaftlichkeit in der Medizin: Seriosität und Qualität in der medizinischen Forschung" der Medizinischen Fakultät der Universität Heidelberg, Februar 8, 2001.
11. Bensch F, Trautwein W. Wissenschaftstheorie. Patmos: Düsseldorf; 1975.
12. Deutsche Forschungsgemeinschaft. Vorschläge zur Sicherung guter wissenschaftlicher Praxis. Wiley-VGH, Weinheim, 1988.
13. Office of Research Integirty (ORI), U.S. Department of Health and Human Services (n.d.) . http://ori.dhhs.gov.
14. Bauer AW. Ethische Argumente im Diskurs über medizinische Forschung – Funktion und Funktionalisierung. Vortrag im Rahmen des Kolloquiums "Wissenschaftlichkeit in der Medizin: Seriosität und Qualität in der medizinischen Forschung" der Medizinischen Fakultät der Universität Heidelberg, 2001.
15. Jaspers K. Einführung in die Philosophie. München: Piper; 1971.

# Addendum: Epilepsy in the Mirror of Arts

*Art does not imitate, but interpret—Giuseppe Mazzini*

As mentioned by the medical historian Schadewaldt, art and medicine seem to represent two opposite positions. Art is unique, unrepeatable, individual, and subjective. Contrarily, medicine postulates objectivity, general applicability, and repeatability. Yet, there is an area in medicine (which is also named as healing arts), where the maxims of art apply: the patient–physician relationship [1, 2]. In this personal area, the principles of art—uniqueness, individuality, subjectivity—play a decisive role. The medical historian von Engelhardt emphasized three functions that shape the relationship between medicine and art: (1) medicine gives factual hints for understanding phenomena of health, illness, and therapy in the art, (2) the representations in art give hints on the state of medicine and its position in society and culture, and (3) art influences people's attitude towards illness, doctors, and treatment [3].

Among the various diseases, epilepsy has received special attention in art. This is partly because epilepsy is a relatively common disease, for which no effective treatment was available until the middle of the nineteenth century, but especially because the major epileptic seizure is a phenomenologically impressive event. It is therefore not surprising that epilepsy frightened and fascinated people at the same time, and that this disease was related to metaphysics and transcendence beyond the pure biological phenomenon. This is already expressed in the eponymics of epilepsy: Hiera nosos, morbus sacer, morbus comitialis, and morbus lunaticus in ancient times (antiepileptic drugs such as antisacer, comital, and epilunal remind of these interpretations), Schedelnde Gottesstraf and St. Valentine's disease in the Middle Ages, and morbus major, the falling evil, and the falling sickness in modern times [4, 5, 6].

The primary task of art is not to present medical facts, but to interpret them. As von Goethe stated in his maxims and reflections: "Art is the mediator of the unspeakable" [7]. Over the centuries, different connotations of epilepsy in arts have evolved: epilepsy as the supernatural (as a divine disease predisposing to prophecy and enlightenment), epilepsy as the threatening (in the sense of unpredictability, violence, delinquency), epilepsy as a symbol (for vulnerability, humanity, sensitivity), and epilepsy as an experienced disease (in the sense of shame, exclusion, but also chance and claim). Examples from the performing arts, literature, film, and music may illustrate and substantiate those interpretations [3, 5].

## Epilepsy as the Supernatural

In the Christian Middle Ages, there were four main reasons for the existence of illness: original sin, guilt, possession, and divine testing. Questions about another "why" or "from where" were therefore pointless. The same applied to the treatment of an illness: Since God sends or at least permits suffering, it can only be cured by him or with the help of an advocate, a saint [8]. This view based on the Christian faith led to a wealth of representations of epilepsy in sacred


J. Zentner, *Surgical Treatment of Epilepsies*, https://doi.org/10.1007/978-3-030-48748-5

art, e.g., in the book of hours of the Duke Jean de Berry of Burgundy, a passionate art collector, in the Bernulphos Codex of the Reichenau, or by other painters (Figs. A.1–A.3).

The epilepsy term "mal des prophetes" reflects the close relationship between epilepsy and prophecy in literature [9]. The first book of Samuel in the Old Testament of the Bible reports how Saul was blessed by the prophet Samuel and anointed the first king of Israel: "The Spirit of God came upon Saul, and Saul fell into prophetic rapture in the midst of them." Although there is no clear evidence, this statement may indicate that the first king of Israel suffered from epilepsy. Johann Kuhnau, predecessor of Johann Sebastian Bach in the position of the Thomas-Cantor in Leipzig, composed six biblical sonatas at the end of the seventeenth century. The second sonata deals with Saul's epilepsy and David's attempts to heal him by playing the harp [10].

Dostoyewsky is one of the best-known epileptic patients. Decisive experiences of the young Dostoyewsky were his arrest and internment for revolutionary activities in April 1849 and his sentencing to death by shooting in December of the same year. Dostoyewsky was already eye to eye with the soldiers of the firing squad for execution at the stake on Semyonov Square in St. Petersburg when he was informed of the Tsar's pardon for 4

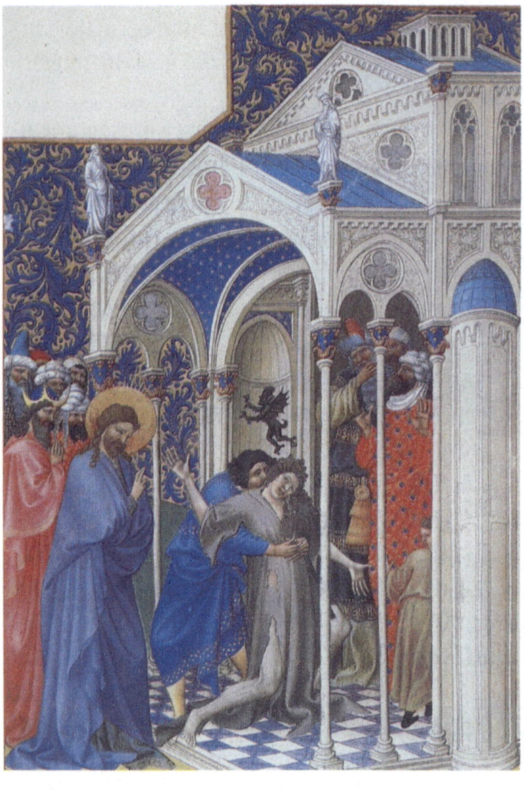

**Fig. A.1** Brothers of Limburg: Christ heals a possessed (epileptic), from the book of hours of the Duc de Berry ("Les Très Riches Heures du Duc de Berry"), around 1415. In contrast to the splendid colorful garments of Christ and the surrounding persons, the dress of the epileptic concerned is in a colorless gray and torn at several places. This depiction is intended primarily to point to the bad social situation of the sick person, which noticeably contrasts to that of the other persons. The fact that Christ's healing was successful is demonstrated by the little winged demon that escapes from the mouth of the now healed person (from Epilepsy in Picture, Geigy-Pharma, Wehr 1985; Museum Condé, Chantilly; Photo: Giraudon, Paris)

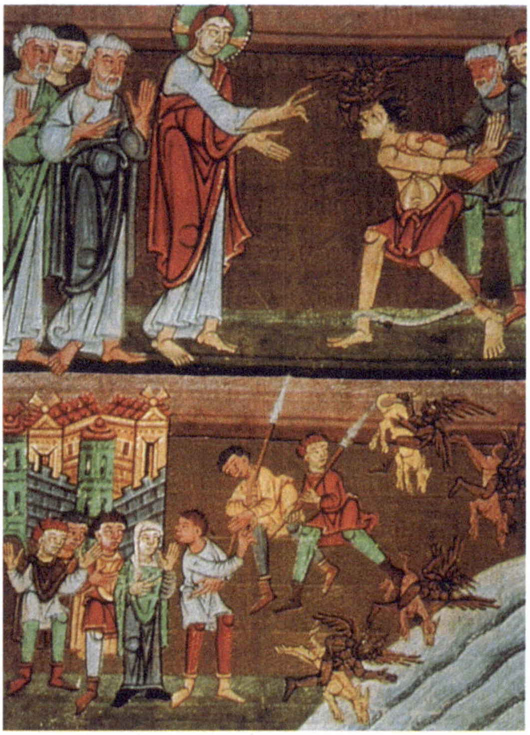

**Fig. A.2** The Healing of the Possessed (Bernulphos Codex, Reichenau, around 1050; Utrecht Rijksmuseum). In the upper scene, Christ beholds the sick (epileptic) man, whose arms and legs are bound, and orders the demons to leave his body. The scene below shows the demons jumping on pigs into the lake. Shepherds between the arriving people of the city and the fleeing demons threat with their weapons (from Heitmann [11])

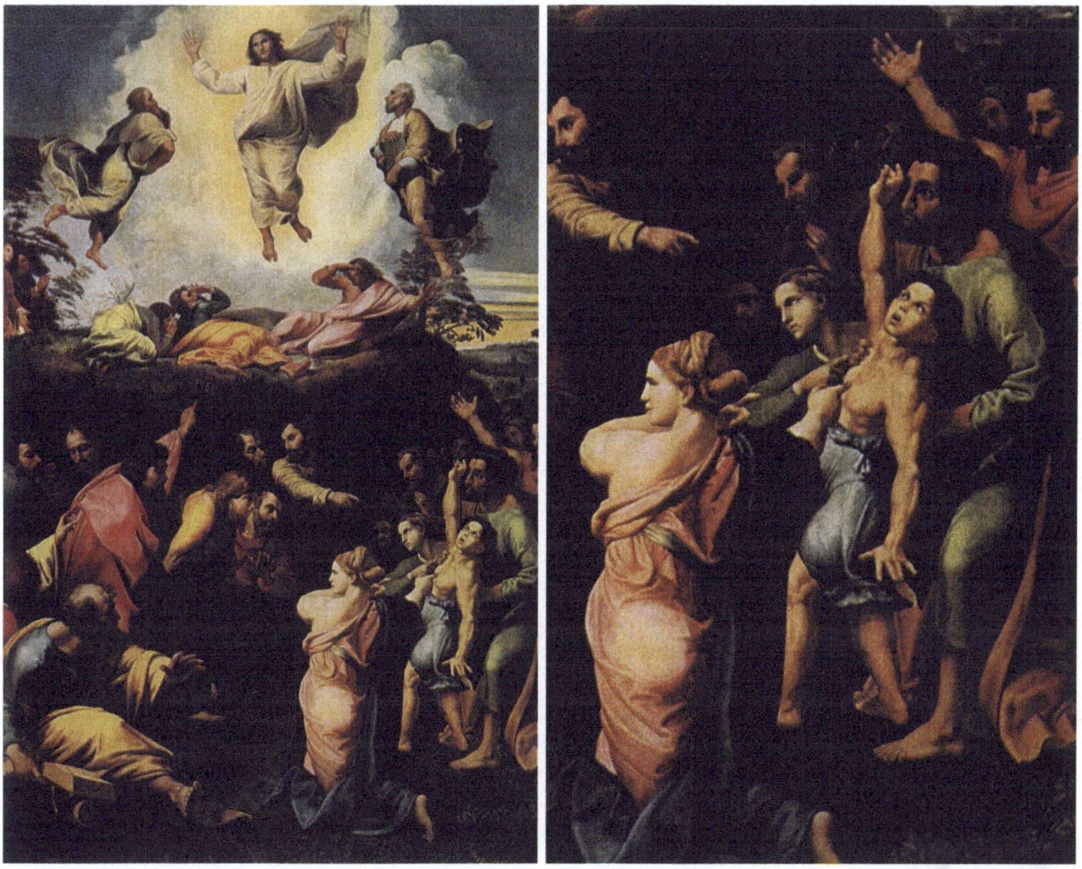

**Fig. A.3** Raffael: The Transfiguration of Christ (1516–1520; Rom, Vatican Museum). Left side: overview; right side: The epileptic boy of the left side is shown in detail. In the upper level on the left side, the divine splendor of Christ and illumination to his disciples at the Mount Tabor is shown. The movements of figures in the lower part contrasts to the glory of transfiguration. The man in the middle of the lower part points to an epileptic boy (from Heitmann [11])

years of forced labor in Siberia. Stefan Zweig has thematized this dramatic event in a poem entitled "Heroic Moment" and he puts this moment into the symptoms of an epileptic seizure, thus providing an association of epilepsy with enlightenment and clairvoyance [12].

In his novel "The Idiot," Dostoyevsky gives the autobiographically presented epileptic prince Myshkin feelings and sensations of enlightenment. In the short moments before his great seizures, Myshkin is filled with a euphoric blissful attitude to life: "The feeling of life, the self-confidence was increased almost tenfold in these lighting moments. Spirit and heart were illuminated by an unusual light, all his emotions, all doubts, all restlessness were all at once soothed, dissolved into a cheerful calm filled with clear, harmonious joy and hope. But he could not doubt that it was really beauty and prayer, really the supreme synthesis of life, nor could he leave any doubt" [13]. The significance of epilepsy as a supernatural sign, its connotation with genius, is expressed in Vincente Minelli's van Gogh film biography "A Life in Passion" (1956).

## Epilepsy as the Threatening

Even though epilepsy in the art is often associated with a positive way of life, with admirable qualities and genius, there is also a connotation of epilepsy with negative characteristics up to criminal activities. In Dostoyewsky´s novel "The brothers Karamazov," Fijodor Karamazov is murdered by his illegitimate son Pavel Smirdjakov, who is employed in his house as a cook. However, a number of circumstances lead to Dimitri Karamasov being considered the perpetrator, and he was brought to justice and sentenced to 20 years of forced labor in Siberia. Smirdjakov who hanged himself before the trial suffers from epilepsy. His parents are marked by idiocy and alcoholism. The environment in which he grows up is hostile to him. His father does not recognize him as a son. The accumulated hatred first gets air in cruelty to animals: "At that time it was especially fun for him to hang cats and then bury them under mourning ceremonies. For this purpose he put on a bed sheet as a chasuble; then he started howling over the cat carcass and swivelled some vessel to it as an incense burner" [14].

In his novel "La bèté humain," Émile Zola takes up the themes of epilepsy and deviant behavior, epilepsy and hereditary disease, epilepsy and alcoholism: "In some hours he felt this hereditary evil. And finally, he thought that he was probably atoning for the others, for the fathers and grandfathers who had drunk, for the generations of drinkers whose tainted blood was in him. Under the strain, his skull almost burst, caught in the fear of a man who was driven to actions in which his will was turned off and whose motive had disappeared" [15]. This novel has been filmed in 1938 by Jean Renoir with Jean Gabin as the leading actor.

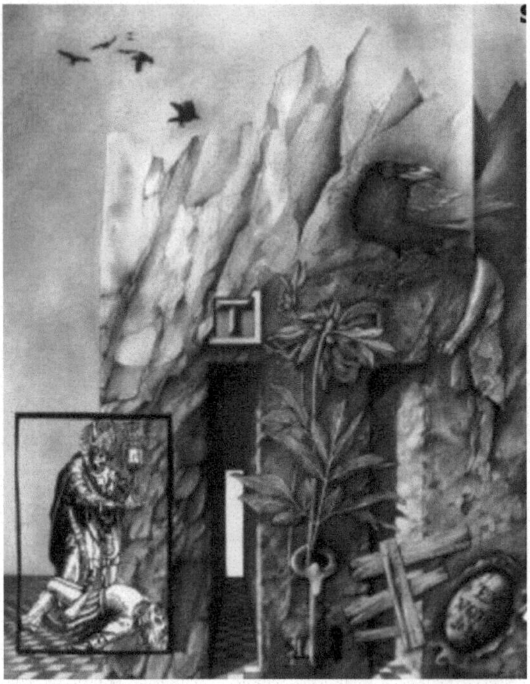

**Fig. A.4** K. Geier: The Symbolism of Epilepsy. Drawing, 1983 [16]. German Epilepsy Museum, Kork. The surreal drawing shows St. Valentine, who bends over an epileptic blessing and healing him. The woodcut is framed by a variety of common epilepsy symbols: ravens, formerly devils, as the embodiment of the evil spirit that had to be cast out; the peony, the blood of a hanged man, as the key to healing (with courtesy of H. Schneble, German Epilepsy Museum, Kork)

## Epilepsy as a Symbol

Many of the epilepsy symbols that have been common for centuries have not been depicted because of their repugnant character. Epileptics were placed under hanged criminals and washed in their blood. Similarly, it was believed that teeth of hanged criminals could perform miraculous healings. Such scenes could only be depicted in symbolism and surrealism in the last century, e.g., in the surreal drawing by Karlheinz Geier (Fig. A.4), or in a plastic of Bodo Wentz (Fig. A.5).

Prince Myshkin, who suffers from epilepsy, knows in Dostoyewsky's "The Idiot" that he would have to withdraw from the entanglements in which he found himself after his return to Russia in order not to succumb to his illness again after the successful cure in Switzerland. Nevertheless, he remains, takes up his suffering and sacrifices himself for his world. The prince reacts with understanding and indulgence to the nasty attacks of Terentyev, who rebels against illness and death, by saying: "Pass us by and forgive our happiness." He is particularly attracted to children, while adults make him uncomfortable. He expresses this with his own words: "I don't like being among adults, among people, I've noticed that for a long time. I don't like it because I don't know how to deal with people.

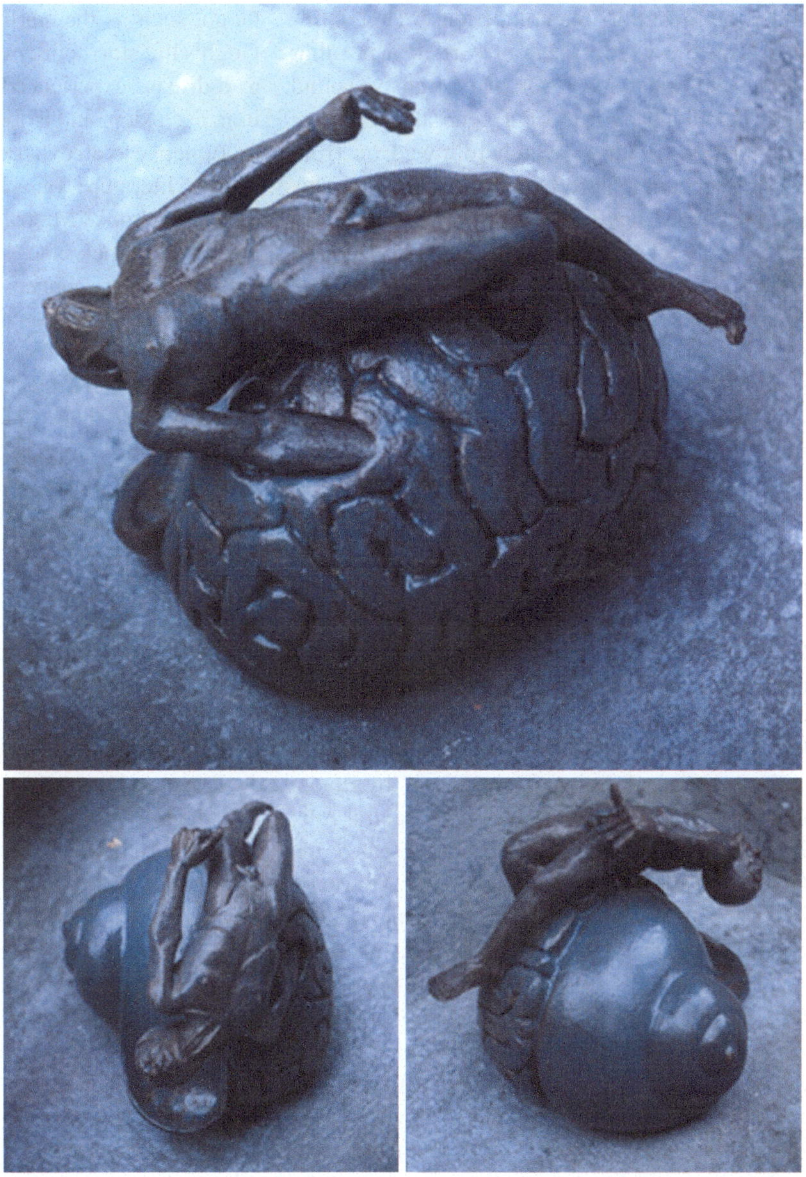

**Fig. A.5** B. Wentz: Falling Sickness. Ceramic, 1983 [17]. German Epilepsy Museum, Kork. The ceramic (above: Total view; below: View from both sides) shows a man with curved limbs, bent fingers and feet, his head thrown back far in the great seizure. This human being grows out of a head-sized form, half of which consists of a snail shell and half of a brain. The brain was chosen as the primarily affected organ. The snail shell symbolizes the social isolation of people suffering from epilepsy (with courtesy of H. Schneble, German Epilepsy Museum, Kork)

Whatever they may tell me, there is always something on me, and I am overjoyed when I can go back to my comrades quite quickly; but my comrades were always the children, not because I am a child myself, but because it always drew me back to the children" [13]. Thus, epilepsy symbolizes devotion, kindness, and humanity.

Disease and medicine has great significance in Thomas Mann's work. In Buddenbrooks, epilepsy symbolizes degeneration and decay. Hanno, the son of the senator, the only child and at the same time the only male representative of the fourth generation "suffered from severe cramps in the earliest period of his life and kept his environment in constant fear." Hanno dies at the age of 15. With the death of his father, the company had already been liquidated, with his own death, the Buddenbrooks' family was extinguished [18].

In his novel "Zauberberg," Thomas Mann writes: "An even new patient, the teacher Popov, a lean and quiet man, proved to be epileptic during the course of dinner, suffering a blatant seizure of this kind, falling to the ground with that cry, the demonic and non-human character of which has often been portrayed, and flapping arms and legs around himself next to his chair under the most horrible contortions." He continues: "But the whole incident carried a peculiar and, in addition to its horror, also offensive sound sign, namely by virtue of a generally intrusive combination of ideas, which followed on from the most recent lecture by Dr. Krokowski." This Dr. Krokowski has just held a series of lectures on the subject of "Love as a disease-forming power." Thomas Mann writes: "This analyst had come to the point of falling sickness in his remarks about love as a disease-forming power just last Monday and had seen this suffering, in which mankind in pre-analytical times alternately saw a holy, even prophetic visitation and a devil obsession, in half poetic, half relentlessly scientific words as the equivalent of the love and orgasm of the brain, in short, in such a sense that its audience had to understand the performance of the teacher Popov, this illustration of the lecture, as a desert revelation and mysterious scandal." Epilepsy here symbolizes ecstasy, rapture and is associated with hysteria [19]. This novel has been filmed by Hans Geissendörfer [20].

In the musical drama "Der Golem" by Eugen dÁlbert, an epileptic seizure plays a central role. Rabbi Loew, a Jewish leader, has created the Golem, an artificial man made of clay. However, he denies his creature language, he wants to keep control. Unexpectedly, his daughter Lea meets the golem and teaches him the language. She teases him. He attacks her. She suffers an epileptic seizure so that the golem shrinks back. Lea´s rigidity during the seizure is a symbol of familiarity and relationship for the golem, which is also rigid. Love is upcoming between the two. Finally, after feeling betrayed by the rabbi's intervention, the golem becomes a destroyer. Lea finds death, and the rabbi takes the life of the golem [21].

## Epilepsy as the Experienced Disease

Van Gogh probably suffered from epilepsy. In his depictions, features are expressed that are considered typical of epileptic painting: Short strokes in a row, the staccato stroke, the garden fence phenomenon, the roof tile phenomenon. These phenomena have been related to the epileptic constitution: Order, regularity, demarcation, convergence. They can be recognized in numerous drawings by van Gogh, such as the starlit night (Fig. A.6). In van Gogh's life story, epilepsy is particularly expressed as a disease experienced in the sense of demarcation, exclusion, and isolation [22].

Epilepsy as an experienced disease is expressed in the literature on self-awareness. In Ursula Schuster's book "Michaels Fall," there is generally no talk of hopelessness and despair. Rather, it is expressed the chance to overcome problems through one's own activity. In this respect, the illness is also understood as a test, the passing of which is experienced as enrichment [23]. In her book "Moritz mein Sohn," Laura Doermer goes beyond overcoming problems through her own activity and criticizes doctors who could not help her son. She writes: "What I don't forgive him (and most of the following doctors), however, is the claim with which they appeared that they alone were in possession of the truth. The current state of scientific knowledge was always the right one, there was never any doubt. My doubts about a drug that obviously helped nothing were wiped aside with a lenient smile [24].

Parents' claim to be able to determine the therapy themselves has been thematized in the film "As long as there is still hope" directed by Jim Abrahams in 1997 demonstrating an extremely negative attitude towards conventional medicine. This film is to be seen in context with the patient rights movement that makes it clear that the doctor–patient relationship has changed dramatically. The first scene shows the condition of the child after conventional medical treatment: The family is financially ruined, but the seizures are more frequent than ever before. The neighboring child, who underwent surgery, has passed away, and so the mother reproaches the attending doctors severely. But the ketogenic diet inaugurated by the mother helped. Patient and parents are happy and content. Significantly, this film ends with the following sentences of the mother to her husband that indicate the main message of the film: "I must always think of how you desperately asked me why the doctors withheld information from us and robbed us of our hopes, and I wonder how our whole health system could go in this wrong direction. We put our son in the care of the doctors. We gave them our trust. And instead of giving us simple information, they abused Robby and almost destroyed all our lives" [25].

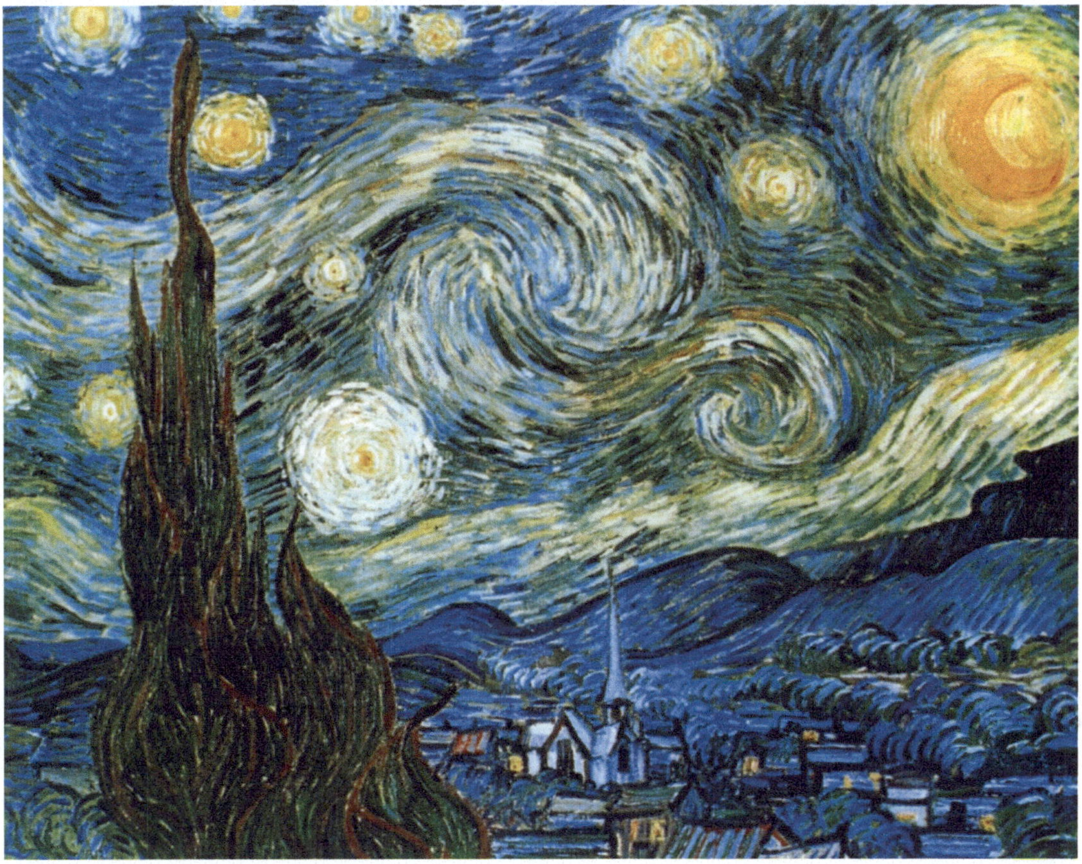

**Fig. A.6** Van Gogh: The Starlit Night (1889). Note the characteristic staccato lines stringed together which have been interpreted to reflect epileptic nature (from In der Beeck [22])

## Conclusions

Representation and interpretation of epilepsy in arts span a wide range. Art is related to science and life, but at the same time has its own reality. The value of arts can therefore by no means be measured solely by its empirical realism or theoretical correspondence with reality. As Paul Klee [26], quoted after [27], pointed it: "Art does not reproduce what is visible, but makes visible". With respect to the relationship doctor–patient–illness, art makes visible how this triangular relationship is weighted and interpreted in its respective time.

In ancient times, epilepsy was regarded as something supernatural—divine or demonic. Accordingly, epilepsy had to be accepted as fate. This view lasted into the last century. Only some decades ago, epilepsy has been seen as a challenge which must be taken in hand and actively dealt with. Artists reminded that health can also mean coping with suffering, and that illness also has a deep sense of understanding human existence. In that era, art opened the view for a reality whose transcendence may reconcile the individual human being with his finiteness, his illness, his death. Today, at the beginning of a new millennium, the transcendent moment in art seems to be receding into the background. The subject emphasizes rights and claims for health.

The example of epilepsy demonstrates how the position of medicine in society and culture has changed during the last century, and how art not only reflects but also influences people's attitudes towards illness, doctors, and treatment—entirely in keeping with the spirit of the times. Hopefully, art and society will return to a balanced relationship with medicine, and maybe art can even contribute to a harmonization between medicine and society through its influence on people's attitudes.

## References


1. Schadewaldt H. Medicine and creative art. Ther Ggw. 1979 Feb;118(2):145–60.
2. Schadewaldt H. Die Krise in der Medizin. Therapeutikon. 1991;6(12):665–8.
3. von Engelhardt D. Sinn und Bedeutung von Epilepisemotiven in der Literatur. Epilepsieblätter. 1996;9(Suppl 1):9–18.
4. Schneble H. Antiepileptische Therapie 1877—Die Behandlung der Epilepsie vor 100 Jahren. Nervenarzt. 1978;49:76–81.
5. Schneble H. Krankheit der ungezählten Namen. Ein Beitrag zur Sozial-, Kultur- und Medizingeschichte der Epilepsie anhand ihrer Benennungen vom Altertum bis zur Gegenwart. Verlag Hans Huber, Bern-Stuttgart-Toronto, 1987.
6. Schneble H. Von der "Heiligen Krankheit" zum "Fallenden Siechtag". Reinbek, Einhorn-Presse, 1987.
7. von Goethe JW. Maximen und Reflexionen. Berliner Ausgabe, 2016.
8. Schadewaldt H. Heilige in der Medizin. Dtsch Ärzteblatt. 1980;77:922–4.
9. Schneble H. Epilepsie und Prophetie in der Literatur. In: von Engelhardt D, Schneble H, Wolf P, editors. "Das ist eine alte Krankheit"—Epilepsie in der Literatur. Stuttgart: Schattauer-Verlag; 2000. p. 123–39.
10. Kuhnau J. Musicalische Vorstellung einiger biblischen Historien in 6 Sonaten. Leipzig, 1700.
11. Heitmann B. Representations of epilepsy as the healing of the possed. In: Lüders HO (ed). Epilepsy Surgery. Raven Press, New York, 1992, p 1–8.
12. Zweig S. Sternstunden der Menschheit. Frankfurt: Fischer; 1997.
13. Dostojewski FM. Der Idiot. Zürich: Ammann-Verlag; 1996.
14. Dostojewski FM. Die Brüder Karamasow. Zürich: Ammann-Verlag; 2003.
15. Zola É. La bèté humaine. Rougon-Macquart, 1926.
16. Geier K. The symbolism of epilepsy. Drawing. German Epilepsy Museum, Kork, 1983.
17. Wentz B. Falling sickness, ceramic. German Epilepsy Museum, Kork, 1983
18. Mann T. Buddenbrooks. Frankfurt: Fischer-Verlag; 1974.
19. Mann TD. Zauberberg. Frankfurt: Fischer-Verlag; 1993.
20. Geissendörfer HW. Der Zauberberg. Film based on the novel of Thomas Mann, 1981.
21. d'Albert E. Der Golem. Musical drama in three acts. Frankfurt, 1926.
22. In der Beeck M. Merkmale epileptischer Bildnerei. Hans Huber, Bern-Stuttgart-Wien, 1982.
23. Schuster U. Michaels Fall: DGVT-Verlag; 1999.
24. Doermer L. Moritz, mein Sohn. C. Bertelsmann, 1990.
25. Abrahams J. As long as there is still hope. Film, 1997.
26. Klee P. Schöpferische Konfession. In: Edschmid K (Hrsg.). Tribüne der Kunst und der Zeit. Eine Schriftensammlung, Band XIII. Reiß, Berlin, 1920, p 28.
27. Schneble H. Epilepsie in der erzählenden Literatur. Epilepsieblätter 1996;9 (Suppl 1): 1.

The manufacturer's authorised representative in the EU is Springer
Nature Customer Service Centre GmbH, Europaplatz 3, 69115 Heidelberg,
Germany. If you have any concerns regarding our products, please
contact ProductSafety@springernature.com

Printed and bound by CPI Group (UK) Ltd, Croydon, CR0 4YY
30/09/2026
02225699-0020